Steffen J. Breusch

Henrik Malchau

The Well-Cemented Total Hip Arthroplasty

Theory and Practice

Steffen J. Breusch (Editor)

Henrik Malchau (Editor)

The Well-Cemented Total Hip Arthroplasty

Theory and Practice

With 521 Figures and 61 Tables

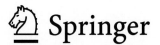 Springer

Breusch, Steffen

M.D., PhD., FRCS Ed

Consultant Orthopaedic Surgeon

Part-time Senior Lecturer

Orthopaedic Department

University of Edinburgh

New Royal Infirmary, Little France

Edinburgh, EH16 4SU

UNITED KINGDOM

Malchau, Henrik

M.D., PhD.

Professor (vis.) at Harvard Medical School,

Co-director:

Orthopaedic Biomechanics and Biomaterials Laboratory

Staff physician,

Adult Reconstructive Unit, Orthopedic Department

Massachusetts General Hospital

55 Fruit Street, GRJ 1126

Boston, Massachusetts 02114-2696

USA

ISBN-10   3-540-24197-3 Springer Berlin Heidelberg New York
ISBN-13   978-3-540-24197-3 Springer Berlin Heidelberg New York

Cataloging-in-Publication Data applied for
A catalog record for this book is available from the Library of Congress.

Bibliographic information published by Die Deutsche Bibliothek
Die Deutsche Bibliothek lists this publication in the Deutsche Nationalbibliografie;
detailed bibliographic data is available in the Internet at <http://dnb.ddb.de>.

Springer Medizin Verlag.
A member of Springer Science+Business Media
springer.de
© Springer Medizin Verlag Heidelberg 2005
Printed in Germany

SPIN 11306535
Cover Design: deblik Berlin, Germany
Typesetting: TypoStudio Tobias Schaedla, Heidelberg, Germany
Printer: Stürtz, Würzburg, Germany
Drawings in this book partly by Dr. Katja Dalkowski, Erlangen, Germany

Printed on acid free paper   18/3160/yb – 5 4 3 2 1

This book is dedicated to the
work and life of Sir John Charnley
and to all patients undergoing total hip arthroplasty

»Those who cannot remember the past are condemned to repeat it«
Santayana

In memoriam Thomas Günther from Springer,
who unexpectedly died during this book project.

He will be greatly missed.

Forewords

In the forty-six years since Sir John Charnley first advanced his a revolutionary concept of a totally artificial hip joint consisting of a metal-to-plastic articulation, literally millions of people have had their lives dramatically and remarkably improved by this seminal innovation.

His brilliance in concept reached successful conclusions only through his relentless dedication, coupled with his outstanding application of his far-ranging commitment to the science and engineering of the issue.

These very unique features of his work were equally matched by his extraordinary persistence. It is interesting to assess, forty-six years later, how close to the mark he was and is. If success is to be measured as standing the test of time, he is exemplary.

Thousands of others have poured these ideas, efforts and experience into this vessel. Understandings have improved and new insights now abound, to augment Charnley's original ideas. It is time, therefore, for a major comprehensive assessment of this entire field of cemented total hip arthroplasty by a broadly based, highly selected group of rigorous scientists and clinicians who have specific skills and knowledge in the multiple aspects of progress in the field.

Such is this book. It is unprecedented in scope, timeliness and quality. It is, indeed, a serious, in depth compilation of the 2005 »state of the art«.

W.H. Harris
Boston, USA

»The surgeon who is less experienced and trained in total joint arthroplasty should predominantly use cement for implant fixation. It is more forgiving and it may be better compensating for insufficient preparation technique«. Surprisingly, it is not long ago, that this opinion was found in many orthopaedic centres. It is based on a fundamental misunderstanding that cement should be used to fill up defects and it ignores all the basics of cemented implant fixation technique, which has been extensively studied and published by Sir John Charnley and other dedicated orthopaedic surgeons. However, many users of cemented total hip replacement are not aware of this fund of well-established knowledge and the status of ongoing research in this field. The same is true for the results of the Swedish and other Scandinavian hip registers. They have clearly demonstrated the benefits of modern cementing technique. However, in many countries as well as many orthopaedic centres the use of modern cementing technique is far from being comprehensive. Limited financial resources are often given as reason. This seems to be an extremely short-sighted way of calculation. Quality in total joint replacement is primarily defined by implant survival. Based on that, a well-cemented total hip arthroplasty remains the golden standard. It is thanks to the editors and contributors of this book that we may learn and understand all about »well-cemented total hip arthroplasty«.

The orthopaedic surgeon, who wants to know, may read the book. The one, who already knows, may also read the book – he will recognise that he did not know everything. The one, who does not want to know, should not read the book – he should also not perform cemented total hip arthroplasty.

V. Ewerbeck
Heidelberg, Germany

Preface

Sir John Charnley stated in his book »Acrylic Cement in Orthopaedic Surgery« (Longman Group Limited, 1970):

»There is no doubt that in orthopaedic surgery acrylic cement is going to be widely used in many different parts of the world; there is equally no doubt that its use by uninformed operators will produce complications which might seriously threaten its reputation and might hold back the progress of science. If criticism of acrylic cement are to come from this type of source, it is important to have available the main references to research in this field, both in favour of and against the main thesis«.

»The Well-Cemented Total Hip Arthroplasty – Theory and Practice« is a contemporary and complete source for the orthopaedic surgeon, fellow or resident performing total hip arthroplasty or other professional groups involved in the treatment of patients operated upon with a total hip.

The content covers topics from clinical aspects such as type of incision, the operative steps in the cementing technique, optimal implant designs, perioperative management and prevention of complications. The basic science aspects include properties of bone cement, mixing and bone preparation. The clinical outcome with different types of implant design is also covered and based on both individual surgeons experience as well as the Scandinavian registries.

We are pleased that today's leading experts, both preclinical and clinical, have contributed with their expertise. The intention from the editors has been to cover as many aspects as possible around the cemented total hip arthroplasty and as broadly as possible. The authors list covers 9 different countries and hopefully a balanced view in the different topics.

It is our hope that the textbook will be informative and serve the clinicians and therefore also improve the clinical results in the coming years.

Summer 2005
Henrik Malchau
Steffen Breusch

Table of Contents

Part I
Approaches and Operative Steps

1 Minimal Incision Approaches to the Hip 2
  M. Lukoschek, S.J. Breusch
1.1 General Aspects 2
1.2 The Posterior Approach 3
1.3 The Antero-Lateral Approach 6
1.4 The Anterior Approach 12

2 Operative Steps 16
2.1 Acetabulum 16
  S.J. Breusch, H. Malchau, J. Older
2.2 Femur 28
  S.J. Breusch, H. Malchau
2.3 The Dysplastic Hip 37
2.3.1 Acetabular Roof Graft 42
2.3.2 Femoral Reconstruction 45
  C. Howie

Part II
Basic Science

3 Properties of Bone Cement 52
3.1 What is Bone Cement? 52
  K.-D. Kühn
3.2 The Mechanical Properties of Acrylic
  Bone Cement 60
  C. Lee
3.3 Testing and Performance of Bone Cements 67
  P.T. Spierings
3.4 Extreme Differences in Properties of Successful
  Bone Cements 79
  A.U. Daniels, D. Wirz, and E. Morscher
3.5 Antibiotic-Loaded Cement 86
  L. Frommelt, and K.-D. Kühn
3.6 The Three Interfaces 93
  K. Draenert, and Y. Draenert
3.7 Which Cement Should we Choose
  for Primary THA? 103
  O. Furnes, B. Espehaug, and L.I. Havelin

4 Mixing 107
4.1 The Benefit of Vacuum Mixing 107
  J.-S. Wang
4.2 Choice of Mixing System 113
  J.-S. Wang, and S.J. Breusch

5 Bone Preparation 119
5.1 The Importance to Establish
  the Best Cement Bone Interface 119
  C. Lee
5.2 Femur 125
5.2.1 Femoral Preparation and Pulsative Lavage 125
5.2.2 The Optimal Cement Mantle 128
  S.J. Breusch
5.3 Acetabulum 141
5.3.1 Bone Bed Preparation 141
5.3.2 Optimal Cement Mantle? 143
  D. Parsch, and S.J. Breusch

Part III
Modern Cementing Technique

6 Optimal Cementing Technique – The Evidence . . 146
6.1 What Is Modern Cementing Technique? 146
  S.J. Breusch, H. Malchau
6.2 The Important Role and Choice
  of Cement Restrictor 150
  C. Heisel, S.J. Breusch
6.3 Cement Gun Performance Matters 155
  P. Simpson, S.J. Breusch
6.4 Femoral Pressurisation 160
  A.W. McCaskie
6.5 Acetabular Pressurisation 164
  D. Parsch, A. New, S.J. Breusch

7 Implant Choice
7.1 Stem Design Philosophies 168
  N. Verdonschot
7.2 Stem Design – The Surgeon's Perspective 180
  J.R. Howell, M.J.W. Hubble, R.S.M. Ling
7.3 Migration Pattern and Outcome
  of Cemented Stems in Sweden 190
  J.A. Geller, H. Malchau, J. Kärrholm
7.4 In-vitro Rotational Stability
  of Cemented Stem Designs 196
  M. Thomsen, C. Lee
7.5 Flanged or Unflanged Sockets? 206
  D. Parsch, S.J. Breusch
7.6 Rationale for a Flanged Socket 208
  A.J. Timperley, J.R. Howell, G.A. Gie

Part IV
Clinical Outcome

8   Femoral Components
8.1   Cemented Stems for Everybody? 216
           O.N. Furnes, L.I. Havelin and B. Espehaug
8.2   Long-Term Outcome after Charnley
           Low Frictional Torque Arthroplasty 221
           B.M. Wroblewski, P.D. Siney, P.A. Fleming
8.3   Long-Term Success with a Double Tapered
           Polished Straight Stem. 228
           M.J.W. Hubble, A.J. Timperley, R.S.M. Ling
8.4   Outcome with the MS-30 Stem. 235
           E.W. Morscher, M. Clauss, G. Grappiolo
8.5   Outcome with a Tapered, Polished,
           Anatomic Stem. 242
           L.J. Taylor, G. Singh, M. Schneider
8.6   The French Paradox. 249
           G. Scott, M. Freeman, M. Kerboull
8.7   Cemented Stems with Femoral Osteotomy 254
           C. Howie

9   Acetabular Components
9.1   Is It Justified to Cement All Sockets? 260
           A.J. Timperley, G.A. Gie, R.S.M. Ling
9.2   Long-Term Success of a Well-Cemented Flanged
           Ogee Cup 268
           J. Older
9.3   Long-Term Survival of Cemented Sockets
           with Roof Graft 273
           C. Howie

10   What Bearing Should We Choose? 279
           C. Heisel, M. Silva, T.P. Schmalzried

11   The Evidence from the Swedish Hip Register 291
           H. Malchau, G. Garellick, P. Herberts

Part V
Perioperative Management,
Complications and Prevention

12   We Need a Good Anaesthetist
           for Cemented THA. 302
           A. Dow

13   Perioperative Management – Rapid Recovery
           Protocol 307
           A.V. Lombardi, K.R. Berend, T.H. Mallory

14   Prevention of Infection 313
           L. Frommelt

15   Pulmonary Embolism in Cemented
           Total Hip Arthroplasty 320
           M. Clarius, C. Heisel, S.J. Breusch

16   How Have I Done It? Evaluation Criteria. 332
           E. Morscher

17   Mistakes and Pitfalls with Cemented Hips. 340
           G. von Foerster

18   Revision is Not Difficult! 348
           T. Gehrke

Part VI
Future Perspectives

19   Economic Evaluation of THA 360
           M. Ostendorf, H. Malchau

20   The Future Role of Cemented Total
           Hip Arthroplasty 367
           H. Malchau, S.J. Breusch

List of Contributors

Editors

Breusch, Steffen
M.D., PhD., FRCS Ed
Consultant Orthopaedic Surgeon
Part-time Senior Lecturer
Orthopaedic Department
University of Edinburgh
New Royal Infirmary, Little France
Edinburgh, EH16 4SU
UNITED KINGDOM

Malchau, Henrik
M.D., PhD.
Professor (vis.) at Harvard Medical
School,
Co-director:
Orthopaedic Biomechanics
and Biomaterials Laboratory
Staff physician,
Adult Reconstructive Unit,
Orthopedic Department
Massachusetts General Hospital
55 Fruit Street, GRJ 1126
Boston, Massachusetts 02114-2696
USA

Authors

Berend, Keith R.
M.D.
Joint Implant Surgeons, Inc.
New Albany Surgical Hospital
Clinical Assistant Professor
Dept. of Orthopaedics
The Ohio State University
720 East Broad Street
Columbus, Ohio 43215
USA

Breusch, Steffen
M.D., PhD., FRCS Ed
Consultant Orthopaedic Surgeon
Part-time Senior Lecturer
Orthopaedic Department
University of Edinburgh
New Royal Infirmary, Little France
Edinburgh, EH16 4SU
UNITED KINGDOM

Clarius, Michael
Dr. med.
Oberarzt
Stiftung Orthopädische Universitäts-
klinik Heidelberg
Schlierbacher Landstr. 200 A
69118 Heidelberg
GERMANY

Clauss, Martin
Dr. med.
Assistenzarzt
Rheinstrasse 26
Kantonsspital Liestal
4410 Liestal
SWITZERLAND

Daniels, A.U. Dan
Professor, PhD.
Laboratory for Orthopaedic
Biomechanics (LOB)
University of Basel
Felix-Platter-Spital
Burgfelderstr. 101
4055 Basel
SWITZERLAND

Dow, Alasdair
MB ChB, MRCP, FRCA
Consultant in Intensive Care
and Anaesthesia
Department of Anaesthetics
Princess Elizabeth Orthopaedic Centre
Royal Devon and Exeter Hospital
Foundation Trust
Barrack Road
Exeter, Devon, EX2 5DW
UNITED KINGDOM

Draenert, Klaus
Professor Dr. med.
Leiter des Zentrum für Orthopädische
Wissenschaften
Gabriel-Max-Str. 3
81545 München
GERMANY

Draenert, Yvette
Dr. med.
Zentrum für Orthopädische
Wissenschaften
Gabriel-Max-Str. 3
81545 München
GERMANY

Espehaug, Brigitte
M.Sc., PhD.
Statistician
The Norwegian Arthroplasty Register
Department of Orthopaedic Surgery
Haukeland University Hospital
5021 Bergen
NORWAY

Ewerbeck, Volker

Professor Dr. med.
Direktor der Abteilung Orthopädie I
Vorsitzender des Vorstandes
Stiftung Orthopädische Universitäts-
klinik Heidelberg
Schlierbacher Landstraße 200a
69118 Heidelberg
GERMANY

Fleming, Patricia A.

Research Assistant
The John Charnley Research Institute
Wrightington Hospital, Hip Center
Hall Lane, Appley Bridge
Wrightington Wigan, WN6 9EP
UNITED KINGDOM

von Foerster, Götz

Dr. med.
Departmentleitung Hüft-
endoprothetik
Endo-Klinik Hamburg
Holstenstr. 2
22767 Hamburg
GERMANY

Freeman, Michael

Professor, BA, MB BCh, MD, FRCS
Visiting Professor
University College London
Honorary Consultant Orthopaedic
Surgeon
Royal London Hospital
Whitechapel
London E1 1BB
UNITED KINGDOM

Frommelt, Lars

Dr. med.
Endo-Klinik Hamburg
Holstenstr. 2
22767 Hamburg
GERMANY

Furnes, Ove N.

M.D., PhD.
Orthopaedic Surgeon
Head of the Norwegian Arthroplasty
Register
Department of Orthopaedic Surgery
Haukeland University Hospital
5021 Bergen
NORWAY

Garellick, Göran

M.D., PhD.
Joint Replacement Unit
Orthopaedic Department
Sahlgrenska University Hospital
413 45 Göteborg
SWEDEN

Gehrke, Thorsten

Dr. med.
Leiter des Hüftdepartments
Ärztlicher Direktor
Endo-Klinik Hamburg
Holstenstr. 2
22767 Hamburg
GERMANY

Geller, Jeffrey A.

M.D.
Assistant Professor
Orthopaedic Surgery
Columbia University College
of Physicians and Surgeons
622 West 168th Street, PH 11
New York, New York 10032
USA

Gie, Graham A.

MB BS, FRCS Ed (Orth)
Consultant Orthopaedic Surgeon
Princess Elizabeth Orthopaedic Centre
Royal Devon and Exeter Hospital
Barrack Road
Exeter, Devon, EX2 5DW
UNITED KINGDOM

Grappiolo, G.

M.D.
Hip Surgery Unit
Santa Corona Hospital
Via XXV Aprile 128 - 17027
Pietra Ligure (SV)
ITALY

Harris, William H.

Professor, M.D.
Director Emeritus of Orthopaedics,
Biomechanics and Biomaterials
Laboratory
Massachusetts General Hospital
55 Fruit Street
Boston, MA, GRJ-1126
USA

Havelin, Leif I.

M.D., PhD.
Professor, Head of Department
of Orthopaedic Surgery
Haukeland University Hospital
5021 Bergen
NORWAY

Heisel, Christian

Dr. med.
Stiftung Orthopädische Universitäts-
klinik Heidelberg
Schlierbacher Landstr. 200a
69118 Heidelberg
GERMANY

Herberts, Peter

M.D., PhD.,
Professor Emeritus,
Orthopaedic Department
Sahlgrenska University Hospital
413 45 Göteborg
SWEDEN

Howell, Jonathan R.

MB BS, MSc, FRCS (Tr&Orth)
Consultant Orthopaedic Surgeon
Princess Elizabeth Orthopaedic Centre
Royal Devon and Exeter Hospital
Barrack Road
Exeter, Devon, EX2 5DW
UNITED KINGDOM

Howie, Colin

B.Sc., MB ChB, FRCS Orth
Consultant Orthopaedic Surgeon
Orthopaedic Department
University of Edinburgh
New Royal Infirmary, Little France
Edinburgh, EH16 4SU
UNITED KINGDOM

Hubble, Matthew J.W.

MB BS, FRCSI, FRCS (Tr&Orth)
Consultant Orthopaedic Surgeon
Princess Elizabeth Orthopaedic Centre
Royal Devon and Exeter Hospital
Barrack Road
Exeter, Devon, EX2 5DW
UNITED KINGDOM

Kärrholm, Johan
Professor, MD, PhD.
Orthopaedic Department
Sahlgrenska University Hospital
413 45 Göteborg
SWEDEN

Kerboull, Marcel
Professor, M.D.
Institut Marcel Kerboull
39 Rue Buffon
75005 Paris
FRANCE

Kühn, Klaus-Dieter
Dr. rer. nat (D. Sc)
Heraeus-Kulzer GmbH
Philipp-Reis-Str. 8-13
61273 Wehrheim
GERMANY

Lee, Christoph
Dr. med.
Stiftung Orthopädische Universitäts-
klinik Heidelberg
Schlierbacher Landstrasse 200a
69118 Heidelberg
GERMANY

Lee, Clive, A.J.
BSc, PhD., CEng, MIPEM, FRSA
Honorary University Fellow,
University of Exeter
Honorary Consultant Clinical Scientist,
Royal Devon and Exeter Hospital
Department of Engineering,
Computer Science and Mathematics,
University of Exeter
Harrison Building
North Park Road
Exeter, EX4 4QF
UNITED KINGDOM

Ling, Robin S.M.
Professor, OBE, MA, BM (Oxon),
Hon. FRCS Ed, FRCS
Consultant Orthopaedic Surgeon
Princess Elizabeth Orthopaedic Centre
Royal Devon and Exeter Hospital
Barrack Road
Exeter, Devon, EX2 5DW
UNITED KINGDOM

Lombardi, Adolph V. Jr.
M.D., FACS
Joint Implant Surgeons, Inc.
President-Elect, Medical Staff Services
New Albany Surgical Hospital
Clinical Assistant Professor
Dept. of Orthopaedics and
Dept. of Biomedical Engineering
The Ohio State University
720 East Broad Street
Columbus, Ohio 43215
USA

Lukoschek, Martin
Professor Dr. med.
Vincentius AG
Orthopädische Klinik
Untere Laube 2
78462 Konstanz
GERMANY

Malchau, Henrik
M.D., PhD.
Professor (vis.) at Harvard Medical
School,
Co-director:
Orthopaedic Biomechanics
and Biomaterials Laboratory
Staff physician,
Adult Reconstructive Unit,
Orthopedic Department
Massachusetts General Hospital
55 Fruit Street, GRJ 1126
Boston, Massachusetts 02114-2696
USA

Mallory, Thomas H.
M.D., FACS
Joint Implant Surgeons, Inc.
New Albany Surgical Hospital
Clinical Professor
Dept. of Orthopaedics
The Ohio State University
720 East Broad Street
Columbus, Ohio 43215
USA

McCaskie, Andrew W.
M.D., FRCS
Professor of Trauma and Orthopaedic
Surgery
University of Newcastle upon Tyne,
The Freeman Hospital, High Heaton,
Newcastle upon Tyne, NE7 7DN
UNITED KINGDOM

Morscher, Erwin
Professor em. Dr. med.
former Chairman of the Dept. of
Orthopaedic Surgery of the University
of Basel
Laboratory for Orthopaedic
Biomechanics (LOB)
Felix-Platter-Spital
Burgfelderstr. 101
CH-4012 Basel
SWITZERLAND

New, Andrew
BEng, PhD., AMIMechE
Bioengineering Science Research
Group
School of Engineering Sciences
University of Southampton
Southampton, SO17 1BJ
UNITED KINGDOM

Older, John
MB BS, BDS, FRCS, FRCS Ed
Consultant Orthopaedic Surgeon,
King Edward VII Hospital, Midhurst
West Sussex GU29 0BL
UNITED KINGDOM

Ostendorf, Marieke
M.D., PhD.
Dept. of Orthopaedics
University Medical Center Utrecht
P.O.Box. 85500
3508 GA Utrecht
THE NETHERLANDS

Parsch, Dominik
Priv.-Doz. Dr. med.
Leitender Oberarzt
Stiftung Orthopädische Universitäts-
klinik Heidelberg
Schlierbacher Landstr. 200a
69118 Heidelberg
GERMANY

Schmalzried, Thomas P.
M.D.
Associate Medical Director
Joint Replacement Institute at
Orthopaedic Hospital
2400 South Flower Street
Los Angeles, CA, 90007
USA

Schneider, Michael
Dr. med
Department of Traumatology
Katholisches Klinikum Mainz
St. Vincenz- and Elisabeth Hospital
An der Goldgrube 11
55131 Mainz
GERMANY

Scott, Gareth
MB BS, FRCS
Royal London Hospital
Whitechapel
London E1 1BB
UNITED KINGDOM

Silva, Mauricio
M.D.
Visiting Assistant Professor
UCLA / Orthopaedic Hospital
Department of Orthopaedics
David Geffen School of Medicine
University of California Los Angeles
Los Angeles, CA, 9007
USA

Simpson, Philip M.S.
BSc Hons, MB ChB, MRCS Ed
Orthopaedic Registrar
Orthopaedic Department
University of Edinburgh
New Royal Infirmary, Little France
Edinburgh, EH16 4SU
UNITED KINGDOM

Siney, Paul D.
BA
The John Charnley Research Insitute
Wrightington Hospital, Hip Center
Hall Lane, Appley Bridge
Wrightington Wigan, WN6 9EP
UNITED KINGDOM

Singh, Gyanendra
MS (Orth), FRCS, M.Ch. (Orth)
Trust Registrar
Orthopaedic Department
St. Richard's Hospital
Spitalfield Lane
Chichester, West Sussex PO19 6SE
UNITED KINGDOM

Spierings, Pieter T.J.
M.D., MSc.
Spierings Medische Techniek B.V.
Madoerastraat 24
6524 LH Nijmegen
THE NETHERLANDS

Taylor, Lee J.
MB, FRCS
Consultant Orthopaedic Surgeon
Orthopaedic Department
St. Richard's Hospital
Spitalfield Lane
Chichester, West Sussex PO19 6SE
UNITED KINGDOM

Thomsen, Marc
Priv.-Doz. Dr. med.
Leitender Oberarzt
Stiftung Orthopädische Universitäts-
klinik Heidelberg
Schlierbacher Landstr. 200a
69118 Heidelberg
GERMANY

Timperley, A. John
MB ChB, FRCS Ed
Princess Elizabeth Orthopaedic Centre
Royal Devon and Exeter Hospital
Wonford Road
Exeter, EX2 5DW
UNITED KINGDOM

Verdonschot, Nico
PhD.
Orthopaedic Research Laboratory
Radboud University Nijmegen
Medical Centre
Theodoor Craanenlaan 7 P.O. Box 9101
6500 HB Nijmegen
THE NETHERLANDS

Wang, Jian-Sheng
M.D., PhD.
Dept. of Orthopedics
Lund University Hospital
221 85 Lund
SWEDEN

Wirz, Dieter
M.D.
Laboratory for Orthopaedic
Biomechanics (LOB)
University of Basel
Felix-Platter-Spital
Burgfelderstr. 101
4055 Basel
SWITZERLAND

Wroblewski, Michael B.
Professor, MD, FRCS
The John Charnley Research Institute
Wrightington Hospital, Hip Center
Hall Lane, Appley Bridge
Wrightington Wigan, WN6 9EP
UNITED KINGDOM

Part I   Approaches and Operative Steps

Chapter 1   **Minimal Incision Approaches** – 2
M. Lukoschek, S.J. Breusch

Chapter 1.1   **General Aspects** – 2

Chapter 1.2   **The Posterior Approach** – 3

Chapter 1.3   **The Antero-Lateral Approach** – 6

Chapter 1.4   **The Anterior Approach** – 12

Chapter 2   **Operative Steps** – 16

Chapter 2.1   **Acetabulum** – 16
S.J. Breusch, H. Malchau, J. Older

Chapter 2.2   **Femur** – 28
S.J. Breusch, H. Malchau

Chapter 2.3   **The Dysplastic Hip** – 37

Chapter 2.3.1 **Acetabular Roof Graft** – 42

Chapter 2.3.2 **Femoral Reconstruction** – 45
C. Howie

Minimal Incision Approaches to the Hip

Martin Lukoschek, Steffen J. Breusch

1.1 General Aspects

Minimal invasive surgery (MIS) or better minimal incision surgery of the hip has gained specific interest within the arthroplasty surgeon community, mainly in the US as documented on the American Academy of Orthopaedic Surgeons (AAOS) 70th Annual Meeting in New Orleans 2003. In Europe the discussion about the length of skin incision was regarded with some curiosity, because skin incisions for total hip arthroplasty (THA) already tended to be around 10 to 15 cm, a length that is defined in the US as minimal invasive [7]. In the US, incision lengths up to 40 cm seemed not to be unusual [16]. Others and our experience however showed, that it is possible to get adequate exposure via incisions of 10 cm length or even less [2, 4, 8, 10, 12, 13] without the need for any special instruments. It has been suggested that with MIS techniques and instruments the advantages were seen in lower morbidity [16], minimal soft-tissue trauma [10], reduced blood loss [4, 6, 14], faster rehabilitation [6] and even the possibility of performing THA day-surgery [1].

In the authors opinion the advantage of minimal invasive surgery is mainly the patient's satisfaction with the small incision. In our own study (first author) we could not find statistically proven differences in blood loss comparing incision lengths of an average 7.5 cm in the MIS-group (n=30) to 15 cm of length in the regular approach group (n=30) in total hip arthroplasty, each group by using conventional implantation instruments. Although a trend is seen in reduction of blood loss, rehabilitation time, and less morbidity – as others –, we could not find differences in analgesia requirements, blood loss and rehabilitation time after the operation [4, 15]. If anything, we found even higher postoperative analgesia requirements in the MIS group. With MIS techniques the potential of component

malposition is given [8] and probably increased. Complications specific to minimal invasive approaches as acetabular malposition and wound complications [15] have been reported. In over 100 MIS hips we have seen 4 times higher healing problems when skin incision length was less than 5 cm. These important complications (not only to the patient) are less frequent in conventional approach THA.

The interest in minimal invasive approaches to the hip is fairly young, but already discussed in public. It has to be remembered, that so far all studies are short-term and do not tell about the consequence of long-term outcome.

Despite lack of evidence, MIS has been promoted not only by some surgeons, but in particular by some companies with surprising vehemence. It is even more intriguing that some surgeons have changed their fixation philosophy from cemented to cementless, for which MIS surgery seems naturally more suited. Regarding some techniques proposed for minimal invasive THA some concerns may arise, such as how a cemented hip can be done by techniques operating under fluoroscopic view where the exposition for eyesight is not given [1].

For these reasons, the authors feel the need to describe and document that MIS techniques can also be safely done in cemented THA. For the cemented hip, the view of the acetabulum and into the proximal femur is essential, therefore three principal single incision techniques are described that allow minimal incision approaches (under 10 cm, 3 inches), but good visualisation of the operating site.

In general, it can be postulated that the technique is the same as for the longer incision, but with aid of some few modified instruments, patient positioning and leg manipulation and, most importantly, by good and accurate placement of the skin incision, minimal incision reconstructive hip surgery allows perfect view and handling space also for cemented THA. It is recommended to shorten the incision step by step to get a better feeling for soft-tissue handling, instruments and positioning. It is not a technique suitable for all patients and not for surgeons performing less than 20 hips a year. The main goal should be the long-lasting hip which requires perfect view and implantation technique. The surgeon shoul perform a longer incision if required. The patient will be grateful still 15 years later when the length of skin incision is already forgotten.

One of the authors performed the antero-lateral approach for more than 10 years using not more than 10 cm incisions, but changed to the posterior approach 3 years ago, because postoperative full-weight bearing is easier for the patients and rehabilitation is faster. For some time now, additionally the anterior approach has been compared to the posterior, but subjectively no differences are seen in recovery between the anterior and posterior approach so far. The anterior approach is faster because no muscle has to be reattached. No experience can be offered with a two incision-technique, as none of the authors see the rational for this.

The position of the patient is in a lateral position for all described approaches, but could be done in supine for the antero-lateral and anterior approach. The supine position, however, is not recommended for the anterior approach by the authors. Exposure of the femur is more difficult than in lateral position and potential damage of the gluteus medius muscle by stretching has to be contemplated.

In the lateral position the pelvis of the patient is stabilised by a support clamp fixing the os pubis and further support clamps on the os sacrum and posterior thoracic wall. It is regarded important to avoid any pressure on the lumbar spine to prevent postoperative back pain. Before the incision is made, place the legs in slight flexion of the hip and in 90° flexion of the knees and place the ankles on top of each other. Evaluate the preoperative leg length at the patella and the tibia. Mark the anatomical landmarks in the initial phase (this in itself will help to reduce the length of incision). The position of both femora, which should be ideally superposed, gives additional information if the patient is in real lateral position or if the pelvis is tilted. Beware of adduction contracture and spinal deformities. Radiographic preoperative planning may be more accurate, particularly in this patient group.

1.2 The Posterior Approach

Exposure

The position of the incision is critical to accomplishing the minimal approach. Palpate the tip of the greater trochanter while flexing and rotating the leg. In obese patients it is difficult to palpate, but the tip of the trochanter can be localised with a needle. The incision is made at the posterior rim of the greater trochanter extending from

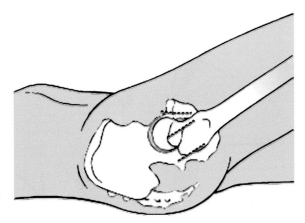

Fig. 1.1. Schematic diagram to illustrate the exact placement of the skin incisions for anterior (*top*), antero-lateral (*mid*) and posterior approach (*bottom*). *Note: All diagrams show a right hip as viewed from above with the patient being in left lateral decubitus position (top is anterior)*

3 cm distal of the tip of the greater trochanter cranially (Fig. 1.1). The incision follows the axis of the femur at the posterior rim. In slim and small patients the incision is about 5 cm (2 inches).

Incise through the subcutaneous tissue to the facia of the gluteus maximus. With a raspatorium mobilise the subcutaneous tissue from the facia in the direction of your skin incision. Incise the facia with a scalpel and lengthen the cut with scissors, taking care not to cut into the vastus lateralis muscle beneath. The cut into the facia is almost twice the length of the skin incision. Gently spread the gluteus muscle cranially by blunt finger dissection. Position a self-retaining retractor to separate the facia and the muscle of the M. gluteus maximus. A Charnley frame-type retractor is usually sufficient. In larger patients a deep self-retaining retractor is useful.

The view should be free to the posterior rim of the greater trochanter. Place the leg in maximal internal rotation. The bursa trochanterica is divided and the fat pad behind the greater trochanter pushed dorsally with a swab. The external rotators and small vessels should now come into vision, from the quadratus femoris to the superior gemellus. The attachment of the musculus piriformis can normally not be seen, because it is well posterior to the greater trochanter in this position. Coagulate any feeding vessels of the short rotators. With a curved Bovie cautery cut the external rotators beginning at the rim of the quadratus femoris making the cut cranial behind the greater trochanter. Ensure to cut carefully and as close as possible to the attachment of the muscles, thus also cutting through the capsule as a single layer at the same time (Fig. 1.2).

With this technique the sciatic nerve does not need to be identified and is protected by the muscular-capsular flap (Fig. 1.2b). Feel the bony curvature of the neck of the femur with your finger and diathermy. At the most

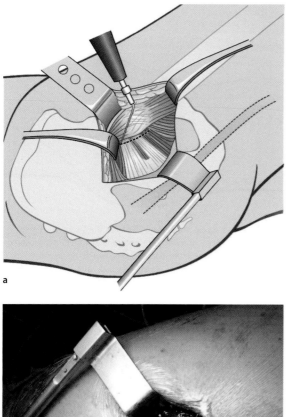

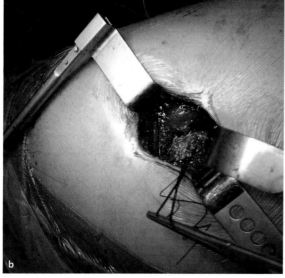

Fig. 1.2a,b. The incision of the short rotators and capsule is carried out in a single layer with a needle diathermy maintaining bone contact. A musculo-capsular flap is created (**b**), which is secured with a stay suture

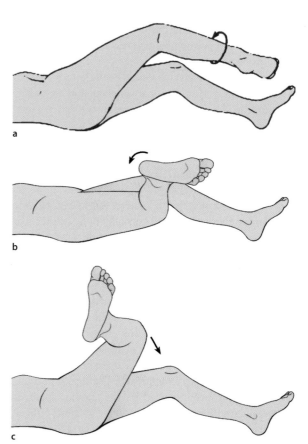

Fig. 1.3a–c. Schematic drawing of right hip illustrating the leg position, which is adjusted by the assistant to aid gradual exposure of the posterior capsule and then dislocation by gradually increasing internal rotation

upper point of the neck femur junction cut the capsule along the neck towards eleven o'clock in right hips (one a clock in left hips) until the bony rim of the acetabulum is felt. Internal rotation is gained while releasing the external rotators and the capsule. Possibly, a Langenbeck retractor is needed to retract the gluteus medius to be able to cut towards the bony rim of the acetabulum. Coagulate any vessels that are cut in the capsule and the external rotators. Pass the curved diathermy at the cranial rim of the neck of the femur towards the fossa piriformis, cut the piriformis and the cranial capsule to complete a T-shape capsular opening. With flexion, adduction and internal

rotation the femoral head is dislocated (**Fig. 1.3**). Eventually incise the quadratus femoris to gain view of the complete neck of the femur. Position the femur in the axis of the operating table, internally rotate so that the tibia is vertical and the knee flexed in 90° (**Fig. 1.3b**).

Palpate the lesser trochanter and measure the cutting distance for the neck. Place Hohmann retractors around the neck and cut it at the angle desired. Orientation is easy holding the femur parallel to the axis of the table (the patient) and the tibia vertical. A saw cut is performed and the neck cut is completed with an osteotome. It is important not to cut into the piriformis fossa to avoid inadvertent avulsion of the tip of the greater trochanter. With the diathermy or periosteal elevator remove any attached soft tissue to free the head (use a cork screw to manoeuvre and finally remove the head).

Remove the Charnley retractor, if the patient is not obese. The leg is positioned from extreme to moderate internal rotation (**Fig. 1.3a**). With a hook retractor the neck is pulled anteriorly and with the finger the posterior rim of the acetabulum is palpated. At the inferior-posterior edge of the acetabulum a Steinmann pin is ham-

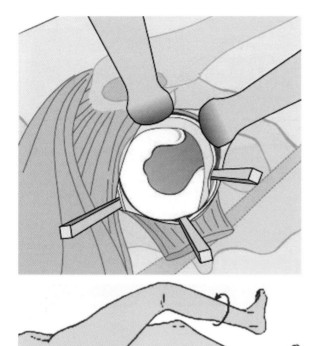

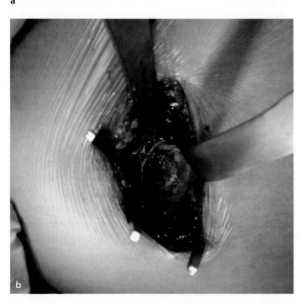

Fig. 1.4a,b. After removal of the head-neck segment the femur is retracted anteriorly and three Steinman pins are positioned as described in the text. This allows good exposure of the acetabulum

mered posterior to the commonly present and palpable osteophyte. Direct the pin cranially to be sure to drive it into ischial bone and not into the obdurator foramen. The second pin is placed directly at 9 o'clock (3 in left hips) almost vertically. The third pin is positioned strictly cranial to the acetabulum pushing the gluteus minimus and the capsule away (**Fig. 1.4**).

Acetabular Technique

With a scalpel clean the rim of the acetabulum from remnant labrum to fully expose the acetabular rim. No or very little capsule should be resected. With a long raspatorium palpate the ventral rim of the acetabulum and elevate or split the capsule with the raspatorium to be able to place a Hohmann or slim curved retractor around the anterior acetabular wall, thus taking the greater trochanter with it. In very tight hips a release cut of the inferior capsule may be necessary to allow adequate anterior transposition of the femur. Complete the view to the acetabulum by putting a second Hohmann retractor inferior-dorsally into the acetabular notch (incisura acetabulae). It is now preferred to change to the other side of the operating table to prepare the socket, as the view into the acetabulum is better from ventral. The acetabulum is then prepared in the usual manner. The angulated acetabular reamers, available now from all companies, have been tested, but they have been found to be more difficult to control (keep interior) than the standard straight instruments. Using a smaller (straight) acetabular reamer as a burr the acetabular roof can be prepared (▶ chapter 2.1).

Using modern cementing techniques described later in this book (▶ chapters 2.1, 5.3 and 7.6), the cup is cemented in place. Use the posterior and anterior walls for orientation to achieve 15–20° anteversion. After removal of any remnant cement and any acetabular rim osteophytes, the Hohmann retractors and the Steinman pins are removed.

Femoral Technique

The leg is internally rotated and a forked, modified Hohmann retractor is placed next to the lesser trochanter around the medial calcar, a larger Hohmann retractor is placed behind the neck cut and a third is placed behind the greater trochanter to retract the gluteus maximus. Now the leg is flexed, internally rotated and adducted, the underlying leg is pushed into extension to allow maximal adduction. It is the same movement pattern and leg position used to dislocate the hip (see **Fig. 1.3c**). The tibia is held vertically with the knee being flexed. The patella points down towards the operating table. The view into the femur is free (**Fig. 1.5**). The fossa piriformis can be seen and palpated to prepare the femur for the stem. The femoral preparation, cementing technique and stem implantation are carried out in the routine manner utilising modern cementing techniques (▶ chapters 2.2 and 5.2). An image intensifier can be utilised for more accurate imaging to check rasp positioning (i.e. stem orientation) and leg length after trial reduction.

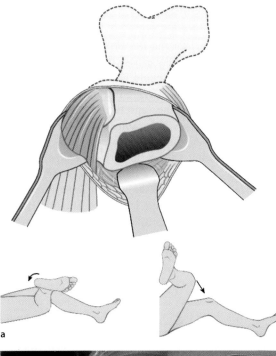

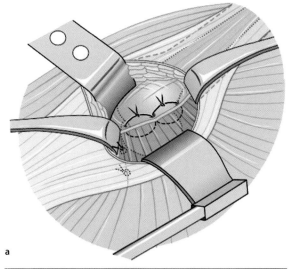

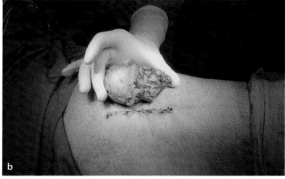

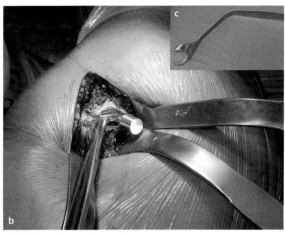

Fig. 1.5a–c. For the femoral preparation the leg is positioned in the same way the hip is dislocated. Three retractors are placed to allow adequate exposure. A forked, modified retractor is useful to expose the medial calcar (*top*). Using modern cementing techniques the stem is implanted

Fig. 1.6. a The musculo-capsular flap is reattached with strong, transosseous sutures. **b** The wound is closed and the resected femoral head is shown over the short incision

Closure

After the cement has cured, reduce the hip with the definite femoral head and put the two legs in the position the leg length was previously measured prior during positioning. Once the definitive implants are in place, close the capsule at the rim of the acetabulum with thick No 2 vicryl sutures. To gain stable fixation and prevent posterior dislocation reattach the external rotators by passing the suture through drill holes of the greater trochanter (**Fig. 1.6**). Use thick resorbable sutures (2×2 metric vicryl) and avoid non-resorbable sutures, as the knots may lead to bursa irri-

tation at the trochanter. Care should be taken to catch and reattach the previously prepared musculo-capsular flap marked with a stay suture (see **Fig. 1.2**). Palpate for the sciatic nerve when passing the needle through the rotator muscles and the capsule. This is the only moment during the operation, when the nerve is at risk. Fixation should be performed in neutral rotation and neutral adduction to allow postoperative internal rotation. For neutral position a large cushion is placed between the legs. The wound is closed in layers (see **Fig. 1.6**).

1.3 The Antero-Lateral Approach

Positioning

The position of the patient may be supine or lateral. However, a lateral patient position is preferred for two reasons. Firstly, a smaller incision is possible as the fat tends to automatically fall anterior and posterior, whereas in the supine position the anterior soft tissues become more prominent and are more difficult to retract. Secondly, in a lateral position a true intracapsular approach is possible. In contrast, with the patient supine an anterior capsulectomy is required – otherwise the tension on the anterior soft tissues commonly causes the retractor, which is placed around the anterior acetabular rim, to fracture the anterior wall, then making a minimal incision procedure virtually impossible. If the supine position is preferred, the sacrum should be elevated by a cushion to allow fat and muscle to fall dorsally. The knee is slightly flexed over a cushion to relax anterior femoral structures. Otherwise, the operative steps are almost identical in lateral or supine position, only the leg positions vary during the preparation.

Although this approach can easily be done with a short incision, it is not minimally invasive by definition, as a subperiosteal elevation of the anterior vasto-gluteal sleeve is necessary.

Exposure

The skin incision is placed just virtually in midline, just slightly towards the anterior rim of the greater trochanter, starting 1–2 cm cranial to the tuberculum innominatum extending over the tip of the greater trochanter (see ◻ Fig. 1.1). The cut follows the axis of the femur (the hip is slightly flexed!). Beware that if the skin incision is too anterior, the skin will not allow getting the femur exposed for the femoral preparation. If angulated acetabular reamers should be used, the incision can be placed slightly more cranially, which eases femoral preparation. After the subcutaneous tissue is cut and the fascia is exposed with a raspatorium, incise the facia with a scalpel in the midline directly over the greater trochanter and lengthen the cut with scissors taking care not to cut into the vastus lateralis muscle beneath. The cut into the facia is almost twice the length of the skin incision and once again follow the long axis of the femur. Retract the facia to free the view of the attachment of the vastus lateralis and the gluteus medius. With a Bovey diathermy needle cut onto bone to detach the gluteus medius and vastus lateralis in one sleeve from the greater trochanter in a subperiosteal manner. Leave enough tissue (white tendon substance) at the anterior rim for later reattachment. This often results in a slightly curved incision (◻ Fig. 1.7).

The gluteus medius fibres are only incised at their trochanteric insertion within the tendineous portion. Then pass a finger armed with a swab into the cut and onto the underlying gluteus minimus fascia (◻ Fig. 1.8). Spread

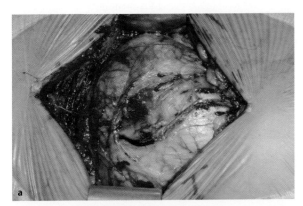

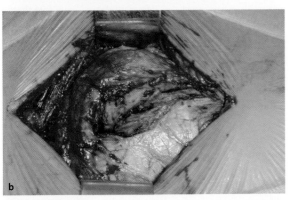

◻ **Fig. 1.7a,b.** The vastus lateralis and gluteus medius are incised at their tendineous origin, usually in a slightly curved fashion (**a**). Then the anterior sleeved is freed by subperiosteal elevation (**b**). *Note: All diagrams show a right hip as viewed from above with the patient being in left lateral decubitus position (top is anterior, left cranial)*

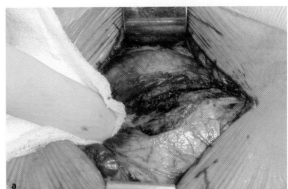

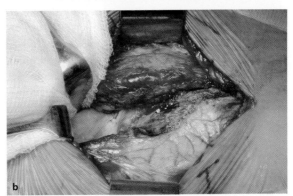

◻ **Fig. 1.8a,b.** Using a finger and a swab the medius fibres are split in line with the muscle fibres (**a**). By sweeping away the intergluteal fat, which contains the superior gluteal neurovascular bundle, the gluteus minimus fascia comes into view (**b**)

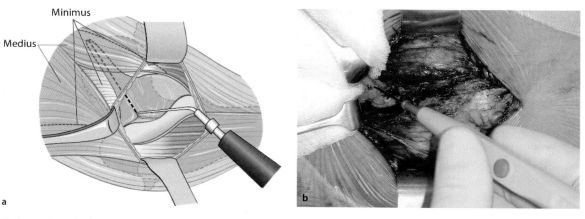

☐ **Fig. 1.9a,b.** Under direct vision the gluteus minimus is divided with the underlying hip capsule in a single layer cutting onto the femoral neck

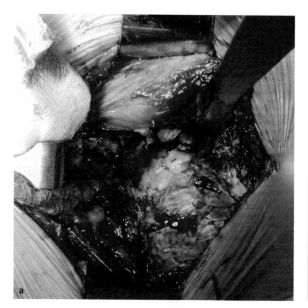
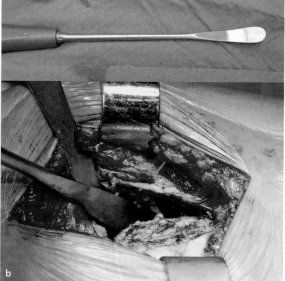

☐ **Fig. 1.10a,b.** A Hohmann retractor is placed around the anterior femoral neck (**a**) to improve traction on the anterior capsule, which is then stripped of the femur with a Wagner periosteal elevator (**b**)

the muscle of the gluteus medius in line with the muscle fibres, which is invariably in an antero-lateral direction. Using the swab as a blunt dissector, the intergluteal fat with its containing neurovascular bundle is swept proximally. The attachment of the muscle gluteus minimus will be seen more clearly once two Langenbeck retractors have been inserted (see ☐ Fig. 1.8). This is a critical step of this approach to protect the superior gluteal nerve, which can run just 1.5 cm above the trochanteric tip.

Then palpate for the femoral neck with the leg being in mild hip flexion and neutral rotation. Incise the gluteus minimus fascia and the underlying hip capsule in one layer using a diathermy needle in an antero-lateral direction, starting from the acetabular rim towards the piriformis fossa (☐ Fig. 1.9). Using a scalpel and cutting onto the femoral neck, the joint is opened and an L-shaped anterior musculo-capsular flap is created. Whilst externally rotating the leg, this

flap is then elevated in a subperiosteal manner and joined to the anterior vasto-gluteal sleeve shown in ☐ Fig. 1.8.

A finger is then placed around the anterior femoral neck and a Hohmann retractor is inserted, which allows better traction and easier further anterior inferior subperiosteal release of the capsule, which is best elevated using a long-handed Wagner raspatorium (☐ Fig. 1.10). It is important to completely strip the antero-medial capsule of the femur, to improve the mobility of the proximal femur, which will be retracted posteriorly and to release any fixed flexion contracture, which is common. The anterior musculo-capsular sleeve containing gluteus minimus, hip capsule, gluteus medius and vastus lateralis should now be loose enough to feel for the lesser trochanter and the transverse ligament.

It is helpful to make small capsular release cut in the superior-posterior aspect of the hip capsule to aid dislo-

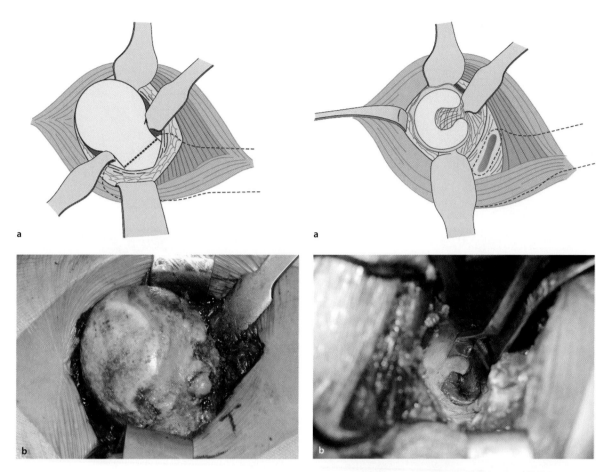

⬛ Fig. 1.11a,b. After hip dislocation the femoral neck cut can be performed under direct vision

⬛ Fig. 1.12a,b. A cobra type retractor is placed into the acetabular notch to expose the inferior aspect of the acetabulum. A Hohmann retractor is placed around the anterior rim osteophyte. Either a posterior curved retractor is placed around the posterior acetabular rim (**a**) or a self-retainer (**b**) may be sufficient to push the femur posteriorly and gain adequate exposure

cation (⬛ Fig. 1.11). Also it is then easier to place a self-retainer into the posterior capsular flap, which protects against too vigorous retraction and traction damage to the superior gluteal nerve. The hip is dislocated by external rotation and adduction.

Acetabular Technique

After the head has been resected, the leg is placed in slight adduction, flexion and external rotation. If the capsule has been adequately stripped off the medial calcar and proximal femur, a cobra retractor can be inserted in the acetabular notch. A self-retainer is used to distract the anterior and posterior portion of the capsule and a Hohmann retractor is placed around the anterior acetabular rim osteophyte (⬛ Fig. 1.12). Alternatively to the cobra retractor, a sharp-pointed curved retractor can be inserted around the posterior-inferior acetabular rim after a short posterior

capsulotomy to accommodate the tip of the retractor. If this is preferred, then commonly a release cut in the inferior capsule is necessary to allow for appropriate posterior transposition of the proximal femur. An additional Steinman pin, hammered into the ilium proximally and posteriorly, can be useful to further improve acetabular exposure.

The acetabulum is then prepared in the usual manner (▶ chapter 2.1). The angulated acetabular reamers, available now from all companies, have been tested, but they have been found to be more difficult to control (keep inferior) than the standard straight instruments. Using a smaller (straight) acetabular reamer as a burr, the acetabular roof can be prepared. It is often useful to temporarily remove the inferior retractor to aid acetabular bone preparation (⬛ Fig. 1.13) and decrease the tension on the inferior corner of the skin incision.

Using modern cementing techniques, described later in this book (▶ chapters 2.1, 5.3 and 7.6), the cup is cemented in place (see ⬛ Fig. 1.13). After removal of any

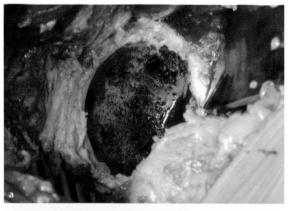

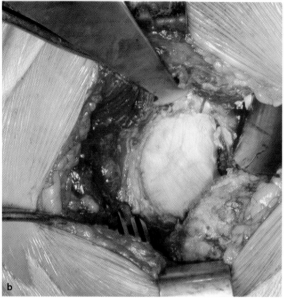

□ **Fig. 1.13a,b.** Even with minimal skin incision excellent exposure for bone preparation (**a**) and cement pressurisation (**b**) can be achieved if an adequate subperiosteal capsular release has been performed

remnant cement and any acetabular rim osteophytes, all retractors and the Steinman pins are removed.

Femoral Technique

If the operation is done in lateral decubitus position, which the authors prefer, the leg is now placed into a sterile leg bag made of a folded drape. Adduct, flex and slide the leg into the bag so that the tibia is at least perpendicular or – even better – in further external rotation, bringing the tibia up almost horizontal (□ Fig. 1.14). This will bring the proximal neck cut into perfect view. Similar to the posterior approach, a lipped or tongued retractor is placed around the medial femoral calcar and the piriformis fossa is freed from soft tissue (□ Fig. 1.15). Femoral preparation and cementing technique are carried out in the exact manner described in ▶ chapters 2.2 and 5.2.

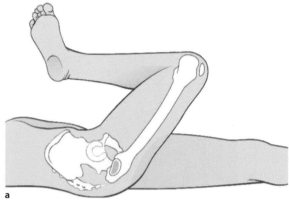

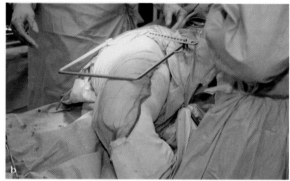

□ **Fig. 1.14. a** For femoral access the leg is placed into a folded sterile drape (leg bag) and placed in hip flexion, adduction and external rotation to gain optimal access (see □ Fig. 1.15). in Fig. 14b the leg position is viewed from the other side of the operating table

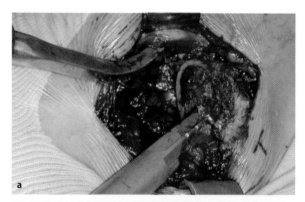

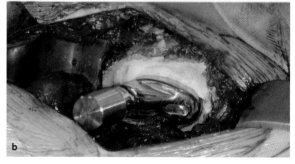

□ **Fig. 1.15a,b.** With the leg externally rotated the neck osteotomy comes into view and excellent access can be gained to the piriformis fossa (**a**). If the exposure of the femur is perfect, the posterior abductor muscle bulk will not infer with correct stem implantation (**b**)

Closure

After the cement has cured, reduce the hip with the definite femoral head after having previously ensured appropriate leg length. The important principle of the closure and soft tissue reconstruction, developed by the authors, is a transosseous reattachment of both capsule and gluteals. The authors regard the capsule as a ligament complex, as is the case in the knee. Therefore, subperiosteal release, preservation and closure of the capsule are essential; in particular as the gluteals also generate abductor force from the capsular origin. Using this technique on more than 500 THAs, no Trendelenburg weakness beyond 3 months has been caused and the postoperative recovery has been enhanced.

As the first step, two parallel drill holes are placed for transosseous refixation from the anterior trochanter into the piriformis fossa (◘ Fig. 1.16), where the L-shaped flap had been released during exposure (see ◘ Fig. 1.9). Then, using a strong transosseous suture, the posterior and anterior capsular flaps are transfixed in a U-shape technique to allow reattachment into the piriformis fossa. The gluteus minimus/capsular flaps are then closed with interrupted

sutures (◘ Fig. 1.17). Then the deep transosseous capsular suture is tied to regain tension on capsule and minimus. The suture ends are not cut, but used in the same fashion as a suture anchor to reattach the anterior vasto-gluteal sleeve, which is then repaired using additional strong No. 2 vicryl sutures (see ◘ Fig. 1.17). It is considered important to place the knots anteriorly and not onto the smooth posterior part or the greater trochanter to avoid local irritation of bursa and fascia lata. The wound is closed in layers and subcuticular skin closure is preferred.

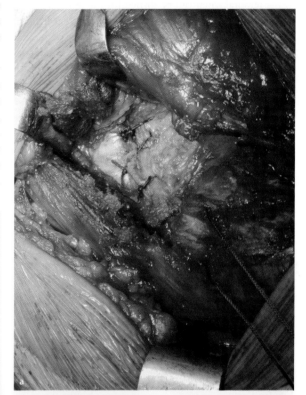

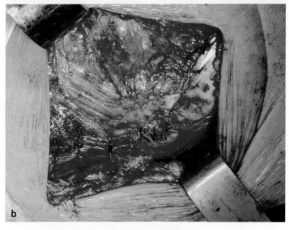

◘ **Fig. 1.17a,b.** Before the transosseous capsular U-suture is tied the gluteus minimus/capsule is repaired with interrupted vicryl sutures (a). Then the deep transosseous suture is tied and used to reattach the anterior gluteal tendon portion in a suture anchor fashion. The remaining vasto-gluteal sleeve is repaired with further vicryl sutures (b)

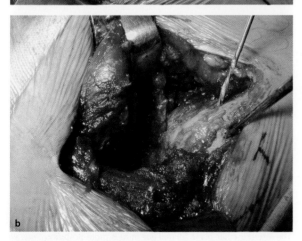

◘ **Fig. 1.16a,b.** After two transosseous drill holes aiming for the piriformis fossa, the anterior and posterior capsular flaps are transfixed (see ◘ Fig. 1.17a)

1.4   The Anterior Approach

Positioning

The classic anterior approach uses the intermuscular plane that is known as the Smith-Peterson approach. A potential to damage the lateral femoral cutaneous nerve is given. The technique described here uses the intermuscular plane known as the Watson-Jones approach. As the exposure of the acetabulum through the anterior approach is of no problem in supine position, the exposition of the femoral canal can be difficult if the femur can not be hyper-extended enough, or the contralateral leg can not be lowered enough to allow the leg, that is operated on, to pass over the leg without anteversion. Some surgeons use an inflatable cushion that is positioned beneath the sacrum and that is inflated during femoral preparation, others put the leg in a traction devise by use of a fracture table. Different techniques are possible with the patient supine, but exposure of the femur remains critical in supine position without damaging the gluteus medius muscle (»minced meat approach«).

However, the main difference to the aforementioned techniques and the real trick of the technique described here [3] is, that the patient is positioned in lateral decubitus with the posterior half of the operating table removed to allow the leg to be dropped down posteriorly into a hyper-extended position (◘ Fig. 1.18).

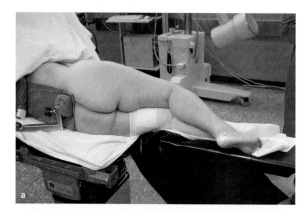

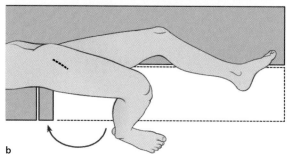

◘ **Fig. 1.18a,b.** For the single incision anterior approach the patient is in a lateral decubitus position with the posterior part of the operating table removed (**a**) to allow to drop and hyper-extend the leg (**b**)

Exposure

As in other minimal incision approaches the position of the skin incision is critical to stay within the minimal incision limits of 10 cm. It is useful to identify and mark the anatomical landmarks prior to the skin incision (◘ Fig. 1.19). Start the incision 2 cm caudal of the anterior superior iliac spine and finish at the anterior superior rim 2 cm below the tip of the greater trochanter (see ◘ Fig. 1.19). To begin with, it is recommended to use X-ray to position the incision directly above the neck of the femur. After dissecting the subcutaneous tissue, the facia of the tensor facia lata is seen. Care should be taken to find the right intermuscular plane between tensor and gluteus muscles, which is not evident, because the intermuscular space of the tensor and rectus may mislead. Dissect the facia at the lateral border of the tensor muscle. Extend

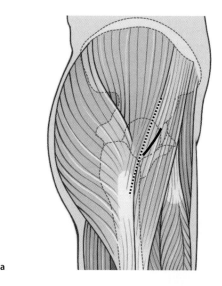

a

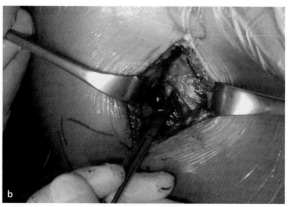

b

◘ **Fig. 1.19a,b.** The skin incision runs in the direction of the anterior superior iliac spine (ASIS) towards the tip of the greater trochanter. The intermuscular plane (*dotted line* in **a**) is more posterior. *Note: All diagrams show a right hip as viewed from above with the patient being in left lateral decubitus position. In the operative photographs anterior is to the right. As landmarks the ASIS and the trochanter have been marked*

the incision of the facia to twice the length of the skin incision. Free the tensor fascia latae in the intermuscular plane from the gluteus medius muscle with the palpating finger used as a blunt dissector. The ascending branch of the lateral femoral circumflex arterial between the muscles has to be divided (see ◘ Fig. 1.19b). The anterior lateral aspect of the hip capsule can be palpated.

With a rasparatorium free the capsule from soft tissue and place two Hohmann retractors. The cranial Hohmann retractor holds back the gluteus medius and minimus. The caudal Hohmann retractor retracts the tensor facia lata and the ileopsoas tendon. The reflected head of the rectus femoris is eventually seen covering the anterior rim of the acetabulum. The caput reflexum has to be cut to be able to reach the acetabulum. After stripping all soft tissue with a Wagner rasparatorium, place an »easy rider« (curved Hohmann) retractor at the anterior rim of the acetabulum. The capsule is opened in a T-shape manner (◘ Fig. 1.20), beginning below the easy rider following the superior aspect of the neck and completing the T-bare by cutting the capsule at the anterior-cranial and anterior-caudal intertrochanteric line. Caudally, the lesser trochanter should be palpable. Eventually, the femoral circumflex vessels have to be cut and coagulated. The capsule has to be detached from the femur until the fossa piriformis can be palpated.

Reposition the extracapsular Hohmann retractors now around the neck within the capsule (◘ Fig. 1.21a). Although dislocation of the hip is possible prior the neck cut by external rotation, adduction, traction and hyperextension (using a cork screw placed in the anterior neck), it is advised to cut the neck in situ. It is preferable to perform a double cut (◘ Fig. 1.21b) that allows removing a slice of the neck to ease the head extraction with a cork-screw [3].

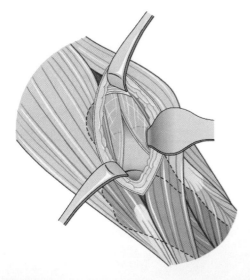

a

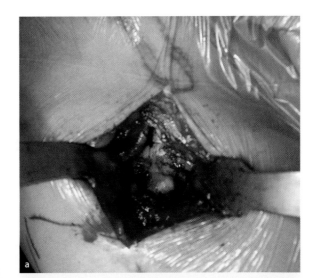

a

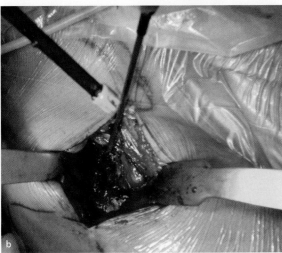

b

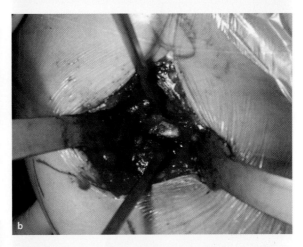

b

◘ **Fig. 1.20a,b.** After blunt division of the intermuscular plane the anterior hip capsule is incised

◘ **Fig. 1.21. a** The hip capsule has been fully incised in line with the femoral neck. The ASIS and the femur have been marked on the skin. **b** Two parallel neck cuts have been performed and the slice is freed and removed using two flat osteotomes

Acetabular Technique

Place a curved Hohmann retractor at the posterior rim of the acetabulum. Eventually, the posterior capsule has to be split with a diathermy to allow the retractor the pass behind the acetabulum. One Cobra retractor is placed inferior in the acetabular notch. This gives adequate exposure for preparation and cementation of the socket (◘ Fig. 1.22). In this anterior approach angulated or curved reamers and cup introducer should be used to minimise the stress on soft tissues.

Femoral Technique

After the cup is in place, the leg is maximally hyper-extended, externally rotated and adducted. Prior to surgery the posterior half of the operating table should have been taken off or lowered to allow the leg to get dropped posteriorly in the position illustrated in ◘ Fig. 1.18. Good anaesthetic relaxation is useful to minimise stress on the muscles.

For good exposure of the proximal femur place an angled tongued retractor behind the greater trochanter to help elevate the proximal femur. With this retractor the

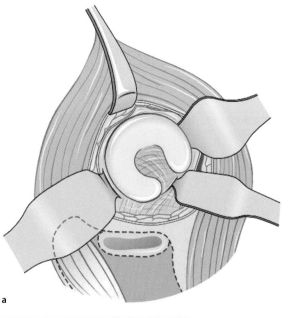

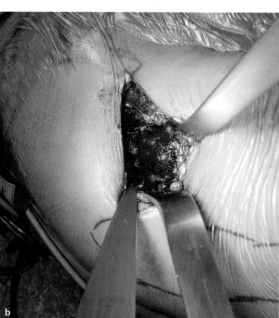

◘ **Fig. 1.22a,b.** Three Hohmann retractors are use to full expose the acetabulum (**a**) and routing acetabular bone preparation can be down, but using angulated and curved instruments (**b**)

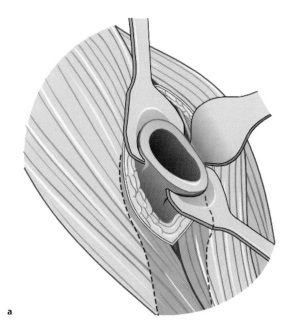

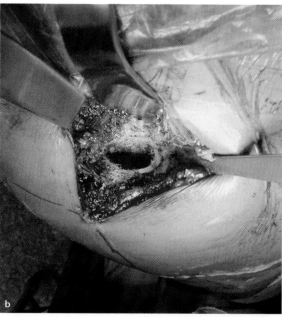

◘ **Fig. 1.23a,b.** The leg is dropped posteriorly in marked hyperextension and adduction and delivered out of the wound to gain maximum access (**a**). Note how vertical the leg is positioned (**b**)

proximal femur is pushed vertically out of the wound. To minimise stress on the greater trochanter (fracture risk, osteoporosis) this manoeuvre is helped by a bone hook that is placed into the neck of the femur. Often the tension of the facia from the tensor, the posterior capsule and the external rotators do not allow to mobilise the proximal femur far enough. Posterior capsular release using a Wagner periosteal elevator or knife is then necessary to gain further hyper-extension. The femur is also pushed up from the knee by the assistant to further expose the femur, but also to relax the gluteus muscle in order to avoid damage during femoral preparation. A second tongue retractor is placed around the medial calcar (◘ Fig. 1.23).

For straight stem designs the release of the external rotators near the fossa piriformis and a release posterior to the greater trochanter seems necessary for the introduction of a straight stem to minimise the risk of varus malaligment. Eventually a Hohmann retractor is placed lateral to slip the facia of the tractus ileotibialis behind the greater trochanter. Curved reamers and anatomically adapted stem designs (preferably in both planes) are better suited and preferable for the anterior approach. In tight hips even with full release straight instruments are very demanding and may be impossible to use. Femoral rotation is checked by using the femoral neck as guide and by palpating the patella.

Closure

Closure in this approach is the easiest and fastest. After final reduction the anterior capsule is closed with thick vicryl sutures. Transtrochanteric sutures are not required. The facia, subcutis and cutis are closed in layers. Subcuticular skin closure provides the best cosmetic result.

References

1. Berger RA, Duwelius PJ. The two-incision minimally invasive total hip arthroplasty: technique and results. Orthop Clin N Am 2004; 35: 163–172

2. Berger RA. Minimal incision total hip replacement using an antero-lateral approach: technique and results. Orthop Clin N Am 2004; 35:143–151

3. Bertin KC, Röttinger H. Anterolateral mini-incision hip replacement surgery: a modified Watson-Jones approach. Clin Orthop 2004; 429: 248–255

4. Chimento GF, Pavone V, Sharrock N, Kahn B, Cahill J, Sculco TP. Minimally invasive total hip arthroplasty: a prospective randomized study. In Proceedings of the 70th Annual Meeting AAOS New Orleans 2003, 637

5. Chimento GF, Sculco TP. Minimal invasive total hip arthroplasty. Operative Tech Orthop 2001; 11(4): 270–273

6. DiGioa AM, Plakseychuck AX, Levison TJ, Jaramaz B. Mini-incision technique for total hip arthroplasty with navigation. J Arthroplasty 2003; 18(2): 123–128

7. Goldstein WM, Branson JJ, Berland KA, Gordon AC. Minimal-incision total hip arthroplasty. J Bone Joint Surg 2003; 85A: 33–38

8. Howell JR, Masri BA, Duncan CP. Minimal invasive versus standard incision anterolateral hip replacement: a comparative study. Orthop Clin N Am 2004; 35: 153–162

9. Irving JF. Direct two-incision total hip replacement without fluoroscopy. Orthop Clin N Am 2004; 35: 173–181

10. Kennon RE, Keggi JM, Wetmore R, Laurine E, Zatorski LE, Huo MH, Keggi KJ. Total hip arthroplasty through the minimally invasive anterior surgical approach. J Bone Joint Surg 2003; 85A: 39–48

11. Ranawat CS, Ranawat AS. Minimally invasive total joint arthroplasty: Where are we going? J Bone Joint Surg. Am 2003; 85: 2070–2071

12. Sherry E, Egan M, Henderson A, Warnke PH. Minimally invasive techniques for total hip arthroplasty. J Bone Joint Surg 2002; 84A: 1481–1482

13. Swanson TV, Hanna RS. Advantages of cementless THA using mini-incision surgical technique. Proceedings of the 70th Annual Meeting AAOS New Orleans 2003, 369–370

14. Wenz JF, Gurkan I, Jibodh SR. Mini-incision total hip arthroplasty: a comparative assessment of perioperative outcomes. Orthopedics 2002; 25(10): 1031–1041

15. Woolson ST, Mow ChS, Syquia JF, Lannin JV, Schurman DJ. Comparison of primary total hip replacements performed with a standard incision or a mini-inccision J Bone Joint Surg 2004;86A: 1353–1358

16. Wright JM, Crockett HC, Delgado S, Lyman S, Madsen M, Sculco TP. Mini incision for total hip arthroplasty – a prospective, controlled investigation with 5-year follow-up evaluation. J Arthroplasty 2004; 19(5): 538–545

Take Home Messages

- Cemented THA can be safely performed with MIS techniques.
- Even with limited incisions, modern cementing techniques can be implemented.
- The exact placement of the incision is of critical importance.
- Only some »MIS« instruments offered by the companies are actually helpful.
- Each approach requires particular tricks to minimise exposure.
- Special patient positioning and modification of the operating table are required for the anterior approach.
- Capsular preservation and closure are important for posterior and antero-lateral approach to minimise the risk of dislocation and limp, respectively
- If in doubt, make the incision/approach more extensive.
- A well-performed operation is much more important than a short incision.

Operative Steps: Acetabulum

Steffen J. Breusch, Henrik Malchau, John Older

Summary

In this chapter the operative technique for the cemented socket is described in detail in a step-by-step manner. Technical considerations, tips and tricks are given to enhance the understanding for this demanding procedure. Particular emphasis is given to restoration of the anatomical centre of rotation, meticulous bone preparation and cementing technique. The indications and techniques for acetabular floor and roof graft are outlined.

Introduction

Despite some excellent long-term results cemented acetabular fixation has become less popular over the years in continental Europe, although it remains the most common procedure in the UK and Scandinavia. In the vast majority of US patients cementless designs are used and indeed in many teaching centres the technique of cemented socket fixation is not part of the trainee's curriculum anymore.

Numerous cementless cup designs are available on the market despite the lack of published data and long term track record. If all reoperations, including liner exchange (wear), bone grafting (osteolysis) and dislocation are included, the overall revision rates (which matter to the patient) for most cementless sockets do not favourably compare with those of well-cemented components (▶ chapter 9.1). Hence there has been a swing back to cemented acetabular fixation in Norway and Sweden.

It is important to realise, that cemented socket fixation remains an extremely successful procedure, particularly if performed well. Long term implant survival rates of more than 95% after 10 years can be achieved and even longer term implant survival can be expected (▶ chapter 9.1, 9.2).

It has become very clear over the last decade that the quality of bone preparation and the cementing technique are the decisive factors influencing outcome significantly more than implant choice (as is the case with femoral components), although the quality of polyethylene is also of particular importance.

The same principles, which are accepted for femoral fixation (▶ chapter 2.2, 5.1, 5.2, 6.4) also apply to the socket (▶ chapter 5.3). Modern cementing techniques aim to improve the mechanical interlock between bone and cement in order to establish a durable interface at the time of surgery. With increased depth of cement penetration the strength of the cement-bone interface is enhanced. It is extremely important to accept, that only meticulous bone bed preparation, thorough bone bed cleansing with pulsatile lavage and sustained cement pressurization, as well as accurate implant positioning, will ensure long term success of a cemented acetabular component.

In the following the authors preferred operative technique is outlined on a step-by-step basis.

Surgical Technique

Hypotensive anaesthesia with spinal or epidural injection is preferred. A low systolic blood pressure (<80–90 mmHg) at the time of cement application is considered essential to minimize the extent of bleeding at the interface. In the authors view an anaesthesist with particular arthroplasty interest and experience will significantly contribute to a successful operative procedure.

Technical Considerations

Containment

It is a cardinal rule, that the acetabular component (cup) should be completely contained under the roof of the acetabulum. This usually requires the acetabulum (socket) to be deepened a variable amount, thus ensuring medial component placement. If the acetabular roof is deficient or dysplastic an acetabular roof graft is necessary (◘ Fig. 2.2b, Fig. 2.4a,b, ► see chapter 2.3.1).

Transverse Deepening

It is of importance to understand the anatomical and biomechanical consequences of preparing and reaming of the acetabulum. ◘ Figure 2.1a outlines the scenario of too later-al cup placement due to inadequate medial deepening. The most common mistake, however, is made not infrequently by reaming the acetabulum in the natural 45° axis of the acetabulum, which will create a concentric, hemispherical cavity, which is good for cement pressurisation, but unfortunately will automatically put the centre of the cup (and rotation) higher than the anatomical level, as simulated in ◘ Fig. 2.1b and documented radiographically in ◘ Fig. 2.2.

This is particularly the case when lateral femoral head subluxation is present, which can lead to erosion of the superior lip. This subluxation with outward and upward femoral head migration commonly occurs in advanced OA, and is usually in association with a large central osteophyte (◘ Fig. 2.3) and developmental dysplasia of the hip (DDH, ◘ Fig. 2.4 a,b).

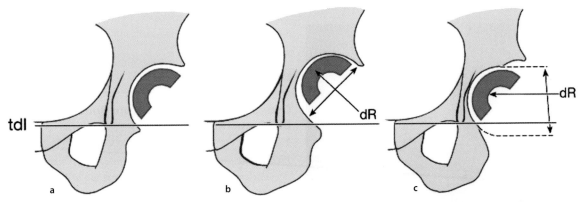

◘ **Fig. 2.1.** *TDL* = tear drop line, *dR* = direction of Reamer
a A too lateral cup placement is simulated due too inadequate medial deepening. Note failure to remove central osteophyte lateral to tear drop (true inner floor of pelvis)

b Common mistake of concentric deepening with reamers kept at 45° thus raising the anatomical centre of rotation
c Correct transverse deepening keeps anatomical centre or rotation, but not infrequently renders socket cavity eccentric, which makes cement containment and pressurisation more difficult

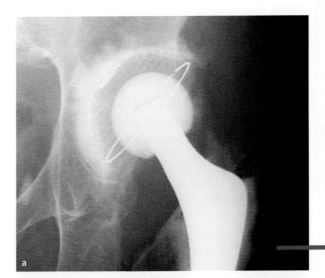

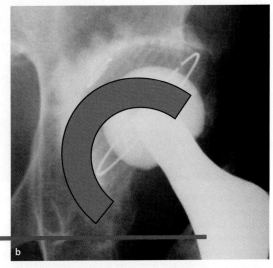

◘ **Fig. 2.2a,b.** This postoperative radiograph (*left*) shows 2 cardinal mistakes: Firstly the transverse deepening was not carried out sufficiently and due to reaming only in 45° direction the hip centre is significantly raised (note: relation to tear drop figure!). Secondly, the cup was not inserted medially first, but pushed superiorly, which has led to a (too) thin cement mantle in DeLee and Charnley Zone I. On the right (**b**), the correct cup position is superimposed

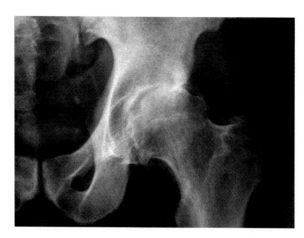

Fig. 2.3. Lateral subluxation and large central osteophyte in osteo-proliferative OA

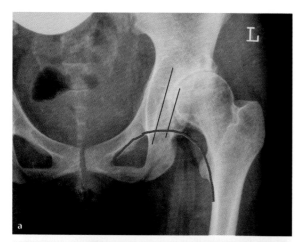

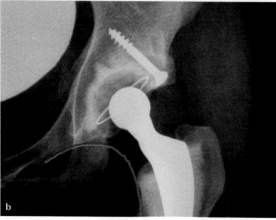

Fig. 2.4. a Acetabular dysplasia with lateral-superior subluxation and bony (distance between two parallel lines) obliteration of the acetabular fossa. The preoperative radiograph provides a good guide for the true depth of the fossa. Note subluxation using the Menard-Shenton line as reference. **b** Postoperative radiograph shows autogenous roof graft and inferior cup placement in correct anatomical position with restoration of the Menard-Shenton line. In contrast to **Fig. 2.2** adequate medial deepening/reaming ensured correct anatomical cup position. This technique will reveal more clearly a roof graft required to archieve full containment.

In **Fig. 2.1c** the correct method of transverse deepening is shown. The reamers are directed horizontally to keep the anatomical centre and level of rotation inferior, thus ensuring preservation of limb length restoration of normal soft tissue tension. Both are important factors for preventing postoperative dislocations.

These circumstances can be mimicked preoperatively by using a hemispheric cup template, which is superimposed on the preoperative radiograph of the pelvis (**Fig. 2.2**), thus giving a good preoperative understanding of any anatomical difficulties to be encountered. Normally a cup size according to the femoral head size (contralateral hip if deformity is present) or smaller is chosen and placed in the desired anatomical position with adequate medial placement, so that a normal centre of rotation and full containment is achieved. An eroded or deficient roof will be brought to light (see **Fig. 2.1c,** 2.2b) by this simple manoeuvre. In difficult circumstances a preoperative drawing is recommended.

Operative Steps

Deepening of Acetabulum and Bone Bed Preparation

Please note: In all intraoperative photographs superior (i.e. acetabular roof) is right and anterior is top of the images.

Exposure and Access to the Socket

Regardless of which approach is used (► chapter 1), three retractors are ideally positioned to allow adaequate access to the socket (**Fig. 2.5**). An angulated Cobra type retractor is placed in the acetabular notch. A narrow, sharp pointed Hohmann and a further curved lever are positioned around the anterior and posterior acetabular margin. If the inferior capsule has not been adequately released access may be difficult.

Rim Osteophytes

To ensure inferior cement containment it is best to preserve the transverse ligament. In cases where this is ossified, this has to be recognised as a too vertical cup placement may result if this inferior osteophyte is used a reference for cup alignment.

For the same reason, i.e. for improved cement containment acetabular rim osteophytes should be preserved until the cup has been cemented. However, in some cases with very large osteophytes these have to be partially removed early to facilitate access to the socket.

Identification Inner Floor of Pelvis

It is recommended and considered important to always identify the true inner floor (lamina interna). If the ligamentum teres is not ossified, it can be excised to reveal

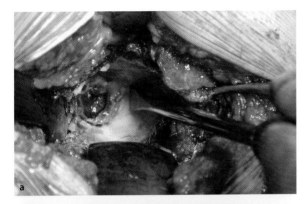

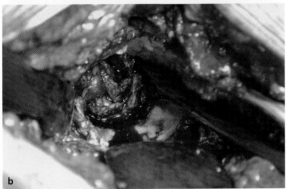

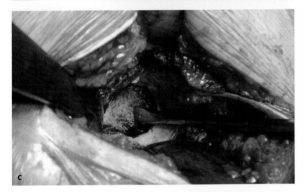

the fossa acetabuli. However, the ligamentous fibres are invariably overgrown by central osteophyte formations and in the extreme case the fossa will be completely obliterated and buried (◘ Fig. 2.3). By resecting the central overhanging osteophyte (◘ Fig. 2.5) prior to reaming using an osteotome (a) and a sharp curette (b), all soft tissue and bone can be easily removed thus exposing the true floor (c). This will ensure adequate roof coverage and medialisation of the component (◘ Fig. 2.4). In the average patient a step of 0.5 to 1 cm between the fossa and the facies lunata will then be revealed. In large men this distance may be greater than 1.5 cm.

Deepening of Acetabular Cavity

It is a sound principle always to deepen the socket sufficiently to contain the cup under the acetabular roof. After the inner floor has been identified, the first small reamer (usually 42–46 mm Ø) is placed horizontally in the unroofed acetabular fossa and directed medially (◘ Fig. 2.6 and 2.11a) until the inner floor is reached.

Once the inner floor is reached, the cancellous bone of the facies lunata becomes flush with the cortical surface of the floor, which corresponds radiographically to the lateral border of the tear drop figure. In the average patient the depth may vary between 0.5 to 1 cm. The reamer is kept inferior in close contact to the transverse ligament. In cases with advanced OA and significant peripheral inferior-posterior osteophyte overgrowth, it sometimes is difficult to identify the inferior aspect and removal of the inferior osteophyte may be necessary first. However, as a rule peripheral osteophytes, which enhance cement containment and aid cement pressurisation, are only removed after having cemented the component. The exception to this rule is the very tight and contracted hip, where only removal of peripheral osteophytes will allow appropriate access to the socket.

◘ **Fig. 2.5a–c.** Three retractors ensure adequate exposure of the socket. The central osteophyte and lig. teres are resected prior to reaming using an osteotome (**a**) and a sharp curette (**b**). All soft tissue and bone can be easily removed thus exposing the true floor – a step is then visible between the floor and the facies lunata (**c**) osteotome on acetabular floor after removal of lig. teres and central osteophyte

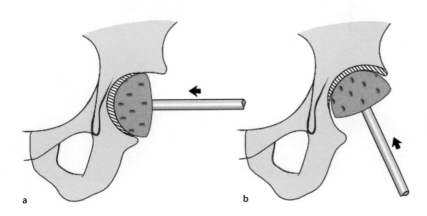

a   b

◘ **Fig. 2.6.** The first reamer is directed transversely to reach to the inner floor (**a**), before the cavity is enlarged and the superior sclerosis is addressed to expose bleeding cancellous bone. Note that an eccentric cavity will result (which is normal!). If immediate upwards reaming is done (**b**) superior and lateral cup placement (see ◘ Fig. 2.2) with inadequate containment will result

2

❗ Cave

Beware of the large man with osteoproliferative OA. In these patients a central osteophyte of more than 1.5 to 2 cm can obliterate the inner floor and it may be prudent to plan for deliberate conservation of deepening, as full deepening may lead to excessive component medialisation and loss of offset, thus increasing the risk of dislocation (preoperative planning!). Also it is important to recognise a protrusio type socket.

Protrusio Acetabuli

In protrusio acetabuli (◘ Fig. 2.7) no central osteophyte is present and the step of transverse deepening should be avoided to prevent perforation of the thinned lamina interna. In these cases a floor graft from the femoral head (◘ Fig. 2.8, Fig. 2.9) is essential to lateralise the cup to restore the anatomy (◘ Fig. 2.7b). Failure to do so, may result in early loosening and migration (◘ Fig. 2.10a–c).

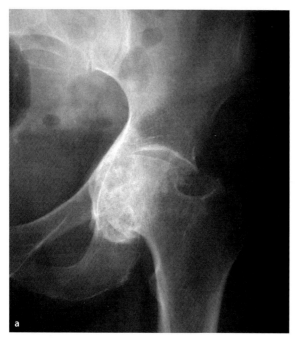

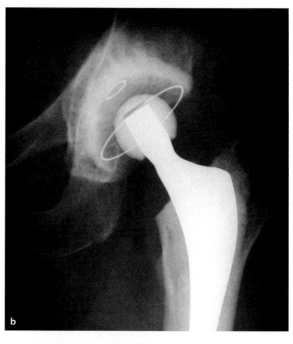

◘ **Fig. 2.7a,b.**
a Protrusio acetabuli with central migration of the femoral head. Note the femoral head is medial to tear drop line

b The postoperative radiograph shows restoration of anatomy with the use of autogenous floor graft from femoral head: Morcellised bone is impacted onto the sclerosed lamina interna, followed by a structural bone slize (◘ Fig. 2.8)

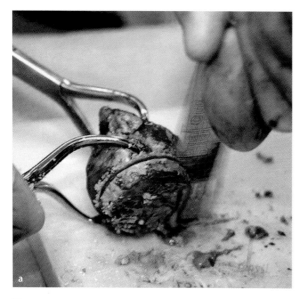

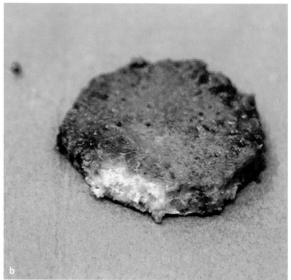

◘ **Fig. 2.8a,b.** Structural autograft taken from femoral head

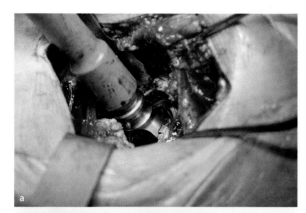

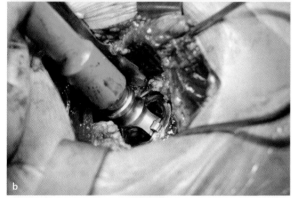

◻ Fig. 2.9a,b. Depth of reamer before (**a**) floor graft in protrusio acetabuli and after (**b**) impaction of morcellized and structural graft (Fig. ◻ 2.8b) confirms adequate intraoperative lateralisation. *Cave: In protrusio the first reamer is not medialised to avoid perforation of the (thinned) sclerotic lamina interna*

Enlarging the Socket and Roof Preparation

A large and sharp curette or two handed Volkmann spoon is used to remove all remaining cartilage and to scrape the roof sclerosis. In some cases with soft bone this instrument may be sufficient to roughen the ebonated bone of the roof. However, more commonly a reamer is necessary.

After transverse deepening and medial reaming (◻ Fig. 2.6, Fig. 2.11a) the next reamers are directed superiorly (◻ Fig. 2.11b) to enlarge the cavity, but no attempt is made to remove the eburnated roof sclerosis. Only partial preservation of the subchondral bone plate will leave the structural support intact.

❶ Cave
> Beware of too superior reaming: this may result in loss of roof cover and superior component positioning (high hip centre, ◻ Fig 2.2).

The final reamer size relates to the anterior-posterior diameter of the acetabulum. If the inferior-superior diameter is larger and a corresponding reamer size is used, overreaming may result in thinning or destruction of the anterior and posterior wall.

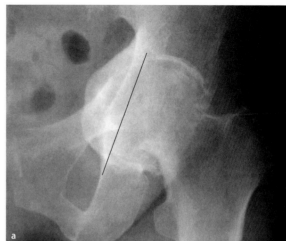

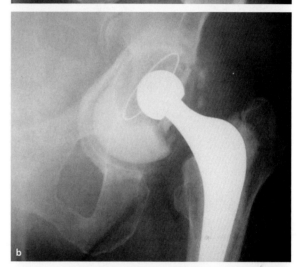

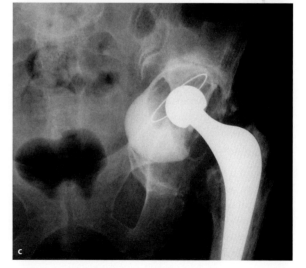

◻ Fig. 2.10. a Protrusio acetabuli. Note medial head migration well beyond tear drop line. No central osteophyte is present and a floor graft is necessary to lateralise the cup to restore the anatomical centre of rotation and prevent early failure (see ◻ Fig. 2.10c)
b Immediate postoperative situation with failure to address the pathology. Note the absence of a floor graft and a very poor cementing technique. **c** Early failure with central and superior en-bloc migration after 18 months

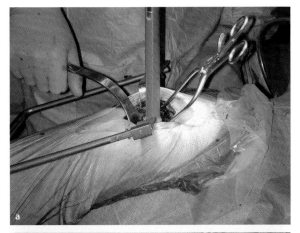

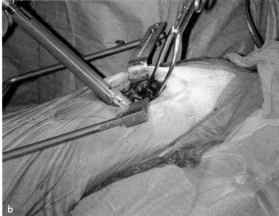

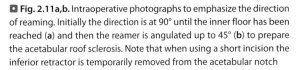

■ **Fig. 2.11a,b.** Intraoperative photographs to emphasize the direction of reaming. Initially the direction is at 90° until the inner floor has been reached (**a**) and then the reamer is angulated up to 45° (**b**) to prepare the acetabular roof sclerosis. Note that when using a short incision the inferior retractor is temporarily removed from the acetabular notch

As a rule of thumb, the largest and final reamer size should only exceed the ap-diameter by 2–4 mm and intends to roughen the anterior and posterior bone surfaces. To prepare the roof, finally, a **smaller sized** reamer, which can easily be manoeuvred in all directions like a burr, is then used to roughen the roof sclerosis to bleeding bone.

> Note: It is the governing principle that cement = cancellous bone. Bone cement cannot bond to a smooth cortical surface (see also ■ Fig. 2.12c), but can only maintain long-term function when interdigitated with the cancellous framework (▶ chapter 3.6, 5.2 and 5.3).

Anchoring Holes

Multiple 6–10 mm anchoring holes of approximately 10 mm depth are made in the roof (■ Fig. 2.12) using a flexible drill. Care has to be taken not to perforate the thin anterior and posterior walls. In these areas only grooves and dimples are made with the drill or a sharp small gauge. We do **not** recommend the traditional large holes made in

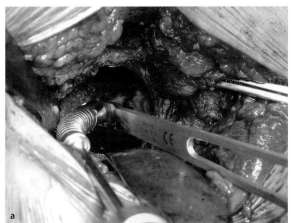

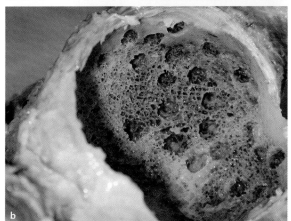

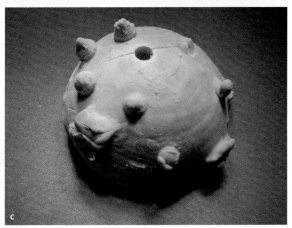

■ **Fig. 2.12. a** A flexible drill with drill guide allows the most accurate placement of the anchoring holes. Partial preservation of subchondral plate is considered beneficial in cases with significant sclerosis (▶ see chapter 5.3). **b** Multiple small drill holes are shown for better clarity in a cadaver specimen. Please note exposed cancellous bone despite partial preservation of bone plate. **c** Inadequate roughening of the sclerosis carries the risk of radiolucent lines and earlier failure, despite multiple drill holes

the pubis and ischium as the cup is loaded in compression and therefore fixed to the roof! Inferior cement pegs are loaded in tension and will commonly debond from the bone interface with time, causing unnecessary bone loss.

Having made the anchoring holes, frequently subchondral cysts will become apparent, especially after pulsatile lavage (◘ Fig. 2.13). In cases with radiologically evident cysts, these must be found and removed. Smaller cysts can be simply curetted, but the pericystic sclerotic wall must always be removed to gain access to the adjacent cancellous honeycombs. A gauge is better than a drill doing this. This may sometimes leave a significant defect, which should then be grafted using the cancellous bone from the femoral neck and head.

Pulsatile Lavage

Bone Bed Cleansing

The single most important step is copious and thorough pulsatile lavage (◘ Fig. 2.14a). Irrigation not only renders white strands of any soft tissue remnants visible, but also effectively removes blood and bone marrow from the bone intersticies, thus aiding cement penetration. (► chapter 5.2.1). A very clean bone bed will result (◘ Fig. 2.14b). This step is commonly repeated several times

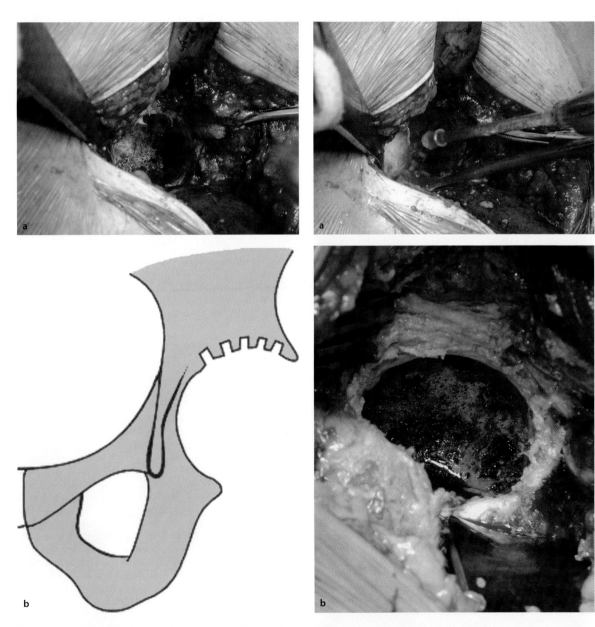

◘ **Fig. 2.13a,b.** Multiple anchoring holes have been made and a large roof cysts has been revealed. A sharp, thin walled gauge is best suited to remove the pericystic sclerotic wall. Failure to do so will result in cement pegs with no interdigitation into cancellous bone. Larger cysts should always be bonegrafted

◘ **Fig. 2.14. a** Prior to cement application, again copious lavage is used. Some further bone preparation may be necessary at this stage. Lavage is repeated and the acetabulum is packed with 3–5% H_2O_2 soaked ribbon gauze. **b** Immediately prior to cement application the socket is irrigated again thoroughly and packed with dry swabs between the steps of bone preparation to facilitate visualisation. Prior to the last wash, a H_2O_2 soaked swap is firmly packed into acetabulum to reduce bleeding and blood loss.

Some surgeons still prefer to use a rotatory brush with stiff nylon bristles. These are particularly useful to remove loose bone and remnant fibrous tissue. However, some bristles may brake from the brush, and since the modern pulsatile lavage is equally powerful in terms of cleansing capabilities, there value is questionable, in particular as no added benefit on long term outcome could be shown (► chapter 6.1).

Cement Application and Pressurization

In contrast to the femur a higher cement viscosity at the time of cement application and cup implantation is preferred to reduce the risk of blood laminations at the interface (► chapter 5.1). In the acetabulum the cement is applied en bloc, so immediate pressurisation can be implemented (Fig. 2.15). Timing is critical and the bone bed should be as clean and dry as possible, even if further lavage and dry swabs are necessary.

Immediately after insertion of the cement ball, pressurisation is commenced manually using a sterile glove filled and padded with a swab (Fig. 2.16a). This ensures prompt (counter)pressure to resist the aectabular bleeding pressure and cement penetration. The tips of the flat fingers should touch the acetabular floor (Fig. 2.16b) thus ensuring, that no cement can escape inferiorly during pressurisation.

After manual pressurisation of approximately one to two minutes, a well designed pressurizer (Fig. 2.17) is positioned, so that it touches the acetabular floor and seals the entire rim of the acetabulum.

If a simple design is used (Fig. 2.17a), its diameter should exceed the acetabular diameter at least 4 mm to allow for appropriate sealing and pressurisation. If the water-inflatable Exeter balloon pressurizer is used (Fig. 2.17b), often wider access to the socket is required to accommodate the device and furthermore some osteophytes may need to be trimmed.

Regardless of what design is used it is important to implement sustained pressurisation (► chapter 5.1 and 6.5) until the cement has sufficiently penetrated and reached a high enough viscosity, so it cannot be displaced by the

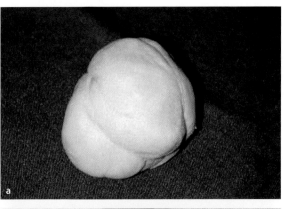

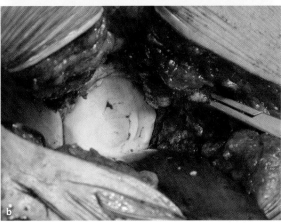

 Fig. 2.15a,b. After further lavage and drying, typically the cement is applied at 3,5 to 4 minutes (for Palacos) as a lump en bloc. For the large socket two mixes may be necessary. For the socket cement in a state of higher viscosity is preferred compared to the femur

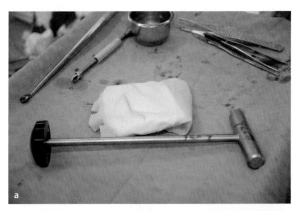

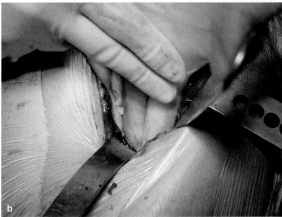

 Fig. 2.16a,b. Immediate manual cement pressurisation is commenced using a padded steril glove before the acetabular pressurizer is positioned

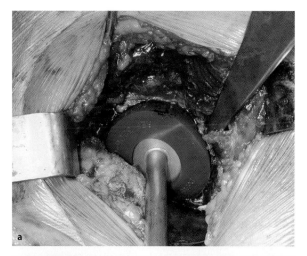

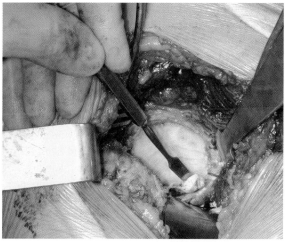

□ **Fig. 2.18.** After successful and adequate pressurisation the pressurizer is removed and at approx. 6–7 minutes no further bleeding will occur. Excess inferior cement is removed from the acetabular floor and notch with a MacDonalds dissector to prevent inferior cement escape during cup insertion

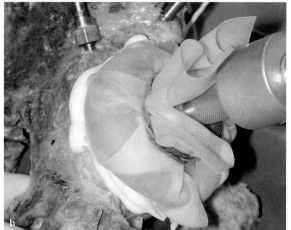

intraosseous bleeding pressure. Care has to be taken, not to bottom the pressurizer, which would lead to a breakdown of the pressurisation process.

As a general rule in socket sizes (largest reamer size used!) up to 54 mm one mix of 40 g bone cement may suffice, but in larger socket sizes 60–80 g will be necessary to guarantee effective pressurisation and enough cement to fix the acetabular component.

After cement pressurisation and increase of cement viscosity, the pressurizer can be removed. Commonly no backbleeding at the cement-bone interface will occur (□ Fig. 2.18). The remaining excess inferior cement is removed with a McDonald dissector (□ Fig. 2.18) and the cement is lifted slightly from the sclerotic acetabular floor to place a thin autogenous floor graft from the last reamings.

Cup Implantation

Depending on the surgeons's preference either a standard or a flanged type acetabular component is implanted. In this chapter the technique with an unflanged cup is described, but in ► chapter 7.6 a detailed description of the rationale and technique with a flanged cup is given. The use of cups with extended posterior lips is generally not advised as these carry the risk of neck-taper impingement, which is associated with a higher risk of polyethylene wear and dislocation.

An acetabular cup size of at least 4 mm smaller in diameter than the largest reamer used, is chosen to ensure a minimum (pure) circumferential cement mantle thickness of 2 mm. PMMA spacers may prevent cup superiori-

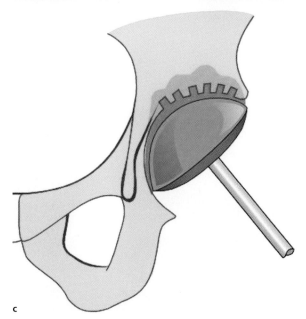

□ **Fig. 2.17a–c.** Cement is then more effectively pressurised with a well designed pressurizer for a minimum period of 60–120 seconds, depending on the cement type, the timing of cement application and the cement viscosity. *Note: Care has to be taken not to bottom the pressurizer to avoid insufficient pressurisation and cement mantle defects*

sation and thin cement mantles in DeLee and Charnley zone I. However it must be realised that these spacers may engage within the trabeculae. Further pressurisation and cup positioning may then become difficult.

After removal of the excess cement (◘ Fig. 2.18) the acetabular component is inserted either by hand or using a cup holder. Applying the same principle when preparing the socket, the cup is inserted horizontally and pushed fully medially first, before gradually angulated to the desired inclination of 45° (◘ Fig. 2.19 and 2.20). Then a cup pressurizer with a ball is inserted to maintain pressure on the cement without the risk of rocking the component. Also good visualisation of the cup position is possible. By holding and rotating the cup pressurizer perpendicular to the cup surface a very accurate account of implant alignment can be judged without the use of special alignment rods or jigs.

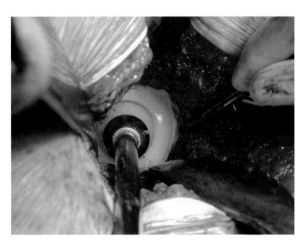

◘ **Fig. 2.20.** An acetabular component with a minimum PE thickness of 8 mm is used. The implant should be downsized at least 4 mm from the last reamer (e.g. Ø 48 mm cup and Ø 52 mm reamer) to guarantee a minimal circumferential cement mantle thickness of 2 mm. Depending on the cup/reamer relation a minimum cement mantle of 2 mm should be visible. This prevents thin cement mantles in Gruen Zone 1 (▶ chapter 6.5).

The component orientation can be assessed by rotation of the ball headed introducer, using the introducer rod as orientation in space. Alternatively, a cup inserter with orientation guides can be used initially

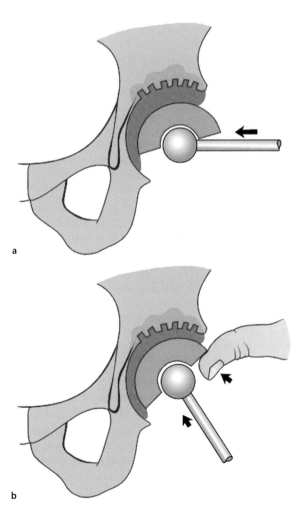

a

b

◘ **Fig. 2.19.** Schematic drawing of cup implantation. With reference to the transverse ligament the component is inserted horizontally and pushed fully medially first, before gradually angulated to the desired inclination of 45°. Pressurisation is maintained using the ball-headed introducer

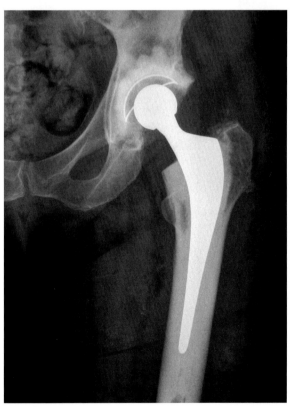

◘ **Fig. 2.21.** Postoperative radiograph with correctly implanted acetabular component. Note the absence of a lucent lines and the adequate degree of cement interdigitation

Using an unflanged component the proximal cement mantle is not only visible to ensure an adequate thickness of >2 mm, but can also be accessed and pressurised during final cement curing to prevent a shrinkage gap at the roof interface.

Finally, all remnant cement and all cementophytes are removed with an osteotome to prevent the risk of third body wear. As a last step all acetabular rim osteophytes are removed flush to the component rim to reduce the risk of anterior and posterior femoro-acetabular impingement leading to dislocation.

Take Home Messages

- Preoperative planning is recommended (e.g. to establish the need for a roof or floor graft and to achieve a normal hip centre).
- Complete containment under the acetabular roof should be achieved.
- This usually requires transverse (medial) deepening to the acetabular floor.
- Meticulous bone preparation with exposure of the cancellous bone is essential.
- Pulsatile lavage for bone bed cleansing is mandatory.
- Sustained cement pressurisation (acetabular pressuriser) ensures adequate cement interdigitation.
- The size of the acetabular component should be at least 4 mm smaller in diameter than the largest reamer used to guarantee a minimal cement mantle thickness of 2–3 mm.
- The acetabular component is positioned in the high viscosity, late phase of cement polymerisation. (The cup should not be regarded as a pressuriser)
- All osteophytes are finally removed to avoid dislocation secondary to impingement.
- It is the surgeon at the time of cup implantation who will determine the success of a cemented socket.

Operative Steps: Femur

Steffen J. Breusch, Henrik Malchau

Summary

In this chapter the operative technique for the cemented femoral stem is described in detail in a step-by-step manner. Bone preparation is considered of particular importance to achieve good stem alignment with a non-deficient cement mantle, but also to ensure a sound cement interlock. The three key features, which have a significant influence on stem survival, are the use of an intramedullary plug, thorough bone cleansing with pulsatile lavage and sustained pressurization with a proximal femoral seal.

Introduction

Cemented THA remains an extremely successful procedure, particularly if performed well. Long-term implant survival rates of more than 95% after 10 years can be achieved. It has become very clear over the past decade that it is the quality of the cementing technique which determines the outcome significantly more than implant choice. Modern cementing techniques aim to improve the mechanical interlock between bone and cement in order to establish a durable interface at the time of surgery. With increased depth of cement penetration the strength of the cement-bone interface is enhanced. Cement interdigitation not only depends on meticulous bone preparation with preservation of strong cancellous bone, but also on lavage and mode of cement application. Thorough cleansing of the bone bed by the use of pulsatile jet lavage, of a distal intramedullary plug and a proximal seal (representing cement pressurization) reduce the risk for revision approximately 20% each. The use of pulsatile lavage is considered of paramount importance to achieve excellent cement penetration and also to reduce the risk of fat embolism. Its use should be considered mandatory in cemented total hip arthroplasty.

In the following the authors' preferred operative technique is outlined on a step-by- step basis.

Surgical Technique

Hypotensive anaesthesia with spinal or epidural injection is preferred (▶ chapter 12). A low systolic blood pressure (<80–90 mmHg) at the time of cement application is considered essential to minimise the risk of bleeding at the interface. In the authors view, an anaesthesist with particular arthroplasty interest and experience will significantly contribute to a successful operative procedure.

Either a posterior or a modified intracapsular Hardinge approach with transosseus refixation of the capsule and Mm. gluteus minimus and medius is performed (▶ chapter 1). Minimally invasive techniques or limited incision surgery are indeed possible, as the femoral access is not problematic.

Operative Steps

Femoral Bone Bed Preparation

Identification of the Piriformis Fossa

The hip is dislocated and the piriformis fossa identified. The entry point should be made postero-laterally in order to facilitate the correct direction of reaming (◘ Fig. 2.22 and 2.23). This will avoid placing the femoral component in varus and reduces the risk of thin cement mantles in Gruen zones 8/9 (▶ chapter 5.2).

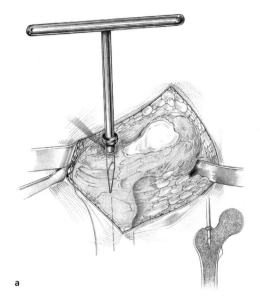 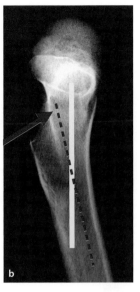

a

b

Fig. 2.22a,b. It is important to identify the piriformis fossa to facilitate femoral preparation and in order to avoid stem malalignment. Note the natural proximal femoral bow at the neck-shaft junction (▶ chapter 5.2) on the lateral radiograph in **b**. The *red arrow* highlights the calcar femoral and emphasizes, how posterior the piriformis fossa is. The *dotted red line* shows the correct direction of canal entry. In contrast the *yellow line* mimics the most common mistake of incorrect femoral canal entry via the direction of the femoral neck

Femoral Head Resection

Resection of the femoral head is carried out in the routine manner approximately 1.5–2 cm above the lesser trochanter. The exact osteotomy level is not critical if a collarless, tapered stem design is favoured. But a relatively high neck cut at level with the piriformis fossa and at approximately 35° to the femoral shaft axis is considered benefical, as partial preservation of the distal neck increases rotational stem stability.

> Note: In contrast, if a collared femoral stem design is used, the neck resection should be made according to the preoperative planning utilising the special instrumentation provided. Depending on the system/instrumentation, final adjustment of the neck length may have to be done as a later step, once the correct leg length has been determined.

Canal Entry

The cortical bone of the piriformis fossa is breached using an initial trochar awl (Fig. 2.22a and 2.23a). Alternatively, a small osteotome or bone nibblers may be used (Fig. 2.23b).

It is regarded a cardinal mistake to enter the femur via the femoral neck, as invariably the instruments are guided in the false direction hitting the posterior femur (Fig. 2.22b).

Opening the Medullary Canal

A »T«-handle canal finder with a blunt distal section (to preserve distal cancellous bone and prevent disruption of arterial blood supply) is rotated and inserted, maintaining posterior calcar bone contact (Fig. 2.24). This should be easy to do and the instrument tip should not

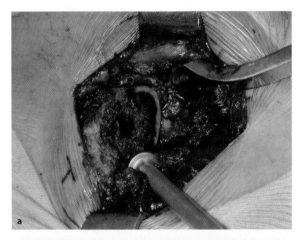

a

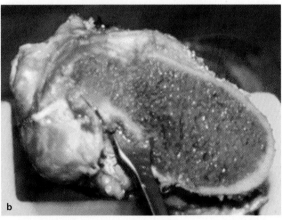

b

Fig. 2.23a,b. Intraoperative photograph of left femur (antero-lateral approach; *top:* medial calcar) showing the correct point of canal entry in the piriformis fossa in **a** using a sharp pointed trochar awl. A prominent posterior bone spike (i.e. the posterior extension of the femoral calcar = *red arrow* in Fig. 2.22b) is partially resected prior to broaching. **b** The manoeuvre is demonstrated in a cadaver specimen, where an osteotome has been placed to partially remove the calcar femorale to ensure posterior canal preparation

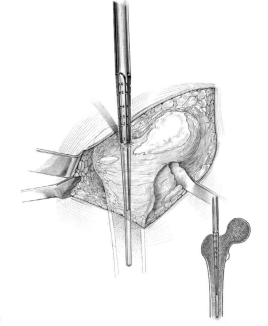

a

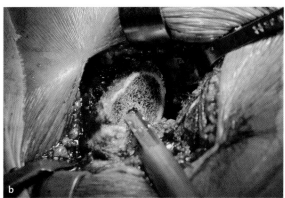

b

make cortical bone contact during advancement of the canal finder into the distal medullary canal.

Preserved anterior cancellous bone and posterior position of the canal finder (see ◘ Fig. 2.24) are good intraoperative signs for correct technique (◘ Fig. 2.25).

> **❶ Cave**
> Opening of the intramedullary canal and exact choice of the point of entry are of crucial importance for the further operative steps and for later stem alignment. If it is difficult intraoperatively to advance the initial canal finder, then commonly the point of entry is incorrect. In too medial placement a varus entry will result with the instrument tip hitting the lateral diaphysis, but more commonly the canal finder is positioned too anterior thus hitting the posterior endosteum as mimicked in ◘ Fig. 2.22b. This problem is more common in obese patients and in particular when using an anterior or anterolateral approach, as there is a tendency for all instruments to be pushed forwards, i.e. anterior by the soft tissues.

Preparation of the Proximal Femur

It is not recommended at this point to start broaching the femur. This would cause compaction and obliteration of cancellous bone interstices. Using a U-shaped offset gouge or a box osteotome, a wedge of cancellous bone parallel to the calcar is removed, but at least 3–5 mm of strong medial cancellous bone should be preserved (◘ Fig. 2.26).

If a stem design is used with a prominent lateral shoulder, flaring out into the greater trochanter, then the cortical bone lamella from the lateral extension of the femoral neck should be removed with an osteotome prior to broaching. Depending on the stem design very lateral canal preparation may be necessary (◘ Fig. 2.27).

◘ **Fig. 2.24. a** The schematic drawing illustrates the first step of opening the medullary canal prior to neck resection. **b** The femoral head has been resected first and the entry hole created with the canal finder. Note the preserved medial and anterior cancellous bone confirming correct alignment and opening of the medullary canal

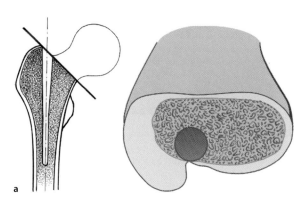

a

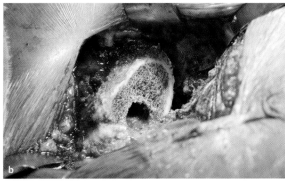

b

◘ **Fig. 2.25a,b.** The schematic (**a**) and intraoperative (**b**) illustrations demonstrate the typical intraoperative appearance after removal of the canal finder, which confirms a correct technique

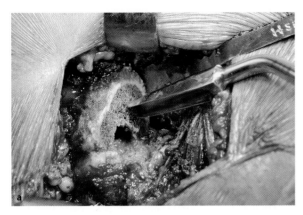

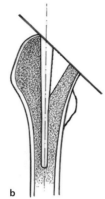

☐ **Fig. 2.26a,b.** Using a U-shaped gauge or a box osteotome, a wedge of medial cancellous bone is removed, but preserving at least 3–5 mm strong cancellous bone adjacent to the medial calcar

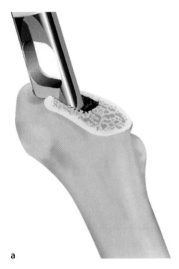

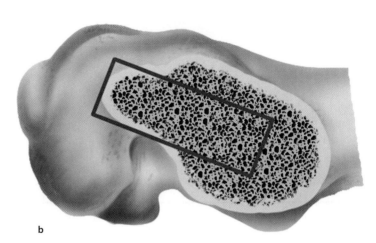

☐ **Fig. 2.27a,b.** A more lateral canal preparation with removal of the lateral neck extension is required when straight stems with a prominent lateral shoulder are implanted to prevent varus malalignment

❶ **Cave**

If this dense cortical structure is not removed prior to broaching, then the broaches will be driven too medial and a varus positioning can easily result. When using a box osteotome in the lateral area of the greater trochanter, this should be done carefully, to prevent intraoperative fractures.

Broaching

The modular broaches are inserted into the medullary canal sequentially. It is important to direct pressure laterally and posteriorly on the broach handle (☐ Fig. 2.28a). This will assist in preserving anterior and medial cancellous bone thus preventing stem malalignment (▶ chapter 5.2).

❯ Note: If the true anatomical calcar causes the resected neck to narrow posteriorly, it should be resected further before reaming (see ☐ Fig. 2.23b).

The final broach size should correspond to the pre-selected, templated stem size. In most stem design systems this means overbroaching one size to create a gap of 2 mm as a minimum cement mantle thickness.

❶ **Cave**

It is a common mistake to insert the largest broach size possible. This may be prudent for cementless stem designs, which seek cortical bone contact. For cemented stems it is of significant importance to preserve a rim of strong cancellous bone (▶ chapter 5.2).

It is a good intraoperative guide to try and aim for preservation of at least 3 mm cancellous bone medially and anteriorly. This can be easily visualised when the broach is left in situ (☐ Fig. 2.28b). The appropriate trial head/neck is selected in order to facilitate assessment of leg length and stability. If stability, stem size and leg length are correct, it is necessary to overbroach one size (see ☐ Fig. 2.28b) to allow for the appropriate cement mantle. If the lining cancellous bone becomes too sparse or if in doubt, downsizing of the stem is recommended.

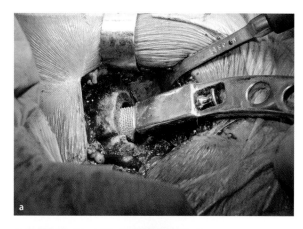

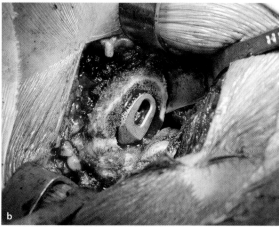

Fig. 2.28. a The photograph emphasizes broaching with maintaining postero-lateral bone contact, trying to preserve the rim of anterior-medial cancellous bone. **b** The broach size, corresponding to the pre-selected stem size, is left in situ. This confirms an adequate distance to the medial and anterior cortex, leaving enough space for a thick cement mantle. The next broach size will create the space for a pure cement mantle of 2 mm minimal thickness, but enough cancellous bone will be preserved for additional cement interdigitation

Final Preparation of Femoral Canal

Prior to the introduction of the cement, the medullary canal is cleansed with copious pulsatile lavage (◘ Fig. 2.29a). Commonly 1 litre of irrigation is used per femur. Ideally this should even be done before templating for the cement restrictor to reduce the risk of fat embolism (▶ chapter 15). Then a cement restrictor is introduced (◘ Fig. 2.29b) to a depth of 1.5–2 cm distal to the expected tip of the prosthesis; this will allow a 2 cm cement column. Usually a restrictor size is used 2 mm larger than the largest olive tip that can be passed to the isthmus.

Whilst the cement is prepared, the canal is packed to minimise backbleeding from the interface. The systolic blood pressure at this point should ideally be below 100 mmHg.

❯ Note: The authors prefer to pack the canal with a H_2O_2-soaked haemostatic ribbon gauze. If this is done, it is important to leave a sucker tube within the canal to prevent possible air embolism from the oxygen liberated. If gelatine based cement restrictors are used, it is important to realise that H_2O_2 can dissolve this material. This may then jeopardize the restrictor stability (▶ chapter 6.2).

Cement Mixing

The surgeon should use a cement with a good track record (▶ chapters 3.4 and 3.7). It is also considered important to be familiar with the »behaviour« of the cement used under operating condition, i.e. the polymerisation characteristics. Both timing and technique of the entire cementing procedure are essential contributing factors for a successful cemented THA and long-term outcome.

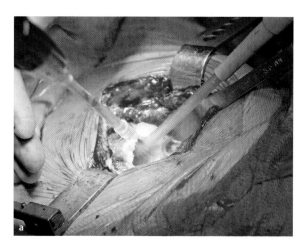

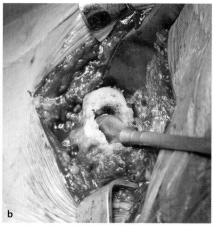

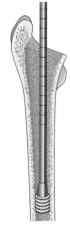

Fig. 2.29a,b. Copious pulsatile lavage ensures removal of bone marrow and blood from the cancellous bone. In the metaphysis the short lavage nozzle with direct water jet is the most effective means of bone cleansing (**a**). Lavage should be done prior to templating and insertion of the intramedullary cement restrictor (**b**). The restrictor is placed 1.5–2 cm below the expected stem tip

The authors prefer to use cement which is mixed under vacuum (▶ chapter 4). The person, who is mixing the cement, should understand the underlying science for this process. Untrained staff may produce a poor mixture, which then may me be to the disadvantage of the patient.

For the average femur, two mixes of cement, i.e. 80 g, are required to allow for extra cement for sufficient pressurization (▶ chapter 6.4). In the large stove pipe femur (Dorr C, ▶ chapter 5.2) with a wide canal more cement (120 g) is required. This has to be taken into account when choosing the mixing vessel and the cement gun-cartridge size. Some, but not all mixing systems provide special sizes for this.

Cement Application

Prior to cement application further meticulous pulsatile bone lavage is done until the cancellous bone appears »white« (■ Fig. 2.30a) and the irrigation fluid is clear. This cleansing technique with pulsatile lavage is essential to achieve optimum cement penetration into the surrounding cancellous bone. Manual lavage is ineffective, reduces the risk of fat embolism and is regarded inappropriate (▶ chapter 5.2). When using a pulsatile lavage, a long nozzle should be used for the larger femur, with the water jet pulsing at 90° angle to clean the endosteal surface (■ Fig. 2.30b).

The exact timing will depend on the preference and experience of the surgeon, the ambient theatre temperature and humidity and on the cement type/formulation. The authors prefer a medium cement viscosity at the time of gun introduction. Cement of too low viscosity is difficult to control and contain (leakage). It also carries the risk of cement intravasation (▶ chapter 15) and higher rates of failure (▶ chapter 3.7).

After having reached the preferred viscosity, the cement is then rapidly applied in a retrograde fashion via a cement gun under pressure (■ Fig. 2.31a). A narrow venting tube placed distally above the cement restrictor will remove trapped air and blood. During cement application from distal to proximal, the nozzle must not be pulled back, otherwise cement laminations and blood entrapment will result. In the authors experience, this manoeuvre is best done (virtually) one-handed, concen-

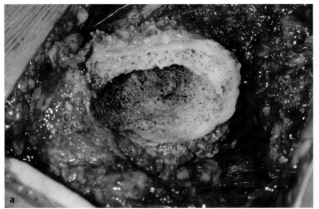
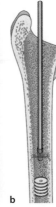

■ Fig. 2.30. a Intraoperative photograph of adequately lavaged and dried bone immediately prior to cement application. b A long lavage nozzle with perpendicular jet outlet is useful in large femora to clean the diaphysis

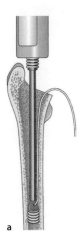
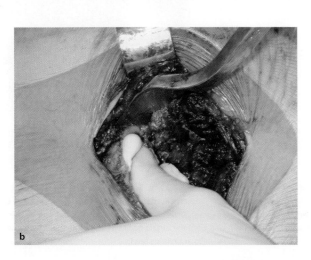

■ Fig. 2.31. a The cement is applied rapidly in retrograde fashion (see text). The venting tube should be removed before the canal is completely filled with cement. It is important to commence immediate cement pressurization using a thumb (b) to resist the bleeding pressure, whilst the nozzle is cut and the proximal seal is mounted

trating on extruding the cement from the gun as fast as possible and only supporting the gun with the other hand. The cement should automatically »drive« out the cement nozzle and gun from the canal.

At the final stages of filling the surgeons thumb (■ Fig. 2.31b) should seal the medial calcar area to immediately generate pressure. The thumb is left in place generating pressure whilst the nozzle is cut and the proximal seal mounted. It is important to apply immediate counterpressure to resist back bleeding at the interface in the early phase (► chapter 6.4).

The nozzle is cut short (■ Fig. 2.32a) and the femoral seal is mounted (■ Fig. 2.32b). Without shortening of the nozzle, no appropriate pressure can be applied, as the nozzle will slip through the seal.

The proximal femoral canal opening is occluded with a seal. Sustained cement pressurization is implemented for at least 2–3 minutes (■ Figs. 2.33 and 2.34). This (and good cement intrusion) is achieved by slow and steady trigger pulls. *It is important not to do this too quickly to avoid running out of cement during this crucial phase.* If cement pressurization is effective, no back-bleeding at the interface will occur. This can be visualised at the neck osteotomy (■ Fig. 2.35b). It is inevitable and normal that some cement will escape from the seal-bone junction. However, as long as pressure is maintained by delivering more cement for pressurization, the intramedullary pressure curve does not drop (■ Fig. 2.34). As positive intraoperative feedback for good technique bone-marrow extrusion should be apparent at the exposed proximal femoral cortex (■ Fig. 2.33b). This will still occur with good pressurization technique, even if 1.5 litres pulsatile lavage have been used.

Femoral Stem Insertion

If pressurization was adequate and the timing (viscosity) is correct, then full cement penetration can be achieved at this point. It is a mistake to rely on the stem to generate pressure for cement intrusion – the implant is merely positioned in place. The definitive femoral stem is inserted slowly in line with the longitudinal axis of the femur using sustained manual pressure (■ Fig. 2.35). The entry point remains lateral and posterior as outlined for canal

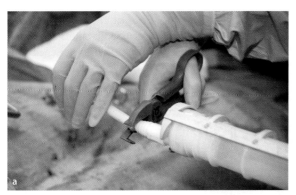

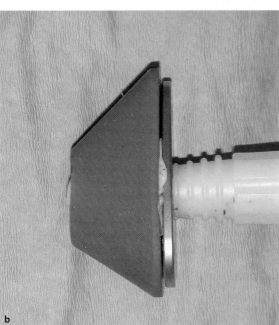

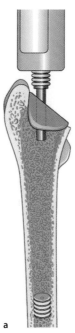
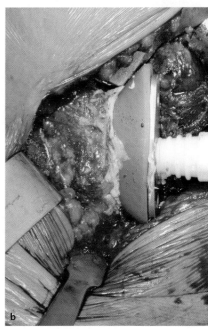

■ **Fig. 2.32a,b.** Whilst the surgeons or assistants thumb is generating pressure, the nozzle is cut (**a**) and the proximal femoral seal mounted. Then sustained cement pressurization via proximal femoral seal is commenced and maintained for at least 2–3 minutes, depending on the viscosity of the cement

■ **Fig. 2.33. a** Sustained cement pressurization via proximal seal is implemented for a minimum of 2–3 minutes (see ■ Fig. 2.34). The seal is supported with a metal base plate to improve pressurization and to prevent the nozzle from slipping. Note the fat extrusion from femoral femur (**b**) as positive feedback for adequate quality of cement penetration

preparation above. Ideally the stem introducer should give rotational control, but should not have a rigid fixation to the stem, as this may result of movement of the stem by the surgeon's unsteady hand (or inadvertent leg movement). During the insertion process slight posterior pressure, directing the stem tip anteriorly to achieve good component alignment, is applied. This will also aid in centralising the stem. The stem should be inserted slowly feeling the counter pressure of the polymerising cement; this provides good additional cement pressurization. It is important that the stem is *not* hammered into position.

Polished stems can be inserted later than matt or textured stems, as the cement stem interface is not disrupted by the polished surface sliding downwards. However, larger stem sizes require slightly earlier stem insertion as more bone cement will need to be displaced.

When centralizers are used, then the stem should not be inserted too late, as the centralizer will otherwise disrupt the cement and can cause voids and laminations.

Routinely, a blood-free femoral neck cut will be visible with all cancellous bone filled with cement plus an additional (bone-free) pure cement mantle (◘ Fig. 2.35b). The overall composite cement mantle (▸ chapter 5.2) at the medial calcar should be at least 5 mm thick. If the technique described above is followed, excellent postoperative

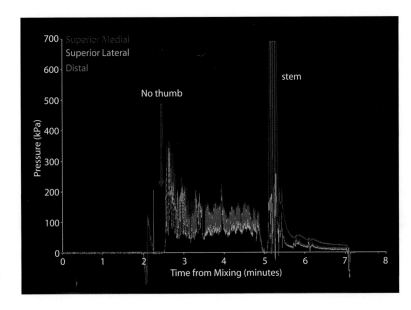

◘ **Fig. 2.34.** A pressure-tracing curve recorded intraoperatively outlines the timing of the pressurization process. Note how the pressure curve immediately drops to zero if no thumb pressure is applied. The proximal pressurization via seal creates higher and prolonged pressure at the proximal transducers, whereas the stem is more effective distally

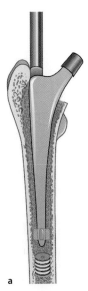

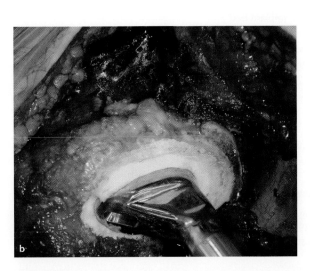

◘ **Fig. 2.35. a** In the schematic drawing, the straight line of stem implantation is shown. At the medial calcar a composite cement mantle of 5 mm should be aimed for. **b** The intraoperative photograph demonstrates the absence of back bleeding at the cement bone interface. Also the composite cement mantle of a layer of pure cement around the stem and a layer of cancellous bone (from ◘ Fig. 2.30a) complete filled with cement

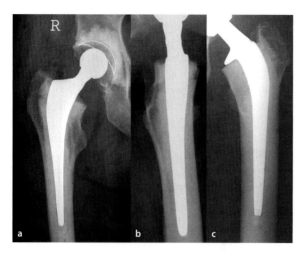

◘ Fig. 2.36a–c. Postoperative radiographs demonstrating the effect of good cementing technique with a »white out« Barrack A cement grading. Note an adequate cement mantle thickness in all a.p. and lat. Gruen zones and in particular in zone 7 at the medial calcar

radiographic results can be expected with a Barrack A cement grading »despite« preservation of cancellous bone (◘ Fig. 2.36).

Take Home Messages

- Preoperative planning is recommended. Ideally a lateral radiograph should be available to appreciate the femoral anatomy.
- A stem size should be pre-selected using templates to guarantee a minimum cement mantle of 5 mm at the medial calcar and 2–3 mm more distally.
- Identification of the piriformis fossa and strict posterior canal preparation are of critical importance to minimise the risk of thin cement mantles in the lateral plane (which cannot be seen on a.p. films!).
- Careful canal preparation should be implemented to preserve strong cancellous bone (a rim of anterior and medial cancellous bone will improve overall stem alignment).
- Pulsatile lavage is mandatory to clean implant bed and facilitate cement interdigitation.
- It is recommended to use a well-documented bone cement pre-loaded with AB. Vacuum mixing seems beneficial.
- Cement is applied at medium viscosity in a retrograde manner via a gun.
- Sustained pressurisation of at least 2–3 min via proximal seal is of utmost importance to resist bleeding pressure and to achieve optimal cement penetration.
- Femoral stem insertion is done slowly against the increasing cement viscosity.
- It is the surgeon at the time of stem implantation who will determine the long term success.

Operative Steps: The Dysplastic Hip

Colin Howie

Summary

In this chapter we will review the indications and problems of hip replacement in the presence of developmental dysplasia of the hip (DDH). The principles of total hip replacement for DDH are similar to those for routine total hip replacement; reconstruction of a near normal soft-tissue envelopes carried out to relieve pain. We are attempting to recreate normal joint biomechanics by restoring the centre of rotation, placing the trochanter lateral to the hip joint, thus improving the lever arm of the abductors, which will reduce the joint reaction force and Trendelenburg dip. We require small implant components and will attempt to insert the largest offset available. We should be able to perform acetabular augmentation and femoral osteotomy to restore the soft-tissue balance around the hip. We should be familiar with anterior and posterior approaches to the hip joint and comfortable with mobilising major neurovascular structures that may be encased in dense fibrosis due to previous surgery in childhood. We will present a system of assessment and reconstruction for the acetabulum and femur we have followed for 10 years (the results of which are recorded in later chapters ▶ chapters 8.7, 9.3), which can be used to resolve the many and varied problems.

Indications for Arthroplasty

Pain

For most patients with osteoarthritis secondary to developmental dysplasia of the hip, replacement is carried out for the same indications as for routine hip replacement, pain. However, often the pain radiates further down to the front of the knee and can be associated with a reasonable range of motion, particularly when the hip was completely dislocated.

Disability

In most cases, surgery is undertaken for pain. However, disability, reduced walking distance, difficulty dressing and mounting stairs can be a major feature in younger patients. Because developmental dysplasia predominantly affects young females, there can be other functional difficulties resulting from reduced abduction leading to problems with personal hygiene and sexual intercourse, particularly when the condition is bilateral.

Where there is significant leg length discrepancy or deformity (◘ Fig. 2.37), long-leg arthritis can develop in the contralateral knee. In these circumstances, it is often wise to perform total hip replacement on the abnormal hip before undertaking total knee replacement in the more normal, longer leg because the knee replacement would work at a mechanical disadvantage; this would lead to premature failure of the knee replacement.

Occasionally patients with longstanding fixed adduction deformity of the hip will present with valgus OA of the ipsilateral knee. Knee replacement in these patients will accentuate their scissoring gate and lead to premature failure of the TKR if the adduction deformity of the hip is not addressed first.

Where leg-length discrepancy is longstanding and the patient has developed a compensatory scoliosis, it is important to ensure that the scoliosis is correctable (by examining the back sitting) before attempting to fully correct any leg-length discrepancy.

Gait

Many patients with osteoarthritis secondary to DDH, or DDH itself, present with a waddling gait (abductor lurch). Developmental dysplasia can be regarded as a field change around the hip that includes the soft tissues as well as the bony anatomy. By reconstructing near normal hip biomechanics with hip replacement, the waddling gait

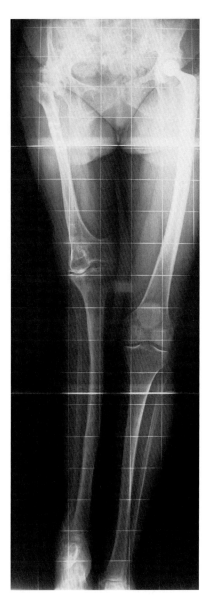

Fig. 2.37. Long-leg films showing knee arthritis, the presenting feature in this woman with surgically induced leg-length discrepancies

will improve. However, even with perfect reconstruction of the hip, many patients will continue to waddle post surgery. All patients should be warned of the possibility of the abnormal gait continuing.

Leg Length

Most patients with unilateral DDH will have significant leg-length discrepancy and may feel this to be a cosmetic problem. When assessing leg length it is important to ensure that the leg-length discrepancy is entirely due to the dislocated hip or abnormal posture. Occasionally, particularly when previous surgery has been carried out, a limb will overgrow below a dysplastic hip such that if the normal hip anatomy is restored, the leg with be over-lengthened. This can be disabling for the patient.

Back Pain

Many older patients will have walked for many years with a significant leg-length discrepancy developing secondary osteoarthritis in the lumbar spine. During clinical examination it is important to assess this by examining the sitting posture to ensure that the spinal deformity will be correct. While correction of leg-length discrepancy may improve long-term back problems in the dysplastic patient, this cannot be guaranteed. Over-correction of the leg length stressing the spinal deformity may lead to or increase back pain.

Conservative Treatments

Prior to considering surgery all conservative treatments, shoe-raises, simple analgesia, injection of steroids and – if insufficient – operative treatment including arthroscopic debridement of labral tears and realignment osteotomies, pelvic or femoral osteotomy (or both) should be considered. However, if these have been tried or are thought not suitable, then total hip replacement may be the only solution. These predominantly young patients present considerable technical problems. However, a successful, total joint replacement will relieve their pain and increase their mobility.

Grading and Planning

A variety of grading systems can be used to try to define the extent of surgery necessary (and the possible problems and outcomes). Unfortunately, most documented grading systems are used to describe the combined acetabular and femoral deformities, e.g. Eftekhar's elongated, intermediate, high, false, or no contact descriptions [3] and Crowe's grading system [2] based on migration of the femoral head in proportion to the height of the pelvis. Crowe's system is particularly difficult to apply routinely when limited views of the pelvis are taken. Perhaps clinically most useful is the grading system of Hartofilakidis [4] (Figs. 2.38 to 2.40) describing the hips as

– **dysplastic:** those with an acetabular segmental defect that is contained with a large medial osteophyte as a consistent feature (Fig. 2.38);
– **low:** those with an overlapping false acetabulum resulting in reduced depth (Fig. 2.39a);
– **high:** a false shallow acetabulum, that is rim deficient and anteverted (Fig. 2.39b).

However, all three systems ignore femoral geometry and problems related to the reconstruction of leg length. They also fail to take into account the increased difficulty of surgery when previous femoral or pelvic osteotomies have been carried out.

To be useful, a grading system should predict surgical difficulties and long-term outcome. Hence, we use the following system to plan surgery.

Dysplasia Type 1

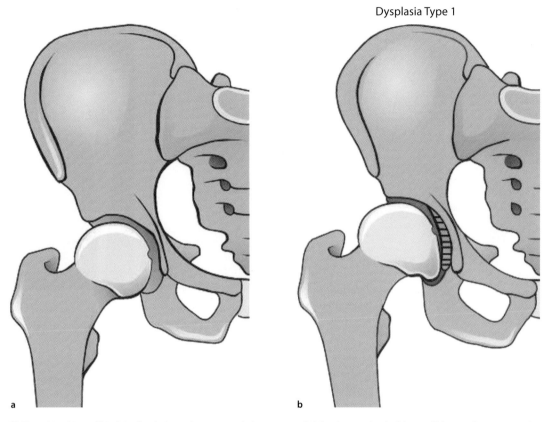

a   b

Fig. 2.38. a Normal hip. **b** In dysplasia grade 1 an acetabular segmental defect is contained with a medial osteophyte as a consistent feature

Dysplasia Type 2

Dysplasia Type 3
(High dislocation)

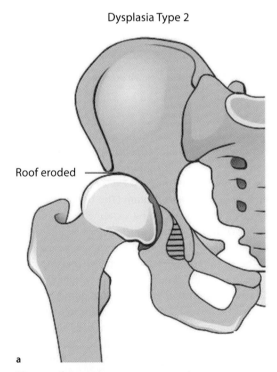

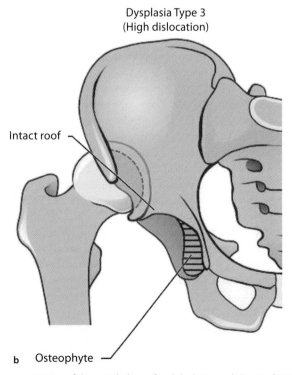

Roof eroded

Intact roof

a   b   Osteophyte

Fig. 2.39a,b. Dysplasia type 2, i.e. low dislocation (**a**) with erosion of the superior roof. In contrast, in type 3 with high dislocation (**b**) note preservation of the acetabular roof and the large medial osteophyte, but good acetabular depth

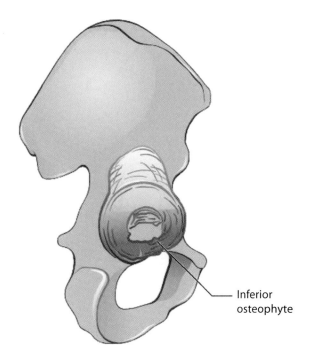

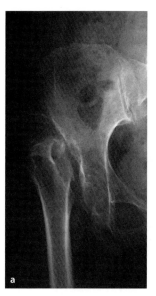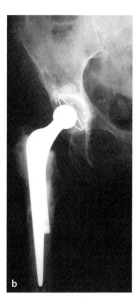

■ **Fig. 2.41a,b.** High dislocation (good acetabulum – bad femur) treated by routine acetabulum and femoral osteotomy

■ **Fig. 2.40.** Lateral view of pelvis in DDH emphasizing the encroaching osteophytes front and back and inferiorly at the level of the true acetabulum

When considering the acetabulum and its problems alone these can be considered as

- **A I: Dysplastic acetabulum (The Good)** (■ Figs. 2.38b and 2.39b): Those with a small segmental defect, but the acetabulum is largely contained and often a medial osteophyte can be removed to increase depth. These reconstructions should have a normal survival compared with routine hip replacements as they will not require grafts.

  In the »high« type 3 Hartofilakidis group, the true acetabulum is nearly always dysplastic, perhaps with a small segmental defect but a large medial osteophyte that can be removed. Grafting is rarely required. After identifying the teardrop, the acetabulum can be excavated and the smallest dimension is the AP diameter of the acetabulum itself. Therefore, the Hartofilakidis »high« group can be regarded as dysplastic. This is evident from comparing ■ Figs. 2.38b and 2.39b, which show a good true acetabular roof and anterior and posterior walls, and ■ Fig. 2.41, which shows a high dislocation treated with a standard cup in the true acetabulum without graft. In his most recent paper Hartofilakidis [5] noted the acetabular results to be similar for these two grades and better than his type 2.

- **A II: Low dislocation acetabulum (The Bad)** (■ Fig. 2.39a): Dislocation where the head lies on and deforms the superior margin of the acetabulum, which results in an overlapping false acetabulum of inadequate depth or roof. This type will always require some form

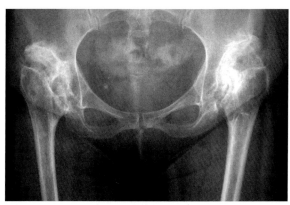

■ **Fig. 2.42.** The bad acetabulum (or low dislocation) which will require roof graft

of graft or support. Clearly, this adds to the complexity of surgery and reduces the likelihood of long-term survival (see later). This group corresponds with the »low« Hartofilakidis group (■ Fig. 2.42).

- **A III: Post-surgical acetabulum (The Ugly):** The post-surgical acetabulum can be extremely difficult. In these cases the soft tissues will be deformed increasing the risk of nerve damage, and the acetabular anatomy may be distorted. Therefore, detailed imaging may be necessary. This group should be subdivided into A IIIa post surgical that does not require grafting. This group will have higher complications perioperatively, but because the acetabulum does not require grafting, the long-term results will be similar to the type 1 dysplastic group. The A IIIb acetabulae will require grafting, the long-term results will be similar to the low dislocation type A II acetabulae.

On the femoral side, a similar grading system can be applied.

- **F I: Dysplastic femur (The Good):** Those with a degree of anteversion and up to 2 cm of apparent shortening, require no specific measures to be taken other than perhaps small-sized implants. These femoral components should have the same long-term results as routine hip replacement. See ◘ Fig. 2.39a and ◘ Fig. 2.43 with bad acetabulum, but good femur.

- **F II: High femur (The Bad):** Those femora where the dislocation is greater than 2 cm or there is extensive anteversion (occasionally retroversion), which requires correction. This extreme rotational abnormality of the proximal femur is important to correct in order to improve the lever arm of the abductors, to reduce joint reaction force and improve gait by placing the trochanter lateral rather than posterior to the hip. This second group requires a rotational and/or shortening osteotomy. As with the type-2 acetabulum this increases surgical complexity and therefore the risk of complications (◘ Fig. 2.44).

- **F III: Post-surgical femur (The Ugly):** Those that have undergone surgical intervention prior to the hip replacement (◘ Fig. 2.45). These can be subdivided into:
  a: no malformation these can be regarded and treated as dysplastic type I femora;

b: gross malformation which can be treated as type II femur;

c: retention of metalwork: In this group the metalwork may be ignored or a major problem, however, it is difficult to categorise as each case will be different. In each case the complexity of surgery increases. Proper imaging including biplanar imaging is mandatory (◘ Fig. 2.46).

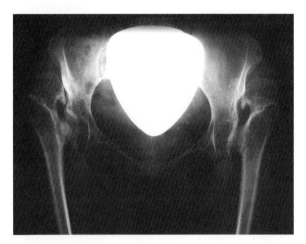

◘ **Fig. 2.44.** Good acetabulum, but bad (high) femur which will require shortening/rotational osteotomy

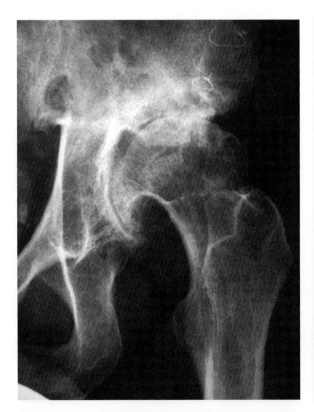

◘ **Fig. 2.43.** Ugly post surgical acetabulum requiring graft, but good femur

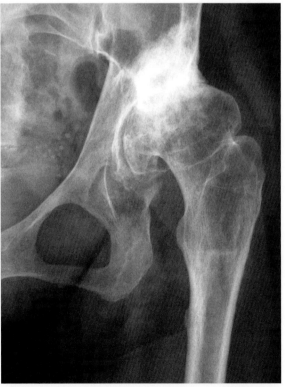

◘ **Fig. 2.45.** Ugly acetabulum (requiring graft) and ugly femur (type F IIIa, previous osteotomy) requiring investigation but probably normal femur and implant

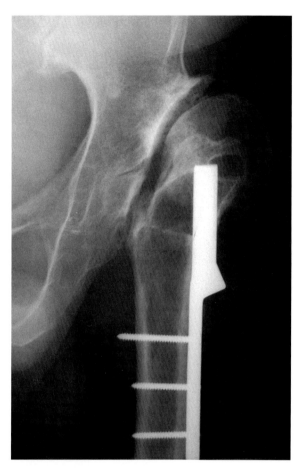

Fig. 2.46. Ugly femur (type 3C) with retained metalwork requiring osteotomy and removal of metalwork

Operative Treatment – Approach

The surgeon should be familiar with both anterior and posterior approaches to the hip joint. The exact approach used should take into account previous surgeries to the hip itself and the surgeons' preference. Previous approaches or osteotomies may cause considerable scarring around the proximal femur and periarticular soft-tissue structures. It is particularly important to identify the sciatic nerve when pelvic osteotomies have been carried out as the nerve may be accidentally damaged by traction over the previous osteotomy site or bound down in dense scar tissue. A posterior approach gives the best opportunity to visualise the sciatic nerve, however, where previous surgery has been carried out, it is important to use an extensive incision and be willing to approach the hip from both front and back to facilitate dislocation and obtain good tissue balance.

Whatever approach is used, extensive release of adhesions to mobilise the hip will be necessary. Many authors have described a trans-trochanteric approach for DDH. We prefer to keep the vasto-gluteal sling intact and if necessary use an extended trochanteric osteotomy to approach the hip. While this may well reflect our inex-

perience with re-attachment of the trochanter, these are difficult cases and re-attachment is not reliable.

Our routine approach is a posterior one supplemented by anterior release either directly over the front or indirectly from the back through the hip. Intra-operative dislocation is usually posterior, however, occasionally anterior dislocation is necessary followed by a posterior approach.

2.3.1 Acetabular Roof Graft

Acetabular Considerations

John Charnley [1] noted that acetabular bone stock was best in the true acetabulum. However, in the high false acetabulum, while the superior cover was better high, the anterior and posterior aspects of the acetabulum were often formed by osteophytes. The depth of the false acetabulum is limited by the thickness of the wing of the ilium.

In the true acetabulum of the high dislocation category (in the Caucasian population), there is often sufficient AP width to insert an implant of 40 mm outside diameter with no need for superior rim graft. Crowe [2] pointed out that when the acetabulum is over-reamed to prepare an elongated false acetabulum then the anterior and/or posterior wall is reamed away leading to instability and early failure of the acetabulum. Therefore, it must be anticipated in most cases of DDH that small implants will be required, which are sized to the AP diameter of the true acetabulum (■ Fig. 2.47).

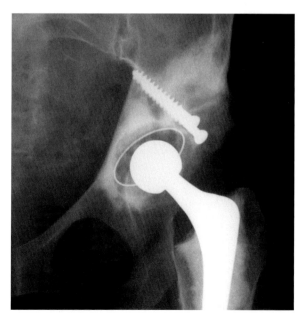

Fig. 2.47. Post-operative film of ugly acetabulum and femur earlier (see ■ Fig. 2.45) showing autogenous graft, adequate cup medialisation and restoration of centre of rotation

In this chapter, we will describe the technique we use to reconstruct the true acetabulum. The rationale for this choice is laid out in ▶ chapter 9.3.

The author's preferred technique is to augment the acetabular defect with bone from the patient's own femoral head by placing the graft back into the defect from which it came screwing the graft into position. Wolfgang [6] described the technique in 1990.

Technique of Acetabular Roof Graft

Pre-operative planning (and templating) for the type-A II defect will suggest that a roof graft will be required. It is often difficult to be sure of the degree of defect prior to surgery but at operation, once the acetabulum has been cleared and the true acetabulum identified with the transverse ligament and teardrop displayed, the encroaching anterior and posterior osteophytes can be removed with crank gouges. The true anterior and posterior walls should be identified and the acetabulum reamed usually to 40–44 mm AP diameter. By placing a trial cup in position (or last reamer in the correct orientation) the defect immediately becomes apparent (◘ Fig. 2.48). The last reamer size corresponds to the given AP socket diameter and should be kept inferior at the level of the acetabular notch (◘ Fig. 2.49b). This will reveal the full extent of the roof defect. Caution should be exercised at this stage as a false sense of cover can be obtained in »minor« cases by opening the cup too much, dislocation will occur.

If the defect is less than 10% this can be safely ignored and the acetabulum dealt with in the usual manner for a primary implant. If the defect is up to 20%, again this can be dealt with in the usual manner, but the author's preference is to use a flanged cup to cover the defect. Where the defect is greater than 20%, graft augmentation would be required using block autograft from the femoral head.

Having mobilised the femur (and cut the femoral neck), identified the anterior and posterior walls of the acetabulum and reamed the true acetabulum to its maximum AP diameter, the defect is identified and any pseudo-cartilage removed from the defect area. The femoral head is then placed back in the defect which it created and the section of the femoral head which fills the defect marked either with a sterile marker pen or with diathermy.

This often amounts to an orange segment shaped wedge after preparation (◘ Fig. 2.50). Prior to cutting the

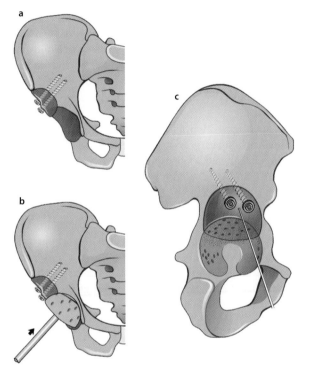

◘ **Fig. 2.49a–c.** Diagrams showing insertion and reaming of graft. **a** The graft is temporarily fixed with a K-wire, but secured with two cancellous lag screws. As shown in the lateral projection (**c**) the direction of the screw placement is posterior towards the sacroiliac joint. When the overhanging bone of the roof graft is reamed, the reamer must be kept inferior (**b**). Multiple anchorage holes are made for cement interlocking

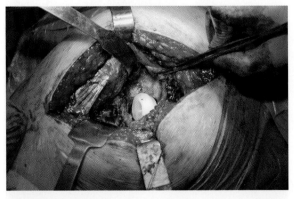

◘ **Fig. 2.48.** Acetabular trial in place highlighting superior defect (*on right*)

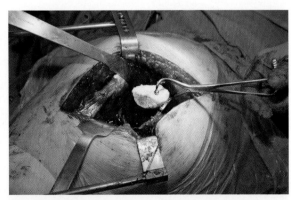

◘ **Fig. 2.50.** Orange segment wedge from femoral head cut to rough size

wedge, the fibro-cartilage is removed with the saw acting as a rasp such that there is no fibro-cartilage left on the head (the subchondral bone is preserved). The orange segment wedge is then cut. It is wise to cut a thicker wedge than required at this stage and trim after insertion of the definitive cup. Attempts to make the correct size at this stage will result in graft fracture when drilling or tapping the graft.

Prior to application of the graft, 3 small pits are created into the true acetabulum, one into the ischium, one into the pubic ramus and one up behind the cortical plate at the level of the defect into host bone. Acetabular reamings from the true acetabulum are then gathered together and compressed in a swab to remove all excess blood and marrow (◻ Fig. 2.51). This gives a very firm, soft, collection of fine bone fragments which can be pressed over the acetabular defect, to which the wedge-shaped graft is applied.

Good apposition and conformity can be obtained. Other techniques previously described have taken the femoral head and applied cancellous bone to the defect rather than cortex to cortex described here. The author has no experience of this, but good results have been reported. Once the orange segment femoral head wedge has been placed in position, a wire is drilled in centrally to temporarily hold the wedge in position (see ◻ Fig. 2.49).

The surgeon should identify the sciatic notch and sciatic nerve as it passes into the pelvis at this stage to orientate the direction for his screws (◻ Fig. 2.49c). With a large 4.5 mm drill bit the graft is over-drilled, then with a 3.2 mm drill the host pelvis is drilled to take the definitive cancellous screw. Drilling is performed using a gentle balloting technique to ensure that the drill does not penetrate the pelvis unexpectedly or deeply. Before measuring screw length the graft should be countersunk to subchondral bone. Screw length can vary considerably and great care should be taken particularly when screw length appears to be greater than 70 mm. The hole is tapped for a large cancellous screw and the definitive screw inserted but not over-tightened. A second screw is similarly inserted. Counter sinking is used to obtain good grip on the sub-chondral bone and place the screw-heads away from the maximum diameter of the acetabulum. This is such that when the reamer is inserted to complete the preparation, it does not get damaged by the screw-heads (using this technique washers are usually not required to spread stress).

With the graft in place and held by 2 screws, the K wire is removed and the screws tightened. Any residual blood in the morsellised graft when placed between the block wedge graft and the pelvis, will squeeze out. Originally 3 screws were used, however, this often caused fracture at the anterior or posterior edge and now 2 screws are used routinely.

The true acetabulum is then reamed with a one size smaller reamer than the final reaming then, using the definitive sized reamer, the true acetabulum is reamed down to the original position (◻ Fig. 2.49b). This final reaming reshapes the inside of the wedge graft to give an almost perfect finish to the internal surface. The surgeon can now more accurately estimate the amount of graft cover created.

It is important to maintain the graft at quite a large size at this stage to prevent fracture. Further trimming can be done after the acetabulum has been cemented in place.

The new acetabulum is now cleaned and dried in the standard manner and standard modern cementing techniques are used with the insertion of an All-Poly acetabular component (◻ Fig. 2.52).

Definitive trimming of the outer surface of the graft can now be carried out without fear of splitting the construct. Post-operatively, the patient is encouraged to mobilise partial weight-bearing for 6 weeks and then mobilise full weight-bearing thereafter.

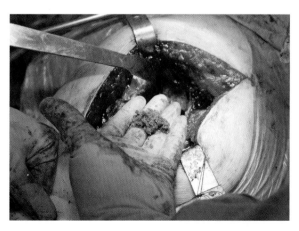

◻ **Fig. 2.51.** Acetabular reamings before compression into graft bed

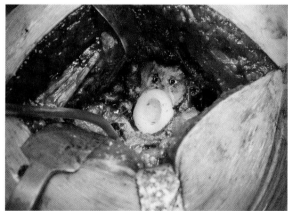

◻ **Fig. 2.52.** Cup and graft in situ

2.3.2 Femoral Reconstruction

Femoral Considerations

The principal aims of femoral reconstruction are
- to restore anteversion and thus reduce the risk of dislocation,
- to reposition the trochanter in a lateral position,
- to restore offset (to improve the abductor lever arm and reduce joint reaction force),
- to restore leg length. To attempt to improve cosmesis and function.

Type F I (The Good)

In these femora it is important to have a variety of stem sizes that will fit the femur. Pre-operative assessment will often reveal significant disparities in the AP and mediolateral dimensions of the femur. Careful pre-operative planning may suggest that one of the reduced stems currently available for the Asia-Pacific countries may be suitable for the conventional DDH in the Caucasian population. These have the benefit of short-stem length, but relatively reduced offset to improve the lever arm and the ready availability of implants. These small implants should be available when attempting to do any surgery in a patient with DDH as the curvature of even a normal looking femur may be such that it precludes insertion of a routine implant. Minor degrees of shortening (less than 3 cm) or rotational abnormalities can be dealt with, by simple positioning of the femoral component and perhaps a low neck cut.

Type F II (The Bad)

In these femora the abnormalities will fall into two categories: length and rotation. Where there is considerable leg-length discrepancy due to a high riding femur (greater than 3 cm), it may be necessary to remove a considerable section of the femur to bring the trochanter down and tension the abductors correctly and yet not overstretch the structures leading from the pelvis to the knee (neuromuscular bundles and adductor muscles.). In high dislocations the abductor mechanism has often been displaced posteriorly and at least the anterior fibres of gluteus medius and minimus will be lengthened. Therefore, bringing the trochanter down, unless there has been previous surgery causing scarring, is not usually an issue. Despite removing a subtrochanteric section of bone, this procedure will often lengthen the leg considerably, if not fully, and improve the patient's disability. Severe rotational abnormalities, particularly in the high dislocations should be corrected to reduce dislocation post surgery and restore the lateral position of the greater trochanter.

Type F III Post-Surgical Femur (The Ugly)

Where the femur has been subjected to previous surgery there may be considerable deformity. True bi-planar films should be obtained of the proximal femur in all cases where femoral surgery has been performed around the hip (◧ Fig. 2.53).

Type F IIIa (No Persisting Deformity) ▸ Following investigation and imaging, the surgeon may be able to insert a standard hip replacement, particularly when all met-

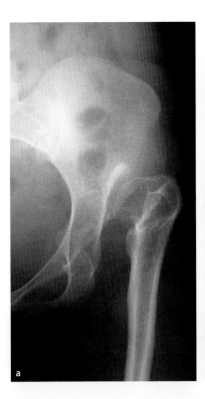
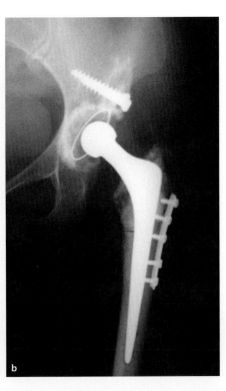

◧ **Fig. 2.53a,b.** Pre- and post-operative radiograph of the high femur type FIII post-surgical femur (The Ugly)

alwork has been previously removed and there has been no gross displacement (◘ Fig. 2.54). These femora should have the same results as the type-1 femur.

Type F IIIb (Persisting, Post-Surgical Deformity) ▶ In these situations, osteotomy should be carried out at the site of maximum deformity (◘ Fig 2.55). Often there will be a degree of size mismatch when the deformity has been corrected, particularly if large rotational abnormalities are corrected.

Type F IIIc (Retained Metalwork) ▶ It is often stated that metalwork should be removed as a separate procedure to reduce the risks of fracture and infection. Unfortunately, if plates have been inserted and not removed in childhood, these may become overgrown and migrate within the medullary canal. Removal of these incarcerated implants will lead to loss of almost half the cortical structure of the femur; at the time of later hip replacement, these defects have not always healed.

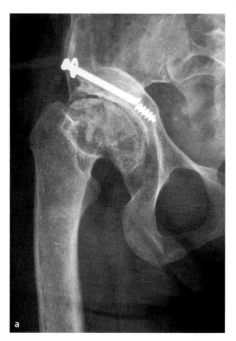
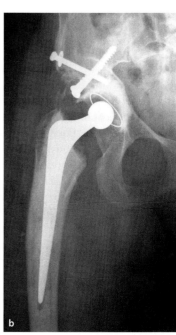

◘ **Fig. 2.54a,b.** Ugly femur with minimal persisting deformity and acetabulum treated with standard femoral component and acetabular grafting

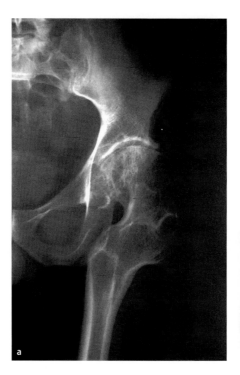
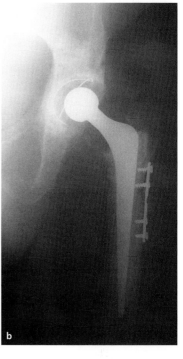

◘ **Fig. 2.55a,b.** Deformed ugly, post surgical proximal femur before (**a**) and after (**b**) osteotomy (not carried out for DDH)

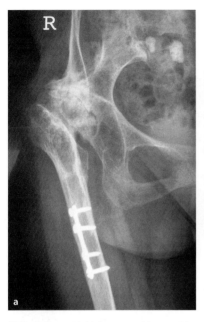
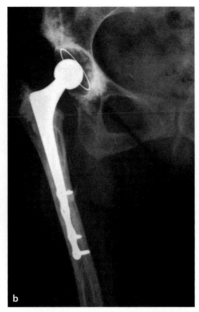
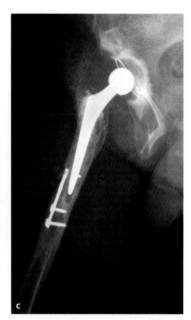

Fig. 2.56a–c. Multiply operated femur with retained metalwork, which (after careful planning) was treated with a standard small implant. Note the plate is encased in bone

It is not always necessary to remove the superficial plates, if the screws can be removed and an implant inserted the plate can be left in situ (**Fig. 2.56**). Occasionally, the screws may have been placed eccentrically and can be ignored. Some screws are notoriously difficult to remove and may fracture on removal due to poor head design or the use of titanium for the implant, which then becomes ingrown. Experience would suggest that when over-drills (tube saws) have been used to remove screws with a broken head, this creates a large cortical defect that does not fill in with time. There may be a number of these large defects leading to a series of holes that can act as a significant stress riser leading to periprosthetic fracture at a later date.

Where necessary, our plan is to remove obvious metalwork, then perform a subtrochanteric osteotomy and remove any residual problematic screws from within the femur using a carbide burr under direct vision. Plates that are encased in the cortex can be cut during osteotomy in situ using carbide discs and left rather than guttering the femur. It is recommended that screws should be removed prior to the attempted osteotomy as this makes stabilisation of the work easier for screw removal.

Technique of Shortening Osteotomy

Although a number of authors recommend a sub-trochanteric osteotomy prior to preparation of the acetabulum, we find that acetabular preparation and insertion should be carried out before the osteotomy as this gives easy control of the femur for acetabular preparation.

The proximal end of the femur is prepared in the standard way to accept the implant prior to osteotomy. With the exception of rasping, much preparation is carried out manually, which can be difficult in a small proximal fragment once sectioned.

Femoral Osteotomy Rasping Proximal Femur

The vasto-gluteal sling should be kept intact, but the psoas and all soft tissue and capsule attached to the femoral neck proximal to the psoas should be removed. The osteotomy is carried out perpendicular to the true shaft of the femur just below the lesser trochanter and proximal to any deformity as a planar osteotomy.

The proximal fragment preparation is then finished and the preparatory rasp inserted through the proximal fragment, but not into the distal fragment (**Fig. 2.57**).

A trial reduction of the proximal fragment is carried out to ensure that the abductors allow normal positioning of the femoral component. With the trial component in situ, through the proximal fragment, the distal femoral shaft is then pulled into normal alignment parallel to the proximal fragment and the femoral resection marked with a sterile pen or diathermy (**Fig. 2.58**), based on the overlapping segment.

> Note: The resection length will often be one half the distance between the existing centre of rotation and the true (desired) centre of rotation of the femoral head as evidence on the pre-operative X-ray, though this may vary due to scarring from previous surgery.

It is always wise to remove slightly less bone in the first instance and the cut should be made perpendicular to

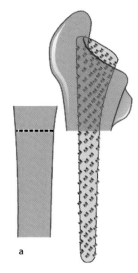

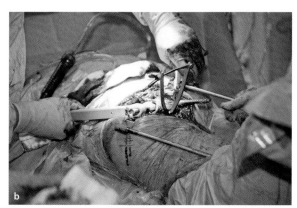

Fig. 2.57a,b. The final rasp is placed through proximal fragment and parallel to shaft, but not entering the distal fragment

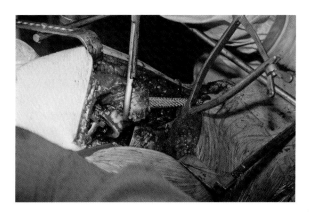

Fig. 2.58. By pulling the leg out to length and having the proximal fragment reduced with the trial rasp, the level of the femoral osteotomy can be marked. The amount of overlap will determine the resection level

the shaft of the femur, where possible parallel to the first cut on the proximal fragment. Before preparing the distal segment, the correct distal rotation should be checked and the rotational alignment noted.

The distal femoral fragment is then prepared with the true normal 10–15° of anteversion. This can sometimes be difficult because of abnormality in the shape of the femur at this level. Occasionally, high-speed burrs may be used to improve the internal morphology of the femur. The rasp is removed from the proximal fragment and used to finish preparation of the distal fragment in the correct degree of anteversion (**Fig. 2.59**).

A cement restrictor is placed down the distal fragment and a trial reduction carried out by placing the rasp through the proximal fragment into the distal fragment, closing the osteotomy and reducing the hip. If reduction is not possible, a further section of bone can be removed from the distal fragment.

If reduction is possible, the osteotomy is examined for its planar qualities and if it is thought not to be correct, further trimming of the osteotomy can be planned to obtain two planar surfaces. Leg length, abductor tension, tension in the sciatic nerve can then be all assessed.

With the preparatory rasp in situ the osteotomy is usually held very firmly (**Fig. 2.59b**). Clearly, when this is removed, for purposes of cementing and insertion of the definitive implant, the osteotomy will displace. This is prevented by placing a uni-cortical plate, usually a 5-hole semi-tubular plate, on the posterior aspect of the femur with the proximal screws going lateral to the rasp through two cortices in the trochanter and uni-cortical distally (**Fig. 2.60**). This will give some rotational stability and the plate is further held with two bone-holding forceps. The anteversion of the femoral component is checked to ensure that the trochanter has been placed laterally and the preparatory broach is removed.

The femoral osteotomy is held in position by the assistant's finger curling round the femur and the plate (occasionally a second plate may be used to obtain full stability, but the second 2-hole plate should be removed).

Some surgeons then attempt to perform internal impaction grafting of the osteotomy site. In our series, we have ignored the osteotomy and proceeded with standard cementing techniques (pulsatile lavage, gun and pressurisation) with the insertion of a standard CDH cemented stem to bridge the osteotomy site. The position is then held until the cement is completely set. The osteotomy is then examined (after allowing the cement to set and removing the assistant's finger from around it!) and with a sharp osteotome excess cement is cracked off. This usually removes most of the cement from the site of the osteotomy. Residual cancellous bone graft from the femoral

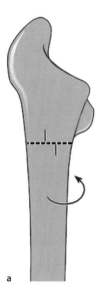

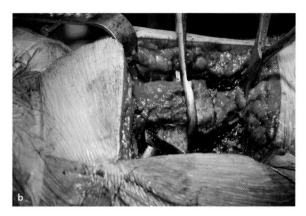

a   b

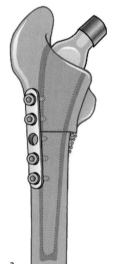

a   b

■ **Fig. 2.59a,b.** The distal femoral segment is rotated into the correct position (**a**) and the femoral rasp is advanced across the osteotomy (**b**)

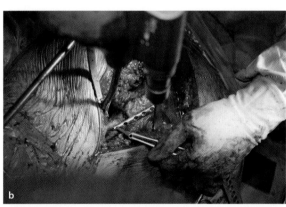

■ **Fig. 2.60a,b.** The correct rotation and alignment at the femoral osteotomy is secured with a short 1/3 tubular plate and unicortical screws

head is then placed around the osteotomy site. The Vastus lateralis is placed back down onto bone and reduction of the hip carried out.

The uni-cortical plate is usually left in situ, the wound is closed in the standard manner and the patient is asked to mobilise partially weight-bearing for 8 weeks.

It is important to note that a femoral osteotomy reduces adductor tension but improves abductor function. It corrects mal-rotation of the femur at the site of deformity and may be performed in the sub-trochanteric region to correct length problems. Where plates have been inserted and cannot be removed without cortical osteotomy, the femoral osteotomy should be carried out through the proximal screw hole to allow internal removal of distal screws. The vasto-gluteal sling should be retained throughout the procedure.

Take Home Messages

- The indications for surgery following DDH are the same as for total hip replacement for other conditions. However, the implications for adjacent joints are more important.
- The aim of reconstruction is to create normal biomechanics.
- Acetabular roof graft and femoral osteotomy should be familiar to the surgeon.
- Reconstruction following previous surgery requires special care and consideration.
- Extensive planning and equipment (e.g. for metal removal) will be necessary, including small implants.

References

1. Charnley J, Feagin JA. Low-friction arthroplasty in congenital subluxation of the hip. Clin Orthop 1973; 91: 98–113
2. Crowe JF. Mani VJ, Ranawat CS. Total hip replacement in congenital dislocation and dysplasia of the hip. J Bone Joint Surg 1979; 61-A: 15–23
3. Eftekhar NS. Principles of total hip arthroplasty. St. Louis, C.V. Mosby, 1978, pp 437–455
4. Hartofilakidis G, Stamos K, Karachalios T, Ioannidis TT, Zacharakis N. Congenital hip disease in adults. Classification of acetabular deficiencies and operative treatment with acetabuloplasty combined with total hip arthroplasty. J Bone Joint Surg 1996; 78-A: 683–692
5. Hartofilakidis G, Karachalios T. Total hip arthroplasty for congenital hip disease. J Bone Joint Surg 2004; 86-A(2): 242–250
6. Wolfgang GL. Femoral head autografting with total hip arthroplasty for lateral acetabular dysplasia. A 12-year experience. Clin Orthop 1990; 255: 173–185

Part II   Basic Science

Chapter 3   Properties of Bone Cement   – 52

Chapter 3.1   What is Bone Cement?   – 52
                K.-D. Kühn

Chapter 3.2   The Mechanical Properties of Acrylic Bone Cement   – 60
                C. Lee

Chapter 3.3   Testing and Performance of Bone Cements   – 67
                P.T. Spierings

Chapter 3.4   Extreme Differences in Properties of Successful
                Bone Cements   – 79
                A.U. Dan Daniels, D. Wirz, and E. Morscher

Chapter 3.5   Antibiotic-Loaded Cement   – 86
                L. Frommelt, and K.-D. Kühn

Chapter 3.6   The Three Interfaces   – 93
                K. Draenert, and Y. Draenert

Chapter 3.7   Which Cement Should we Choose for Primary THA?   – 103
                O. Furnes, B. Espehaug, and L.I. Havelin

Chapter 4   Mixing   – 107

Chapter 4.1   The Benefit of Vacuum Mixing   – 107
                J.-S. Wang

Chapter 4.2   Choice of Mixing System   – 113
                J.-S. Wang, and S.J. Breusch

Chapter 5   Bone Preparation   – 119

Chapter 5.1   The Importance to Establish
                the Best Cement Bone Interface   – 119
                C. Lee

Chapter 5.2   Femur   – 125

Chapter 5.2.1   Femoral Preparation and Pulsative Lavage   – 125

Chapter 5.2.2   The Optimal Cement Mantle   – 128
                S.J. Breusch

Chapter 5.3   Acetabulum   – 141

Chapter 5.3.1   Bone Bed Preparation   – 141

Chapter 5.3.2   Optimal Cement Mantle?   – 143
                D. Parsch, and S.J. Breusch

Properties of Bone Cement: What is Bone Cement?

Klaus-Dieter Kühn

Summary

Bone cements based on polymethylmethacrylate are essential products in joint arthroplasty. Originally developed for dental applications, they have been used successfully in arthroplasty surgery for more than 40 years.

Though they seem to be simple cold curing powder/liquid systems, there are many details in which bone cements can differ leading to significantly varying properties.

Acrylic Bone Cements – Bone Cements Based on Polymethylmethacrylate

History

Polymethylmethacrylate (= PMMA) was known in 1902 by the chemist Otto Röhm. As »Plexiglas«, a glass-like hard material, it has been used for many purposes since then. By 1936, the company Kulzer (1936; patent DRP 737058) had already found that a dough can be produced by mixing ground polymethylmethacrylate (PMMA) powder and a liquid monomer that hardens when benzoyl peroxide (BPO) is added and the mixture is heated to 100 °C in a stone mould. The first clinical use of these PMMA mixtures was an attempt to close cranial defects in monkeys in 1938. When these experiences became known, surgeons were anxious to try these materials in plastic surgery on humans. The heat curing polymer Paladon 65 was soon used for closing cranial defects in humans by producing plates in the laboratory and later adjusting the hardened material on the spot [7].

> **Note: Historical Development**
> 1901 Thesis of Otto Röhm »Polymerization products of acrylic acid«
> 1928 Röhm and Haas patented application of PMMA as plastic material
> 1936 Kulzer patented heat-curable dough
> 1943 Kulzer and Degussa patented a cold-curing material
> 1958 Sir John Charnley succeeded in anchoring femoral head prostheses with self-curing cement = bone cement on acrylic basis

When chemists discovered that the polymerization of MMA would occur by itself at room temperature if a co-initiator is added, the companies Degussa and Kulzer (1943, patent DRP 973 590) by using tertiary aromatic amines established a protocol for the chemical production of PMMA bone cements in 1943; this process is still valid to this day. These studies must be considered the hour of birth of PMMA bone cements.

Judet and Judet [6] were the first to introduce an arthroplastic surgical method. Soon, however, it became apparent that the PMMA (Plexiglas) prosthesis used could not be integrated in the body (for biological and mechanical reasons). In 1958, Sir John Charnley first succeeded in anchoring femoral head prostheses in the femur with auto-polymerizing PMMA [2]. Charnley called the material »bone cement on acrylic basis«. His studies described a totally new surgical technique [3].

PMMA bone cements originally were only cold-polymerized materials based on methyl methacrylate, whereas for some years the term has been used for bone substitute materials, too, hoping to substitute the biologically inert polymethylmethacrylate by biologically active materials.

Chapter 3.1 · Properties of Bone Cement: What is Bone Cement?

53 **3**

Clinical Use and Function

Bone cements are used for the fixation of artificial joints. The cements fill the free space between the prosthesis and the bone and constitute a very important zone. Owing to their optimal rigidity, the cements can evenly buffer the forces acting against the bone. The close connection between the cement and the bone as well as cement and the prosthesis leads to an optimal distribution of the stresses and interface strain energy.

The transfer of the forces bone-to-implant and implant-to-bone is the primary task of the bone cement. The ability to do so reliably for a long time is crucial for the long-term survival of the implant. An adequate cement interdigitation/interlock and reinforcement of the spongious bone are of utmost importance. If the continuous stress from outside exceeds the capability of the bone cement to transfer and absorb forces, a fatigue break is possible [8].

Antibiotic-loaded bone cements are also drug-delivery systems. It is well known that artificial implants are especially susceptible to bacterial colonisation on their surfaces because the germs can then escape the natural protection via the body and cause a periprosthetic infection. When applying antibiotics locally, bone cements can have the function of the carrier matrix.

> Note: Functions of Bone Cements
> ▬ Fixation of artificial joints
> ▬ Anchoring of the implant to the bone
> ▬ Load transfer from the prosthesis to the bone
> ▬ Optimal stress/strain distribution
> ▬ Release of antibiotics

Composition

PMMA bone cements are offered as two-component systems (powder and liquid). The polymer powder component consists of PMMA and/or methacrylate copolymers (◘ Figs. 3.1 and 3.2). Additionally, it contains benzoyl peroxide (BPO) as initiator of the radical polymerization being included in the polymer beads or simply admixed to the powder. The powder also contains a radiopacifier and optionally an antibiotic (◘ Fig. 3.3).

In the liquid phase methyl methacrylate (= MMA) is the main ingredient and sometimes other methacrylates such as butyl methacrylate (◘ Fig. 3.4).

In order to be used for bone cements the methacrylates must be polymerizable. As a pre-condition for that they must bear a C=C double bond. As an activator for the forming of radicals the liquid contains an aromatic amine, such as N,N-dimethyl-p-toluidine (DmpT). Additionally, it contains an inhibitor to avoid a premature polymerization during storage and optionally a coloring agent (e.g. chlorophyll with Palacos).

Methyl methacrylate (MMA)

$$H_2C = \overset{\overset{\displaystyle COOCH_3}{\displaystyle |}}{\underset{\underset{\displaystyle CH_3}{\displaystyle |}}{C}}$$

Clear colourless liquid of intense odour
Ester of methacrylic acid: CO-O-CH₃
Stabilized by hydroquinone or hydroquinone derivatives
Polymerizable C=C double bond

Boiling point:	100 °C
Density:	0.943 g/cm³ at 20 °C
Vapour pressure:	38 hPa at 20 °C
Molecular weight:	100 g/mol
Odour threshold:	0.2 ppm

◘ **Fig. 3.1.** Methyl methacrylate

Polymethylmethacrylate

R – (CH₂ – C – CH₂ – C – CH₂ – C -)ₙ – R   chemical formula
with CH₃ and COOCH₃ side groups

- material marketed under many brands
- fine powder (polymer beads)
- bead diameter: 1-125 µm
- soluble in monomer
- density: 1.18 g/cm³
- molecular weight: 800.000 Da

◘ **Fig. 3.2.** Poly(methyl methacrylate)

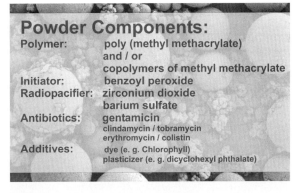

Powder Components:

Polymer:	poly (methyl methacrylate) and / or copolymers of methyl methacrylate
Initiator:	benzoyl peroxide
Radiopacifier:	zirconium dioxide barium sulfate
Antibiotics:	gentamicin clindamycin / tobramycin erythromycin / colistin
Additives:	dye (e. g. Chlorophyll) plasticizer (e. g. dicyclohexyl phthalate)

◘ **Fig. 3.3.** Powder components

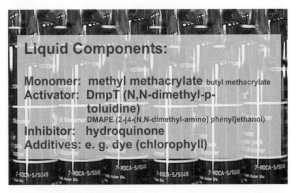

Liquid Components:

Monomer:	methyl methacrylate butyl methacrylate
Activator:	DmpT (N,N-dimethyl-p-toluidine) DMAPE (2-[4-(N,N-dimethyl-amino) phenyl]ethanol)
Inhibitor:	hydroquinone
Additives:	e. g. dye (chlorophyll)

◘ **Fig. 3.4.** Liquid components

Radiopacity

As radiopacifier zirconium dioxide or barium sulphate are added to the bone cements. Both are not integrated in the polymer chains but remain evenly distributed in the polymer matrix. Animal studies as well as recent cell culture studies show significantly higher osteolytic changes with barium sulphate as compared to the more radiopaque zirconium dioxide [8]. In spite of the low solubility of barium sulphate toxic barium ions can be set free whereas zirconium dioxide has a higher abrasive potential. These dangerous properties, however, can only come into play if the implant loosens or if loose cement particles can gain access the joint articulation.

> **Note:**
>   ▬ Zirconium dioxide = ZrO_2
>   ▬ Barium sulfate = $BaSO_4$
>
>   Radiopacifiers are needed
>   ▬ for monitoring
>   ▬ for identification of failures

Initiator System for the Polymerization

Mixing of powder and liquid results in a reaction between the initiator benzoyl peroxide and the activator DmpT forming radicals already at room temperature. For that purpose the DmpT (liquid) causes the decomposition of the BPO (powder) in a reduction/oxidation process by electron transfer resulting in benzoyl radicals. These are reactive, short-living chemical entities being able to start the polymerization by adding themselves to the reactive C=C double bond of the MMA (◘ Fig. 3.5).

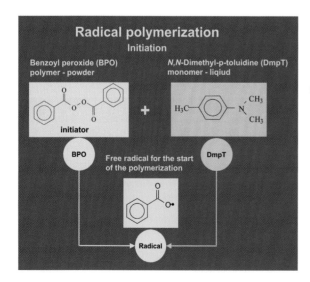

◘ Fig. 3.5. Initiation

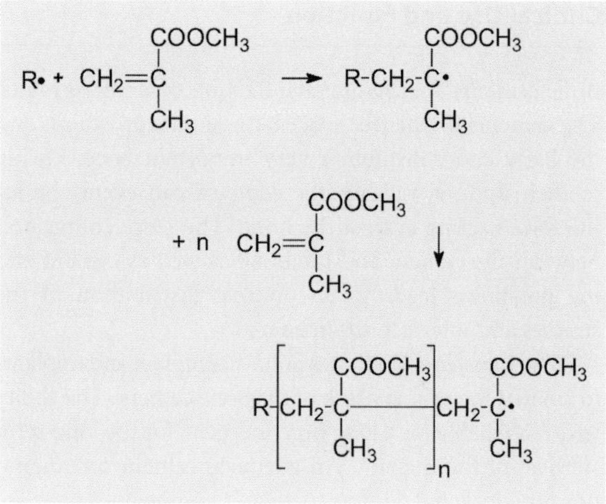

◘ Fig. 3.6. Chain growth

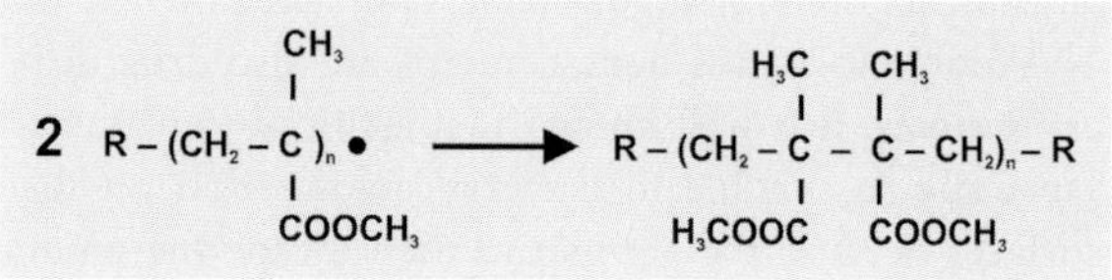

◘ Fig. 3.7. Chain recombination

Because of the large amount of radicals a big number of rapidly growing polymer chains are generated, reaching molecular weights of 100,000 to 1,000,000. With the increasing viscosity of the dough the mobility of the monomer is reduced. By recombination of two radical chains the system depletes of radicals and the polymerization dies down (◘ Figs. 3.6 and 3.7).

Polymerization Heat

The radical polymerization is an exothermic chemical reaction. So with the proceeding polymerization and consequently also growing dough viscosity the temperature increases, as 57 kJ of polymerization heat are generated per mole MMA.

> Note: Radical polymerization of MMA to PMMA = exothermic reaction
> Heat of polymerization: 57 kJ (13.8 kcal) per mole MMA

The peak temperature being observed only for a short time period during the curing of the cement was mentioned many times as the main reason for aseptic loosening by heat necrosis. Especially connective tissue reactions at loose implants were interpreted as a result of a primary heat damage to the bone bed. However, the peak temperatures recorded *in vitro* do not correspond with those actually reached *in vivo* (◘ Fig. 3.8). Clinical tests showed significantly lower intraoperative peaks

Chapter 3.1 · Properties of Bone Cement: What is Bone Cement?

55   3

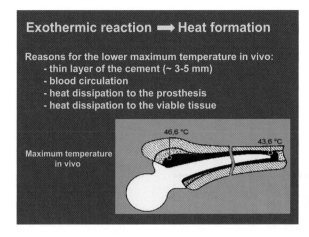

Fig. 3.8. In vivo temperatures

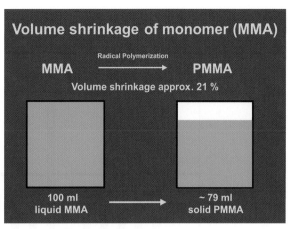

Fig. 3.9. Volume shrinkage

(40–46 °C) at the bone-cement interface. The upper limit is supposed to be reached only in pure cement layers of 3 mm or thicker without cancellous interdigitation [1].

With adequate operative technique with preservation of the spongiosa it seems to be unlikely that the protein coagulation temperature is exceeded, particularly because of the heat dissipation of the system via the implants and local blood circulation. The temperature peak can only be influenced slightly (e. g. by liquid composition, different powder/liquid ratio or radiopacifier content). Those changes will, however, result in quite different working properties and, usually, a significant reduction in mechanical stability.

Polymerization Shrinkage

Bone cement cannot be produced from monomer methyl methacrylate (MMA) alone; polymerization would take much too long, and the polymerization shrinkage would be extremely high. In addition, the heat occurring during the polymerization of the monomer could not be controlled.

During the polymerization, many monomer molecules combine to few long polymer molecules. Those approach to one another and an inevitable volume shrink is observed. Pure MMA shrinks by 21%, that means that 1 litre of MMA results in 790 ml PMMA (Fig. 3.9).

By using the pre-polymerized powder component, the share of MMA in the system is reduced to 1/3. The theoretical shrinkage is 6–7% then. In reality it is lower due to the cement porosity. That is why hand-mixed cements tend to shrink a little less than vacuum-mixed cements. *In vivo* a major part of the volume shrinkage is compensated by water uptake of the cement.

Molecular Weight

The molecular weight of the cured cement depends mainly on the molecular weight of the polymer in the powder component and its sterilization method. The molecular weight has a significant influence on the swelling property, the fatigue properties, the cement viscosity and the working time. Contrary to ethylene sterilization the gamma irradiation leads to a reduction of the molecular weight. The advantage is the high penetration depth allowing the material to be sterilized in the final package.

> Note: Factors influencing the polymer's molecular weight:
> - Molecular weight (MW) of the raw materials used in the polymer
> - Sterilization method of the polymer powder (sterilization by irradiation results in a reduction to approx. 50% of the MW)
> - Molecular weight of the monomer
> - Concentration of the initiator system or ratio initiator/activator, respectively
> - Progress of the temperature in the reaction
> - Presence of regulators

However, it is also known that the irradiation causes changes of the properties of plastic materials. The highly energetic rays clearly reduce the initial molecular weight of the polymer in the powder. Thus, one can assume that irradiated polymers must have had a much higher molecular weight before the sterilization (Fig. 3.10).

Because of the different polymer structure the handling properties of cements are quite different before and after irradiation.

Ethylene oxide (EO)-sterilization is very complex and more sensitive. The residual EO also has to be desorbed from the powder using a valid process.

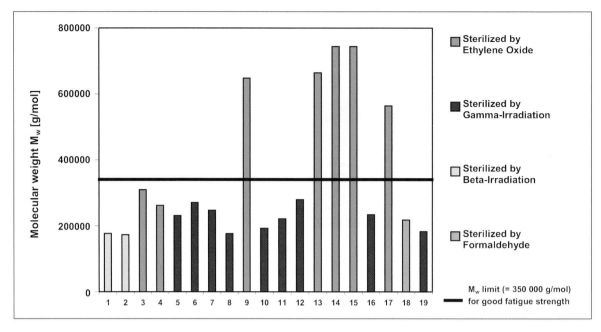

Fig. 3.10. Methods of sterilization

Residual Monomer and Blood Circulation Reactions

On the radical polymerization of MMA a 100% conversion can never be reached, as the mobility of the monomer molecules decreases dramatically with the increasing dough viscosity. Hence, there is always an amount of 2–6% of residual monomer in a cement matrix right after setting [5] (■ Fig. 3.11). This amount decreases within 2–3 weeks to about 0.5%, mainly (about 80%) by slow post-polymerization. The minor part of the residual MMA enters the blood circulation and then leaves the body by simple respiration or being metabolized via the Krebs cycle.

Ever since bone cements have been introduced, some negative effects on the cardiorespiratory system have been observed during the operation, even rarely leading to a patient's death. Although these phenomena have often been attributed to MMA, it is now well established that the intramedullar increase of pressure during cement and prosthesis insertion is the main pathological mechanism [4] leading to embolisation of bone marrow and fat as shown during with the use of transoesophageal, two-dimensional echocardiography.

Glass Transition Temperature

Plastics change their physical state with rising temperature from glass-like/brittle to rubber-elastic. The temperature range in which this change occurs is characterized by the so-called glass transition temperature. It depends on the chemical nature of the polymer and the presence of addi-

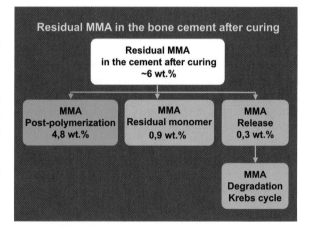

Fig. 3.11. Residual monomer

tives. Water-uptake has a decisive influence on the softening of a plastic and thus on the glass transition temperature (■ Fig. 3.12). The softening effect is due to the upcoming micro-Brown movement and leads to changed elasticity modulus, heat conduction and thermal expansion.

In a dry state, PMMA bone cements have a relatively high glass transition temperature (about 90–100 °C) compared to the body temperature. After its setting, the cement is brittle with a high elasticity modulus and high cohesiveness. After the implantation into the body with its liquids at 37 °C, the cement will be water-saturated within a few weeks. Thus by the plasticizing effect the glass transition temperature drops.

The difference between dry and water-saturated samples of bone cements is about 20 °C. Since the glass

Chapter 3.1 · Properties of Bone Cement: What is Bone Cement?

57   **3**

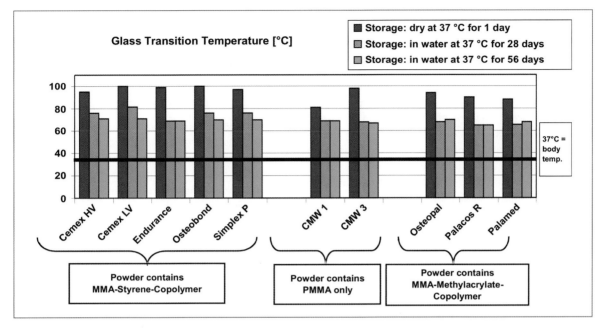

Fig. 3.12. Glass transition temperature

transition temperature is only a measure for the transition range, polymers can already slump below that temperature. With the growing rubber-elastic properties the cements show a higher tendency to creep, and so the implants may „sink" deeper into the cement mantle. The common bone cements on the market show a glass transition temperature of about 70 °C after water saturation. With this temperature clearly above the body temperature a safe use of the cements is assured [5].

Creep Behaviour

Acrylic bone cements also show plastic properties. So it is physically possible that they intrude slowly into cavities after their curing and seal them. This important property gives them a high flexibility in the bone. Therefore, the creep behaviour is taken as an additional criteria for bone cement testing.

The interfaces between bone and bone cement as well as bone cement and prosthesis are mechanical boundaries. The bone cement as the central part functions as an elastic buffer.

Mechanical Tests

Unfortunately, a lot of literature data about the mechanics of bone cements cannot be compared because of the lack of information about preparation and storage of the test specimens and the test method. According to the internationally accepted standard ISO 5833, compres-

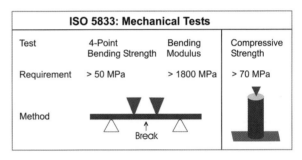

Fig. 3.13. ISO 5833 mechanical tests

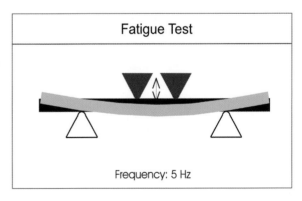

Fig. 3.14. Fatigue test

sive strength, bending strength and bending modulus are tested (Fig. 3.13).

Beside these static tests dynamic studies are performed, too, such as fatigue testing (Fig. 3.14). Different variants are possible: tensile, compression or bending.

Mostly, the fatigue testing is done by bending as the necessary equipment is relatively simple. Such studies are very time-consuming, being done until 1,000,000 or better 10,000,000 cycles are reached. To get a correlation to the practical life, one assumes an annual number of 1,000,000 double steps (= 2,000,000 steps). Thus, 10,000,000 reached cycles would be equivalent to a time period of five years. Anyway, such tests can only give a rough idea of the quality of a cement especially as their properties change under physiologic conditions (body temperature and fluids) and in so far the clinical relevance of test standards must be challenged [8].

Working Behaviour and Viscosity

After mixing of the powder and the liquid components, a doughy mass is formed by swelling and dissolution. Because of the initiated radical polymerization the viscosity increases continuously until the complete hardening/curing of the cement. The user must have detailed knowledge about the viscosity course to plan the operation optimally.

> Note: Working properties
> — The viscosity is the most important handling property for the surgeon
> — The viscosity increases continually during the working period
> — The timing for the injection of the cement is important for the success of the surgery

The progression of the viscosity depends on the cement composition, the powder/liquid mixing ratio, the humidity and especially on the temperature of the dough and the surroundings.

On the use of bone cements different phases are distinguished: mixing phase, waiting phase, application phase and setting phase:

— **mixing phase:**
  – wetting and polymerization,
  – cement relatively liquid (low viscous),
  – few chains, very movable;
— **waiting phase:**
  – chain propagation,
  – cement less liquid,
  – more chains, less movable;
— **working phase:**
  – chain propagation,
  – reduced movability,
  – increase of viscosity
  – heat generation;
— **setting phase:**
  – chain growth finished,
  – no movability,
  – cement hardened,
  – high temperature.

Already in the mixing phase great differences are observed for different cements. Some are mixed easily, others are hard to mix because of a high initial viscosity. As a consequence, many air bubbles can be incorporated into the dough at this early stage leading to a high porosity of the cement endangering the mechanic stability.

 Note: ISO 5833 requirement
»It is suggested that a graphical representation of the effect of temperature on the length of the phases in cement curing, prepared from experimental data on the particular brand of cement, be provided.«

The design of the mixing vessel and spatula as well as the mixing speed and number of strokes per minute also influence the homogeneity of the dough. The longer and the more vigorously it is mixed the more porous it becomes. The waiting phase allows the cement to come to a non-sticky consistency ready to use. It is then that the porosity can be reduced significantly by smooth manual kneading.

During the application phase the surgeon brings the dough into the bony cavity. The dough must be of moderate viscosity and non-sticky if manually inserted. The differences between the cements in this context are considerable. It must be mentioned, however, that regardless of the manufacturer's classification as low, medium or high viscous all cements start with a low-viscous phase changing to higher viscosity more or less rapidly, depending on the viscosity type.

> Note: Factor influencing the viscosity
> — Swelling and dissolution behaviour of the polymer powder in the liquid monomer
> — The ratio of the powder and the liquid
> — The temperature of
>   the powder and the liquid
>   the mixing equipment
>   the operating room
>   = Result in low- and high-viscous cements

Using mixing systems, the phases can change significantly because the user does not need to wait for the dough to loose its stickiness. Nevertheless, the viscosity at the beginning of the application phase must not be too low. Otherwise the inserted dough might not withstand the bleeding pressure in the femur with the consequence of blood entrapment within the cement representing potential areas of weakness with increased fracture risk. This phenomenon is the main problem when applying low viscosity cements with their short application phase too early. Normal or high viscosity cements in this regard seem to be more user-friendly and forgiving resulting in better long-term performance [1, 9].

Chapter 3.1 · Properties of Bone Cement: What is Bone Cement?

59

3

Pre-Chilling of Cement Components

The chilling of components or low ambient temperature slow down the polymerization and reduce the viscosity and vice versa. Pre-chilling as well as the application of vacuum mixing reduce the cement porosity and improve the mechanics of the cured cement. Such mixing systems (▶ chapter 4) consist of a mixing cartridge with a mixing element and the vacuum equipment with pump, tubing and charcoal filter to absorb the MMA vapours. The mixing cartridge is also the application unit so that the cement need not be transferred to another unit. The dough is injected with an appropriate cement gun.

Vacuum mixing systems can have a positive influence on the cement quality and thus on the durability of cemented prostheses. The basic requirement, however, is the correct usage of the system. With poor handling leading to insufficient mixing or low vacuum, the quality of the cement may be poor. Also the correct mixing sequence (of powder and liquid) must be regarded which does not always seem to be the case (◻ Fig. 3.15).

If the vacuum equipment is insufficient or used incorrectly, no positive effect on the porosity can be expected. A vacuum pressure too high or applied for too long, on the other hand, may cause the monomer to boil already at room temperature as its vapour pressure at 23 °C is 38 kPa. Boiling MMA of course leads to bubbles/pores in the cement.

A variety of different vacuum mixing systems are offered on the market. Standard systems come empty and have to be filled with the desired cement components. A new trend are the pre-packed systems: semi-pre-packed systems contain only the powder component whilst full-pre-packed also contain the liquid in a special construct. The latter systems avoid that the user comes in direct contact with the cement components. Vacuum mixing systems have proven of value for most surgeons nowadays. Newer studies show the systems with horizontal mixing screw to be superior and favour the collection of the dough under vacuum.

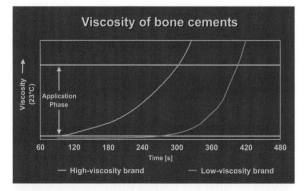

◻ **Fig. 3.15.** Viscosity curves

Take Home Messages

- Acrylic bone cement is used for implant fixation and local release of antibiotics.
- Bone cements mainly consist of PMMA or copolymers in the powder and methyl methacrylate in the liquid.
- Added zirconium dioxide or barium sulphate provide radiopacity.
- Benzoyl peroxide (powder) and N,N-Dimethyl-p-toluidine (liquid) are the initiators of the polymerization process.
- The polymerization heat of the exothermic radical polymerization of methyl methacrylate is 57 kJ per mole.
- The polymerization shrinkage of acrylic bone cements is about 3–5%.
- Working behaviour and fatigue properties depend on molecular weight (the higher the molecular weight the better).
- As the radical polymerization is never complete, residual monomer remains in the hardened cement. Serum traces of MMA are respired or metabolized rapidly in the Krebs cycle.
- Static properties according to ISO 5833 as well as dynamic properties (fatigue) provide important mechanical data.
- Many factors, especially the temperature, influence the dough viscosity and the working properties, which are most important to the user.

References

1. Breusch SJ (2001) Cementing technique in total hip replacement: Factors influencing survival of femoral components. In: Walenkamp GHIM, Murray DW (eds) Bone cements and cementing technique. Springer, Berlin Heidelberg New York Tokyo
2. Charnley J (1960) Anchorage of the femoral head prostheses of the shaft of the femur. J Bone Joint Surg 42 Br: 28–30
3. Charnley J (1970) Acrylic cement in orthopaedic surgery. Williams and Wilkins, Baltimore
4. Crout DMG, Corkill JA, James ML, Ling RSM (1979) Methylmethacrylate metabolism in man. Clin Orthop Rel Res 141: 90–95
5. Ege W, Kühn KD, Tuchscherer C, Maurer H (1998) Physical and chemical properties of bone cements. In: Walenkamp GHIM (ed) Biomaterials in surgery. Georg Thieme, Stuttgart
6. Judet J, Judet R (1956) The use of an artificial femoral head for arthroplasty of the hip joint. J Bone Surg 32 B: 166
7. Kleinschmitt O (1941) Plexiglas zur Deckung von Schädellücken. Chirurg 13: 273
8. Kühn KD (2000) Bone cements. Springer, Berlin Heidelberg New York Tokyo
9. Kühn KD (2001) Handling properties of polymethacrylate bone cements. In: Walenkamp GHIM, Murray DW (eds) Bone cements and cementing technique. Springer, Berlin Heidelberg New York Tokyo

Properties of Bone Cement: The Mechanical Properties of PMMA Bone Cement

Clive Lee

Summary

This chapter describes the mechanical properties of PMMA bone cement, dividing them into two parts – short-term and long-term properties. Short-term properties show that bone cement is weak in tension and strong in compression. Long-term properties (creep, stress relaxation and fatigue) are considered in more detail as they can significantly affect the transmission of load into bone over the expected life of a total hip arthroplasty. The effects of the body environment in which the cement functions, and the design characteristics of the device being implanted, on the function of the bone cement are described. The overall mechanical properties of bone cement are shown to be able to lead to long-term stability of the replacement joint.

Introduction

A significant number of papers have been written describing the mechanical properties of PMMA bone cements [9, 11, 13, 17]. These papers have, in most cases, been published in the »Biomaterials« literature and not in the »Clinical« literature; in consequence, knowledge of cement properties and their clinical significance is poor among many orthopaedic surgeons. This chapter is an attempt to address that partial lack of knowledge and to put into perspective the relative importance of the various properties – short and long term – of bone cement.

Why are the properties of bone cement so important? The function of bone cement in a cemented hip arthroplasty is to locate the implant components in the bony skeleton and to transmit loads through the joint into the bone and muscle surrounding the joint over very long periods of time. In order to carry out this function, bone cement must be compatible with the tissues it contacts and have adequate strength. Since the forces transmitted through the hip joint are high [2, 3] – about 3 times body weight when walking, rising to 8 times body weight when stumbling – bone cement is subjected to high stresses and has to function in the relatively aggressive environment of the body. The various strength properties of bone cement will be examined in the following paragraphs, with comments on how these properties affect the function of implant components *in vivo*.

Requirements of ISO 5833:2002 for Bone Cements

In order to control the properties of bone cement a standard is used – the current standard is ISO 5833:2002 Implants for surgery – Acrylic resin cements [4]. The standard specifies requirements for the liquid (appearance, stability and accuracy of ampoule contents), for the powder (appearance and accuracy of contents) and for the dough (hardening characteristics and intrusion). There are numbers of special requirements concerning packaging and, finally, requirements for set and cured cement. There are just three requirements for set and cured cement: compressive strength (minimum of 70 MPa), bending modulus (minimum of 1800 MPa) and bending strength (minimum of 50 MPa). The compressive strength is tested on cylindrical samples of bone cement 24 ± 2 hours after forming and storage in dry air at 23 °C. The strength is calculated from fracture load, 2% offset load or upper yield point load, whichever occurs first. The bending modulus and bending strength is measured using a four point bending test on beam specimens of bone cement 24 ± 2 hours after forming and storage in dry air at 23 °C. Formulae are given for the calculation of bending modulus and bending strength.

All bone cements that are commercially available – and Kühn [8] lists 24 plain cements and 18 antibiotic cements as commercially available – must satisfy the requirements of ISO 5833. Users of bone cement – patients and surgeons – need to be satisfied that compliance with the requirements of the international standard is sufficient to ensure that the cement being used will have satisfactory long term performance. The author suggests that this is not the case.

In 2002 the Swedish National Hip Arthroplasty Register [15] stated that the most common cause of revision of a total hip joint is aseptic loosening of an implant component, with or without focal osteolysis. Since 93% of the total replacement hip joints in Sweden are reported as being cemented, it can be concluded that aseptic loosening is the most common cause of failure of cemented implants. Aseptic loosening of a cemented implant most commonly indicates failure by shear or tension of the bone/bone cement interface, or failure following the production of wear debris (cement, metal, polyethylene, etc.) coupled with hydraulic effects within the joint, causing osteolysis. Very rarely, if ever, is failure due to compression or bending of bone cement. Consequently, the requirements of the international standard, while being useful for quality control, are not sufficient to ensure that bone cements are fit for purpose.

The following paragraphs describe tests and properties of bone cements, both short-term and long-term, that should be assessed before a cement is used in a patient.

Short-Term Strength of PMMA Bone Cement

Five properties of bone cement should be measured by testing cement samples in the laboratory. These are: tensile strength, shear strength, compressive strength, bending strength and modulus of elasticity. Results from Saha and Pal [17], from Lewis [11] and from Kühn [8] give the following average values:

- tensile strength   35.3 MPa
- shear strength   42.2 MPa
- compressive strength   93.0 MPa
- bending strength   64.2 MPa
- bending modulus   2552 MPa

These values are averaged over a large number of samples reported in the three papers referenced above and any particular cement will have characteristic properties that will vary according to the age, environment, porosity, etc. of the sample. The book by Kühn [8] gives the characteristics of individual cements in the most easily understood form.

It can be seen from the strength properties listed above that cement is weak in tension, strong in compression and has a low bending modulus of elasticity (modulus of elasticity for stainless steel or cobalt chrome alloy is about 200×10^3 MPa, for cortical bone about 20×10^3 MPa and for PMMA about 2×10^3 MPa). In consequence, bone cement should be loaded in compression wherever possible. It should be supported by cortical bone to allow the compression to be generated and to restrict tensile stresses.

Long-Term Strength of PMMA Bone Cement

Bone cement has to function effectively for very long times in hip replacements – clinical experience of more than thirty years has now been reported [6]. Bending modulus of elasticity and Knoop hardness of cement samples recovered from patients after 15 to 24 years *in-vivo* use is reported to be comparable to that of 1-year-old laboratory made cement [14]. Coupled with long-term clinical success of hip replacements, these results give users confidence that bone cement will remain fully functional over very long times in patients.

In addition to the simple elastic mechanical properties described above, there are three long-term viscoelastic properties that are of importance when considering long-term function – creep, stress relaxation and fatigue. The viscoelastic properties are described below after a comment about the nature of the environment in which testing takes place.

PMMA bone cement is a thermoplastic polymer and, as such, has properties that change with ambient temperature. If bone cement is tested at room temperature (18–20 °C) and is also tested at body temperature (37 °C), it will be found its properties change as temperature changes – there is a mechanical state change, the beta transition, between room temperature and body temperature [1, 5]. Because cement has this characteristic, it is necessary to test at body temperature. Like most polymers, bone cement will react to the environment surrounding it, for example, cement will absorb water from its surroundings; the water will act as a plasticiser and change the characteristic properties of the cement [9]. Consequently, bone cement must be tested in an environment that replicates the body environment as far as possible, it is particularly important that this is done when the long-term viscoelastic properties of cement are considered [13].

Creep of Bone Cement

Creep is defined as the change in strain with time in a sample held at constant stress [13]. Creep in metals only becomes important at temperatures greater than about

0.4 times the absolute melting temperature (i.e. above about 400 °C for stainless steel) and, in consequence, creep of metal components of no concern in orthopaedics. On the other hand, creep in polymers is significant at body temperature and must be considered when designing a cemented implant system or when describing the clinical performance of such a system (◘ Fig. 3.16).

A number of creep tests have been carried out in the author's laboratory and have been reported previously [10, 13]. ◘ Figure 3.17 gives a typical graph of the central deflection versus time of a beam under constant load in four point bending in saline at body temperature for various bone cements. It can be seen that all bone cements creep. Curves, similar to those of ◘ Fig. 3.17, could be drawn for tensile test specimens and would show creep occurring at rates dependent on the environment (◘ Fig. 3.18). ◘ Figure 3.18 shows that the strain rate of cement in saline at room temperature is well defined. The strain rate of cement in saline at body temperature is higher and less well defined (the distribution curve of strain rate values is spread) and the strain rate of cement in fat extracted from the medullary canal of a patient

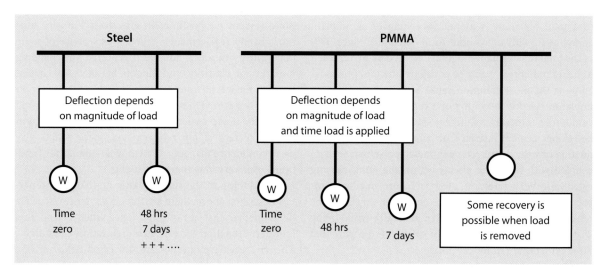

◘ **Fig. 3.16.** Creep of metals and polymers at 37 °C

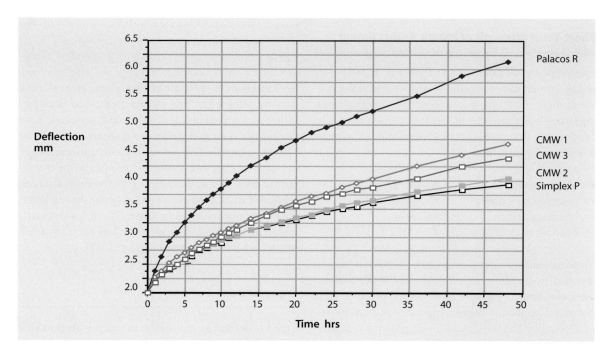

◘ **Fig. 3.17.** Creep of various bone cements – four point bending, 7 day old cement, central deflection vs. time, body temperature

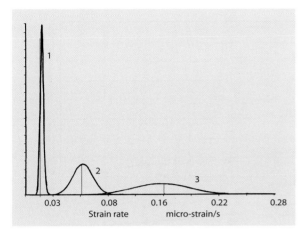

Fig. 3.18. Normal distribution of strain rates of 5 day old specimens (1) in normal saline at room temperature, (2) in normal saline at 37 °C, (3) in fat at 37 °C

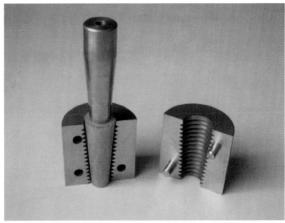

Fig. 3.19. Conical cement shell inside a grooved constraint before testing

undergoing hip replacement is even higher and even less well defined. The conclusion from these curves is that cement properties vary considerably with the environment surrounding the cement; a conclusion that is true for all properties of cement, not just tensile properties. Bone cement under compression or shear will creep, but at a much reduced rate.

The results discussed above were of specimens of cement prepared for standard laboratory tests and do not represent the shell-like shape of cement as used in hip replacement. In order to better illustrate the way in which cement can behave when formed into a shell with internal loading, a further series of tests were carried out. In these tests the specimens were formed into conical shells and loaded, inside metal constraints, by compression on a polished metal taper that fitted inside the cement shell (**Fig. 3.19**). The whole loading apparatus was held in a water bath at 37 °C. The constraints had a number of grooves on the inside surface, the cement specimens were initially smooth on the outside surface. After testing, it can be seen that the shell appeared to have a number of bands on its outside surface (**Fig. 3.20**). These bands were formed by the cement creeping outwards into the grooves of the metal constraint, illustrating how creep of cement can cause the cement to move in directions other than that of the load.

After all the creep tests had been carried out, it was concluded that:

- all PMMA cements creep,
- creep can produce movement of cement in any direction,
- creep rate reduces with age of the cement,
- creep rate is influenced by the environment of the cement,
- creep rate increases with temperature,
- creep rate increase with stress level.

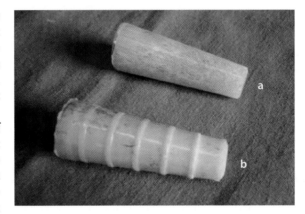

Fig. 3.20. Conical cement shells (**a**) before testing (**b**) after testing showing »bands« caused by outward creep of cement

Stress Relaxation of Bone Cement

Stress relaxation is defined as the change in stress with time under constant strain (deformation) [5]. Just as with creep, stress relaxation is important for polymers at body temperature, not important for metals. A number of stress relaxation tests have been carried out in the author's laboratory and are reported in detail elsewhere [7, 10, 13]. **Figure 3.21** gives a typical graph showing stress relaxation of beams of bone cement held at constant central displacement, under four point bending in saline at 37 °C. All PMMA bone cements stress relax. Stress relaxation in bone cement takes place by a similar molecular relaxation process within the polymer as that which causes creep. The effects of age, environment, temperature and stress level as observed for creep are repeated for stress relaxation. Although stress relaxation will occur under compressive, shear and tensile stresses, it should be noted that it is the high tensile stresses in cement that preferentially reduce as time goes by.

3

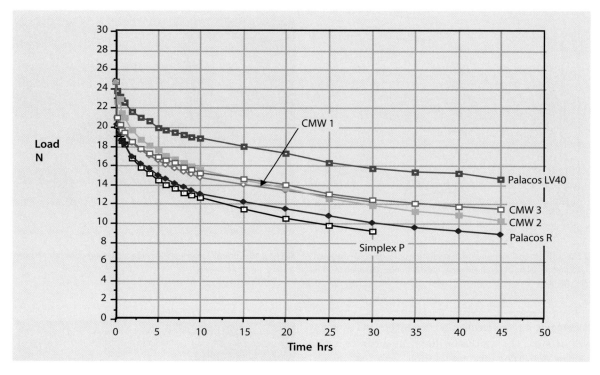

■ **Fig. 3.21.** Stress relaxation of various bone cements – four point bending, 7 day old cement, load to maintain central deflection vs. time, body temperature

Fatigue of Bone Cement

Fatigue is the effect of repeated load cycles below the level needed to fail the material in a single load application [5]. Many metals have an endurance limit – that is, a level of stress below which the material will not fail no matter how many times the stress is repeated. Polymers do not have such a limit – they will always fail after sufficient load cycles have been applied no matter how low is the stress produced by the load cycle (■ Fig. 3.22). A patient with a replacement hip joint will take about one million walking steps every year; i.e. will put about 10^6 load cycles on their hip each year. Fatigue failure would therefore seem to be inevitable for bone cement after it has been loaded in a patient for a number of years. How then does a replacement hip joint survive for long times in patients? It is known that fatigue failure normally originates at points of high tensile stress concentration [7]. As noted above, tensile stresses in bone cements can stress relax rapidly if the conditions are favourable: it is this stress relaxation that provides a form of self-protection for bone cement in patients (see below).

The Clinical Significance of Long-term Properties of Bone Cement

The clinical significance of the long-term properties of PMMA bone cement is described in detail in a previously published paper [12]. As was stated in that paper, long-term properties of bone cement are particularly important when the performance of polished, collarless, tapered and cemented femoral stems are concerned. Such a stem is the Exeter stem designed and developed by the author and Professor R.S.M Ling, together with numerous other colleagues, since 1970. The mechanism of load transfer of the Exeter stem will be described briefly in the following paragraphs.

When a patient has a replacement hip joint, that patient loads the joint according to his/her activity (■ Fig. 3.23). In general terms, significant loads are applied to the joint when the patient is awake (about 16 hours per day) and loads are reduced to almost zero when the patient is asleep (about 8 hours per day). When a load is applied to a replacement joint, the joint structures (implant, cement, bone and muscles) must develop strain energy sufficient to support the loads put upon them (strain energy is a measure of the work done in deforming the structures). Therefore, during daily activity the joint structures develop the relatively high levels of strain energy needed to support activity loads. With a tapered, collarless, polished femoral implant component, a significant part of the necessary strain energy is produced by engagement (subsidence) of the tapered part of the stem within the bone cement, inducing radial compression, hoop tension and shear stress into the cement. When the patient goes to bed at night, the loads

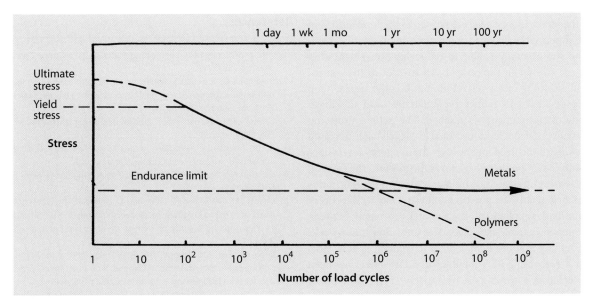

■ **Fig. 3.22.** Fatigue of metals and polymers

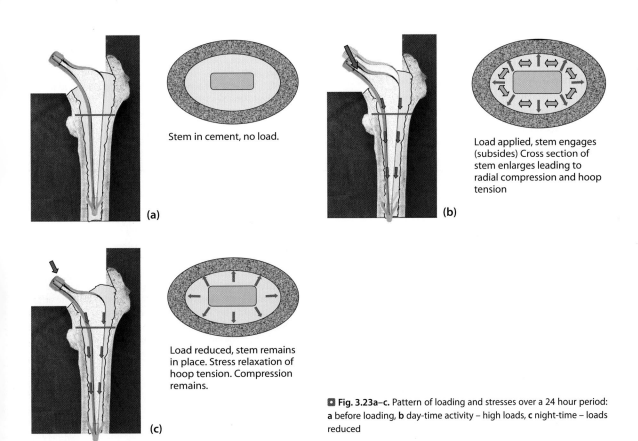

Stem in cement, no load.

Load applied, stem engages (subsides) Cross section of stem enlarges leading to radial compression and hoop tension

(a)

(b)

Load reduced, stem remains in place. Stress relaxation of hoop tension. Compression remains.

(c)

■ **Fig. 3.23a–c.** Pattern of loading and stresses over a 24 hour period: **a** before loading, **b** day-time activity – high loads, **c** night-time – loads reduced

on the joint are significantly reduced; consequently, the strain energy needed within the joint structures to support these loads is also reduced. The tapered, collarless, polished femoral implant component is self-retaining within the cement (the stem taper acts in a similar way to the self-retaining of the femoral head on the conical taper of a modular stem). With the stem remaining in position in the cement, the strains induced in the cement are the same as before the loads were reduced – thus the stresses are the same as before the loads were reduced. This leads to the state where the cement has excess strain energy (i.e. the amount needed to support the high activity loads)

3

– the strain energy needs to reduce to the level sufficient to support the reduced night-time loads on the joint. The strain energy is able to reduce by stress relaxation of the stresses in the cement. All stresses in the cement will reduce by stress relaxation, but it is the tensile hoop stresses that will reduce preferentially until the lower state of strain energy is reached. The patient wakes up the next morning and load (activity levels) are increased leading to the need for the high strain energy levels once more. The stem therefore moves further into the cement, increasing stresses and strain energy until equilibrium is reached again. The process is repeated day by day. Every time load is applied, sub-microscopic movement between stem and cement takes place. It is only after many weeks of activity that the stem/cement movement is detectable on X-rays; using RSA about 0,7 mm movement has been detected at 4 weeks post-operatively [16]. The amount of movement of the stem in the cement gets smaller as time passes because engagement of the stem in the cement produces ever tighter constraint around the stem, the viscoelastic creep property of the cement changes with time to produce lower creep rates and stress levels in the cement are evened out to produce a lower but more uniform distribution of stresses around the stem. Nevertheless, the stem continues to move for very long times, movement has been detected in clinical reviews of patients at an average follow-up of 33 years. The overall stress situation in the cement after many years clinical use is one of dominance of compressive stress. The tensile stress generated within the cement is reduced by stress relaxation each night and never normally reaches the levels needed to initiate fatigue failure – the »self-protection« mechanism referred to before.

Take Home Messages

- ▬ Bone cement has mechanical properties that influence the function of a replacement hip joint. It is strong in compression, relatively weak in tension and has a low bending modulus of elasticity.
- ▬ Bone cement is not a simple elastic material, but is a viscoelastic polymer subject to the long-term properties of creep, stress relaxation and fatigue. The importance of fatigue may be reduced by stress relaxation during periods of relative unloading.
- ▬ The effect of the body environment on the properties of cement is very important to the long-term function of the material.
- ▬ With a tapered, collarless, polished femoral stem, the end result of stem movement (subsidence), creep and stress relaxation is to increase the compressive stress in the cement and at the cement-bone interface which leads to long-term stability of the total replacement hip joint.

References

1. Ashby MF, Jones DHR. Engineering Materials 2. Pergamon Press, 1988, pp 218–232
2. Bergmann G, Graichen F, Rohlmann A. Hip joint loading during walking and running, measured in two patients. J Biomechanics, 1993, vol. 26 no.8 p969–90
3. Berme N, Paul JP. Load actions transmitted by implants. J Biomed Eng. 1979, 1 p 268–272
4. British Standards Institution. International Standard ISO 5833 Implants for surgery – Acrylic resin cements. 2002
5. Callister WD. Materials Science and Engineering. John Wiley & Sons, 2000
6. Charity JAF, Gie GA, Hoe F, Timperley AJ, Ling RSM. The Exeter polished stem in the long-term: a survivorship study to the 33rd year of follow-up and a study of stem subsidence. Hip International 2004; 14: 83
7. Eden OR, Lee AJC, Hooper RM. Stress relaxation modelling of polymethylmethacrylate bone cement. Proc Instn Mech Engrs, 216, Part H: J Engineering in Medicine, 2002, p195–199
8. Kühn K-D. Bone cements. Springer, Berlin Heidelberg New York Tokyo, 2000
9. Lee A J C, Ling RSM, Vangala SS. Some clinically relevant variables affecting the mechanical behaviour of bone cement. Arch Orthop Traumat Surg 1978; 92: 1–18
10. Lee AJC, Perkins RD, Ling RSM. Time-dependent properties of polymethylmethacrylate bone cement. In Older J (Ed). Implant Bone Interface, Chapter 12. Springer, Berlin Heidelberg New York Tokyo, 1990
11. Lewis G. Properties of acrylic bone cement: state of the art review. J Biomed Mater Res 1997; 38: 155–182
12. Lee AJC. The time-dependent properties of polymethylmethacrylate bone cement: the interaction of shape of femoral stems, surface finish and bone cement. In: Learmonth ID (ed) Interfaces in total hip arthroplasty, Springer, Berlin Heidelberg New York Tokyo, 2000, p 11–19
13. Lee AJC, Ling RSM, Gheduzzi S, Simon J-P, Renfro RJ. Factors affecting the mechanical and viscoelastic properties of acrylic bone cement. J Mater Sci – Mater in Med, 2002, 13: 723–733
14. Lee AJC. The mechanical properties of recovered PMMA bone cement. Hip International 2004; 14 2 p79
15. Malchau H, Herberts P, Garellick G, Söderman P and Eisler T. Prognosis of total hip replacement. Scientific exhibit, 69th annual mtg of the AAOS, Dallas USA, Feb 2002.
16. Ornstein E, Franzén H, Johnsson R, Löfqvist T, Stefánsdottir A and Sundberg M. Does the tapered Exeter stem migrate at the stem-cement interface or/and at the cement-bone interface? Acta Orthop Scand, 1997, Suppl 274: 68
17. Saha S, Pal S. The mechanical properties of bone cement: a review. J Biomed Mater Res 1984, 18: 435–462

Properties of Bone Cement: Testing and Performance of Bone Cements

Pieter T.J. Spierings

Summary

Although all commercially available bone cements are based on polymethylmethacrylate and other acrylic co-polymers, they all differ in their precise chemical formulation and composition. This results in different physical properties like viscosity, heat release, and mechanics. These differences affect surgical handling and clinical outcome. Various testing methods of bone cement are discussed in this chapter. Clinically most relevant is fatigue testing and traditional cements perform best.

Introduction

General

All cements which found widespread use in orthopaedic surgery are based on polymethylmethacrylate (PMMA). This acrylic resin is used now for over 50 years for the fixation of orthopaedic implants. The first published artificial joint implantations occurred in 1949 at Copenhagen by M.S. Kiaer and in 1951 in the hospital for Joint Diseases at New York by E. Haboush [5]. The first commercially available bone cements were released to the market in the beginning of the seventies. Since then many types and makes of bone cement have been introduced. Only few stood the test of time.

Alternative Cements

Many attempts have been made to improve the physical properties of bone cements and many alternatives for acrylic were tested, like:

- glass-ionomeric cements,
- bioactive glass cements,
- resorbable cements.

The main advantages of ionomeric bone cements are the absence of heat generation during polymerization and its adhesive properties to bone. The main disadvantage is its low mechanical strength which makes it unsuitable for load bearing applications. Bioactive glass cements are a composite of bioactive calcium-phosphate (CaP) powder and a high molecular weight acrylic matrix. The mechanical strength is 2 to 3 times higher than of acrylic cement. It has less heat generation and less shrinkage during polymerization. Main disadvantage is its high rigidity and brittleness. It is weak in tensile fatigue loading. Resorbable cements like CaP and polypropylene-fumarate cements all suffer from brittleness and insufficient strength in load bearing applications [3].

Improvement of acrylic cements has been tried (▶ chapter 3.6) in many ways like:

- addition of CaP powders,
- addition of artificial fibres,
- modification of the curing mechanism,
- modification of the radiopacifier.

By addition of CaP powders as a filler material to cement, one has tried to enhance bony ongrowth to the cement surface and bony ingrowth into the cement mantle. Simultaneously, it would decrease the exotherm reaction. To obtain ingrowth high amounts up to 30 to 50 w/w% of CaP powder are needed to obtain a sufficient open structure. This open structure weakens the strength of the cement considerably. In the Far East such cements have been applied for the fixation of endoprotheses.

Addition of artificial fibres is meant to increase the mechanical strength. Fibres will increase the static fracture strength, the modulus of elasticity and the fatigue strength. Creep is diminished and fracture toughness is increased. Many fibres like Kevlar, carbon, glass and PET have been tested in a magnitude of 1 to 2 w/w%. The major drawback of artificial fibres is the long term biological effect of small wear particles. Many materials which are fully biocompatible as block material will give rise to tissue reactions if they are released on a microscopical scale. No artificial filler materials are at present applied clinically.

Test Standards

ISO standard 5833, which was first released in 1979 and latest revised in 2002, is a standard which describes a number of test methods and minimal requirements for acrylic bone cements [6]. All commercially available cements have to fulfill the requirements set forth in this standard. Unfortunately, the test methods and requirements are set on a low level and can be easily met. Therefore, this »standard« is not capable to discriminate whether a cement is suitable for clinical application or not. The ISO 5833 would for example find a setting time of just 3 minutes acceptable for a doughy cement. Even Boneloc cement, which had dramatic clinical results, fulfilled all requirements of the ISO 5833 standard.

In particular, a straight forward tensile test is missing in ISO 5833. Bone cement is remarkably weak in tension, but relatively strong in compression. It is also much more brittle in tension than in compression. In the 1992 version of this standard a bending test was added. Bending does include a tensile component, but the requirements of this bending test will be easily passed by all available cements. Most importantly there is not any type of fatigue testing in the ISO standard. This type of testing was recently described in ASTM standard F2118–2001 [1]. This standard accurately describes a method for a fully reversed tensile and compression cyclic loading test of acrylic bone cement. Unfortunately, the test does not state a minimum requirement.

Running a fatigue test is a very time-consuming procedure and therefore expensive test. The test results will highly depend on the mixing conditions (temperature, vacuum) and the resulting porosity of the test specimens. Only very few papers have been published which compare fatigue data of bone cements.

Effect of Chemical Composition

Polymers

The type of polymer powder is the most important factor which characterizes the performance of a particular type of bone cement. The most commonly used polymer powders are methylmethacrylate (MMA) homopolymer, methacrylate (MA) copolymer, butylmethacrylate (BMA) copolymer and styrene copolymer. They are applied in various commercially available bone cements (■ Table 3.1).

The addition of MA in the MMA-MA copolymer results in a change of physical properties as compared to MMA homopolymer. MA is a small molecule which makes the cement more hydrophilic and flexible (■ Fig. 3.24). The hydrophilic nature of MA speeds up the monomer absorption and powder dissolving. Hence the higher the MA concentration the higher the cement's initial viscosity will be. The addition of MA will mechanically result in a more flexible cement with a higher failure strain, relative low compression strength and a relative higher strength and failure strain in tension. Bone cement is a brittle material, which tensile strength is very susceptible for stress risers like air voids. MA cements will be less influenced by porosity due to this flexible behaviour.

Addition of a small percentage BMA, which has a higher molecular weight than MMA, gives the powder a more porous open structure. This may enhance the bond between the polymer matrix chains, which will entangle with the outer surface of the beads. A small percentage of BMA is claimed to result in better mechanical properties [7].

Styrene cements have a more hydrophobic behaviour. The time needed to obtain a homogenous mixture will take longer than for an MMA-MA cement. Addition of styrene copolymers is thought to be beneficial for the fatigue strength. No data exists whether this is true.

■ **Table 3.1.** Types of polymer used in various bone cement powders

Type of Polymer	Cement Brand
MMA homopolymer	CMW1, CMW3, Cemex RX, Cemex System, Zimmer regular+LVC
MMA-MA copolymer	Palacos R, Palamed, Osteopal, SmartSet HV, Versabond
MMA-BMA copolymer	Sulfix-6, Boneloc, Biolos
MMA-Styrene copolymer	Surgical Simplex RO, Osteobond, CMW Endurance

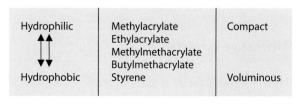

■ **Fig. 3.24.** Properties of various types of acrylic molecules

Monomers

The types of monomer molecule in the cement's liquid are of particular importance for the amount of heat generation. By reducing the number of molecules per gram of powder, the exotherm can be reduced. This can be accomplished by increasing the powder/liquid (P/L) ratio or by using high molecular weight monomers like BMA (M=140) or even isobornylmethacrylate (M=223) and n-decyl methacrylate (M=226). This method is applied by various manufacturers, who wish to market a reduced temperature bone cement, like e.g. Boneloc, Sulfix-6 and Cemex RX (Table 3.2).

By partially replacing methylmethacrylate (M=100) liquid molecules by a higher molecular weight monomer, the total number of monomer molecules is reduced. This results in less heat generation. A similar effect can be obtained by increasing the P/L ratio, which normally is 2.1 w/w. By increasing the P/L ratio to 3 w/w, the number of molecules and the amount of heat generation is reduced by 30%. From a chemical point of view a P/L ratio of 3 is acceptable. From a handling point of view it will become more difficult to obtain a homogeneous mixture.

Radiopacifier

To make cement visible on a radiograph it is needed to add a radiopaque element to the cement. Commercially used are $BaSO_4$ and ZrO_2. The advantage of ZrO_2 is that a relatively better contrast can be obtained than with a similar weight amount of $BaSO_4$. Another advantage of ZrO_2 is that it has no tendency to cluster like $BaSO_4$ (Fig. 3.25). Clustering leads to inclusions in the cement mass which may decrease the mechanical properties. Attempts have been made to diminish the mechanical drawback from including a radiopacifier. Experiments showed that adding a radiopacifier of submicron size significantly increased the fatigue strength of bone cement [8]. Other attempts were made to replace the addition of a radiopaque powder by building iodine into the polymer molecules [2]. Such cement also showed a remarkable increase in fatigue strength. Due to risk of iodine allergy this development was never commercialized.

Handling

Handling is the most critical parameter for cement use in the theatre. In particular when applying modern cementing techniques like vacuum mixing and cement pressurization more working time is needed (Table 3.3). The working time of a cement can be extended by applying a no-touch technique in which case the cement is handled immediately after the start of mixing inside a mechanical

Table 3.2. Traditional and low temperature bone cements and their types of liquid and powder/liquid ratio

Cement Brand	Monomer	P/L Ratio w/w
Palacos R, Palamed, Osteopal, Surgical Simplex, CMW1+3, Zimmer regular + LVC	100% MMA	± 2.1
Boneloc	50% MMA + 20% isobornylMA + 30% n-decylMA	2.3
Sulfix-6, Duracem 3	85% MMA + 15% BMA	2.3
Biolos 1	86% MMA + 14% BMA	2.8
Cemex RX	100% MMA	3.0

Table 3.3. First, second and third generation of cementing technique

Generation	Method	Year
First	Mixing with bowl and spatula	1965
	Cement kneading	1965
	Finger packing	1965
Second	Cement gun and syringe	1970
	Bone plug	1975
	Retrograde injection	1975
	Pressurization	1980
	Bone lavage	1980
	Low viscosity cement	1980
Third	Vacuum mixing	1985
	Prosthetic positioning by spacers	1987

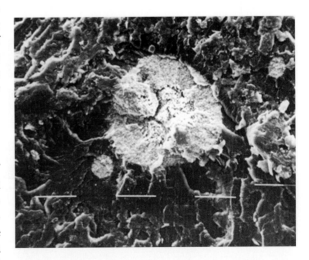

Fig. 3.25. SEM of clustered $BaSO_4$ in fracture surface of tensile specimen (*white line* = 100 μm.)

3

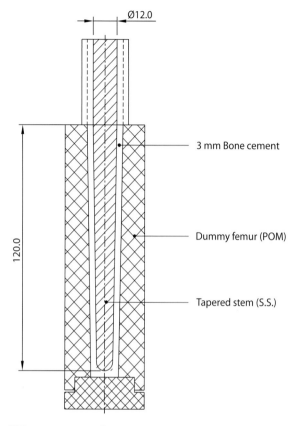

Ø12.0

120.0

3 mm Bone cement

Dummy femur (POM)

Tapered stem (S.S.)

Fig. 3.26. Test setup for a simulation hip implantation test

mixing system. If even then the working time is not sufficient, the polymerization process can be slowed down by pre-cooling the cement and mixing system.

Manual handling of cement can be divided in various stages: Mixing until homogeneous, doughing stage, kneading, working period and hardening. A time schedule for such a procedure can be derived from simulation hip implantation tests at specific ambient temperatures. **Figure 3.26** shows a test set up which can be used for such an experiment.

Manual mixing in an open bowl generally takes 30 seconds for a hydrophilic MA cement and up to two minutes for a hydrophobic styrene cement. Doughing stage is the period during which the cement polymerizes until it can be picked up by hand. Then the cement is kneaded to a roll and filled in a syringe to be extruded into the bony cavity. During the working period the cement can be extruded, pressurized and a prosthesis must be inserted. The hardening period is the time needed to complete polymerization. **Figure 3.27** shows a time schedule of non-cooled Palacos R for such a procedure, at various ambient temperatures. **Figure 3.28** shows a time schedule for cooled Palacos R cement mixed in a Cemvac syringe vacuum mixing system. Mixing time is longer than for bowl mixing. Still the working period is much longer because there is no doughing time. The setting time is extended two minutes due to cooling of cement.

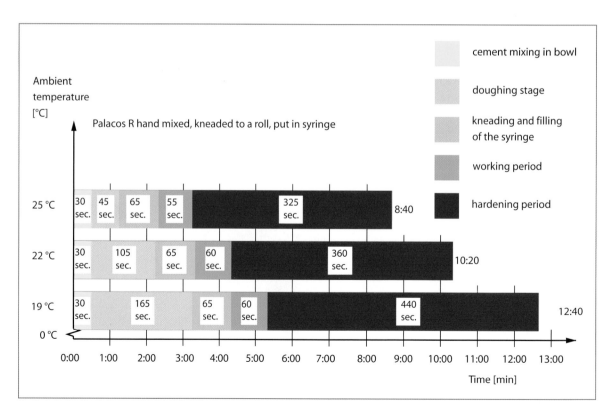

Fig. 3.27. Time schedule for manual kneading and syringe extrusion of non-cooled Palacos R bone cement at various ambient temperatures.

Note the short working time of non-cooled high viscosity cement if used in a syringe application. The dummy femur was pre-heated to 30 °C

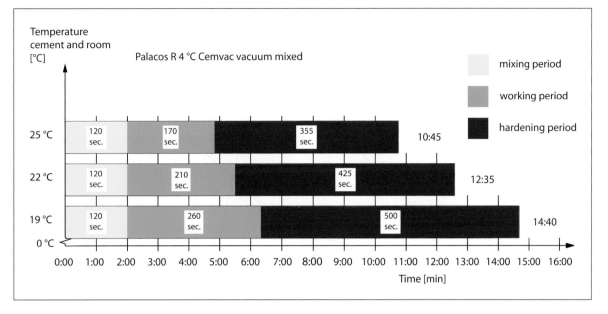

Fig. 3.28. Cooled Palacos R mixed in a Cemvac vacuum mixing system. Note the increased setting time compared to Fig. 3.26 as a result of cement cooling to 4 °C. The dummy femur was pre-heated to 30 °C

Viscosity

General

Viscosity is defined as the resistance of a fluid to shear deformation (■ Fig. 3.29):

$$\eta = \frac{\tau}{\dot{\gamma}}$$

The higher the viscosity of a bone cement is, the more difficult it will be for a surgeon to extrude the cement through a nozzle or to insert a prosthesis into the cement mass. Hence the development of the cement's viscosity during the polymerization process is an important parameter determining the handling of the cement.

When cement polymerizes it transforms from a fluid to a solid material. At the beginning of the polymerization process, cement is predominantly a fluid with viscous properties, at the end it is transformed to a solid phase with elastic properties. During the transformation, bone cement has both viscous and elastic properties and hence it is called a visco-elastic material with both viscous energy dissipating properties and elastic energy storage properties. This transformation can be demonstrated by measuring the dynamic visco-elastic properties with a rheogoniometer. In ■ Fig. 3.30 the dynamic viscosity development is shown for Sulfix-6 bone cement. In the beginning, when the mixed cement is more or less a suspension of polymer beads in the monomer fluid, the elastic properties are minor. During the polymerization process, the monomer will form elastic chains and they

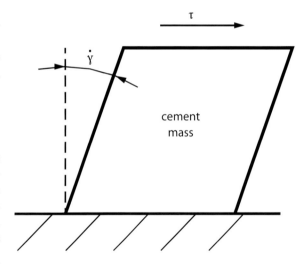

Fig. 3.29. Viscosity η (Pa.s) is defined as shear stress τ (Pa) divided by the resulting shear rate γ̇ (rad/s)

will integrate with the dissolved outer surface of the polymer beads. Simultaneously, it will become more difficult to shear the cement. This results in an increase of the elastic and viscous properties. When the matrix of newly formed chains is more or less complete and the cement starts behaving as an elastic material, the dynamic viscosity drops again and can no longer be measured. Finally, a solid material with elastic properties remains. What rests from the fluid behaviour are the creep or so called cold flow properties. They are, however, measured on a much larger time scale.

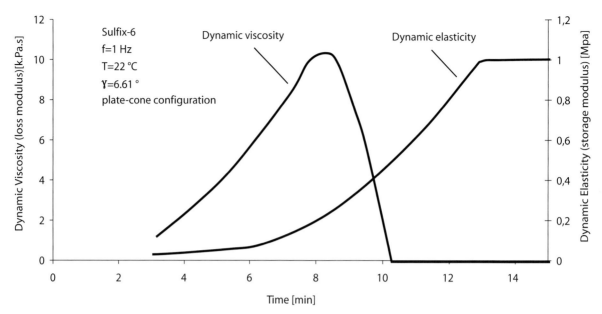

Fig. 3.30. Dynamic viscosity of Sulfix-6 bone cement. The graph shows the development of the viscous energy dissipating modulus and the elastic energy storage modulus as a function of time after mixing. The graph is measured with a Weissenberg rheogoniometer with cone-plate configuration at a frequency of 1 Hz

Apparent Viscosity

When cement viscosity is measured during simple shear at a constant shear rate, no distinction can be made between viscous and elastic properties. The measured viscosity then is called apparent viscosity. Cements are often named and characterized by the height of their apparent viscosity, to wit: high, medium or low viscosity. High viscosity cements are those which were originally developed for manual application, such as Palacos R and CMW-1. These cements can easily be rolled and kneaded and applied manually. They exhibit a high initial viscosity (**Fig. 3.31**). The high initial viscosity enables rapid manual handling. If high viscosity cements have to be used in a syringe system, cooling is recommended. Such cooling does not have to be at refrigerator temperature. Cooling to 15 or 18 °C already lowers the viscosity sufficient to enable syringe application.

Most low viscosity cements were developed much later for ease of handling in syringes with long thin nozzles for retrograde cement injection. Well known low viscosity cements are: CMW3, Sulfix-6, Osteopal, Palacos E-flow, Zimmer LVC, Cerafix and others. In **Fig. 3.31** it is shown that the starting viscosity of these cements is very low. This makes it impossible to handle them manually in an early stage. As all cements polymerize roughly in the same time span, it means that the working time for low viscosity cements is less than for medium or high viscosity cements. They are difficult to contain if they are extruded too early and they polymerize more rapidly at

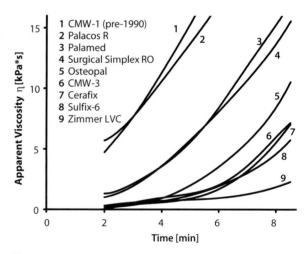

Fig. 3.31. Apparent viscosity of various types of bone cement as a function of time after mixing. Note the difference in starting viscosity of high (1, 2), medium (3, 4) and low (5, 6, 7, 8, 9) viscosity cements

the end of the working stage. **Figure 3.31** shows a more exponential viscosity increase for low viscosity cements and a more linear viscosity increase for high viscosity cements. In general the behaviour of low viscosity cement is therefore more critical to ambient temperature and time schedule.

A few cements exist with an intermediate viscosity development. Examples of these medium viscosity cements are: Surgical Simplex RO and Palamed. Their viscosity enables both manual application and syringe application in an early stage. Even if one needs more working time for vacuum mixing and pressurization, these cements can be applied without the need for cooling.

Factors Affecting Viscosity

The speed of the polymerization process is temperature dependent. Therefore ambient temperature affects the viscosity development and setting time. ◘ Figure 3.32 shows the effect of ambient temperature on the apparent viscosity as a function of time after mixing. Roughly 1 °C ambient temperature increase results in ½ minute reduction of working and setting time.

Cooling cement prior to surgery will change its handling properties. The viscosity development slows down and the setting time increases. ◘ Figure 3.33 shows the effect of cooling Palacos R to 4 °C. Its viscosity curve now has moved to the medium viscosity area. If not only the cement but also the environment is cooled to 4° C, than this high viscosity cement behaves like a low viscosity cement.

Viscosity is determined by the speed at which the powder is dissolved in the monomer. Variables which affect this process are for example the amount of outer surface of the beads, the amount of hydrophylic molecules and the powder/liquid ratio. A hydrophylic molecule like MA will rapidly absorb the monomer and increase the cement's viscosity. The main difference in the Palacos cement family is the amount of MA as part of the total

cement mass. By decreasing the amount of MA from 10% to 5% w/w, the behaviour is modified from high viscosity cement to a low viscosity cement (◘ Fig. 3.34).

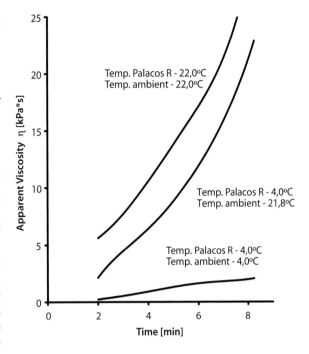

◘ **Fig. 3.33.** Apparent viscosity of Palacos R cement as a function of time after mixing at various cement and ambient temperatures.

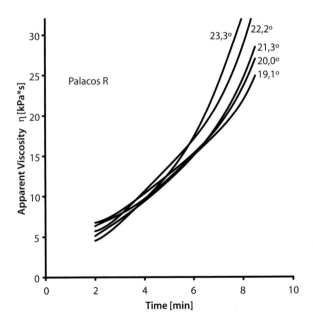

◘ **Fig. 3.32.** Apparent viscosity of Palacos R bone cement as a function of time after mixing at various ambient temperatures. Test shear rate = 0.358 s⁻¹, cone-plate configuration

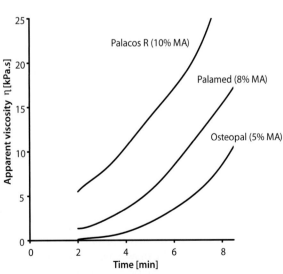

◘ **Fig. 3.34.** Apparent viscosity development for 3 bone cements which differ in their MA copolymer concentration

Thermal Properties

General

During curing of acrylic bone cement, the liquid component consisting of mainly MMA monomer molecules polymerizes to a solid mass of MMA polymer chains. This process is accomplished by the C=C double bond of each monomer which opens up to form a –C-C-C-C- polymer strain. Opening of the C=C double bond is accompanied by the release of heat. For one gram of pure MMA monomer 588 Joule of heat is generated. In comparison, 420 Joule is sufficient to increase the temperature of 1 gram of water from 0 °C to 100 °C. This heat release results in a temperature rise of the curing cement mass and its environment. The speed of this process is temperature-dependent and the heat release results in a self accelerating polymerization rate and subsequent temperature increase. This is called the Tromsdorff effect and can be demonstrated by measuring the temperature of a curing cement mass. In this chapter the thermal behaviour of various types of cement will be discussed.

Heat Generation

The amount of heat generation is determined by the number of monomers per gram of bone cement. However, not all monomers have the same molecular weight and not all cements contain the same amount of monomer liquid. Therefore, not all cements experience a similar temperature increase. Various bone cements were developed in particular to decrease the cement's temperature increase. Various methods have been used by manufacturers to reduce the amount of heat generation (⬚ Table 3.4).

Methods 1 to 3 of ⬚ Fig. 3.28 all result in less heat generation. Method 4 is distinctively different because the same amount of heat per gram cement is generated, but released at a slower rate. One can measure the temperature rise of a cement mass with a thermocouple. If the cement mass is large enough and isolated, the temperature in the centre will rise to an adiabatic steady value which equals the amount of heat generation divided by the specific heat value of the cement. Assuming that all cements have the same specific heat, the centre peak temperature will resemble accurately the amount of heat generation. ⬚ Figure 3.35 shows the test setup for such an adiabatic temperature measurement. The measured adiabatic temperature rise for a number of bone cements is listed in ⬚ Table 3.5.

Traditional bone cements based on MMA monomer and a P/L ratio w/w of 2:1 show a temperature increase of ±104 °C. It means that starting at an ambient temperature of 22 °C, a peak temperature of 126 °C will be measured. The low temperature cements generate less heat and a temperature rise between 71 °C and 94 °C is measured. Reduction

⬚ **Table 3.4.** Methods to decrease the amount of heat generation

1. High Powder/Liquid (P/L) ratio (Cemex RX, Sulfix-6)
2. Use of high molecular weight monomers (Boneloc, Sulfix-6)
3. Addition of water to the liquid (Implast)
4. Decrease the polymerization rate (Palacos)

⬚ **Table 3.5.** Adiabatic temperature rise representing the amount of heat generation of low temperature and of traditional »normal temperature« types of bone cement

Type of Cement	Temperature Rise [°C]
Boneloc	71
Implast	76
Biolos 1	86
Cemex RX	90
Sulfix-6	90
Biolos 3	94
Zimmer LVC	104
Palacos R	104
Osteopal	104
CMW 3	105
Surgical Simplex Ro	105

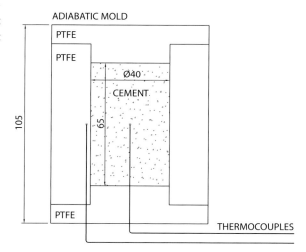

⬚ **Fig. 3.35.** Test setup for adiabatic temperature measurement

of heat generation will reduce heat-induced bone-tissue injury. In this way less bone would have to be remodelled after cemented arthroplasty and the surgical reconstruction might have a better survival. This philosophy behind the development of low temperature cements has never been proven clinically. What has been proven is the clinical failure of some low temperature cements. The use of high molecular weight monomers in Boneloc has led to a very low modulus of elasticity and a high creep rate. Implast which had 20% w/w of its monomer replaced by water, was after polymerization a highly porous cement which results in a low fatigue strength [4]. Reducing the amount of liquid may lead to difficult wetting of the powder. In tensile fracture surfaces of Cemex RX undissolved powder beads can be found (◘ Fig. 3.36). Reduction of heat generation is always at the expense of other cement properties. The best clinical results are still obtained with normal temperature cements.

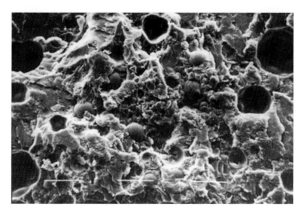

◘ **Fig. 3.36.** SEM of fracture surface of tensile specimen made of Cemex RX cement. P/L ratio of 3 results in inhomogeneous wetting of powder and undissolved powder beads in fracture surface

ISO 5833 Temperature Test

In the ISO 5833 standard a temperature measurement test is described for a cement mass of ø 60×6 mm thickness. In the centre of the cement mass the temperature development during polymerization is measured with a thermocouple. ◘ Figure 3.37 shows the test setup and a resulting cement mould. The outcome of this test is very susceptible for accurate placement of the thermocouple. ◘ Figure 3.38 shows a graph of an ISO 5833 temperature test.

The temperature rise will be less than for an adiabatic test because during polymerization heat will flow to the colder environment. ◘ Table 3.6 shows the temperature rise and setting time for a number of bone cements. The setting time is defined as the time as half the temperature rise is attained. This is during the self accelerating polymerization stage just prior to reaching maximum temperature. ISO 5833 temperature rise is lowest for Boneloc with 36 °C and highest for Surgical Simplex RO with 69 °C.

A similar temperature rise in an adiabatic test does not mean that a similar temperature rise is measured in an ISO 5833 test. Palacos R and Surgical Simplex Ro with roughly the same heat generation have a 13 °C difference

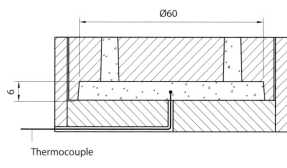

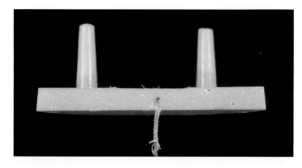

◘ **Fig. 3.37.** Test setup of temperature test according ISO 5833. Important is very accurate placement of thermocouple in the middle of the 6 mm thickness

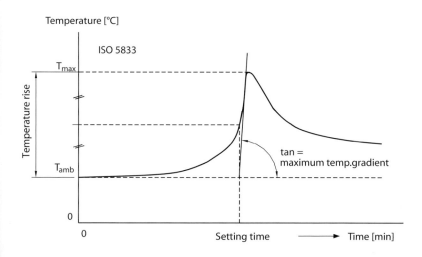

◘ **Fig. 3.38.** Temperature graph measured in an ISO 5833 temperature test. Setting time is defined as time when temperature is middle between ambient and maximum temperature. Max. gradient is attained just before reaching maximum temperature

3

in the ISO 5833 temperature rise. A closer look at the ISO-temperature graph reveals that there is a high difference in polymerization rate during the self accelerating polymerization step. Palacos R has a maximum temperature gradient of 60 °C/min and Surgical Simplex Ro of 179 °C/min (◘ Table 3.7). This means that in case of Palacos the generated heat has more time to flow to the environment and thereby reducing peak temperature.

◘ **Table 3.6.** Maximum temperature rise and setting time for various types of cement measured in an ISO 5833 temperature test

Type of Cement	Temperature Rise [°C]	Setting Time [min:sec]
Boneloc	36	11:00
Cemex RX	44	13:20
Sulfix-6	48	10:50
Zimmer LVC	52	11:50
Palacos R Genta	56	10:40
SmartSet Genta	56	9:50
Osteopal	58	12:10
CMW Endurance	63	12:10
CMW 3	65	10:50
CMW 1 Genta	67	9:10
Surgical Simplex Ro	69	11:50

Mechanical Properties

Introduction

In vivo bone cement is subjected to a complex and varying load pattern. It is impossible to simulate experimentally such loading conditions in order to obtain information about the mechanical properties of specific types of bone cements. However regardless the complexity of the loading situation, only 3 modes of mechanical stress do exist: tensile, compression and shear stress. Rather than performing a complex loading simulation test, one can perform a much simpler test to establish the properties for each stress mode separately. Originally, the ISO 5833 standard only described a compression test at 24 hours after mixing. In the 2002 version a bending test at 24 hours after mixing was added.

One may question the validity of a test at 24 hours after mixing. There is a considerable amount of residual monomer after curing of bone cement and afterpolymerization will take several weeks. The effect of afterpolymerization in a compression and in a tensile test can be seen in ◘ Tables 3.8 and 3.9. Palacos R was submitted to a compression test at 2 hours, 2 days and 28 days after mixing. The stress at failure, strain at failure and the modulus of elasticity showed an increase of resp. 48%, 15% and 30% over a 4 week period. In tension there is no effect from

◘ **Table 3.7.** Different maximum ISO temperature rise despite similar amount of heat generation due to difference in self accelerating polymerization rate

Type of Cement	ISO 5833 Test		
	Adiabatic Temp. Rise	Maximum Temp. Gradient	Maximum ISO Temp. Rise
Palacos R Genta	104 °C	60 °C/min	56 °C
Surgical Simplex Ro	105 °C	179 °C/min	69 °C

◘ **Table 3.8.** ISO 5833 compression test of Palacos R at various intervals after mixing

Compression Test Palacos R	2 Hours	2 Days	28 Days	Increase
Stress at failure [MPa]	73	86	108	48%
Strain at failure [%]	6.8	7.1	7.8	15%
Modulus of elasticity [MPa]	1920	2170	2500	30%

◘ **Table 3.9.** Tensile testing of Palacos R at various intervals after mixing. Specimen shape according to DIN 53455 and crosshead speed of 25 mm/min

Tensile Test Palacos R	2 Hours	2 Days	28 Days	Increase
Stress at failure [MPa]	52	53	52	0%
Strain at failure [%]	2.9	2.7	2.6	−9%
Modulus of elasticity [MPa]	2720	3050	3020	11%

afterpolymerization on the strength and a limited effect on strain and elasticity. Beyond 4 weeks no major change in mechanical properties has to be expected *in vitro* or *in vivo*. Therefore, mechanical testing should better be performed at 4 weeks after mixing than after 24 hours.

The tensile strength of cement is 2–3 times lower than in compression. This is a result of air voids and other inclusions which act as stress risers in this brittle material. This effect is much higher in tensile and outweigh the effect of the afterpolymerization. In this chapter we describe tensile, compressive and shear properties in quasi-static tests.

In vivo cement is subjected to cyclic loading, but because of the time consuming aspect and high costs involved in fatigue testing, only few papers have been published on fatigue data.

Compressive Properties

An overview of several bone cements and their compression properties are seen in ◘ Table 3.10. Cements based on more brittle PMMA polymers seem to have a higher compressive strength and modulus of elasticity than cements like Palacos and Boneloc which are based on more flexible molecules. Cements with a low monomer concentration (P/L ratio of 3) like CEMEX RX exhibit less strength increase due to afterpolymerization than cements with a regular monomer concentration (P/L ratio of 2) like CMW 3 (◘ Table 3.11). In all cases, the compression strength is much higher than physiological compressive stress levels which are in the order of 5 MPa.

Tensile Properties

There is no specific standard for a quasi-static tensile test of bone cement. General standards for tensile testing of plastics, however, do exist, like DIN53455 and ASTM D638. ◘ Table 3.12 shows the results of tensile testing of specimens made according to DIN53455, stored in air at ambient temperature, and tested at 28 days after mixing with a crosshead speed of 25 mm/min. All specimens with voids of ø 1.5 mm or more at the fracture site are discarded. The failure stress varies between 29 and 52 MPa. There is a clear effect from the chemical formulation on the mechanical properties (◘ Fig. 3.39). The cements based on copolymers with ductile MA-molecules (SmartSet, Palacos, Palamed) show the highest tensile strength, while the more brittle cements based on copolymers with styrene molecules or PMMA homopolymers show the lowest tensile strength. Note that Boneloc has a normal tensile strength but the lowest modulus of elasticity, which resembles its high creep rate. The more ductile MA-copolymers have a strain to failure of ± 2.1% which doubles

Elasticity	Molecule	T_{glass} [°C]
Brittle	Styrene	120
↑	Methylmethacrylate	105
	Ethylmethacrylate	65
↓	Butylmethacrylate	20
Ductile	Methylacrylate	6

◘ Fig. 3.39. Mechanical properties of various types of acrylic molecules

◘ Table 3.10. Compressive properties of bone cements derived from a compression test according to ISO 5833

Type of Cement	Compression Tests at 24 Hours after Hand Mixing, According to ISO5833		
	Failure Stress [MPa]	Failure Strain [%]	Modulus of Elasticity [MPa]
CEMEX RX	101.8	7.1	2608
CMW 3	101.7	7.1	2518
CMW 1 Genta	96.5	7.0	2147
SULFIX-6	96.3	6.9	2461
CMW 3 Genta	95.9	6.9	2177
Palacos R Genta	80.7	6.2	1993
Boneloc	80.0	6.5	2177

◘ Table 3.11. Increase of compressive failure stress due to afterpolymerization of bone cements with various P/L ratios. Higher liquid portion gives more strength increase

Type of Cement	Compressive Failure Stress at 24 Hours [MPa]	Compressive Failure Stress at 28 Days [MPa]	Increase of Failure Stress [%]	P/L Ratio w/w
CMW 3	101.7	122.3	20.3	2.1
SULFIX-6	96.3	110.4	14.6	2.3
CEMEX RX	101.8	113.0	11.2	3.0

◻ Table 3.12. Tensile properties of bone cements derived from a tensile test at 28 days after mixing. Specimens made according to ISO 53455, specimens stored in air at room temperature, crosshead speed 25 mm/min

Type of Cement	Tensile Tests at 28 Days after Hand Mixing		
	Failure Stress [MPa]	Failure Strain [%]	Modulus of Elasticity [MPa]
SmartSet HV	51.7	2.2	3068
Palacos R	49.8	2.1	3176
Palamed Genta	48.2	2.0	3283
Palacos R Genta	46.4	1.8	3300
SULFIX-6	40.7	1.6	2949
CMW 1 Genta	35.5	1.3	3031
Boneloc	35.4	0.9	2360
Surgical Simplex Ro	33.9	1.2	3017
CEMEX RX	30.7	1.1	3098
CMW 3 Genta	28.9	1.0	3050

the failure strain of ± 1.1% of the weaker and more brittle Styrene-copolymers and MMA homopolymers.

Shear Properties

Unfortunately, shear strength cannot be measured accurately experimentally. To design an experiment which causes an even shear stress distribution on the fracture site is very difficult, if not impossible. So called push out tests which are often used for shear testing will not generate an even shear stress. The best experimental setup to determine the shear strength is possible an AIA model [9]. However, even after extensive testing with this model we did not succeed to develop a well functioning shear test for bone cement.

Take Home Messages

- The ISO5833 standard is not suitable for cement quality assessment.
- The ASTM F2118 fatigue-test standard lacks a minimum strength requirement.
- Low viscosity cements have no surgical or patient benefits.
- Low temperature cements have no surgical or patient benefits.
- Medium viscosity cements can be handled in a syringe without cooling.
- Flexible MMA-MA copolymer cements perform best in tensile.
- Stiff PMMA and Styrene cements perform best in compression.
- The most important pre-clinical cement test is a fatigue test.
- The most important clinical cement property is handling.
- Traditional cements perform best.

References

1. ASTM F2118–2001.Test method for constant amplitude of force controlled fatigue testing of acrylic bone cements materials. ASTM International, USA, 2001
2. Bellare A, Lee Y-L, Fitz W, Thornhill TS. Using nanotechnology to increase the fatigue life of acrylic bone cement. Transactions 51st Annual Meeting ORS, Washington, February 20–23 2005, p 288
3. Caywood GA, Gunasekaran S, Kharas GB. Synthesis and preclinical evaluation of a fast curing bioresorbable composite bone cement. Transactions of the Fifth World Biomaterials Congress, Toronto, Canada, May 29-June 2 1996, p 911
4. De Wijn JR. Porous polymethylmethacrylate cement. Dissertation University of Nijmegen, Nijmegen, The Netherlands, January 1982
5. Haboush EJ. A new operation for arthroplasty of the hip based on biomechanics, photoelasticity, fast-setting dental acrylic and other considerations. Scientific Exhibit, AAOS, Chicago, January 1952
6. ISO5833:2002. Implants for surgery-Acrylic resin cements. International Standardization Organisation, Switzerland, 2002
7. Jacobs CR. Bone cement compositions. World patent PCT/US99/05497, WO99/45978.The Penn State Research Foundation, 1999
8. Kruft MAB. New radio-opaque polymeric biomaterials. Dissertation University of Technology Eindhoven, Eindhoven, The Netherlands, April 1997
9. Mahanian S, Piziali RL. Finite element evaluation of the AIA shear specimen for bone. J Biomechanics 1988; 21: 346–356

Properties of Bone Cement: Extreme Differences in Properties of Successful Bone Cements

A.U. Dan Daniels, Dieter Wirz, Erwin Morscher

Summary

In clinical registries, use of two acrylic bone cements correlates especially highly with longevity of total hip replacement: Palacos R and Simplex P. However, the cements are markedly different. Palacos R is based on a high molecular weight starting powder that is chemically sterilised, while Simplex P employs a different polymer formulation of much lower molecular weight that is radiation-sterilised. In the lab, Palacos R is high in strength, toughness and fatigue resistance, and Simplex P is not. In a long-term clinical retrieval study, Palacos R molecular weight declined but remained high, while Simplex P molecular weight began low and continued to decline. Lower molecular weight cements are inherently more prone to creep and stress relaxation. It seems clear that the basis for excellent clinical performance of each of these cements must be different. Our analysis implies that cements which emphasise strength and durability may be the best choice for hip stems designed to provide interlock, and cements which emphasise controlled creep and stress relaxation may be preferable with stems designed to allow subsidence.

Purposes of this Chapter

Our purpose is to present and support three ideas:
- Clinically successful acrylic bone cement formulations can differ extremely in formulation and mechanical properties,
- changes in cement over time must be considered more carefully in trying to understand cement clinical performance, and
- the above factors plus consideration of cement dynamic mechanical properties suggest that the best cements may be different for stems designed to provide interlock, versus stems designed to allow subsidence.

Clinically Successful Bone Cements Can Differ Extremely in Composition and Properties

A clinical conundrum: Analyses of the Swedish and Norwegian hip registries [3, 9] showed that the choice of cement correlates better with hip femoral component longevity (time until required revision) than does choice of hip stem. In addition, the two cements which best correlate with high longevity are Palacos R and the cement in longest clinical use, Simplex P. It is not meant to imply that these are the only two satisfactory bone cements. Instead, comparing and contrasting these two very different cements is used here as a means for attempting to increase our understanding of the relationships between bone cement composition, mechanical properties, stem design and clinical performance.

Compositions of Palacos R and Simplex P

One might then expect that these two similarly performing cements would exhibit similar composition and structure – or at least similar key mechanical properties – and thus provide a model that all cements should emulate. Unfortunately, the absolute converse is true. As we have found, and stated previously in several publications, »bone cement does not equal bone cement« [12]. First, as shown in ◻ Table 3.13, the two cements are extremely different in composition. As indicated, they contain differing amounts of different radio-opacifiers. More importantly, not only are the two cements based on different polymer formulations, but the starting powder molecular weight of Simplex P is among the lowest reported, and that of Palacos R is the highest reported. As discussed later, the method of powder sterilisation is also completely different (chemical vs. radiation), and this has potential effects on composition changes with time.

Mechanical Properties of Palacos R and Simplex P

One might hope that in spite of these compositional differences, these two clinically successful bone cements would exhibit similarities in key mechanical properties, thus demonstrating that they just represent different materials-based paths to the same mechanical solution. Unfortunately, this is not the case either, as shown in ◻ Table 3.14 and discussed below.

Among 22 cements tested [5], Simplex P was among the lowest in quasi-static bending strength, and Palacos R was one of the highest (> 20% above Simplex P). One might expect that the two cements instead exhibit similarities under dynamic conditions which better reflect the environment in which they must operate. Unfortunately, it is again the converse that is true. In Kühn's fatigue tests [5] of 12 cements, the residual strength of Simplex P after 10^7 cycles was 25% below Palacos R, even though Palacos R is a high viscosity cement during mixing and thus more prone to development of defects that affect fatigue performance. A low viscosity version of Palacos R (i.e., Osteopal) exhibited the highest residual strength of all cements tested (~ 83% higher than Simplex P). The same was true in another test, that we think is important, due to the cyclic impact loads that cements receive during gait. Among 22 cements tested by Kühn for dynamic impact strength (i.e., toughness), Simplex P was below average, and Palacos R was highest of all (~ 92% higher than Simplex P).

Wear Phenomena

Another mechanical approach to finding an explanation for differences in bone cement clinical performance is the laboratory study of wear at the cement/metal interface under carefully simulated implantation conditions. In a recent study [11, 12], two of the authors of this chapter (Wirz, Morscher) paid particular attention to creating a proper simulation. They developed a wear-test machine and environmental protocol which produced wear patterns on metal (S30 steel) surfaces that closely resembled those found on clinically retrieved cemented hip stems that had become loose in the cement mantle. They evaluated four different acrylic cements with a principal aim

◻ **Table 3.13.** Comparison of Palacos R and Simplex P – main constituents of solid starting materials. Minor constituents (e.g. initiators, etc.) are omitted for clarity. Note that the liquid component employed with both cements is the same (methyl methacrylate) and the solid/liquid ratios are virtually the same (data from Kühn [5])

Cement	Palacos R	Simplex P
Radio-opacifier	6.13 g zirconium dioxide	4.0 g barium sulfate
Polymer powder	33.55 g poly (methyl acrylate, methyl methacrylate)	29.4 g poly (methyl methacrylate, styrene) 6.0 g poly (methyl methacrylate)
Molecular Weight	~ 740 k Daltons	~ 230 k Daltons
Sterilization method	Ethylene oxide	Gamma radiation

◻ **Table 3.14.** Comparison of Selected Mechanical Properties for Palacos R and Simplex P. (Data from Kühn, [5]; values read from figures (approximate), or taken from tables)

Selected Mechanical Properties	Palacos R	Simplex P	Units
Initial bending strength	87	72	MPa
Residual strength after 10^7 cycles	17.8	14.2	MPa
Dynamic impact strength	7.5	3.9	kJ/mm^2

of investigating the effects of opacifiers on wear (presence or absence of opacifier, use of $BaSO_4$ vs. ZrO_2). The use of ZrO_2 was of particular concern, since it is a ceramic used as an abrasive. However, neither cement nor metal-weight loss correlated with opacifier variables. Also, none of the four cements caused both a high loss of cement weight and a high loss of metal weight. The only cement which resulted in both a low cement weight loss and low metal weight loss was one (of two) containing ZrO_2 opacifier: Palacos R (+ Gentamycin). Also, Palacos R burnished the metal surface to a much greater extent than any of the others (~ surface reflectance values 5–6 times higher). Simplex P was not among the other cements studied. However, a pure cement having a similar amount of the same opacifier ($BaSO_4$) but without styrene was among those evaluated.

Clearly, the explanation for why Palacos R and Simplex P are among the best performers clinically does not lie in their similarities. For Palacos R, the data reviewed above suggest that the reasons for its good clinical performance are mostly conventional ones. Mechanically (compared to other acrylic bone cements), Palacos is above the norm in strength, toughness and fatigue resistance. Also in our wear study (which ruled out the effect of opacifiers), it was mechanically and chemically durable enough to polish stem metal without increased metal or cement wear. Chemically, the Palacos R situation is analogous to that now known for conventional forms of UHMWPE. That is, Palacos R has a high molecular weight and is not radia-

tion-sterilised. Both these factors improve resistance to chemical degradation of polymers, and thus help maintain structure and mechanical properties for a longer term.

> **Note:** Conversely, the data suggest that the excellent clinical performance of Simplex P may be related instead in someway to its low molecular weight and susceptibility to further changes after implantation.

Bone Cements Change After Implantation

Clinical Changes in Molecular Weight

Alterations in acrylic bone cement composition have not been widely documented over time, other than loss of residual monomer soon after polymerization. Lack of documentation of long-term changes after implantation is particularly unfortunate since such changes are a logical source of changes in both cement mechanical properties and cement mechanical behaviour (e.g. amount of creep) under applied loads. However, a recent paper [4] provides unequivocal evidence that the composition of acrylic bone cements around hip stems can change significantly during years of clinical implantation. As shown in ◘ Fig. 3.40, the molecular weight of both Palacos R and Simplex P specimens was lower than freshly mixed and analyzed control specimens at all times of retrieval (~4 years or more). The apparent mean decrease for Palacos R (5 specimens)

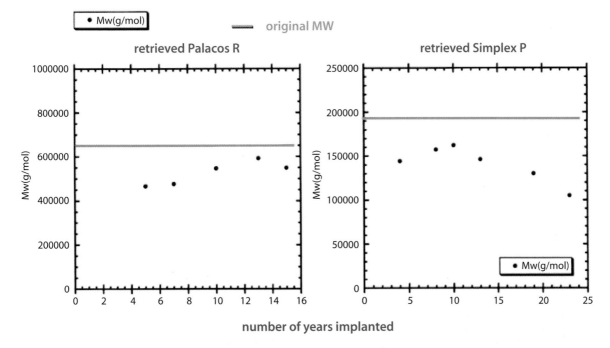

◘ Figure 3.40. Molecular weight of acrylic bone cement specimens retrieved from around femoral stems. Original MW = molecular weights of cements of the same brand freshly prepared at the time the retrieved specimens were studied. (Adapted from Hughes [4])

over periods of 4 to 15 years was from 620,000 g/mol (i.e., 620 kD) to 526 kD or ~15%. For Simplex P (4 specimens) over a similar period (4 to 13 years), the mean decrease was from 194 kD to 152 kD or ~22%.

The data also suggest that Simplex P not only starts with a molecular weight less than 1/3 that of Palacos R, but may exhibit a greater continuing decline with time. The maximum decrease exhibited for Simplex P (at 23 years) was from 194 kD to 105 kD or 46%.

In the same paper, Hughes et al. [4] also reported companion laboratory studies of the degradation of both cements under accelerated oxidative conditions (at 60 °C in 30 vol.% hydrogen peroxide, replenished daily for 12 weeks). Simplex P molecular weight declined 14% and Palacos R declined 6%. This suggests that the observed substantial difference in clinical degradation between the two cements was to be expected. Overall, the results also point up the fact that Palacos R remains a relatively high molecular weight material over years of implantation while Simplex P remains (and perhaps becomes increasingly) a low molecular weight material. For example, comparing the mean molecular weights for the 4–15 year Palacos R specimens and the 4–13 year Simplex P specimens, the molecular weight of implanted Palacos R remained ~3.4 times higher.

Radiation Sterilization of Cement Starting Powders

This continuing decline in Simplex P molecular weight could be due to sustained activity related to radiation-induced free radicals and/or a molecular weight threshold effect. That is, once the molecular weight is low enough, clinical environmental factors (e.g., pulsatile cyclic gait loads, water, ions, lipids, enzymes) may combine to cause polymer chain scission. Recent work we performed [1] using an entirely different method also supports what is broadly implied by the findings of Hughes et al.– i.e. that changes in Simplex P with time can be expected to occur much more rapidly than in Palacos R. The method we

used was isothermal microcalorimetry (IMC) – measurement of heat flow in the microwatt (mW) range at constant temperature. All chemical reactions or physical changes of state either produce heat or consume heat, and the resultant heat flow rate is directly proportional to the aggregate rate of the reactions taking place. Because of its sensitivity, micro- (and now nano-)calorimetry provides a means for measuring and comparing the rates of solid-state reactions (e.g. chain scission, oxidation, crystallization) in small solid specimens (~0.5 to 5 g). This can be accomplished in a matter of hours, even if the reactions are occurring very slowly; i.e. with a half life in the range of 20 years.

Using IMC, we briefly assessed the stability of three bone cement starting powders, looking for effects of both molecular weight and sterilisation method. IMC heat flow rate provided a measure of the overall exothermic activity taking place in each acrylic bone cement powder specimen. Likely reactions taking place include chain scission and oxidation of the polymer, and breakdown of initiators or plasticizers. Heat flow confirms that there are on-going physico-chemical processes, and relative heat flow rates offer a relative measure of the aggregate physico-chemical stability of each powder. Results are summarized in ◘ Table 3.15.

As shown, Palacos R starting powder was the most stable and ~4 times as stable as Simplex P. Duracem has about the same low starting molecular weight as Simplex P but is ethylene oxide sterilized rather than radiation sterilized. Its stability was intermediate between Palacos R and Simplex P, suggesting that part of the lower stability of Simplex P is due to its low molecular weight and part to free radicals created by radiation sterilization. We concluded that overall stability was substantially influenced by the combination of polymer molecular weight and radiation sterilization. Also, it should be remembered that the results do not indicate that Simplex P powder is grossly unstable, but rather just the least stable among three relatively stable materials. A recent overview of the use of microcalorimetry in studying implant materials is available [6].

◘ **Table 3.15.** Microcalorimetric comparison of heat flow rates at 25 °C in air from 5 g of acrylic bone cement starting powders. Results are extrapolated from mean heat flow rates measured during the interval from 15–20 hours after specimens were placed in the calorimeter [1]

Cement (Powder)	Polymers*	MW (kD)	Sterilization (Method)	Heat Flow (Extrapolated) (J/g, First 5 Years)
Simplex P	MMA-Sty	230	Radiation	6.7
Duracem	MMA-BMA	220	Ethylene Oxide	3.6
Palacos R	MA-MMA	740	Ethylene Oxide	1.8

MMA methyl methacrylate, *Sty* styrene, *BMA* butyl methacrylate, *MA* methacrylate.

There are other studies which suggest radiation sterilization is a major factor in determining both bone cement molecular weight and durability. As prepared for clinical use, Palacos R is ethylene oxide sterilized. However, Lewis and Mladsi [7] showed that 2.5 Mrad of radiation sterilization of Palacos R powder reduced the molecular weight from 754 kD to 315 kD – a drop of more than 50% – while ethylene oxide sterilization caused no significant change. The estimated tensile fatigue limits (cyclic stress below which failure is unlikely) for ethylene oxide sterilized and radiation-sterilized Palacos R after polymerisation were 9.32 and 4.61 MPa, respectively. The differences are roughly proportional to the differences in molecular weights.

Evidence seems strong that both lower molecular weight and radiation sterilization are factors which decrease long-term stability of acrylic bone cements. Conventional wisdom is that these changes are deleterious. A further implication of the molecular weight degradation with time is obvious – fatigue resistance of implanted cement will also become lower at the same time that the number of load cycles continues to increase. Given this double effect, one must then ask why hip stems cemented with Simplex P do not seem to be routinely subject to catastrophic cement failures at long implantation times. As discussed next, it seems possible that the answer lies in viscoelastic effects and perhaps their increase over the long term.

Cement Dynamic Properties and Implications for Choosing Cement/Stem Combinations

Viscoelasticity

Acrylic bone cements (indeed all polymeric solid materials) are viscoelastic to varying degrees. This means their mechanical behaviour lies between essentially elastic materials (e.g., titanium alloys, alumina ceramics) and slow-flowing liquids (e.g., lubricating oils, solutions containing high concentrations of high molecular weight polymers). Consequently, acrylic bone cements exhibit four interrelated viscoelastic phenomena pertinent to their clinical performance; stress relaxation, damping, creep and the dependence of mechanical properties on the rate at which the material is deformed (► chapters 3.1, 3.2, 3.3).

Brittleness

The potential importance of viscoelastic effects arises from the fact that acrylic bone cements are relatively brittle polymeric materials. For example, the reported range of elongation to failure in conventional tensile tests is only 0.8–2.5% [13]. For comparison, the range for UHMWPE is 200–350%. This difference is in great part due to the fact that at body temperature, UHMWPE is above its polymeric glass transition temperature and acrylic cements are below their transition temperature, meaning that they are in a semi-crystalline (i.e. more brittle) state. Factors which lower the glass transition temperature of acrylic cements, bringing it closer to body temperature, are discussed later.

Any tensile component of cyclic strain is the source of crack growth (fatigue) in materials. Unfortunately, some regions of the hip stem cement mantle are subject to bending and shear loads and thus unavoidably experience large components of tensile cyclic stress. Also, high tensile loads can induce enough strain in relatively brittle materials to cause sudden, single-overload failures. The conventional (e.g. Palacos R) approach to minimizing the effects of tensile loads on brittle acrylic cements is to make them innately as strong and tough as possible.

Stress Relaxation and Water Uptake

Stress relaxation can reduce strains in cement as discussed in general in ► chapter 3.2. The focus here is on Simplex P. In a recent study [2] stress relaxation was measured in 3-point bending. Prior to performing the studies, these authors monitored water uptake. It was found that the rate of water uptake of Simplex P is much slower than other cements not containing styrene (which renders acrylic polymers more hydrophobic). After 24 hours at 37 °C, water uptake of Simplex P was only 0.5%. After 530 hours, water uptake was ~2.7% and was still rising rather than reaching an equilibrium value. In spite of this observation, the authors chose to measure stress relaxation after equilibrating with water for a maximum of 168 hours (~1.3% water). De Santis et al. observed 18.1% stress relaxation 1 hour after applying 0.9% strain in 3-point bending.

> Note: It seems likely that the stress relaxation of Simplex P would be even faster if it contained an equilibrium amount of water, as it would after months or years in the body.

Dynamic Damping

Stress relaxation is a measure of the ability of a material to dissipate strain energy as heat, due to internal intermolecular motion and friction, and this energy loss is the basis of stress relaxation. The ability of a material to dissipate energy can also be measured dynamically, and this is perhaps more appropriate in the case of acrylic cements for hip fixation, since they experience dynamic loads during gait. The method is called dynamic mechanical analysis (DMA). A cyclic strain is applied, and the *damping factor*, tan ∂, is measured. Tan ∂ is essentially the dynamic ratio of lost energy to stored energy for a material. An increased damping factor indicates increased ability to dissipate energy, and therefore »damp« the maximum stresses which occur.

Energy dissipation stems from polymer molecular mobility, and according to De Santis et al. [2] »... the stress relaxation test is suitable to depict the effect of the (specimen) conditioning on the mobility of the polymer main chain (and) ... the DMA test better describes the effect ... on the mobility of the polymer side chain.« Therefore, in addition to stress relaxation tests, they also used DMA. For Simplex P at 37 °C (after 168 hours in air at 20 °C plus 168 hours in water at 37 °C) tan ∂ at 1 Hz (similar to gait frequency) was ~0.07 (∂ = ~4 °). However, damping *rose* markedly with frequency, approximately doubling at 10 Hz and almost doubling again at 100 Hz to a value of tan ∂ = 0.23 (∂ = ~13 °). Higher frequencies are of clinical interest because hip joint loading in gait is *not* sinusoidal. Instead (because of heel strike and toe-off) it involves sudden increases in force (high strain rates) and therefore effective frequencies in the range of 20–200 Hz [10].

This increase in damping factor with frequency for acrylic cements is in marked contrast to the behaviour of skeletal system tissues such as articular cartilage [10], in which damping declines with frequency and mechanical behaviour becomes increasingly elastic. De Santis et al. [2] were aware of there unusual finding for bone cements, stating that »the plot of damping factor as a function of frequency indicate a remarkable capacity for energy dissipation at 37 °C.« and that »from the viewpoint of classical linear viscoelasticity, the stress relaxation experiments and the DMA data are not in agreement«.

> **Note:** This increase in damping with frequency may do much to help explain why acrylic cements (which are brittle in quasi-static mechanical strength tests) are able to withstand gait loading as well as they do.

Glass Transition Temperature of Cement

De Santis et al. [2] also recognised that the effect on cement viscoelastic properties of exposure to water at 37 °C) on their viscoelasticity is complex. This is because during initial days of exposure (in lab tests or in the body) methacrylate monomer is being lost (thus decreasing polymer chain mobility and lowering damping) while water is being gained (increasing polymer chain mobility and increasing damping). Part of the effect of water uptake on viscoelasticity can be seen in a reduction of the glass tran-

sition temperature to a level closer to body temperature (see the general discussion in ▶ chapter 3.1). In a study by Kühn [5], the initial glass temperature (after 24 hours at 37 °C in dry air) of Simplex P was ~97 °C – among the highest of 26 cements assessed (range ~65–100 °C). However, after 8 weeks in water at 37 °C, the glass transition temperature of Simplex P was ~70 °C and in the same range as all cements assessed (~65–70 °C).

> **Note:** Of equal importance, the glass temperature of a given polymer declines with declining molecular weight. Therefore, if the molecular weight of Simplex P declines further with time after implantation, so will its glass transition temperature.

As discussed previously, Hughes et al. [4] found that the already low molecular weight of Simplex P in hip stem cement mantles apparently continues to decrease markedly over years of implantation. What, we wonder, is the damping capacity of water-saturated Simplex P after 15–20 years of implantation?

Cement Creep

In addition, if a bone cement exhibits stress relaxation or damping, it exhibits creep, as discussed in some detail in ▶ chapter 3.2. It is interesting to note here, though, the clinical success of Ling, using the Exeter polished, tapered stem and Simplex P cement [8]. Although he observed subsidence of the stems in 93% of his cases, the revision rate for failure of cementation was only 2.54% at 21 years. Creep provides the opportunity for acrylic cement to remodel. Potentially, this maximizes the area of interfacial contact with bone and metal and thus minimizes interfacial stress concentrations. Also, it potentially shifts the balance of internal stresses away from tensile loading and toward compressive loading, the mode in which acrylic cements exhibit maximum strength.

Conclusions

Combining the various findings described above, it seems that acrylic bone cements can perform well for very different mechanical reasons. We believe there is strong evidence that the clinical success of lower molecular weight acrylic bone cements is especially tied to (a) their ability to dissipate energy and moderate internal stress levels that lead to fatigue failure and (b) also remodel via creep, and thus distribute loads at interfaces as uniformly as possible. In addition, the documented continuing decline in molecular weight of Simplex P over a period of years post-implantation suggests that it (and similar cements) may serve increasingly as an energy-dissipating shock absorber as time passes. Perhaps cements like Simplex P should be viewed as »long-term dynamically active bone cements.«

If our analysis is correct, it can affect clinical choice of cement and also lead to further development of cements in two different directions. It suggests that for stems designed to provide mechanical interlocking of the cement mantle, cements which provide toughness and fatigue resistance may be best. Conversely, if a stem is designed for subsidence to redistribute stress, more viscoelastic cements may be preferred. Hip registry or other published longevity data should be examined for correlations between types of stems and types of cements.

Finally, we are just beginning a clinical retrieval programme at our institution that will allow us to assess long-term composition, structural and mechanical changes in bone cements, and we encourage others to engage in similar efforts. Acrylic cements change with time post-implantation, and assessing the changes will allow us to better understand their performance and how it can be improved. To our knowledge, little effort has been made in this direction compared to efforts to study retrieved metal and polyethylene components. This seems ironic in light of two clinical findings: so far, cemented hip stems as a class generally exhibit better clinical longevity than non-cemented ones, and (as discussed at the beginning) choice of cement correlates better with longevity than does choice of stem design.

Take Home Messages

- In clinical registries, use of two acrylic bone cements correlates especially highly with longevity of THA: Palacos R and Simplex P.
- However, the two cements are markedly different. Palacos R starting powder is high in molecular weight and chemically sterilized. Simplex P employs a different polymer formulation of much lower molecular weight that is radiation sterilized.
- In lab studies, Palacos R is high in strength, toughness and fatigue resistance, and Simplex P is not. In a long-term clinical retrieval study, Palacos R molecular weight declined but remained high, while Simplex P molecular weight began low and continued to decline. Lower molecular weight cements exhibit more creep and stress relaxation in lab studies.
- The basis for excellent clinical performance of each of these cements must be different, and this should be considered in connection with stem design.
- Cements emphasising strength and durability may be best for stems designed to provide interlock. Cements emphasising controlled creep and stress relaxation may be preferable with stems designed to allow subsidence.

References

1. Daniels AU, Lewis G, Son Y, Wirz D, Göpfert B, Morscher EW (2003) Possible differences in long-term stability of bone cements, Program 62nd Ann. Mtg. Schweizerische Gesellschaft Orthopädie, p54
2. De Santis R, Mollica F, Ambrosio L, Nicolais L (2003) Dynamic mechanical behavior of PMMA based bone cements in wet environment. J Materials Sci Materials in Med 14:583–594
3. Havelin LI, Engesæter LB, Espehaug B, Furnes O, Lie SA, Vollset SE (2000) The Norwegian Arthroplasty Register: 11 years and 73,000 arthroplasties. Acta Orthop Scand 71(4):337–353
4. Hughes KF, Ries MD, Pruit LA (2003) Structural degradation of acrylic bone cementd due to in vivo and simulated aging. J Biomed Materials Res 65A:126–135
5. Kühn KD (2000) Bone Cements: Up-to-date comparison of physical and chemical properties of commercial materials, Springer, New York, pp 272.
6. Lewis G, Daniels AU (2003) Use of Isothermal Heat-Conduction Microcalorimetry (IHCMC) for the Evaluation of Synthetic Biomaterials. J Biomed Materials Res 66B: 487–501
7. Lewis G, Mladsi S (1998) Effect of sterilization method on properties of Palacos R acrylic bone cement. Biomaterials 19:117–124
8. Ling RS (1992) Clinical experience with primary cemented total hip arthroplasty. Chir Organi Mov 77: 373–381
9. Malchau H, Herberts P, Söderman P, Odén A. Prognosis of total hip replacement: Update and validation of results from the Swedish National Hip Arthroplasty Registry. 67th Annual Meeting of the American Academy of Orthopaedic Surgeons, Orlando, USA, March 15–19, 2000
10. Park S, Hung CT, Ateshian GA (2004) Mechanical response of bovine articular cartilage under dynamic unconfined compression loading at physiological stress levels. Osteoarthritis and Cartilage 12: 65–73
11. Wirz D, Zurfluh B, Göpfert B, Li F, Frick W, Morscher EW (2003) Results of in vitro studies about the mechanism of wear in the stem-cement interface in THR. In: Winters GL, Nutt MJ (eds) Stainless steel for medical and surgical applications, STP 1438. ASTM International, Conshohocken PA, USA, pp 222–234
12. Wirz D, Daniels AU, Göpfert B, Morscher EW (2005) Clinical development and current status: Europe. In: Acrylic cement in the new millenium. D. Smith, Ed., supplement, Orthop Clin N Am 36:63–73
13. Wright TM, Li S (2000) Biomaterials. In: Buckwalter JA, Einhorn TA, Simon SR (eds) Orthopaedic basic science, 2nd edn. American Academy of Orthopaedic Surgeons, USA, pp 181–216

Properties of Bone Cement: Antibiotic-Loaded Cement

Lars Frommelt, Klaus-Dieter Kühn

Summary

In this chapter an overview is given about the rationale for antibiotic-loaded bone cement as a drug delivery system. The characteristics of antibiotic release, the suitability of various antibiotics for admixing and the clinical application and impact are described.

Rationale for the Use of Topical Antibiotics

The topical application of antibiotics is held responsible for inducing bacterial resistance to antimicrobial agents. There are therefore nowadays very few conditions where local application is still justified. One of these conditions is the infection of bone tissue. Due to the fact that bone tissue is mineralized and cannot be expanded, inflammation results in reduced blood flow. Therefore, inflammatory conditions in bone tissue cause a reduced supply of blood and also of drugs transported via blood circulation. That is why bone tissue has to be looked upon as an inferior compartment with respect to pharmacokinetics, comparable to the central nervous system, even though there is no anatomical barrier [12]. Artificial joints are indwelling medical devices intended for long-term presence in bone tissue. These artificial joint replacements are at risk of infection if a small amount of bacteria succeeds in colonising the foreign material. Bacteria stick to the surface and become sessile by forming biofilm. Periprosthetic infection results if some of the bacteria in biofilm convert to planktonic forms and induce infection of the adjacent tissue. Under these circumstances, antibiotics administered systemically by the intravenous route or orally are able to affect planktonic bacteria in soft tissue or bone but not sessile forms in the biofilm [4]. Sessile bacteria are characterised by minimal inhibitory concentration (MIC)

which exceeds those of their planktonic relatives by up to a thousand fold and they are protected from the host defence mechanisms by the biofilm [17]. Eradication of these pathogens therefore needs surgical revision, including radical removal of foreign material and antimicrobial agents. Otherwise, sessile bacteria will survive and are available to act as a reservoir for recurrent periprosthetic infection.

Under these conditions, topical application of antimicrobial agents is useful for both therapy and prophylaxis. It is an option to obtain extraordinarily high levels of antibiotic concentration at the site of infection and prophylactically on the surface of implants at risk for bacterial colonisation.

Polymethylmethacrylate (PMMA) as a Drug Delivery System

The addition of antimicrobial agents to acrylic bone cement was begun as early as 1969. Together with Lodenkämper, Buchholz [3] started investigations on polymethyl-methacrylate (PMMA) bone cement to determine its suitability as a drug delivery system. The observation that acrylic monomers are eluted from the bone cement for a long period of time after the cement has set, gave them the idea that antimicrobial agents might also be released as well. In a letter to the company Kulzer, the supplier of the PMMA brand Palacos in 1969 Buchholz wrote: »… A small percentage of residual monomer left in the bone cement may still be eluted for some period of time after Palacos has set. When investigating this I wondered if it might be possible to achieve an antibiotic depot in the body, perhaps also a depot of sulphonamides, by mixing these with Palacos …«.

In further experiments, antibiotic powder was mixed with the polymer powder of PMMA. The monomeric liquid was then added for polymerisation [3]. Lodenkämper added several antimicrobial agents to PMMA bone cement in the laboratory and found that some of them were released over long periods of time, others were not released at all [2]. Gentamicin, especially, proved to be very effective in producing long-term high-level concentrations.

Buchholz performed one-stage revisions in patients suffering from periprosthetic infection using antibiotic loaded acrylic cement (ALAC) in these early days [2]. Success with this technique encouraged Buchholz and his co-workers to use ALAC not only for revision surgery but also for prophylaxis in primary implantation of artificial joint replacements. By doing so, he was able to reduce the infection rate after primary implantation of artificial joint replacement from about 7% to lower than 1%.

Delivery of Antibiotics from PMMA Bone Cement

PMMA bone cement is a meshwork of PMMA chains. Antibiotics enclosed in these meshes are released by elution from the bone cement. The elution properties of acrylic bone cements correlate directly with the ability to absorb water during bone cement preparation. Lindner [10], as well as Low and co-workers [11], showed that the elution is in compliance with Fick's law and is thus characterised as diffusion. Lindner concluded with respect to the extremely low speed of transportation of the molecules in the bone cement that this is performed by bulk diffusion. Bulk diffusion is a very slow diffusion in areas free of any solvents. Solvent mediated diffusion takes place at the moment when the antibiotic molecules come into contact with water and are dissolved very fast. Whether the conclusion with respect to bulk diffusion is correct or not, it is a fact that the velocity of diffusion within the bone cement is slow and the rapid diffusion from the surface results in the typical pattern of elution of antibiotics from bone cement. When in first contact with solvents, the agents are eluted in a high concentration for an extremely short period of time which is followed by a long period of elution in decreasing concentration. Elution is at its peak within the first minutes as shown by van Sorge and co-workers [15]. These elution characteristics apply not only to antimicrobial agents but to other ingredients in the bone cement as well.

The shape of the elution curve depends on the antimicrobial agents, their combination and the bone cement preparation.

Characteristics of Bone Cement for Delivery of Antimicrobial Agents

All bone cements currently available are based on the same basic compound: methyl methacrylate (MMA). Co-compounds like styrol, ethyl or buthyl methacrylate are used in some preparations. Chemically, MMA is an ester of methacrylic acid, which has the ability to polymerise to PMMA. This material is characterised by a wide variety of different properties depending on the method of preparation. Plexiglas and bone cement are both PMMA. It is therefore not surprising that different bone cement preparations have different elution properties [8].

To prepare bone cements, a dough is made from liquid MMA and PMMA powder. Curing of the dough results from polymerisation of MMA in contact with the pre-polymerized PMMA particles. In the meshwork the »new« PMMA chains a variety of substances, such as antibiotics, may be incorporated.

The elution of water-soluble substances like antimicrobial agents from bone cement depends directly on the ability to absorb water [16]. The absorption of water by bone cements is determined by the hydrophobicity of the components (◘ Fig. 3.41) and the physical configuration of the bone cement resulting in porosity and roughness. ◘ Table 3.16 shows data as presented in a publication by van de Belt and co-workers [14]. Due to the fact that antibiotics are eluted when in direct contact with water,

◘ **Table 3.16.** Hydrophobicity (contact angle) and surface roughness as hint for the porosity of the material. (From [14])

Bone Cement	Contact Angle [°]	Surface Roughness [µm]
PMMA	70–80	no data
CMW 1	70	0.33
CMW 3	75	0.20
CMW 2000	73	0.16
Palacos	76	0.29
Palamed	80	0.49

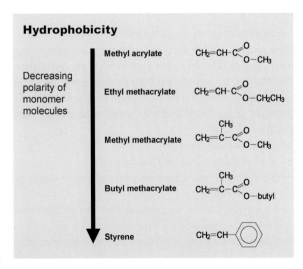

◘ **Fig. 3.41.** Hydrophilic/hydrophobic properties of some monomers used in bone cement. (From [8])

the amount of antibiotics eluted correlates directly with the surface available. In conclusion, porosity, roughness and hydrophobicity determine the absorption of water by the bone cement preparation and thus the elution characteristics.

Adding antimicrobial agents to bone cement alters its mechanical properties. ALAC should comply with the standard specifications of ISO 5833. That means bending strength must exceed 50 Mpa and compressive strength 70 MPa. The decrease of mechanical properties correlates with the quantity of antibiotics added and the homogeneity of the preparation.

Homogeneity of the mixture of polymer powder and crystalline antibiotics and the particle size of the antibiotic powder also play a role elution and mechanical properties [13]. In commercially available preparations homogeneity and particle size are standardised and thus reliable. If antibiotics are added to the bone cement in the operating room, a standardised mixture is not possible. Therefore, if industrial preparations are available, these are preferable. There are some sporadic references in the literature with regard to different elution properties resulting from different methods of bone cement preparation. In contrast to industrial preparations, data are rarely available for substances added to the bone cement in the operating theatre.

In the experience of the Endo Clinic, Hamburg, antimicrobial agents incorporated by hand mixing should not exceed 10% of the bone cement preparation. Studies must be carried out to ensure which portion may be incorporated in bone cement to obtain good elution properties and tolerable loss of mechanical properties of the bone cement.

Characteristics of Antimicrobial Agents Suitable for Preparation of Antibiotic Loaded Acrylic Cement (ALAC)

Antimicrobial agents are added to PMMA bone cement in order to achieve high-level concentrations adjacent to the bone cement. The intention is to control an established infection or to protect medical devices from bacterial colonisation. These antibiotics need a profile of physical-chemical properties that allows them to be eluted from PMMA:

- High solubility in water
- Heat stability during polymerisation
- No chemical interaction with PMMA or mediators of polymerisation
- Low effect on the mechanical strength of the bone cement
- Good release from cured/polymerised bone cement

Most of these properties are not predictable and must thus be determined by carrying out experiments for the different combinations of bone cements and antimicrobial agents. One interesting point is the amount of antibiotic that is eluted in comparison to the content of the antimicrobial agent of the bone cement (◘ Fig. 3.42). Another criterion is the period of elution with respect to the minimal inhibitory concentration (MIC) of the pathogens expected at the site of infection. Adams and co-workers showed in animal experiments that relevant antibiotic elution takes place not only in vitro but also in vivo [1]. In a canine model they showed that the concentration adjacent to implanted ALAC beads exceeded the MIC according to the National Committee of Clinical Laboratory Standards (NCCLS) regulations for a distinct period of time depending on the antimicrobial agent used: cefazolin 14 days, ciprofloxacin 3 days, clindamycin 28 days, ticarcillin 9 days, tobramycin 21 days, and vancomycin 3 days.

Regarding biological properties the antibiotics should be highly efficient against known or suspected bacterial pathogens and have a low rate of adverse drug effects in patients treated by local therapy using ALAC. Antimicrobial agents must be available at the site of infection in an appropriate concentration in their active form. Inactivation is possible, for example, e.g. bonding to plasma protein or metabolism as the bonding of tetracycline to hydroxylapatite of the bone matrix. The »biological« profile should include the following properties:

- Broad antimicrobial action on gram-positive and gram-negative bacteria
- Bactericidal effect on bacteria in low concentrations (exception: clindamycin)
- Low rate of primarily resistant germs
- Low frequency of emerging resistances
- Low frequency of allergic adverse reactions in humans
- Low toxic properties in humans
- Low protein bonding
- No interaction with the adjacent tissue

In cases of infection, the risks and benefits to the patient have to be weighed against each other and it is often impossible to fulfil all criteria. With the exception of clindamycin, antibiotics must have a bactericidal effect on pathogens. In spite of the fact that clindamycin is characterised as bacteriostatic agent, it has a proven efficacy in controlling infections especially in periprosthetic infection.

The elution of antimicrobial agent depends not only on the properties of the bone cement but also on the amount of antibiotics incorporated in the bone cement. It is surprising that not only the amount of antimicrobial agents results in better elution properties but also the combination of antibiotics. In the presence of clindamycin, the elution of gentamicin is much better in contrast to the application of gentamicin alone [8]. A possible explanation may be that high-level elution from superficial enclosures within the first minutes after contact with solvent may lead to an enlargement of the surface area

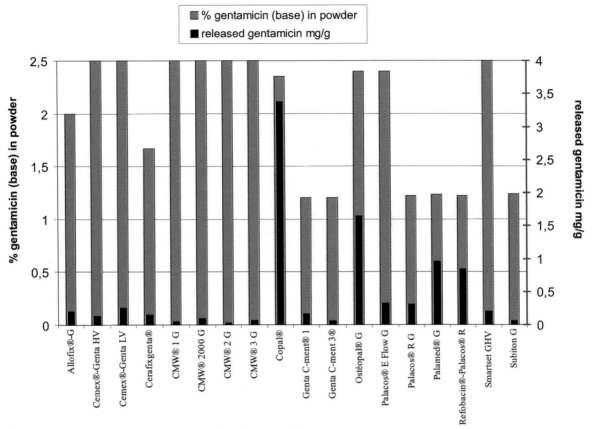

□ Fig. 3.42. Accumulated release of gentamicin within 7 days. (From [9])

[13]. In Copal® bone cement, 2 g antimicrobial agents (clindamycin 1 g and gentamicin 1 g) are incorporated.

If antimicrobial agents are added to bone cement during surgical revision, only antibiotic powder can be used. Antibiotics diluted in water will ruin the mechanical properties of the PMMA and the procedure of elution will be unpredictable.

The choice of antibiotic follows the susceptibility pattern of the individual pathogen and is restricted to agents that are known for their elution properties. The antibiotics must not interfere chemically with the bone cement or other ingredients like accelerators. Such interference leads, for example, to an extremely prolonged setting time if rifampicin is used. Examples for appropriate agents are listed in □ Table 3.18.

Clinical Impact and Possible Use of Antibiotic Loaded Bone Cement (ALAC)

ALAC is used for both prophylaxis and therapy. The requirements for these two purposes are different.

Prophylactic use is determined by the pathogens expected at the site of the prosthesis. These antimicrobial agents must be effective against possible pathogens known from epidemiological data and must be as harmless as possible with respect to adverse drug effects. Gentamicin turned out to be a suitable agent for prophylactic use in ALAC. There is a long tradition in using gentamicin-loaded bone cement for this purpose. Retrospective studies suggest that the combination of systemic prophylaxis with antibiotics and local use of ALAC for fixation of artificial joint replacement has a favourable effect in the prevention of periprosthetic infection [1]. When used for prophylactic purposes only, commercial available standardised preparations should be used in order to minimise the potential risk for patients.

In the prophylactic use of ALAC the surface of the bone cement acts as a substitute for the surface of the prosthesis and the interface between the medical device and the bone is now between the ALAC and the bone tissue. The aim is to prevent bacteria from colonising the surface of the artificial joint replacement [5].

For the therapy of periprosthetic infection the pathogen must be identified prior to revision surgery so that appropriate antibiotics can be selected in advance according to the susceptibility pattern of the individual bacterial strain for application in ALAC. For this purpose it is often necessary to add antimicrobial agents in the operating room because there are very few commercially available

3

antibiotic loaded bone cements which contain the specific antibiotics needed for antimicrobial therapy. In order to obtain safe elution, the characteristics and standardised mechanical properties of industrial preparations should be used whenever possible.

The aim of topical application is to obtain a high-level concentration at the site of infection that cannot be obtained by the intravenous route without adverse toxic drug effects. If ALAC is used for fixation of a prosthesis, another effect is the protection of the surface from colonisation by residual bacteria.

However, if hand-mixing is necessary, the rules of pharmaceutical mixing of powders have to be followed as accurately as possible in the operating theatre (see ◘ Table 3.17). Before mixing, the antibiotics should be ground to a small particle size. Clumps of antibiotics

◘ Table 3.17. Rules for incorporating antimicrobial agents in gentamicin bone cement during surgical procedure

Equipment	Procedure	
Appropriate container (sterile) Spatula (sterile)	Step 1	The whole amount of sterile antibiotic powder is transferred into the container under aseptic conditions
	Step 2	The same amount of PMMA powder is added to the antibiotic powder
	Step 3	Both quantities are mixed well
	Step 4	The same proportion of PMMA powder as it is now in the container is added
	Step 5	Both quantities are mixed well
	Step 6	Steps 4 and 5 are repeated until no PMMA powder is left
	Step 7	MMA Monomer liquid is added and the procedure is continued in compliance with the manufacture's instructions

◘ Table 3.18. Options of appropriate antimicrobial agents for preparation of ALAC in the operating theatre after assessment of susceptibility in the individual (choice)

Antimicrobial Agent	Pathogen	Note
Amikacin	*Pseudomonas aeruginosa*	e.g. in combination with cefoperazon
Ampicillin	*enterococci streptococci anaerobes*	
Cefuroxim	*staphylococci* (MSSA, CNS – methicillin susceptible) *streptococci*	
Cefotaxim	*Enterobacteriaceae*	Combination with gentamicin necessary
Cefoperazon	*Pseudomonas aeruginosa*	Combination with Amikacin or Gentamicin or tobramycin
Clindamycin	*staphylococci streptococci propionibacteria anaerobes*	Commercially available (Combination with gentamicin)
Gentamicin	diverse	Preferred for prophylaxis and combination Several brands available
Ofloxacin	*Enterobacteriaceae Pseudomonas aeruginosa*	
Vancomycin	*staphylococci* (MRSA, CNS – methicillin resistant) – *Corynebacterium amycolatum*	– Poor elution properties – Poor bacteriostatic character – Use only in combination, if possible
General rules	Pathogens must be tested for susceptibility Combination with gentamicin is of benefit for elution of some other antibiotics	

MSSA methicillin-susceptible *Staphylococcus aureus*; *CNS* coagulase-negative *Staphylococci*; *MRSA* methicillin-resistant *Staphylococcus aureus*

present in the bone cement harbour the risk of causing micro fractures in the cured bone cement if exposed to weight-bearing.

ALAC is used as a drug-delivery system with the intention of obtaining high-level concentration of antibiotics in the adjacent tissue. This option applies to beads and to spacers used in revision arthroplasty performed in two or more stages. Another option is the use for fixation of artificial joint replacements: Under these conditions not only the delivery of antibiotics is of importance but protection of the permanently implanted device by preventing the surface from being colonised by bacteria [7].

Conclusions

PMMA bone cement is able to harbour antimicrobial agents, which are eluted from the matrix of PMMA chains if in contact with water. Therefore, PMMA may serve as a drug delivery system for antimicrobial agents.

ALAC may be used for two different purposes: In order to obtain high-level concentrations at the site of infection spacers or beads are used. These carriers are removed after a short period of time when antimicrobial agents are no longer eluted in sufficient concentrations. Mechanical properties are not of high relevance in this option. Another purpose is the use of ALAC for fixation of artificial joint replacements. In these cases ALAC serves as a substitute for the surface of the prosthesis which is impregnated with antibiotics dedicated to preventing bacteria from colonising this surface. This applies to prophylactic use and to treatment of periprosthetic infection by one-stage revision. Mechanical properties are of great importance here because the bone cement is used for fixation of artificial joint replacement and thus permanently implanted and subject to weight-bearing.

When antibiotics are used prophylactically, the mechanical properties of bone cement must be preserved to an adequate degree and must be standardised and fulfil the requirements of the standard ISO 5833. Therefore, only industrial preparations are appropriate for this purpose.

The application of antimicrobial agents to PMMA bone cement in the operating theatre is often necessary in septic revision of artificial joint replacements because no commercial preparations are available. The choice of antibiotics has to correspond with the susceptibility pattern of the individual pathogen causing the periprosthetic infection. In this situation, control of the infection and eradication of the pathogen has priority but the mechanical properties still have to be good and have to be respected as far as possible. If commercial preparations are available, like clindamycin gentamicin PMMA bone cement, these should be used.

Topical application of antimicrobial agents is restricted to a few infections where systemically administered antibiotics fail to obtain sufficient concentrations at the site of infection. Infection of bone tissue with or without foreign material is one of the conditions where local antibiotics are appropriate, but this therapy has to be accompanied by surgical debridement and systemic antibiotic therapy.

Take Home Messages

- Bone cement is frequently used as drug-delivery system in bone infection and in order to prevent artificial joint replacement from becoming infected.
- A variety of antimicrobial agents can be eluted from the PMMA matrix if in high-level concentration and thus act at the site of application on sessile bacteria or to prevent them from becoming sessile in case of prophylactic use.
- Elution of antimicrobial agent depends on the sort of bone cement, the properties of the antibiotics and the way of preparing ALAC. Homogeneity of the mixture and particle seize of antibiotic powder admixed determine the elution properties and the mechanical alteration of the bone cement as well. Standardisation applies only to industrial preparations but not to admixing antibiotics in the operation theatre.
- Admixing of antibiotics by hand should be restricted to conditions where no commercial preparation of ALAC is available and should be exclusively reserved for the therapy of bone tissue infection or/and device related infection but not for prophylactic use.

References

1. Adams K, Couch I, Cierny G, Calhoun J, Mader JT (1992) In vitro and in vivo evaluation of antibiotic diffusion from antibiotic-impregnated polymethacrylate beads. Clin Orthop 278:244–252
2. Buchholz HW, Elson RA, Lodenkämper H (1979) The infected joint implant. In: McKibbin B (ed) Recent advances in orthopaedics 3. Curchhill Livingston, New York, pp 139–161
3. Buchholz HW, Engelbrecht H (1970) Über die Depotwirkung einiger Antibiotika bei Vermischung mit dem Kunstharz Palacos. Chirurg 41:511–515
4. Costerton JW, Stewart PS, Greenberg EP (1999) Bacterial biofilm: A common cause of persistent infections. Science 284:1918–1322
5. Espehaug B, Engesæter LB, Vollset SE, Havelin LI, Langeland N (1997) Antibiotic prophylaxis in total hip arthroplasty. Review of 10,905 primary cemented total hip replacements reported to the Norwegian Arthroplasty Register, 1987–1995. J Bone Joint Surg (Br) 79B:590–595
6. Frommelt L (2000) Periprosthetic infection – bacteria and the interface between prosthesis and bone. In: Learmonth ID (ed) Interfaces in total hip arthroplasties. Springer, London. pp 153–161
7. Frommelt L (2004) Prinzipien der Antibiotikabehandlung bei periprothetischen Infektionen. Orthopäde 33:822–826
8. Kühn KD (2000) Bone cements. Springer, Berlin Heidelberg New York Tokyo, pp 253–262

9. Kühn KD, Ege W, Gopp U (2005) Acrylic bone cements: composition and properties. Orthop Clin N Am 36:17–28

10. Lindner B (1981) Physikalische Analyse des Freisetzungsmechanismus von Chemotherapeutika aus dotiertem Polymethylmethacrylat. Inauguaraldissertation, Kiel

11. Low HAT, Fleming RH, Gilmore MFX, McCarthy ID, Hughes SPF (1986) In vitro measurement and computer modelling of the diffusion of antibiotic in bone cement. J Biomed Eng 8:149–155

12. Mader JT, Adams KR (1988) Experimental Osteomyelitis. In: Schlossberg D (ed) Orthopedic Infection. Springer, New York, pp 39–48

13. Pfefferle HJ, Nies B (2004) Charakterisierung arzneimittelhaltiger Biomaterialien als kundenspezifische Sonderanfertigung. Orthopäde 33:817–821

14. van de Belt H, Neut D, Schenk W, van Horn JR, van der Mei HC, Busscher HJ (2001) Infection of orthopedic implants and the use of antibiotic-loaded bone cements: A review. Acta Orthop Scand 72:557–571

15. van Sorge NM, Yska JP, Blansjaar H, Driessen S, Schepers P, Bovenga SR, van Sorge AA (2000) Gentamicin containing surgical bone cement: in vitro characteristics of Palacos® and Palamed®. 6th Internet World Congress for Biomedical Sciences (INABIS), Poster 67

16. Wahlig H, Hameister W, Grieben A (1972) Über die Freisetzung von Gentamicin aus Polymethymethacrylat. Langenbecks Arch Chir 331:169–212

17. Zimmerli W, Lew PD, Waldvogel FA (1984) Pathogenesis of foreign body infection – evidence for a local granulocyte defect. J Clin Invest 73:1191–1200

Properties of Bone Cement: The Three Interfaces

Klaus Draenert, Yvette Draenert

Summary

In this chapter an overview of the experimentally applied research on the three interface characteristics of bone cement is given. With regard to the polymer-monomer interface, in addition to prechilling and vacuum mixing, pre-pressurisation of cement after mixing has been shown to enhance the homogeneity and the composite strength of bone cement. The influence of vacuum on shrinkage is discussed and underlined by experimental findings. The processing of bone cement under vacuum is considered as a milestone not so much for the strengthening of the material but for the revascularisation process and the bond of bone cement to the metal to ensure equal load transmission. The systematic histomorphological work on animal experiments and human retrieval analysis is presented and the important principle of a viable bone-to-cement interface is outlined.

Introduction

All bone cements used for joint replacements are poly-methylmethacrylates (PMMA) [21]. The powder component consists of linear linked polymer chains in form of beads. The powder is added to the liquid monomer and then mixed. The secondarily polymerising monomer, which consists of methylmethacrylate, is embedding the beads of the powder component. Little is known about this polymer-monomer interface, but it is important to understand the fundamental characteristics of this PMMA composite, which is not only influenced by the homogeneity of the mixture [13], but also by the process of mixing and the so-called pre-pressurising of the mixed bone cement [9].

Inevitably, during polymerisation shrinkage of the cement will occur. The process of cement shrinkage is complex and the effect (of shrinkage) on the bone-to-cement interface is of considerable importance [9].

The bone-to-cement interface has always been considered as the most important tissue reaction with respect to long-term results. For a long time, the »fibro-cartilage« has been considered as the normal tissue found at the cement-to-bone interface [3, 31, 35]. But Draenert et al. [7, 8, 10–13] introduced new laboratory processing techniques, which preserved the PMMA, bone and soft tissue. Histologically, they documented direct contacts between bone and PMMA without fibrous tissue interposition at the interface, even under load in animal experiments and in post-mortem human retrieval specimens.

In this chapter, the effect of cement preparation upon the polymer-monomer interface is discussed, a controversial view is given on the metal-to-bone cement interface and, furthermore, the importance of cement shrinkage for the revascularisation process and the viability and integrity of the cement-to-bone interface are outlined.

The Polymer-Monomer Interface

The Embedding of the Polymer Beads

Little is known about the embedding characteristics of the polymer beads within the monomer matrix. Investigations using Scanning Electron Microscopy (SEM) by Draenert [9] showed that the embedding process is a very sensitive reaction depending on the chemistry and environmental conditions during mixing (◘ Figs. 3.43 and 3.44). These findings have been compared with samples

3

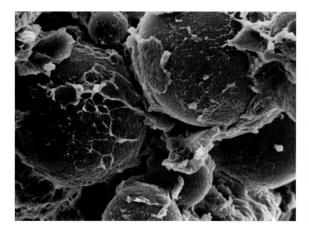

Fig. 3.43. The chemical reaction of the polymerisation process has been stopped in intervals of 60 s using liquid nitrogen followed by a freeze-drying process. After 60 s the polymer spheres are partly covered by the monomer; their surface remains nearly unchanged. SEM

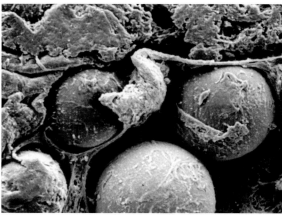

Fig. 3.45. Loosened polymer beads of a cement sample retrieved during revision seven years after primary total hip arthroplasty. The beads present a rather smooth surface; fibrous tissue has been grown in between the polymer beads and the degradation of the monomer matrix is clearly visible. SEM

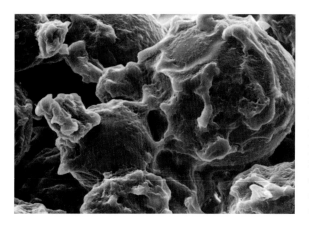

Fig. 3.44. Polymerisation process after 2 min the secondarily polymerising monomer has thickened the coat of the beads; void inclusion are clearly visible The bond of the coat reveals some small gaps clearly indicating that an interface polymer-monomer still exists. SEM

of bone cement retrieved at revision surgery [13], which clearly proved that an interface between polymer beads and secondarily polymerising monomer exists.

As an important phenomenon it became apparent from the retrieval specimen analysis, that the embedding process was often incomplete and the polymer beads were freed and loosened from the surrounding monomer matrix (Fig. 3.45). The chemical etching process revealed a high variance of surface characteristics of the polymer beads and embedding defects. However, such voids, defects and inclusions within the cement composite can reduce the local fracture toughness and fatigue failure resistance [32]. Furthermore, these may be the starting point for cement cracks and further crack propagation within the cement mantle.

Keller and Lautenschlager [20] were the first to try strengthening the bone cement by applying temporary pressure during the polymerisation process. They achieved a significant increase in strength of the material; the pressure, however, could not be applied during the complete polymerisation process. Draenert [13] achieved a significant increase of the polymer embedment and a significantly stronger cement mass with pre-pressurisation of the mixed cement during the first two minutes after mixing. By combining pre-pressurisation and prior vacuum mixing artifact-free samples with complete embedding of the spheres could be achieved (Fig. 3.46).

Vacuum mixing (► chapter 4) was first investigated by Demarest and Lautenschlager [6] and later introduced into clinical praxis by Lidgren et al. [23]. Systematically applied research was then performed by Draenert et al. [13] showing that standard viscosity bone cements have to be chilled before vacuum mixing thus avoiding boiling of the monomer under high vacuum (Fig. 3.47). It is important to differentiate between air bubbles and voids generated by monomer evaporation [27]. Differences in porosity will occur depending on the method of mixing [25].

Homogeneity of the Mixture

The homogeneous and firm embedment of polymer spheres and fillers requires an equal and homogeneous distribution of the polymer in the monomer liquid during mixing. Surprisingly, relatively few studies have been performed in this area. It is important to realise that the polymerisation process starts immediately after the powder has been added to the liquid. Hence, the following considerations for the mixing process should be

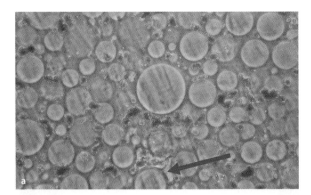 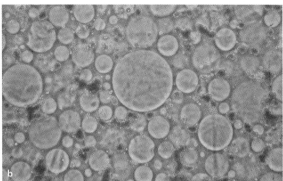

Fig. 3.46. a Cross section of a bone cement sample in the phase contrast: The mixture was exposed two minutes to a pressure acting on it of 3,5 Bar. The included air bubble, visible as a *light blue line*, is deformed (*arrow*). All beads reveal a dense ring around their circumfe- rence thus presenting a firm contact to the secondarily polymerising monomer. Light microscope (*LM*). **b** Vacuum-mixed and pre-pressuri- sed bone cement sample in the phase contrast. The sample is free of pores and reveals closed interfaces of polymer and monomer. LM

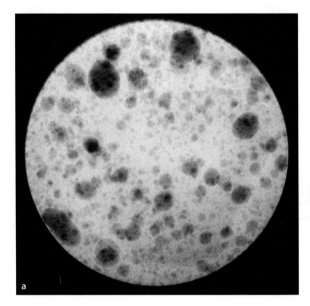 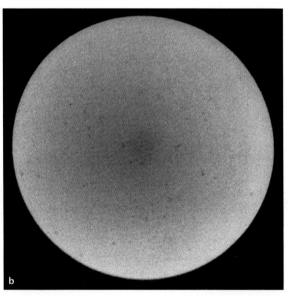

Fig. 3.47. a Radiographic appearance of bone cement sample mixed under vacuum at room temperature. The sample retrieved from the mixing bowl resembles a foamed material due to evaporated monomer. **b** Radiograph of vacuum- mixed sample of pre-chilled bone cement. The mixture is homogeneous and free of pores

made: A turbulent and fast-mixing phase is necessary to ensure rapid distribution of the polymer beads within of the stirring process with reduced frequency is essential to achieve homogeneity and to reduce air inclusions. Draenert et al. [13] showed in their studies of a specific vacuum mixing system (■ Fig. 3.48), that with a diameter of the mixing bowl below 55 mm a homogeneous mixture could not be achieved for 80 g of PMMA bone cement. The homogeneity can be measured precisely using thermal electrodes [13], but more obvious the radiographic evaluation (■ Fig. 3.49) of the samples revealed milky ways (powder with X-ray contrast particles) and dark radiolucent areas (monomer lakes). A prerequisite for all homogeneous mixtures in their studies was the Teflon-coated rod instead of a spatula.

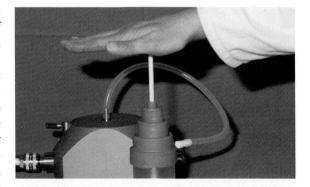

Fig. 3.48. Vacuum-mixing system investigated with ideal-diameter mixing bowl. The Teflon-coated rod does not adhere to PMMA bone cement thus avoiding inhomogeneity of the mixture and air inclusions leading to macroporosity during mixing

3

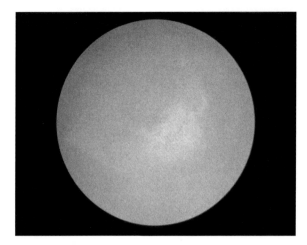

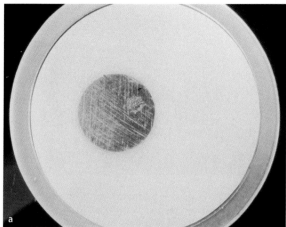

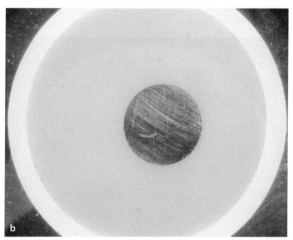

☐ **Fig. 3.49.** Radiographic phenomenon of »milky ways«, correlating to unmixed polymer powder

☐ **Fig. 3.50. a** Vacuum-mixed bone cement shows the shrinkage of the cement mass away from the »cortex«. **b** Conventionally mixed bone cement without shrinkage

Vacuum Mixing and its Influence on Cement Shrinkage

Volumetric changes during setting of the cement had been already observed by Charnley [3], who has studied also basic work in chemistry, where the shrinkage of the monomer was defined with 23%. Charnley [3] had focused mainly on the expansion process during polymerisation, whereas Oest et al. [27] differentiated the complicated process of expansion and shrinkage and determined a shrinkage of about 2% 30 min after the curing process and a calculated value of about 8–10% overall shrinkage as time goes on. Keller and Lautenschlager [20] and Demarest et al. [6] were the first to approach this early phase of polymerisation experimentally using vacuum during mixing and pressurisation during the hardening phase, respectively. They showed a significant increase in strength of the material, but did not consider, however, any change in cement volume. The bead-embedding process is mainly influenced chemically based on the chemical relationship between monomer and polymer, but depends also on environmental conditions such us temperature and vaporisation pressure and air inclusion and water uptake [9].

The influence of cement shrinkage upon the interface characteristics have never been discussed or investigated. Draenert et al. [13] have shown that any shrinkage of the final cement mass can be attributed to the liquid monomer component, thus forming the typical pearl-like appearance of the free cement surface. In contrast, the cement surface adjacent to the metal stem clearly reveals the flat replica of the stem thus indicating compression generated by hoop stresses from shrinking. This phenomenon might explain the pores near the metal interface representing rather evaporated monomer more than a

phenomenon attributable to shrinkage of the cement mass away from the metal due to the fact, that the polymerisation starts earlier at the bony interface. Bone cement of a cement sheath shrinks onto the metal stem and away form a cylindrical bone tube [7, 9, 27]. This can be nicely demonstrated in a simple model (☐ Fig. 3.50).

Bishop et al. [1] achieved a more equally distributed polymerisation process in an experiment with cadaver specimens by pre-heating the stem to 44 °C. The authors found chains of bubbles along the metal-to-bone cement interface and succeeded with their elimination by the described preheating of the stem. In spite of the fact that the cause of bubbles along the metal-to-bone cement interface might be different than that of a simple shrinkage phenomenon of the cement mass, it influences the strength of the bond of bone cement to the metal. The morphology of the bubbles resembles monomer bubbles due to evaporation of monomer in the polymerising cement mass reaching the metal interface at last, thus allowing monomer to evaporate.

Combining vacuum mixing with pre-pressurisation can produce a cement mixture free of pores (see ■ Fig. 3.46b) and the associated cement shrinkage can already be visualised on at least two of the three interfaces. The interface polymer-monomer (interface 1) is documented under phase contrast, the interface metal-to-bone cement (interface 2) and also the interface 3 (cement-to-bone) revealed the difference visible by the naked eye. In the SEM the pearl-like appearance was more pronounced, the surface towards the metal is absolutely flat and the gap between syringe (bone) and the cement mass much more marked. Especially the latter phenomenon contributes enormously to the revascularisation process and thus to the survival of living bone tissue embedded in bone cement.

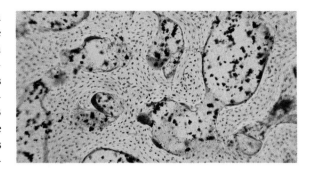

■ **Fig. 3.51.** Cancellous bone of the distal femoral metaphysis of a rabbit embedded in bone cement one year after vacuum applied bone cement filling of the distal metaphysis. The osteocytes represent living bone; the crescent-like red marrow spaces present the secondary medullar cavity. LM: fuchsine staining

The Important Role of Shrinkage

When vacuum-mixed bone cement, which is associated with higher rates of shrinkage than the more porous hand mixed cement, was implanted in animal experiments [8, 13], necrotic bone trabeculae were never found (■ Fig. 3.51), as it had been described by other authors [2, 16, 19, 30].

The process of shrinkage of the cement mass embedding cancellous bone is a rather complicated process and best understood by appreciating that cement shrinks onto a trabeculae and at the same time away from a circumference of 270° of the walls of the cancellous bone honeycombs thus providing space for revascularisation (■ Fig. 3.52). The fast revascularisation can be shown in animal experiments using the polychromatic sequential labelling and the replica technique for presenting the vasculature in the SEM (■ Fig. 3.53).

These histological findings in the animal experiment up to one year after the operation clearly highlight the importance of early revascularisation of trabecular bone stiffened with vacuum-mixed bone cement. In comparison to this very important phenomenon, which has not been described by other authors, the strengthening of the material (cement) by these pore reducing techniques seems to be of minor importance.

For the symbiosis between living bone and bone cement it is of utmost importance that space is given for an early revascularisation. That space given three-dimensionally by the shrinkage of the cement mass is much more pronounced in vacuum-mixed bone cement than under conventional conditions (see ■ Fig. 3.50a,b).

In conclusion, cement shrinkage has been identified to have a significant influence on all three interfaces described and thus also on the load transfer from metal to bone cement [13], but even more importantly on the revascularisation process which takes place in the bone-to-cement interface.

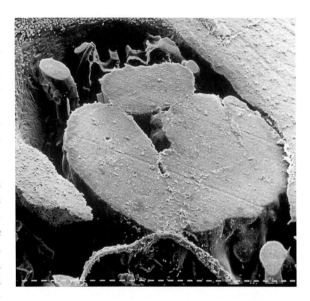

■ **Fig. 3.52.** Marrow space in a monkey's femoral head filled with bone cement: the bone cement (*middle*) has shrunken to the bony trabeculae and at the same time a gap (*top*) has been formed due to its shrinkage around 270° of the honeycombs circumference. In this gap, the pattern of the intact micro-vasculature is revealed by micro cast technique in the SEM

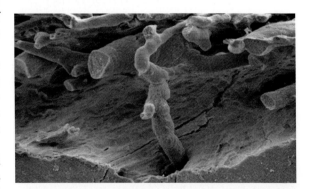

■ **Fig. 3.53.** View upon the gap generated by shrinkage of the bone cement in a cross section of a rabbit femur 8 days after filling the medullar cavity of the femur with cement. Two layers of a newly formed capillary system are revealed. SEM: micro cast

The Metal-to-Bone Cement Interface

The interface metal-to-bone cement was controversially discussed and decisions with respect to stem design and surface finish were made in most cases empirically. In this way, Charnley [4] made the experience that his highly-polished stems had better clinical results than the sandblasted surfaces. Raab et al. [28, 29] tried to strengthen the interface metal-to-bone cement with PMMA pre-coating techniques [17]. Niederer et al. [26] already reported 1978 experimental results on sandblasted and structured stem surfaces to achieve stable load transmission metal-to-bone cement and bone cement-to-bone. Their experiments took the hoop stresses generated by shrinkage of bone cement first mentioned by the group of Stachiewicz et al. [33] into consideration.

The Exeter group of scientists has performed impressive experiments to show the time-dependent cold flow characteristics of cement and how to use it in clinical practice [15, 22]. The authors have demonstrated that bone cement under constant load creeps as time goes on into surface profiles of metallic cones which they have used for their experiments (▶ chapter 3.2). Cold flow characteristics of bone cements [22] allow subsidence of a highly-polished stem within the cement sheath. Verdonschot and Huiskes [34] simulated subsidence using finite element analysis and concluded that subsidence as a result of cement creep is considered rather low. Since human bone and especially cancellous bone adjacent to the cement sheath is deformable, the subsidence of a high-polished stem might be conflicting for the cement mantle. The high-pressurizing technique which has been applied at the same time by the Exeter group [15] counteracts that deformation of bone structures due to the stiffening of the marrow spaces by bone cement. In a human cadaver specimen, the patho-histology of a highly-polished Exeter stem, borne 14 years without complaints reveals fracture-lines in the proximal cement sheath adjacent to the corners of the implant, as well as corrosion of the metal surface (◻ Fig. 3.54).

In the fatigue test considering 50 Hz and an increasing load up to 5-times body weight (0,5–3,5 kN) acting on an high-polished Exeter femoral prosthesis embedded in a 75% cement mantle and held in an environment of 37 °C warm Ringer solution, it could be shown that the cement mantle revealed fracture lines and it could already be detected corrosion of the metal surface, after 3,5 million cycles (◻ Fig. 3.55a); compared to that a smooth undulated surface structured stem embedded in a vacuum mixed cement mantle presented an intact interface even after 55 million cycles (◻ Fig. 3.55b).

The improved load transfer of structured stem surfaces had already been demonstrated by Niederer et al. [26]. There are, however, two different aspects which have to be considered discussing the metal-to-cement interface: 1) the load-transfer conditions and 2) the surface abrasive properties in a loose metal-to-cement interface. It is no question that a high-polished surface is less abrasive than a sandblasted or sandblasted and structured surface, considering load transfer the contrary is valid (▶ chapters 7.1, 7.2). The topic of ideal stem surface remains controversial [17, 24].

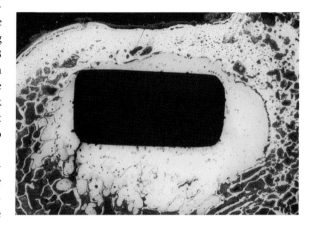

◻ **Fig. 3.54.** Highly-polished Exeter stem in a cross section of a cadaver specimen 14 years after implantation: The cement sheath has been fractured and corrosion of the steel is visible. LM: fuchsine staining

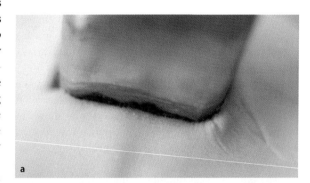

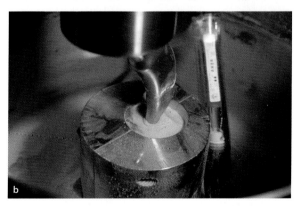

◻ **Fig. 3.55. a** Highly-polished Exeter stem in a fatigue testing machine in Ringer's solution at body temperature. After 3 million cycles corrosion and microfractures of the sheath are visible. The bone cement had been vacuum mixed and pre-pressurised; 50 Hz, 3.5 kN. **b** Undulated stem surface in a vacuum-mixed and pre-pressurised cement mantle in Ringer's solution at body temperature revealing an intact interface after 55 million cycles; 50 Hz, 3.5 kN

The Bone-to-Cement Interface

The first fibrous tissue-free bone-to-cement contacts have been described 1953 by Henrichsen et al. [18], who have investigated bone cements of the »powder and fluid type« experimentally. However, their histological description remained an indirect similar to all other subsequent histological reports [5, 14, 35]: the adjacent tissue was presented in absence of the plastic which has been removed by the processing technique. Introducing new histological technologies Draenert et al. were first to present a bone-to cement interface without fibrous tissue interposition [10]. Since then histopathology has evolved and bone in direct contact to the cement surface has been studied more systematically. Furthermore, in detailed animal experiments and human retrieval and cadaver specimens, the revascularisation process at the bone-to-cement interface and the adjacent cortex, as well as the strain-adaptive bone remodeling phenomena [4, 7, 8, 12] have been evaluated [11, 13].

There are basically two biomechanical phenomena which define the bone response to the cement implant:

1) the smooth surface of all PMMA bone cements and 2) the penetration of the cement mass into the bony honeycombs thus stiffening the scaffolding of cancellous bone and converting cancellous bone to a stiffer compound material which represents a living symbiosis between bone and its PMMA »inlay« (see ◘ Fig. 3.51).

In an animal experiment, primary bone healing along the interface could be found after a press-fit PMMA cylinder implant had been inserted in a standardised cylindrical bone defect, which had been created with a diamond (◘ Fig. 3.56). Morphologically, stable bone support contacts at the cement surface are always formed like an elephant's foot (◘ Fig. 3.57). Relative movements at the interface induce loss of mineral followed by osteoclastic reabsorption and replacement by tangentially oriented fibrous tissue (◘ Fig. 3.58). Accordingly, Charnley's »fibro-cartilage« [3] can be considered to represent demineralised osteoid substance. These contacts, however, are considered to present an unstable steady state under nearly unloaded conditions. Under normal load, as it is given for a cemented femoral stem, bony elephant feet have been found only

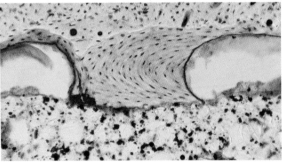

◘ **Fig. 3.57.** Stable elephant-foot contact of cortical bone-to-bone cement in a cross section of a rabbit. The interface resembles an unstable steady state of bony support indicating slight reabsorption where micro-movements occur. LM: fuchsine staining. 1 year after implantation

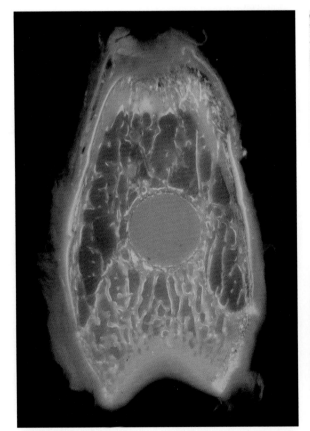

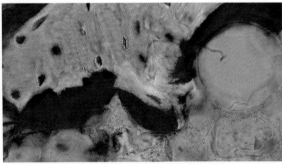

◘ **Fig. 3.56.** Cross section through a compact PMMA cylinder press-fit implanted in the patellar groove of a rabbit: The polychromatic sequential labelling during the first four weeks (first seven days: Oxy tetracycline = *yellow*; second week: Alizarin Complexon = *red*; third week: Calcein blue = *blue* and last week: Calcein green: *green*. Incident fluorescent light: 6 weeks after the operation

◘ **Fig. 3.58.** Bone-to-cement contact in a rabbit's femoral cross section revealing a distinct fibrous tissue free bone contact on PMMA surface (*middle*). On the right a fine layer of fibrous tissue has formed and on the left demineralised bone matrix is visible: LM: stained with basic fuchsine: *red*. 2.5 years after implantation

if the cancellous bone structure has been preserved and has been stiffened with bone cement (Fig. 3.59) [11].

It has been shown, however, that the smooth surface of bone cements does not allow the same bone bonding as known from ceramics, where bone contacts were formed regularly like an elephant's foot [7, 8] indicating interface stability.

The histological appearance changes completely when ceramic particles are rigidly fixed in or at the cement surface [8]. It makes no difference whether an Al_2O_3 particle is fixed in the cement mass with direct contact to the adjacent bone (Fig. 3.60) or the interface is bonded by ceramic particles thus providing stability and the newly formed bone resembles a replica of the pearl-like surface of the cement (Fig. 3.61) or tricalciumphosphate (TCP) or hydroxyapatite (HA) are embedded in the cement surface. In all cases, a tangential bonding of the newly formed bone is found adjacent to the ceramic; tricalciumphosphate is

reabsorbed and followed by bony in-growth (Fig. 3.62); if the cement surface is densely covered by TCP and HA particles the complete surface of bone cement is coated with tangentially oriented mineralising collagen fibres (Fig. 3.63). A combination of PMMA with tricalciumphosphate and hydroxyapatite seems to offer potential benefits over classic PMMA with a smooth surface, but clinical trials will be necessary for further evaluation.

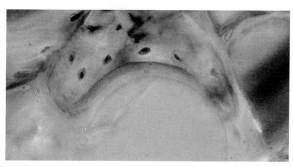

Fig. 3.61. Bone-to-cement contact revealing a replica of the surface without fibrous tissue in a ceramic containing bone cement: Cross section through a rabbit's femur; LM: fuchsine staining. 6 months after implantation

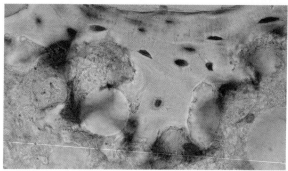

Fig. 3.62. Newly formed bone following the paths of Tricalcium phosphate into the cement mass. Cross section through a rabbit's femur. LM: fuchsine staining. Two years after implantation

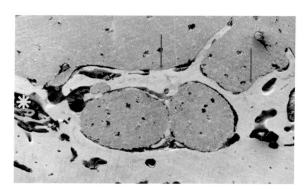

Fig. 3.59. Cross section at the midshaft level through a human femur with a cemented Müller-Banana stem (9y). The cortico-cancellous structures remained preserved and were stiffened with bone cement; elephant-foot contacts (*arrows*) are visible indicating a very stable situation at the interface. New bone formation (*asterisk*) is seen in marrow spaces not filled with cement. Note the typical pattern of direct bone contacts onto cement with adjacent gaps, which are essential for the microcapillary system shown in Fig. 3.52. SEM

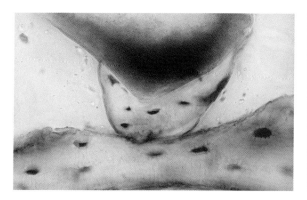

Fig. 3.60. Newly formed bone bonding directly on a ceramic particle adjacent to the bone-to-cement interface. Cross section through a rabbit's femur filled with bone cement containing Al_2O_3 ceramic particles. LM: fuchsine staining. 6 months after implantation

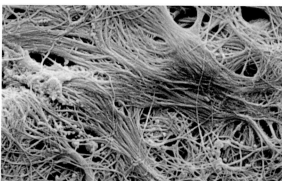

Fig. 3.63. Newly formed tangential fibre layer revealing the growing mineral crystals along the fibres directly on the cement surface. Cross section of a rabbit's femur filled with a ceramic containing bone cement 9 months after the operation. SEM freeze dried specimen

Modes of Cemented Fixation

A comprehensive analysis of cemented fixation of retrieved human femora using high intensity incident fluorescent light microscopy (HIIFL) [7] has revealed important and different histological features [11, 13] with consistent findings depending on the quality of cementing technique and mode of anchorage. Although in the specimens analysed no case with perfect cementing technique could be documented, it became apparent, what characterises a well-cemented stem, which had maintained firm bony anchorage over a long time. This was the case when three features were present (see ▫ Fig. 3.59 and ▫ Fig. 3.64): a complete cement sheath, preserved cancellous bone and interdigitated bone cement within the cancellous frame work [11]. In contrast, in areas where cancellous bone had been removed by the rasp and hence no cement could interlock, fibrous tissue had filled the gaps.

In the concept of self-locking cemented stems, where cement is regarded as a filler and a press-fit fixation with direct metal to bone contact is attempted, inevitably areas of thin and deficient cement mantles result. This so-called cemented press-fit anchorage type [11, 13], however, may lead to destruction of the cement mantle due to micro-motion and subsequent cement degradation (▫ Fig. 3.65) inducing granuloma formation and osteolysis. This mode of anchorage has to be questioned.

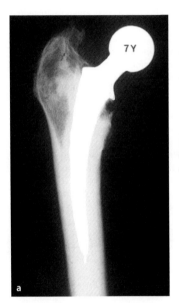

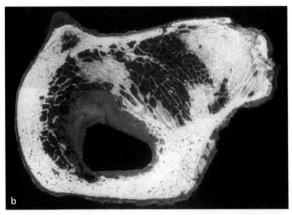

▫ **Fig. 3.64a,b.** Histological analysis of a well fixed femoral stem after 7 years with no radiological signs of loosening (**a**). The cross-section (**b**) at the level of the lesser trochanter shows an intact cement-to-bone interface with an intact cement sheath and fibrous tissue free cement interlocking in preserved cancellous bone. HIIFL microscopy

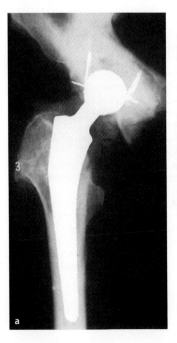

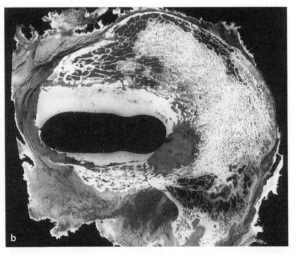

▫ **Fig. 3.65a,b.** Analysis of cemented-press-fit stem 8 years following implantation. Although radiographically (**a**) no obvious osteolyis is detectable, the histological analysis (**b**) of a cross-section reveals cement cracks and destruction of the cement sheath with granuloma formation. HIIFL microscopy

3

Take Home Messages

- Careful mixing of linearly linked PMMA bone cements including mixing high vacuum and pre-chilling has an important impact in homogeneity, porosity reduction and shrinkage.
- Pre-pressurising of cement increases cement homogeneity and improves the monomer-polymer interface.
- Cement shrinkage, often regarded as a disadvantage, has been shown to be of utmost importance for revascularisation of the adjacent bone and load transfer.
- Once revascularised, the adjacent bone has limited possibilities to grow on plastic surfaces.
- »Cemented press-fit« anchorage leads to thin cement mantles and can result in granuloma formation and loosening at the bone-to cement interface.
- Stiffening of preserved trabecular bone with cement is the key for long-term fixation and success with maintaining a viable bone-to-cement interface.

References

1. Bishop NE, Ferguson S, Tepic S. Porosity reduction in bone cement at the cement-stem interface. J Bone Joint Surg 1996; 78B:349–356
2. Bloebaum RD, Gruen TA, Sarmiento A. Interface and bone response to increased penetration of bone cement. Trans Biomaterials 1984; 84:82
3. Charnley J. Acrylic cement in orthopaedic surgery. Livingstone, Edinburgh London; 1970
4. Charnley J. Low friction arthroplasty of the hip: theory and practice. Springer, Berlin Heidelberg New York, 1979
5. Charnley J, Crawford WJ. Histology of bone in contact with self-curing acrylic cement. J Bone Joint Surg 1988; 50B:228
6. Demarest VA, Lautenschlager EP, Wixon RL. Vacuum mixing of acrylic bone cement. Presented at the 9th Annual Meeting of the Society for Biomaterials, Birmingham, Alabama, 1993, p 37
7. Draenert K. Histomorphology of the bone-to-cement interface: remodeling of the cortex and revascularization of the medullary canal in animal experiments. The John Charnley Award Paper. In: The Hip. Proceedings of the ninth open scientific meeting of the Hip Society. Mosby, St Louis Toronto London, 1981, pp 70–110
8. Draenert K. Histomorphological observations on experiments to improve the bone-to-cement contact. Nicholas Andry Award Paper. Paper presented at the thirty-eight annual meeting of the Association of Bone and Joint Surgeons held in Vancouver, 1986; March 27–31. Philadelphia: Lippincott
9. Draenert K. Zur Technik der Zementverankerung. Forschung und Fortbildung in der Chirurgie des Bewegungsapparates 1. Art and Science, München, 1983
10. Draenert KD, Rudigier J, Willenegger H. Tierexperimentelle Studie zur Histomorphologie des Knochen-Zement-Kontaktes. Helv Chir Acta 1976; 43:769–773
11. Draenert KD, Draenert YI, Krauspe R, Bettin D. Strain adaptive bone remodelling in total joint replacement. Clin Orthop 2005; 430:12–27
12. Draenert KD, Rudigier J. Histomorphologie des Knochen-Zement-Kontaktes. Eine tierexperimentelle Phänomenologie der knöchernen Umbauvorgänge. Chirurg 1978; 49:276–285
13. Draenert K, Draenert Y, Garde U, Ulrich C. Manual of cementing technique. Springer, Berlin Heidelberg New York Barcelona Hong Kong London Milano Paris Singapore Tokyo, 1999
14. Feith R. Side effects of Acrylic Cement Implants into Bone. 1975. Dissertation. Nijmegen: Drukkeri Brakkenstein
15. Fowler J, Gie GA, Lee AJC, Ling RSM. Experience with the Exeter hip since 1970. Orthop Clin North Am 1970; 19:477–489
16. Goodman SB, Schatzker J, Sumner-Smith G, Fornasier VL, Goften N, Hunt C. The effect of the polymethylmethacrylate on bone: an experimental study. Arch Orthop Trauma Surg 1985; 104:150–154
17. Harris WH. Is it advantageous to strengthen the cement-metal interface and use a collar for cemented femoral components of total hip replacements? Clin Orthop 1992; 285:67–72
18. Henrichsen E, Jansen K, Krough-Poulsen W. Experimental investigation of the tissue reaction to acrylic plastics. Acta Orthop Scand 1952; 22:141–146
19. Hoy ALS, Bloebaum RD, Clarke IC, Sarmiento A. The dynamic bone response to acrylic implantation. Presented at the 30th Annual ORS, Atlanta, Georgia, 1984; February 7–9
20. Keller JC, Lautenschlager EP. Experimental attempts to reduce acrylic cement porosity. Biomat Med Dev Art Org 1983; 11:221–236
21. Kühn K D. Bone Cements. Up-to-date comparison of physical and chemical properties of commercial materials. Springer, Berlin Heidelberg New York Barcelona Hong Kong London Milano Paris Singapore Tokyo, 2000
22. Lee AJC, Perkins RD, Ling RSM. Time-dependent properties of polymethylmethacrylate bone cement. In: Older J (ed) Implant bone interface. Springer, London Berlin Heidelberg New York Paris Tokyo Hong Kong, 1990, pp 85–90
23. Lidgren L, Drar H, Moller J. Strength of polymethylmethacrylate increased by vacuum mixing, Acta Orthop Scand 1984;55(5): 536–41
24. Ling RSM, Hon F. The use of a collar and precoating on cemented femoral stems is unnecessary and detrimental. Clin Orthop 1992; 285:73–83
25. Macaulay W, DiGiovanni CW, Restrepo A, Saleh KJ, Walsh H, Crossett LS, Peterson MG, Li S, Salvati EA. Differences in bone-cement porosity by vacuum mixing, centrifugation, and hand mixing. J Arthroplasty 2002; 17:569–575
26. Niederer PG, Chiquet C, Eulenberger J. Hüftendoprothesen mit oberflächen-strukturierten Verankerungsschäften. Resultate von statischen Belastungsversuchen. Unfallheilkunde 1985; 81:205–210
27. Oest O, Müller K, Hupfauer W. Die Knochenzemente. Enke, Stuttgart, 1975
28. Raab S, Ahmed A M, Provan J W. The quasistatic and fatigue performance of the implant/bone-cement interface. J Biomed Mat Res 1981; 15:159
29. Raab S, Ahmed A M, Provan J W. Thin film PMMA precoating for improved bone-cement fixation. J Biomed Mat Res 1982; 16:679
30. Shao W R, Foster T. Leland R H, Bachus K N. Atrophy of cancellous bone due to microcasting. 39th Annual Meeting Orthop Research Society San Francisco, 1993, Feb 15–18
31. Slooff TJH. The influence of acrylic cement. An experimental study. Acta Orthop Scand 1971; 42:465–481
32. Soltész U. The influence of loading conditions on the life-times in fatigue testing of bone cements. J Mater Sci Mat Med 1994; 5:654–656
33. Stachiewicz JW, Miller J, Burke DL. Hoop stress generated by shrinkage of polymethyl-methacrylate as a source of prosthetic loosening. Transactions of the 22nd Annual Meeting of the Orthopaedic Research Soc, New Orleans, 1976, p 60
34. Verdonschot N, Huiskes R. Acrylic cement creeps but does not allow much subsidence of femoral stems. J Bone Joint Surg 1997; 79-B:665–669
35. Willert HG, Puls P. Die Reaktion des Knochens auf Knochenzement bei der Alloarthroplastik der Hüfte. Arch Orthop Unfallchir 1972; 72:33–71

Properties of Bone Cement: Which Cement Should We Choose for Primary THA?

Ove Furnes, Leif Ivar Havelin, Birgitte Espehaug

Summary

In total hip arthroplasty (THA), the surgeon should use a well-proven antibiotic-containing cement, like Palacos or Simplex. In addition to antibiotics in the cement, systemic antibiotic prophylaxis should be administered 4 times on the operating day to prevent septic implant loosening. Studies based on data in the Norwegian Arthroplasty Register indicate that the type of cement may be a more important predictor for prosthesis outcome than commonly used prosthesis brands.

Introduction

In the early phases of hip replacement, surgery focus was on the design of the femoral stem, and on bearing surfaces. There was less focus on different types of bone cement. Later, when aseptic loosening became a recognised problem and the term »bone cement disease« was introduced, there was a shift towards more use of uncemented implants and towards new cements like the cold curing Boneloc cement and different low viscosity cements. The Swedish and Norwegian hip implant registers have shown that the type of cement is important for the performance of the hip implant and type of cement may in many ways be more important than the design of the prosthesis. The Norwegian hip implant register has published several reports concerning bone cement.

Results of Bone Cement Studies in the Norwegian Arthroplasty Register

In our first study on bone cement and prosthesis failure in Charnley prostheses, the cold curing cement Boneloc performed inferior to high viscosity cements, and low viscosity cements performed worse than high viscosity cements [5] (◘ Fig. 3.66). CMWIII was the most widely used low viscosity cement and hence the evidence against this cement was strongest. The poor performance of low viscosity cements might in part be explained by the difficult handling characteristic of these cements. In the next study from 1997 we showed that the polished tapered Exeter stem performed better with use of Boneloc cement than did the Charnley stem [4]. This is an interesting perspective and it seems that different prosthesis designs might require different mechanical properties of the cement. A 10-year follow-up of the different cement brands used in Norway showed that the high viscosity cement CMWI performed poorer than the other high viscosity cements Palacos and Simplex [3]. The poor performance of the CMWIII cement was further confirmed. A Charnley prosthesis implanted with CMWI cement had a failure rate of 12% at 10 years, but only 5.9% when used with gentamicin-containing Palacos cement (◘ Fig. 3.67). If you as a surgeon implant 100 Charnley prostheses with CMWI cement, this will lead to 6 extra revisions after 10 years compared to using Palacos or Simplex cement. These findings represent an argument for greater awareness regarding current marketing regulations of medical devices.

Should We Add Antibiotic in the Cement?

In two publications we have addressed the question of whether to use antibiotics in the cement or not, and the influence of systemic antibiotic prophylaxis. We have shown that use of systemic antibiotic prophylaxis gave less aseptic and septic loosening of the implant, and that the addition of antibiotic in the cement gave an added protective effect [2] (◘ Fig. 3.68). A combination of systemic antibiotic and

3

antibiotic in the cement gave four times less septic revisions and two times less aseptic revisions compared to use of systemic antibiotic prophylaxis only. It seems to be important to have high doses of antibiotics locally in the joint to prevent the bacteria to colonise the implant. In a recent study with over 10-years follow-up, the performance of the antibiotic loaded bone cements was still good and the protective effect of systemic antibiotic prophylaxis combined with antibiotic in the cement was maintained both for aseptic and septic loosening. The study implies that the concern of

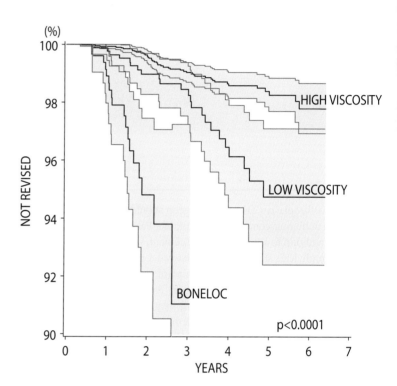

◘ Fig. 3.66. Kaplan Meier survival curves of Charnley femoral prostheses with high viscosity, low viscosity, and Boneloc cement. (Reproduced with permission from [5])

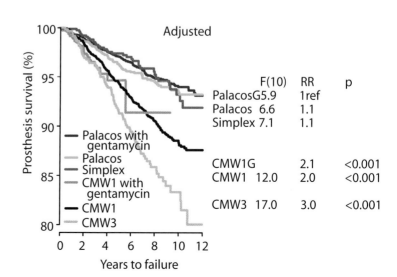

◘ Fig. 3.67. Survival curves calculated for 17,323 Charnley THRs with type of cement as the strata factor and any failure of either component as the endpoint (817 failures). The Cox proportional hazards method was used for adjusted estimates. (Reproduced with permission from [3])

a bio-mechanically weaker bone cement due to added antibiotics does not have any clinical significance, at least not within 10 years [1]. We have further shown that giving four doses antibiotics systemically the operating day resulted in less revisions due to septic and aseptic loosening compared to one, two or three doses, and that there was no additional beneficiary effect of giving the antibiotic prophylaxis for two or three days (■ Fig. 3.69). Most Norwegian surgeons gave either penicillin (Oxacillin, Dikloxacillin) or first and second generation Cephalosporin's in doses of 2 g × 4.

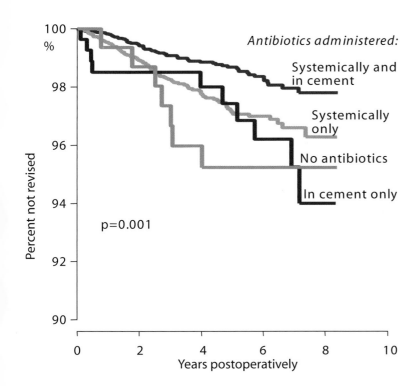

■ **Fig. 3.68.** Cox regression-adjusted survival curves calculated with revision due to any cause as the endpoint and regimen as the strata factor. (Reproduced with permission from [2])

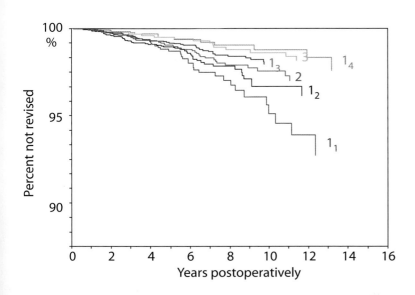

■ **Fig. 3.69.** Cox regression-adjusted survival curves with aseptic loosening as endpoint for THAs receiving antibiotic in the cement and antibiotic prophylaxis systemically for 1 day [with number of doses as subscript-i.e., 1 dose (1_1), 2 doses (1_2), 3 doses (1_3) and 4 dose (1_4)], 2 days (2) and 3 days (3)

3

| **Take Home Messages** | |

- The cement type may be a more important predictor for long term outcome than commonly used prosthesis brands.
- Palacos and Simplex cements are associated with the lowest risk for revision.
- The risk for infection following primary THA is lowest when antibiotic loaded cement is used in combination with 4 systemic antibiotic doses on the operating day.

Acknowledgements. We thank orthopaedic surgeons at all hospitals in Norway without whose co-operation the Norwegian Arthroplasty Register would not be possible. The work of the register is a teamwork and we thank our co-authors Lars B. Engesæter, Stein Emil Vollset, Stein Atle Lie and Norvald Langeland, and our secretaries Adriana Opazo, Ingvan Vindenes and Inger Skar for their accurate registration.

References

1. Engesæter LB, Lie SA, Espehaug B, Furnes O, Vollset SE, Havelin LI. Antibiotic prophylaxis in total hip arthroplasty: effects of antibiotic prophylaxis systemically and in bone cement on the revision rate of 22,170 primary hip replacements followed 0–14 years in the Norwegian Arthroplasty Register. Acta Orthop Scand. 2003; 74:644–651

2. Espehaug B, Engesæter LB, Vollset SE, Havelin LI, Langeland N. Antibiotic prophylaxis in total hip arthroplasty. Review of 10,905 primary cemented total hip replacements reported to the Norwegian Arthroplasty Register, 1987–1995. J Bone Joint Surg (Br) 1997; 79B:590–595

3. Espehaug B, Furnes O, Havelin LI, Engesæter LB, Vollset SE. The type of cement and failure of total hip replacements. J Bone Joint Surg (Br) 2002; 84-B: 832–838

4. Furnes O, Lie SA, Havelin LI, Vollset SE, Engesæter LB. Exeter and Charnley arthroplasties with Boneloc or high viscosity cement. Comparison of 1127 arthroplasties followed for 5 years in the Norwegian Arthroplasty Register. Acta Orthop Scand 1997; 68:515–520

5. Havelin LI, Espehaug B, Vollset SE, Engesaeter LB. The effect of cement type on early revision of Charnley total hip prostheses. A review of 8,579 primary arthroplasties from the Norwegian Arthroplasty Register. J Bone Joint Surg (Am) 1995; 77A:1543–1550.

Mixing:
The Benefit of Vacuum Mixing

Jian-Sheng Wang

Summary

Vacuum mixing of bone cement has been used in cemented hip-joint replacement procedures for over two decades. Although literature on bone cement is voluminous, relatively few studies have reported the effects of vacuum-mixing methods on the cemented hip replacement. While it has been proven that vacuum mixing improves the mechanical properties of bone cement, other effects need to be clarified. This chapter discusses the effects of vacuum mixing on cement quality, cement homogeneity, the cement-prosthesis interface and the operating room environment. It also discussed vacuum mixing in terms of bone-cement shrinkage and antibiotic release in total hip replacements.

Introduction

Until the 1980s, the composition and preparation of bone cement had not changed from the standards introduced by Charnley back in 1959. Then, in the 1980s, techniques for improving cement strength began to be investigated. Closed mixing under vacuum was developed initially for environment reasons, but its benefits in terms of producing homogenous cement, enhancing the mechanical properties of cement, improving cementing technique as well as safeguarding the operating room environment soon became evident.

In order to improve the mechanical properties of bone cement and thereby reduce the risk of cement failure in arthroplasties, substantial efforts have been invested into the development of new techniques for bone cement mixing and delivery applications with the objective of reducing macro- and microporosity. These techniques have the net effect of improving the overall quality of the cement.

Numerous studies have shown that, compared to other mixing methods, vacuum mixing reduces monomer evaporation and exposure in the operating room. Furthermore, it prevents air entrapment in cement, reduces cement porosity, decreases the number of unbounded particles in cement and increases the cement's mechanical strength. Clinical observations have revealed that vacuum mixing of bone cement improves mid- and long-term survival rates of total hip implants [41].

This chapter focuses on the effect of vacuum mixing on the characteristics and the quality of bone cement used in arthroplasty.

The Evolution of Cement Mixing Systems

When bone cement was first used in arthroplasty, it was hand-mixed in a bowl in the operating room and then inserted by hand or transferred and injected into the desired location. Because PMMA comes as a powder composed of prepolymerised particles to be mixed with the liquid monomer, monomer fumes release into the air. Furthermore with hand mixing, a certain amount of porosity in the final material, even in lower viscosity cements, is unavoidable owing to air entrapment.

During the 1980s different vibrating mixing techniques were introduced in the hope of improving mixing and thereby bone cement properties [37]. The results, however, were not convincing. While Burke et al. [9] reported an increase in the cement's fatigue life and ultimate tensile strength when centrifugation was used, a phenomenon they attributed to a reduction in the number and size of pores, Rimnace et al. [49] found no

4

improvement in the static or dynamic properties of several brands of bone cement when mixed by centrifugation. The results seemed to vary significantly depending on the type of centrifugation and cement used, and the cement was not consistently homogenous. Moreover, antibiotics and radiographic contrast media tended to gather in the periphery of the mix, and the upper volume of the cement often became more porous than the rest of the cement.

At about the same time as vibration and centrifugation were being developed and tested, closed mixing under vacuum was introduced [4, 35, 36]. After some refining, it produced better results than centrifugation, which was soon thereafter abandoned in favour of vacuum mixing, particularly because of the ease of delivery when using cartridge mixing. Today, vacuum mixing is widely accepted as the method of choice for achieving homogenous cement, reducing porosity and increasing cement strength, which is why it is an integral part of Modern Cementing Technique [40].

Improvement of Environment

MMA is a toxic, highly volatile organic solvent. Cytotoxic effects on human fibroblasts in culture media have been described and attributed to MMA [57]. It is now known that the adverse effects of working with MMA include local mucosal irritation i.e., irritation of the respiratory system, eyes and skin contact sensitivity that may lead to toxic dermatitis [20, 31, 33, 47]. Indications are headache, nausea and lack of appetite. MMA is not thought to be carcinogenic to humans under normal conditions of use. However, techniques should be employed to reduce medical staff exposure to MMA during cemented implantation. Operating staff should avoid direct contact with MMA, and room ventilation should be optimised.

Monomer exposure is regulated by law in many countries. The exposure limits range from 50–100 ppm in different countries in Europe. The exposure of conventional mixing in open bowl is about 10 ppm in the breathing zone [8]. Vacuum mixing systems reduce the exposure by 50–70% [53] and eliminate contact with bone cement during delivery [6, 8, 12, 19, 53]. The working environment for the operating staff is improved, and the risk of fume-induced headaches, respiratory irritation and allergic reactions becomes minimal.

Improvements in Cement Quality

Porosity

Pores and voids of different sizes in cement are caused by air from the polymer powder. The air becomes trapped in the cement during mixing and transferring from mixing

container to delivery system [11, 43, 62, 69]. Conventional mixing of bone cement produces porosity of 5–16%. Vacuum mixing produces porosity of 0.1–1% [38, 65].

Relationship Between Porosity and Fatigue Property of Cement

Porosity has been found to be the major cause of decreased mechanical strength and fatigue life of bone cement. To ensure its in vivo survival, the cement must be able to withstand the varying loads it endures. Thus fatigue property, which is directly affected by porosity, is as important in determining the long-term survival of a joint replacement as static strength.

Fatigue failure occurs when cement cracks are initiated as a result of defects in the cement mantle. It is the presence of large voids within the cement that leads to a rapid propagation of fracture (◨ Fig. 4.1a). Secondary cracks develop along the small pores (◨ Fig. 4.1b). Such

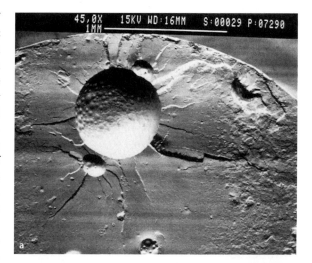

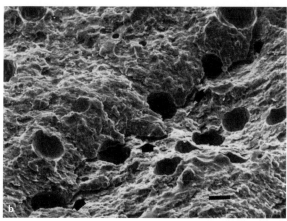

◨ **Fig. 4.1a,b.** SEM micrograph of fatigue fracture surface. **a** A large pore causes stress concentration and initiates crack [27]. **b** Secondary crack associated with pores [56]

fractures are commonly observed in vitro and in vivo [10, 27, 30, 45, 56]. Because of stress concentration, the initial crack is likely to start in an area of weakness or at a void in the material [29]. Evidence of this cracking has been found when examining retrieved cement [30, 56].

The reduction of porosity prevents or at the very least retards the initiation of fatigue propagation. It is known that vacuum mixing of cement increases mechanical properties [4, 5, 13, 35, 36, 38, 69] largely as a result of decreasing micro- and macropores [62, 66]. Numerous studies have confirmed that vacuum mixing enhances the fatigue life of the bone cement [17, 23, 34, 43, 45, 52, 65, 67, 70].

Cement Homogeneity

Bulk form PMMA cement exhibits good biocompatibility when implanted in bone. However, in particulate form, PMMA can evoke a foreign body and chronic inflammatory reaction similar to that seen around loose cemented arthroplasties [1, 22, 32, 55, 68].

Incomplete mixing of the monomer and polymer may lead to partially united and, in some cases, free unbonded cement particles. Vacuum mixing of bone cement not only decreases the number of voids but also improves the microscopic homogeneity of Palacos R cement [64]. Electronic microscopy shows that voids located on the surface of cement as well as on the fracture surface of cement invariably contain partially polymerised PMMA particles and contrast media particles, such as zirconium dioxided particles (■ Fig. 4.2). When cement fracture occurs, less homogeneous cement may release a larger number of PMMA spheres and contrast media particles to the bone-cement interface. These particles may evoke a foreign body response or stimulate osteoclast activity [50 ,51, 68], leading to osteolysis of the surrounding bone.

Cement-Prosthesis Interface

Studies have indicated that mechanical loosening of cemented implants originates at the stem-cement interface [28, 30, 60]. Loosening of the cemented stem further increases stress in the cement mantle [24, 59]. Extensive porosity at the cement-stem interface has been found in retrieved cement mantles and in laboratory-prepared specimens [7, 28] (■ Fig. 4.3).

This interface porosity is caused by entrapment of air at the stem surface during stem insertion and by residual porosity in the cement. A further cause is the cement's shrinkage away from the colder stem surface which produces pores [7]. Although cement curing is chemically initiated, polymerisation is thermally activated. Thus cement curing starts at the warmer bone surface and progresses towards the cooler stem. Resultant pores as well as residual pores in the cement are driven towards the last polymerising region on the stem.

When cement is mixed under vacuum, cement porosity is significantly reduced, producing less porosity at the cement-prosthesis interface [7, 61] (■ Fig. 4.4). Various stud-

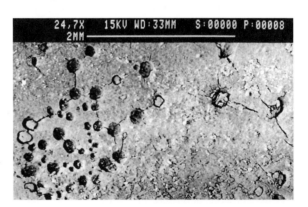

■ **Fig. 4.3.** In SEM numerous small voids are present on the cement surface at the prosthesis interface [30]

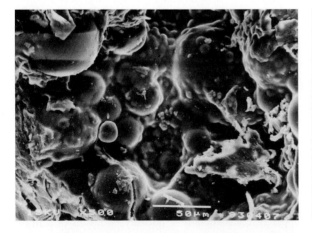

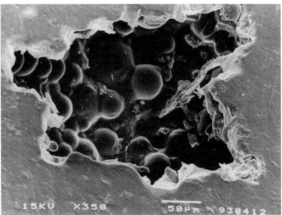

■ **Fig. 4.2.** Void on a fracture surface (*left*) and void located on the surface (*right*) of a Palacos R cement rod prepared at atmospheric pressure. Many partially unpolymerised PMMA particles and zirconium dioxide particles are seen in the voids [64]

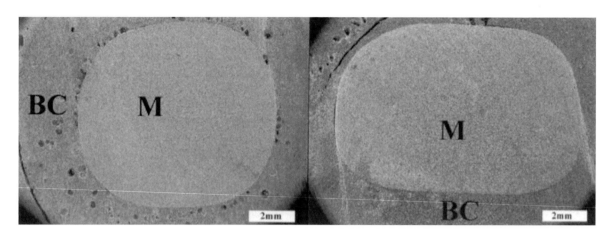

Fig. 4.4. Samples from a cemented implant. The cement was mixed at atmospheric pressure (*left*), and under vacuum (*right*). *M* metal; *BC* bone cement

ies have shown that interface porosity affects the debonding energy of the interface [43], weakens the resistance of the cement to torsional load [15] and decreases fatigue life of the cement-metal interface [26]. Interface porosity has also been linked to the initiation of cement cracks [28, 30, 58]. The evidence is convincing that reduction of interface porosity improves the strength of the interface, thereby increasing the longevity of cemented implants.

Shrinkage

Cement has 3–5% volumetric shrinkage after curing [11]. Concerns over this shrinkage have focused primarily on the stability of the implant. With vacuum mixing, the volumetric shrinkage may be increased from 3–5% to 5–7% in different cements [44]. In a cemented hip stem, for example, the cement grout is along the stem with a long cement mantle (150–200 mm) and thin cement layer (2–4 mm). The shrinkage occurs more along the longitudinal axis rather than diametrically [14], and it is the diametrical shrinkage that may influence the cement interface. Studies have been unable to find differences in diametrical shrinkage or gap formation between cement and prosthesis when a reduced porosity cement is used [14, 63]. Shrinkage, however, within the cancellous bone bed can be regarded as beneficial (▸ chapter 3.6), as some interface gaps allow for re-vascularisation [16]. Vacuum mixing of cement has not been found to negatively affect interface strength between cement and prosthesis. RSA (▸ chapter 7.3) showed a stable cemented implant in early and middle term studies of vacuum-mixed cemented implants [2, 48].

Antibiotic Release

While vacuum mixing reduces the porosity of bone cement, it is thought that the process may adversely affect antibiotic release (▸ chapter 3.1). Surgeons understandably are concerned about the extent to which the mixing procedure affects the release of antibiotics from the cement. Studies have shown that the concentrations of several antimicrobial agents from antibiotic-loaded bone cement exceed those obtained by systemic administration [21] as well as the minimal inhibitory concentrations of several pathogens according to the National Committee for Clinical Laboratory Standards breakpoints lasting from 3–38 days [3]. Vacuum mixing of gentamicin-loaded bone cements has been shown to effectively reduce the number and size of cement pores with only a minor reduction in antibiotic release [46]. The Norwegian Arthroplasty Register [18] documents the best results occurring when antibiotic prophylaxis is administered both systemically and with bone cement containing antibiotics prepared under vacuum.

Clinical Significance

The aetiology of aseptic loosening of total joint arthroplasties appears to be multifactorial, with surgical technique, cementing technique, cement quality, cement viscosity, prosthesis design, wear debris, joint fluid pressure and micromotion all being involved. Although improved surgical techniques have increased the probability of prosthesis survival, reducing or eliminating bone cement fracture by improving its material strength will further enhance the longevity of cemented prostheses.

The affects of porosity reduction on the longevity of the cement mantle and on the survival rate of a joint replacement are still debated. In favour of porosity reduction is the fact that no direct clinical evidence has ever shown an association between reduced survival rates and porosity reduction [39]. Janssen et al. [29] explain the apparent contradiction of porosity by means of a finite element model showing that when stresses are distributed homogenously in cement, pores act as crack initiators;

whereas under inhomogeneous stress conditions, crack formation is governed by local stress intensities. The study suggests that mechanical failure of cemented femoral components is initiated in areas where stress concentrations are generated. Therefore, the effect of reduced porosity on the failure mechanism in these areas will be limited and clinically detectable only in large studies.

It remains clear, however, that with pores located in areas of high stress concentrations, the cement mantle will fail rapidly. The Swedish Hip Register gives a risk ratio of vacuum mixing to revision of 0.74 after five years from implantation [41], suggesting that vacuum mixing improves the mid- to long-term survival rate of THA significantly as compared to hand mixing. With 25 years of clinical experience, Harris [25] indicated that in a cemented total hip replacement, bone cement can be made five times stronger just by porosity reduction. Various studies indicate that macropores increase the risk of fatigue failure, and the current opinion is that efforts should be made to minimise the number and size of macropores.

Take Home Messages

- Vacuum mixing significantly reduces macro- and micropores in bone cement, thereby enhancing the cement's mechanical strength.
- Vacuum mixing also improves cement homogeneity and strengthens the cement-prosthesis interface.
- Closed vacuum-mixing systems reduce the risk of monomer exposure to operating room staff.
- The slight bone cement shrinkage that occurs has not been shown to adversely affect prosthesis stability in any way. Nor does vacuum mixing have a significant effect on effective antibiotic release.
- A well-fixed cemented implant requires strong cement to support the various loads it endures over a prolonged period; only vacuum-mixed cement seems to provide this kind of enduring strength.

References

1. Abbas S, Clohisy JC, Abu-Amer Y (2003) Mitogen-activated protein (MAP) kinases mediate PMMA-induction of osteoclasts. J Orthop Res 21(6):1041–8
2. Adalberth G, Nilsson KG, Kattholm J, Hassander H (2002) Fixation of the tibial component using CMW-1 or Palacos bone cement with gentamicin: similar outcome in a randomized radiostereometric study of 51 total knee arthroplasties. Acta Orthop Scand 73(5):531–8
3. Adam K, Couch L, Cierny G, Calhoun J, Mader JT (1992) In vitro and in vivo evaluation of antibiotic-impregnated polymethylmethacrylate beads. Clin Orthop 278:244–52
4. Alkire M, Dabezies E, Hastings P (1987) High Vacuum As a Method of Reducing Porosity of Polymethylmethacrylate. Othopaedics 10:1533–39
5. Askew MJ, Kufel MF, Fleissner Jr PR, Gradisar Jr IA, Salstrom SJ, Tan J (1990) Effect of vacuum mixing on the mechanical properties of antibiotic-impregnated polymethylmethacrylate bone cement. J Biomed Mater Res 24:573–80
6. Bettencourt A, Calado A, Amaral J, Vale FM, Rico JM, Monteiro J, Castro M (2001) The influence of vacuum mixing on methylmethacrylate liberation from acrylic cement powder. Int J Pharm 219:89–93
7. Bishop NE, Ferguson S, Tepic S (1996) Porosity reduction in bone cement at the cement-stem interface. J Bone Joint Surg (Br) 78(3):349–56
8. Buchhorn GH, Streicher RM, Willert HG (1992) Exposure of surgical/orthopedic operating room personnel to monomer vapors during the use of bone cements--review of the literature and report of experiences. Biomed Tech (Berl) 37:293–302
9. Burke D, Gates E, Harris W (1984) Centrifugation as a method of improving tensile and fatigue properties of acrylic bone cement. J Bone Joint Surg (Am) 66:1265–73
10. Carter DR, Gates EI, Harris WH (1982) Strain controlled fatigue of acrylic bone cement. J Biomed Mater Res 16:647–657
11. Charnley J (1970) Low friction arthroplasty of the hip: theory and practice. Springer, Berlin Heidelberg New York
12. Darre E, Gottlieb J, Nielsen PM, Jensen JS (1988) A method to determine methylmethacrylate in air. Acta Orthop Scand 59:270–1
13. Davies JP, Harris WH (1990) Optimization and comparison of three vacuum mixing systems for porosity reduction of Simplex P Cement. Clin Orthop 254:261–69
14. Davies JP, Harris WH (1995) Comparison of diametral shrinkage of centrifuged and uncentrifuged Simplex P bone cement. J Appl Biomater 6(3):209–11
15. Davies JP, Kawate K, Harris WH (1995) Effect of interfacial porosity on the torsional strength of the cement-metal interface. 41st Annual Meeting Orthopedic Research Society, Orlando, FL, USA, p 713
16. Draenert K, Draenert Y, Garde U, Ulrich C (1999) Manual of cementing technique. Springer, Berlin, Heidelberg, New York, Tokyo, pp 26–28
17. Dunne N J, Orr J (2001) Influence of mixing techniques on the physical properties of acrylic bone cement. Biomaterials 22:1819–26
18. Engesaeter LB, Lie SA, Espehaug B, Furnes O, Vollset SE, Havelin LI (2003) Antibiotic prophylaxis in total hip arthroplasty: effects of antibiotic prophylaxis systemically and in bone cement on the revision rate of 22,170 primary hip replacements followed 0–14 years in the Norwegian Arthroplasty Register. Acta Orthop Scand 74(6):644–51
19. Eveleigh R (2002) Fume levels during bone cement mixing. Br J Perioper Nurs 12(4):145–7, 149–50
20. Fregert S (1983) Occupational hazards of acrylate bone cement in orthopaedic surgery. Acta Orthop Scand 54:787–9
21. Frommelt L (2001) Gentamicin release from PMMA bone cement: mechanism and action on bacteria. In: Walenkamp GHIM, Murray DW (eds) Bone cement and cementing technique. Springer, Berlin Heidelberg New York Tokyo
22. Goodman SB, Fornasier VL, Kei J (1988) The effects of bulk versus particulate polymethylmethacrylate on bone. Clin Orthop (232):255–62
23. Harper EJ, Bonfield W (2000) Tensile characteristics of ten commercial acrylic bone cements. J Biomed Mater Res (Appl Biomater) 53:605–16
24. Harrigan TP, Harris WH (1991) A three-dimensional non-linear finite element study of the effect of cement-prosthesis debonding in cemented femoral total hip components. J Biomech 24(11):1047–58
25. Harris WH (1992) The first 32 years of total hip arthroplasty. One surgeon's perspective. Clin Orthop (274):6–11
26. Iesaka K, Jaffe WL, Kummer FJ (2003) Effects of preheating of hip prostheses on the stem-cement interface. J Bone Joint Surg Am 85(3):421–7
27. James SP, Jasty M, Davies J, Piehler H, Harris WH (1992) A fractographic investigation of PMMA bone cement focusing on the

4

relationship between porosity reduction and increased fatigue life. J Biomed Mater Res 26:651–62

28. James SP, Schmalzried TP, McGarry FJ, Harris WH (1993) Extensive porosity at the cement-femoral prosthesis interface: a preliminary study. J Biomed Mater Res 27(1):71–8

29. Janssen DW, Stolk J, Verdonschot N (2004) Why would cement porosity reduction be clinically irrelevant, while experimental data show the contrary? 50th Annual Meeting of the Orthopaedic Research Society. San Francisco, USA, p 3

30. Jasty M, Maloney WJ, Bragdon CR, O'Connor DO, Haire T, Harris WH (1991) The initiation of failure in cemented femoral components of hip arthroplasties. J Bone Joint Surg (Br) 73(4):551–8

31. Jensen JS, Trap B, Skydsgaard K (1991) Delayed contact hypersensitivity and surgical glove penetration with acrylic bone cements. Acta Orthop Scand 62:24–28

32. Johanson NA, Bullough PG, Wilson PD Jr., Salvati EA, Ranawat CS (1987) The microscopic anatomy of the bone-cement interface in failed total hip arthroplasties. Clin Orthop (218):123–35

33. Leggat PA, Kedjarune U (2003) Toxicity of methyl methacrylate in dentistry. Int Dent J 53(3):126–31

34. Lewis G (1997) Properties of Acrylic Bone Cement: State of Art Review. J Biomed Mater Res (Appl Biomater) 38:155–82

35. Lidgren L, Bodelind B, Möller J (1987) Bone cement improved by vacuum mixing and chilling. Acta Orthop Scand 57:27–32

36. Lidgren L, Drar H, Moller J (1984) Strength of polymethylmethacrylate increased by vacuum mixing, Acta Orthop Scand 55(5):536–41

37. Lindén U (1991) Mechanical properties of bone cement. Importance of the mixing technique. Clin Orthop 272:274–8

38. Linden U, Gillquist J (1989) Air inclusion in bone cement. Importance of the mixing technique. Clin Orthop 247:148–51

39. Ling RS, Lee AJ (1998) Porosity reduction in acrylic cement is clinically irrelevant. Clin Orthop 355:249–53

40. Malchau H, Herberts P (1996) Prognosis of total hip replacement; surgical and cementing technique in THR: a revision-risk study of 134 056 primary operations. 63rd Annual Meeting of the AAOS, February 22–26, Atlanta, USA

41. Malchau H, Herberts P (2000) Prognosis of total hip replacement. 65th Annual Meeting of the AAOS. March 15–19, Orland, USA

42. Mann KA, Damron LA, Race A, Ayers DC (2004) Early cementing does not increase debond energy of grit blasted interfaces. J Orthop Res 22(4):822–7

43. Mau H, Schelling K, Heisel C, Wang JS, Breusch SJ (2004) Comparison of different vacuum mixing systems and bone cements with respect to reliability, porosity and bending strength. Acta Orthop Scand 75:160–72

44. Muller SD, Green SM, McCaskie AW (2002) The dynamic volume changes of polymerising polymethyl methacrylate bone cement. Acta Orthop Scand 73(6):684–7

45. Murphy BP, Prendergast PJ (2002) The relationship between stress, porosity, and nonlinear damage accumulation in acrylic bone cement. J Biomed Mater Res 59(4):646–54

46. Neut D, van de Belt H, van Horn JR, van der Mei HC, Busscher HJ (2003) The effect of mixing on gentamicin release from polymethylmethacrylate bone cements. Acta Orthop Scand 74:670–6

47. Nissen JN, Corydon L (1985) Corneal ulcer after exposure to vapours from bone cement (methyl methacrylate and hydroquinone). Int Arch Occup Environ Health 56(2):161–5

48. Nivbrant B, Karrholm J, Rohrl S, Hassander H, Wesslen B (2001) Bone cement with reduced proportion of monomer in total hip arthroplasty: preclinical evaluation and randomized study of 47 cases with 5 years' follow-up. Acta Orthop Scand 72(6):572–84

49. Rimnace CM, Wright TM, McGill DL (1986) The effect of centrifugation on the fracture properties of acrylic bone cements. J Bone Joint Surg (Am) 68:281–7

50. Sabokbar A, Fujikawa Y, Murray DW, Athanasou NA (1997) Radio-opaque agents in bone cement increase bone resorption. J Bone Joint Surg (Br) 79:129–34

51. Sabokbar A, Murray DW, Athanasou NA (2001) Osteolysis induced by radio-opaque agents. In »Bone cements and cementing techniques« Springer, Berlin Heidelberg, pp 149–61

52. Schelling K, Breusch SJ (2001) Efficacy of a new prepacked vacuum mixing system with Palamed G bone cement. In: Walenkamp GHIM, Murray DW (eds) Bone cement and cementing technique. Springer, Berlin Heidelberg New York Tokyo, pp 97–107

53. Schlegel UJ, Sturm M, Ewerbeck V, Breusch S (2004) Efficacy of vacuum bone cement mixing systems in reducing methylmethacrylate fume exposure: comparison of 7 different mixing devices and handmixing. Acta Orthop Scand;75(5):559–66

54. Schreurs BW, Spierings PT, Huiskes R, Slooff TJ (1988) Effects of preparation techniques on the porosity of acrylic cements. Acta Orthop Scand 59:403–9.

55. Shardlow DL, Stone MH, Ingham E, Fisher J (2003) Cement particles containing radio-opacifiers stimulate pro-osteolytic cytokine production from a human monocytic cell line. J Bone Joint Surg (Br) 85(6):900–5

56. Topoleski LD, Ducheyne P, Cuckler JM (1990) A fractographic analysis of in vivo poly(methyl methacrylate) bone cement failure mechanisms. J Biomed Mater Res 24(2):135–54

57. Vale FM, Castro M, Monteriro J, Couto FS, Pinto R, Toscano G, Rico JM (1997) Acrylic bone cement induces the production of free radicls by cultured human fibroblasts. Biomaterials 18:1133–5

58. Verdonschot N (1995) Biomechanical failure scenarios for cemented total hip replacement. Thesis

59. Verdonschot N, Huiskes R (1997) The effects of cement-stem debonding in THA on the long-term failure probability of cement. J Biomech 30(8):795–802

60. Walker PS, Mai SF, Cobb AG, Bentley G, Hua J (1995) Prediction of clinical outcome of THR from migration measurements on standard radiographs. A study of cemented Charnley and Stanmore femoral stems. J Bone Joint Surg (Br) 77(5):705–14

61. Wang JS, Aspenberg P, Goodman S, Lidgren L (1998) Interface porosity in cemented implants in vitro study. 8th European Orthopeic society Meeting in Armsterdam, The Netherlands, May P, 2

62. Wang JS, Franzén H, Jonsson E, Lidgren L (1993) Porosity of bone cement reduced by mixing and collecting under vacuum. Acta Orthop Scand 64(2):143–46.

63. Wang JS, Franzén H, Lidgren L (1999) Interface gap implantation of a cemented femoral stem in pigs. Acta Orthop Scand 70(3):229–33.

64. Wang JS, Goodman S, Franzén H, Aspenberg P, Lidgren L (1994) The effects of vacuum mixing on the microscopic homogenicity of bone cement. Europ. J. Exper. Musculoskeletal Res 2:159–65

65. Wang JS, Kjellson F (2001) Bone cement porosity in Vacuum Mixing system. In: Walenkamp GHIM, Murray DW (eds) Bone cements and Cementing technique. Springer, Berlin Heidelberg New York Tokyo, pp 81–95

66. Wang J-S, Toksvig-Larsen S, Müller-Wille P, Franzén H (1996) Is their any difference between vacuum mixing systems in reducing bone cement porosity? J Biomed Mater Res (Applied Biomaterials) 33:115–19.

67. Wilkinson JM, Eveleigh R, Hamer AJ, Milne A, Miles AW, Stockely I (2000) Effect of mixing technique on the properties of acrylic bone cement. J Arthroplasty 15:663–7

68. Wimhurst J, Brooks R, Rushton N (2001) The effects of particulate bone cements at the bone-implant interface. J Bone Joint Surg (Br) 83(4):588–92

69. Wixon RL, Lautenschlager EP, Novak MA (1987) Vacuum mixing of acrylic bone cement. J Arthroplasty 2:141–49

70. Yau WP, Ng TP, Chiu KY, Poon KC, Ho WY, Luk DK (2001) The performance of three vacuum mixing cement guns- acomparison of the fatigue properties of Simplex P cement. International Orthopaedics 25:290–293

Mixing:
Choice of Mixing System

Jian-Sheng Wang, Steffen J. Breusch

Summary

Studies have shown that pores in bone cement adversely affect the cement's mechanical strength and that removal of these air inclusions can significantly enhance fatigue properties. Currently, the most popular cement mixing technique is vacuum mixing, and there is extensive evidence that vacuum mixing reduces cement porosity. However, in clinical use vacuum mixing systems and cement brands are arbitrarily combined, precluding conclusive analysis on the effectiveness of the combinations used. This chapter compares various systems in the market and discusses the influence of mixing systems and cements on cement quality and monomer evaporation.

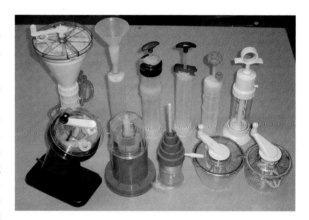

Fig. 4.5. Vacuum mixing systems in the market

Introduction

It is believed that the porosity of bone cement used in orthopaedic surgery influences the long-term mechanical stability and thus the survival of joint prostheses. Extensive evidence (▶ chapter 4.1) has demonstrated that vacuum mixing reduces cement porosity and increases mechanical properties, especially when compared to hand mixing [2, 6, 7, 9, 11, 14–18, 20, 22, 24, 30–32]. Vacuum mixing also reduces the porosity at the interface of cement and prosthesis [4, 12, 28] as well as the number of unbonded cement particles [27]. In addition, vacuum mixing systems reduce monomer evaporation [5, 23].

The vacuum mixing of bone cement was introduced by Lidgren in 1984 [15]. Since then many vacuum mixing systems have been developed, but many have had problems yielding quality cement [6, 29]. There are now about 20 vacuum mixing systems on the market and

employed clinically (◻ Fig. 4.5). Some of these systems are arbitrarily used with different bone cements, making assessments of cement performance and handling difficult. Some of the mixing systems were recently carefully investigated on features, user-friendliness and reliability (◻ Table. 4.1, [18]).

Despite efforts to create more advanced cementing techniques for joint replacement, the variation in bone-cement quality, influenced by mixing procedure, may negate any advances. It might be expected that all cements mixed under vacuum would have low porosity, but Kühn [13] has repeatedly emphasised that not all cements are alike and that the properties of cement are changed by even slight variations in composition. Vacuum-mixing systems allow for different vacuum levels and employ different mixing methods. Thus cured cement may vary in quality, i.e., in terms of porosity and mechanical strength differences, which may substantially influence the long-term clinical results of joint replace-

◨ Table 4.1. Features, user-friendliness and problems with the mixing systems (from [18])

System	Build up	Way of Mixing	Cement Collection	Cement Gun and Extrusion	Problems	Specials
Palamix	stable	Vertical	Dismantling of the stirring rod and collecting the cement requires multiple steps.	The cartridge can be firmly connected to the cement gun via a thread. Long extrusion times from the cement gun due to the low feeding rate		Prepacked system for 60 g of Palamed The air is evacuated separately from the components before vacuum mixing.
Summit	stable	Rotational	Dismantling of the stirring rod is complicated as cement has to be manually wiped off	The cartridge can be firmly connected to the cement gun via a thread. The cement gun requires high forces for cement extrusion due to the high ratio of the plunger to the nozzle diameter	Black streaks from the seal can be intermixed into the cement. The lid was deformed during extrusion of high viscosity cements and cement can leak through the thread	
Cemvac	Wobbly due to its height	Vertical and twisting	Cement is collected manually while the vacuum is still applied	Firm connection to the cement gun. Easy cement extrusion from the cement gun.	Sometimes the narrow filling funnel is blocked by cement powder and has to be freed by shaking before the cartridge is sealed with the plugging rod	The vacuum pump is switched on to suck the components into the cartridge
Optivac	stable	Vertical and twisting	The cement is automatically collected under vacuum	Firm connection to the cement gun. Easy cement extrusion from cement gun	Automatic collection failed twice. With Versabond and Simplex cement monomer was sucked into the vacuum filter	Extensions are available for 120 g polymer
VacuMix Plus	stable	Rotational	Removal of the stirring rod is impractical as the cement has to be manually wiped off	The cement gun has a stable connection and was the most comfortable to use	The »economiser« can break early during cement extrusion with high viscosity cement and the cement cannot be fully extruded. Only 60 g of the more voluminous Simplex P can be loaded into the system	A mechanism called »economiser« is built in to reduce the dead space of the nozzle. After the cement is extruded from the cartridge the driving rod breaks through the lid into the nozzle and extrudes the cement from the nozzle. It is available as a prepack for CMW1 and CMW2000
MixOr	stable	Vertical and twisting	cement is collected automatically under vacuum	The connection to the cement gun is not very stable. Cement gun and cartridge have to be stabilized with both hands. Low feeding rate of the cement gun	The automatic cement collection failed 7 times. With Versabond, Simplex, Palacos and Palamed cement monomer was occasionally sucked into the vacuum filter	It is the only system with an integrated barometer that shows the actual vacuum pressure. Extensions are available for 120 g polymer (90 g Simplex P).

4

ment. Additionally, an improperly used vacuum mixing system may produce an inordinate number of large pores in the cement. It may therefore be said that familiarity with mixing systems is of great importance for clinical success.

Influence of Mixing Systems on Porosity and Mechanical Strength

A hip joint is subjected to forces as great as ten times body weight and functions up to two million times each year. Thus fatigue properties of cement are critical. Porosity has been found to decrease the mechanical strength of bone cement, with pores or other inclusions concentrating stress in the material and initiating fatigue cracks, which may lead to failure.

In the early 1990s both vacuum mixing and centrifugation were shown to reduce the porosity of cement compared to hand mixing. However, while centrifugation eliminated large voids, small pores persisted [6, 14]. As well, centrifuged cement was not consistently homogenous [21]. For its part, vacuum mixing reduced microporosity, but the presence of macropores depended on the vacuum mixing system used [1, 8, 10]. Further study found that large pores were trapped during the collection of high-viscosity cement after vacuum mixing. A later study then showed that after vacuum mixing, if the cement was slowly collected under vacuum until totally compacted, air entrapment was avoided and the number of macropores decreased significantly [27, 29]. Additional studies confirmed that collection under high vacuum notably increased mechanical strength [7, 30]. This method is well recognized and patented in Optivac system.

Mau et al. [18] tested six commercially available vacuum mixing systems in combination with six bone cements. Marked differences were found among the systems with respect to overall porosity depending on the cement used (range 2–18%) as well as among the cements depending on the system used (range 2–17%, ▪ Table 4.2). Several factors seem to influence the porosity and mechanical

strength of bone cement mixed in such systems. The design of the mixing system may be one such factor, as syringe-shaped vacuum mixing systems produce a lower porosity cement with greater density, bending modulus and bending strength than bowl vacuum mixing systems [7, 30]. The type of mixing paddle used also seems to make a difference, with the best results coming from paddles made of a material that does not adhere to bone cement. It also has been noted that axis-rotating mixing paddles are not able to reduce macropores in high viscosity cement [30]. Vacuum level has been shown to directly influence the quality of cement [7], with mechanical strength increasing once the pressure is reduced lower than 80% as compared to a vacuum level around 50% [7, 30]. Studies have shown that mixing and collection of cement under vacuum, such as Optivac system, produces a much lower macroporosity in high-viscosity cement than other vacuum mixing systems [7, 18, 29, 30].

Quality of Different Cements in Various Mixing Systems

The vast majority of cements are based on the same chemical substance: methylmethacrylate. After mixing the liquid and the powder, the final material becomes polymethylmethacrylate (PMMA). But this does not mean that the properties of all bone cements are alike. In addition to containing methylmethacrylate, bone cements may be composed of other methacrylates, radiopacifiers (zirconium dioxide or barium sulphate), varying amounts of initiator and accelerator (which initiate polymerisation and control setting time), powder particles of varying sizes and shapes (influencing volume and viscosity) and antibiotics of various types and amounts. All these variations in a cement's makeup will affect its characteristics.

Several studies investigated the porosity of different cements mixed in the Optivac system, known to be one of the most efficient at porosity reduction [19, 29, 30]. Palacos R, Simplex P, Palamed, Osteopal and Osteobond cements were mixed in different amounts (40 g, 60 g, 80 g and 120 g) in varying sizes of Optivac containers. The resultant number of macroporosity in Palacos R, Palamed and Simplex P was significantly lower than that in Osteobond and Osteopal (▪ Fig. 4.6). The pore area showed no significant differences, indicating that the pores were relatively smaller because of a cement's lower viscosity [26]. No vacuum mixing system can produce optimal results for all cements, in the same way that no single cement gets good results from all mixing systems [18]. Higher viscosity cement, for example, requires a longer mixing time and a higher vacuum level to remove bubbles. Each brand of bone cement will have its own optimal mixing technique.

▪ **Table 4.2.** Total porosity (%) from vacuum mixing systems [18]

Data of Total Porosity [%] from Cylinders

	mean	SD	min.	max.	95% CI
VacuMix	18,4	15,2	1,5	57,4	14,4–22,3
Summit	12,6	11,0	0,0	37,0	9,8–15,4
MixOR	4,9	12,7	0,0	70,0	1,6–8,2
Cemvac	1,8	3,1	0,0	12,6	1,0–2,6
Optivac	4,4	7,0	0,0	33,0	2,6–6,2
Palamix	11,7	7,8	2,4	23,8	6,1–17,2

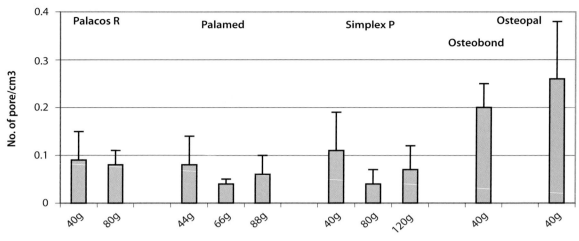

Fig. 4.6. The pore area (%) in different bone cements mixed in Optivac (mean ± SD) [26]

What Level of Vacuum is Optimal in a Vacuum Mixing System?

In 1987, Alkire et al. [1] suggested a high vacuum level for reducing the porosity of bone cement. Subsequently, it was found that observing a minimum vacuum level of –72 kPa improved mechanical properties of the cement [7]. Later it was found [27] that a vacuum level of under 0.2 bar significantly reduced porosity (by 50%) and significantly increased density in a high-viscosity cement such as Palacos R, compared to mixing at atmospheric pressure. However, when the vacuum level increased to 0.05 bar, macropores decreased no more than at 0.2 bar. While the use of a higher vacuum level (0.05 bar) did not decrease macropores in this high-viscosity cement, it did increases the size of pores, owing to air trapped in the cement when the vacuum is releasing. The best solution to minimize macropores, therefore, is continuous mixing and collection of the cement under vacuum [7, 30, 18, 27, 29]. In general, a vacuum level of 0.25 to 0.05 bar is optimal for various kinds of cement.

Porosity Related to Cement-to-Container Volume Ratio

It is still not clear why vacuum mixing produces large variations of macropores. One indicator of this problem is that one package of bone cement produces more macropores than two packages of bone cement mixed in the same size mixing cartridge [6]. Another study found that 40 grams of cement mixed in smaller container yielded a lower pore area percentage than when the same amount of cement was mixed in a larger container (Fig. 4.7), confirming that cement porosity is dependent on the cement-to-container volume ratio [25]. The macropore formation is probably the result of a larger mixing cartridge contain-

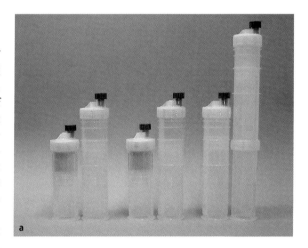

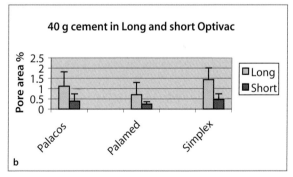

Fig. 4.7. a Pore area (%) of three cements that mixed in different volume mixing cartridge (mean ± SD) [26]. **b** The picture shows volume difference between cartridge and mixed cement. The powder of Simplex P is more voluminous, therefore larger cartridges were used (*left to right:* Palacos, Palamed and Simplex in long and short cartridge)

ing more air than a smaller one, as the vacuum pump does not produce perfect vacuum. Matching the mixing cartridge size to the cement volume used may have significant impact on the quality of the cement (► chapter 3.6). Yet most mixing systems have only one cartridge size.

Failure Mechanisms of Mixing Systems

According to several studies [18, 29, 30], cement quality sometimes varies in a mixing system. Some variation is due to the failure of the mixing system. As we know, vacuum mixing system should be a closed system. If there is leakage in the mixing system, air can easily be entrapped into the cement. Once cement clogs the opening of a vacuum mixing system, it will hinder remaining air from getting out, thus pores will stay in the cement. Failure of collection under vacuum will fail to reduce macropores. Sucking out monomer into the vacuum tube during the mixing may influence the efficiency of the vacuum. These failures of mixing systems will cause the handling problem and increase porosity in the cement, which will reduce the strength of the cement. Therefore, it is important to use vacuum mixing systems properly.

Influence of Mixing Systems on MMA Monomer Release

Vacuum mixing systems are connected to suction units and are expected to minimise exposure to methylmethacrylate (MMA) monomer fumes which evaporate during the mixing procedure [3, 5, 23]. A few studies have been published regarding exposure of nurses to MMA fumes during vacuum mixing and hand mixing of bone cement in arthroplasty. The early studies showed that MMA concentration from vacuum mixing was about 87 ppm over a mixing period of 10 min. During the same mixing period, open bowl hand mixing yielded a result of 200–500 ppm [5]. Recently, Schlegel et al. [23] tested seven commonly used vacuum mixing systems for MMA exposure. The data again showed that most vacuum mixing systems significantly reduce MMA exposure as compared to open bowl hand-mixing. Note also that significant differences of monomer exposure were found among the vacuum mixing systems themselves (◘ Fig. 4.8).

The causes of monomer release from a vacuum mixing system include the following:

- Evaporation of monomer when adding the monomer liquid to the polymer powder in the mixing cartridge,
- increased evaporation of monomer when collecting cement mechanically,
- monomer leakage during mixing.

It is therefore important to keep some distance from the system during mixing. Mixing should remain under vacuum until the cement is collected to the top of mixing cartridge. Eventually vacuum mixing systems with prepacked bone cements will offer an even better solution for environmental protection.

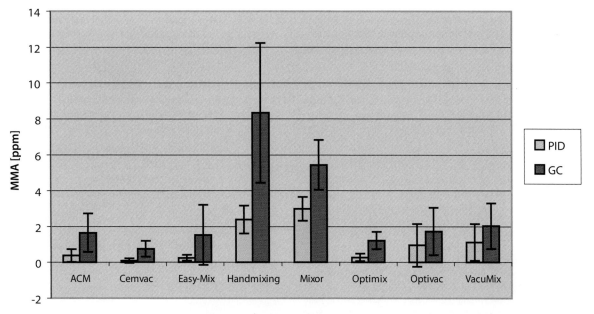

◘ Fig. 4.8. MMA concentrations in different vacuum mixing systems compared to hand mixing [23]

- Vertical paddles are better than horizontal.
- Vacuum levels of 0.25 to 0.05 bar are optimal for various kinds of cement.
- Higher viscosity cement requires a longer mixing time and a higher vacuum level to remove bubbles/pores.
- Each brand of bone cement should have its own optimal mixing technique/system.
- There are better and worse mixing system/cement combinations for a given system and a given cement (mix and match!).
- Smaller container yield a lower porosity.
- Additional cement collection under vacuum is essential step for reduced porosity.
- Keep distance when mixing to avoid fume exposure.

References

1. Alkire M, Dabezies E, Hastings P. High vacuum as a method of reducing porosity of polymethylmethacrylate. Othopaedics. 1987; 10:1533–39
2. Askew MJ, Kufel MF, Fleissner Jr. PR, Gradisar, Jr. IA, Salstrom SJ, Tan J. Effect of vacuum mixing on the mechanical properties of antibiotic-impregnated polymethylmethacrylate bone cement. J Biomed Mater Res. 1990;24:573–80
3. Bettencourt A, Calado A, Amaral J, Vale FM, Rico JM, Monteiro J, Castro M. The influence of vacuum mixing on methylmethacrylate liberation from acrylic cement powder. Int J Pharm. 2001;219:89–93
4. Bishop NE, Ferguson S, Tepic S. Porosity reduction in bone cement at the cement-stem interface. J Bone Joint Surg (Br). 1996;78(3):349–56
5. Darre E, Gottlieb J, Nielsen PM, Jensen JS. A method to determine methylmethacrylate in air. Acta Orthop Scand. 1988;59:270–1
6. Davies JP, Harris WH. Optimization and comparison of three vacuum mixing systems for porosity reduction of Simplex P Cement. Clin Orthop. 1990;254:261–69
7. Dunne N-J, Orr J. Influence of mixing techniques on the physical properties of acrylic bone cement. Biomaterials. 2001;22:1819–26
8. Eyerer P, Jin R. Influence of mixing technique on some properties of PMMA bone cement. J Biomed Mater Res. 1986;20:1057–1094
9. Graham J, Pruitt L, Ries M, Gundiah N. Fracture and fatigue properties of acrylic bone cement: the effects of mixing method, sterilization treatment, and molecular weight. J Arthroplasty. 2000;15(8):1028–35
10. Hansen D, Jensen JS. Mixing does not improve mechanical properties of all bone cements. Manual and centrifugation-vacuum mixing compared for 10 cement brands. Acta Orthop Scand. 1992;63(1):13–8
11. Harper EJ, Bonfield W. Tensile characteristics of ten commercial acrylic bone cements. J. Biomed Mater Res (Appl Biomater) 2000;53:605–16
12. Jafri AA, Green SM, Partington, McCaskie AW, Muller SD. Pre-heating of components in cemented total hip arthroplasty. J Bone Joint Surg (Br). 2004;86:1214–19
13. Kühn KD (2000) Bone cement. Springer, Berlin Heidelberg

14. Lewis G. Properties of acrylic bone cement: state of art review. J Biomed Mater Res (Appl Biomater). 1997;38:155–82
15. Lidgren L, Bodelind B, Möller J. Bone cement improved by vacuum mixing and chilling. Acta Orthop Scand. 1987;57:27–32
16. Lidgren L, Drar H, Moller J. Strength of polymethylmethacrylate increased by vacuum mixing, Acta Orthop Scand. 1984;55(5):536–41
17. Linden U, Gillquist J. Air inclusion in bone cement. Importance of the mixing technique. Clin Orthop. 1989;247:148–51
18. Mau H, Schelling K, Heisel C, Wang JS, Breusch SJ. Comparison of different vacuum mixing systems and bone cements with respect to reliability, porosity and bending strength. Acta Orthop Scand. 2004;75:160–72
19. Müller-Wille P, Wang J-S, Lidgren L (1996) Integrated system for preparation of bone cement and effects on cement quality and environment. J Biomed Mater Res (Applied Biomater) 38:135–142
20. Murphy BP, Prendergast PJ. The relationship between stress, porosity, and nonlinear damage accumulation in acrylic bone cement. J Biomed Mater Res. 2002;59(4):646–54
21. Rimnace CM, Wright TM, McGill DL. The effect of centrifugation on the fracture properties of acrylic bone cements. J Bone Joint Surg (Am)1986;68:281–7
22. Schelling K, Breusch SJ. Efficacy of a new prepacked vacuum mixing system with Palamed G bone cement. In: Walenkamp GHIM, Murray DW (eds) Bone cement and cementing technique. Springer, Berlin Heidelberg New York Tokyo, 2001, pp 97–107
23. Schlegel UJ, Sturm M, Ewerbeck V, Breusch S. Efficacy of vacuum mixing systems in reducing methylmethacrylate fume exposure. Comparison of 7 different vacuum mixing devices and open bowl mixing. Acta Scand Orthop. 2004;75(5):559–566
24. Schreurs BW, Spierings PT, Huiskes R, Slooff TJ. Effects of preparation techniques on the porosity of acrylic cements. Acta Orthop Scand. 1988;59:403–9
25. Wang JS, Kjellson F. The effect of volume of the mixing cartridge on bone cement porosity in vacuum mixing. Combined Orthopedic Research Society Meeting, June1-3, Rhodes, Greece. 2001, P 230
26. Wang JS, Kjellson F. Bone cement porosity in Vacuum Mixing system. In Bone cements and Cementing technique. In: Walenkamp GHIM, Murray DW (eds) Bone cement and cementing technique. Springer, Berlin Heidelberg New York Tokyo, 2001, pp 81–95
27. Wang JS, Franzén H, Jonsson E, Lidgren L. Porosity of bone cement reduced by mixing and collecting under vacuum. Acta Orthop Scand 1993;64(2):143–46
28. Wang JS, Taylor M, Flivik G, Lidgren L. Factors affecting the static shear strength of the prosthetic stem-bone cement interface. J of Mater Science: Mater in Med. 2003;14:55–61
29. Wang J-S, Toksvig-Larsen S, Müller-Wille P, Franzén H. Is their any difference between vacuum mixing systems in reducing bone cement porosity? J Biomed Mater Res (Applied Biomaterials) 1996;33:115–19
30. Wilkinson JM, Eveleigh R, Hamer AJ, Milne A, Miles AW, Stockely I. Effect of mixing technique on the properties of acrylic bone cement. J of Arthroplasty. 2000;15:663–7
31. Wixon RL, Lautenschlager EP, Novak MA. Vacuum mixing of acrylic bone cement. J Arthroplasty. 1987;2:141–49
32. Yau WP, Ng TP, Chiu KY, Poon KC, Ho WY, Luk DK. The performance of three vacuum mixing cement guns- acomparison of the fatigue properties of Simplex P cement. International Orthopaedics. 2001;25:290–293

Bone Preparation: The Importance of Establishing the Best Bone-Cement Interface

Clive Lee

Summary

This chapter describes the interface between bone cement and bone, pointing out that the operating surgeon is responsible for establishing that interface at the time of surgery. If the interface is not well established at the start, the replacement joint has no chance of long-term function. The cement-bone interface is a mechanical interlock between the two materials that can be enhanced by the preparation of the bone surface, pressurising cement into that surface and holding the cement under pressure until its viscosity is such that bone bleeding cannot displace it. Effective pressurisation can only be obtained using suitable instruments. The effect of heating the femoral stem before insertion is described. The surgeon has to be aware of the effect of all the variables in order that the strongest possible interface is obtained at the time of surgery.

Introduction

It has been estimated that aseptic loosening of an implant component causes approximately 75% of failures of cemented total hip arthroplasties [17]. Aseptic component loosening implies that the interface between cement and bone has failed in some degree. Consequently, it is plain to see that establishing the best possible interface between cement and bone should be a primary concern of a surgeon performing hip arthroplasty.

Structure of the Interface Between Bone and Cement

It was pointed out by Ling [16] in 1986 that the interface between any orthopaedic implant and bone is not a simple abutment of bone against implant, but is composed of complex junctional tissues that separate the implant from the host bone. The nature of the junctional tissues depends substantially on mechanical factors, given that the implant itself is basically non-reactive. The junctional tissues can vary between a state of osseointegration, to fibrous tissue and fibrocartilage, and cutting out or early mechanical loosening. The junctional tissues that result at the interface are dependent on a balance between the strength of the initial mechanical interlock between implant and host, and the magnitude of the applied loads. The surgeon is responsible for the strength of the initial interlock, the patient applies the loads during activity after the operation. High interface strength plus relatively low loads can result in osseointegration between implant and bone; low interface strength plus high loads will give a thick soft tissue layer between implant and bone. It is the duty of the surgeon at the time of the initial operation to ensure that the mechanical interlock between cement and bone is as good as it is possible to achieve. The clinical verification of the principle stated by Ling has been shown in a number of papers, as an example, Iwaki et al. [13] showed that, with secure initial fixation, minimal migration of the implant component and no radiolucent lines, then no lytic lesions will develop by five years and no aseptic loosening by ten years. On the other hand, insecure initial fixation shown by more rapid migration and progressive radiolucent lines at two years, leads to lytic lesions at five years and loosening at ten years. They state that the outcome of total hip replacement is determined at the initial operation and may be predicted at two years – loosening is due to failure of the operating technique. Loosening occurred, not because of lysis, but because it represented the end point of a process that had been present subclinically from the time of operation.

Obtaining the Best Mechanical Interlock Between Cement and Bone

Details of the surgical technique that should be used to obtain the best possible mechanical interlock between cement and bone are given later in this chapter and the next. However, a number of factors need to be stated at the outset to 'set the scene'. Bone cement is not a glue or adhesive – it does not bond with any significant strength to implant stem or cup, or to bone. The strength of the interface between cement and bone depends on a mechanical interlock between cement and bone – that is, it depends on the establishment of a bone-cement composite by forcing cement into the spaces in trabecular bone before the cement polymerises in place. The strength of this interlock also depends on the nature of the stresses present at the interface. The interface can resist compressive stresses best, then shear stresses and resists tensile stresses worst. Fortunately, tensile stresses at the interface are relatively small, but shear stresses are significant and shear failure of the interface has to be resisted. Halawa et al. [9] investigated the shear strength of trabecular bone from the femur and some factors affecting the shear strength of the cement-bone interface. They determined that the strongest trabecular bone is to be found close to the cortico-cancellous bone junction (within 3 mm of the cortex). In vitro, the strongest cement-bone interface strength is obtained by exposing strong cancellous bone and thoroughly cleaning it, afterwards forcing cement into the bony spaces under pressure. In-vitro tests showed that for push out tests on matching slices of femur/cement:

- With 2–3 mm of cancellous bone, load at failure was 100% higher than with 5 mm of cancellous bone.
- A cleaned bone surface gave 200% higher load at failure than a not cleaned surface.
- Insertion of cement at 3 minutes gave load at failure 60% higher than insertion of cement at 6 minutes.
- Pressurising cement at 0.3 N/mm^2 gave load at failure 100% higher than pressurisation at 0.15 N/mm^2.
- Difference for load at failure between using the best and worst techniques for establishing the cement-bone interface was 800%.

Consequential Effects of Establishing the Bone-Cement Interface

It is shown above that the strongest bone-cement interface is a composite of bone and cement formed by pressurising cement into the open trabecular spaces of the bone. It is necessary to examine the effects that such techniques may have on the patient at the time of the operation and subsequently.

In order to clean the bony spaces after the cavity has been formed in the bone, pressure lavage is used (see section 5.2.1 below). Following lavage, the bone should be dried and blood flow discouraged at the interface. Ribbon gauze soaked in 10 vol% hydrogen peroxide is often used for this purpose and has been used by the author's surgical colleagues for more than 30 years. The effectiveness of hydrogen peroxiode as a haemostatic agent has been shown by Hankin et al. [10]. They used hydrogen peroxide and saline to treat metaphyseal bone sites in ten mongrel dogs, six sites in each dog. Hydrogen peroxide was used at three sites, saline (control) at three sites and the haemostatic effect of both noted. Post treatment blood loss was significantly less for the hydrogen peroxide treated sites than for the saline controls – for hydrogen peroxide there was a mean reduction in bleeding of 38.7 mg/cm^2/min, saline had a mean increase of 26.0 mg/cm^2/min. When using hydrogen peroxide in the femoral cavity, it is important to have a catheter vent tube in the cavity below the level of the ribbon gauze to allow any oxygen liberated to be vented to atmosphere, preventing the possibility of (air) embolism. When used properly, hydrogen peroxide soaked gauze is a safe and effective way of treating bone before cement pressurisation.

After cleaning the bone, cement is pressurised into its open trabecular spaces. According to Askew et al. [1], bone cement should be maintained at a pressure of at least 76 kPa (0.75 bar) for 5 seconds to achieve adequate penetration of cement into bone. This paper presented results from in-vitro studies, these do not take bone bleeding into account. Bleeding pressure in femora during total hip replacement operations was measured by Heyse-Moore and Ling [11] who reported bleeding pressures of between 0 and 36 cm of saline (0–27 mm of Hg). The effect of bone bleeding was assessed experimentally by Benjamin et al. [2]. They used a simple model to demonstrate the ability of blood to displace bone cement after it has been introduced into the femoral cavity. Their apparatus consisted of a cylinder of Perspex into which 80×1 mm diameter holes had been drilled. Bone cement was introduced into the cylinder and levelled off at the top. An annulus surrounded the cylinder, which could be filled with blood at a known pressure. Blood pressure was controlled by raising or lowering the reservoir containing the blood (◘ Fig. 5.1).

When blood was allowed to surround the cement in the cylinder, at pressures up to the maximum measured in patients, the cement was displaced upwards, out of the cylinder, for times up to six minutes after the start of mixing (Simplex RO cement at room temperature). A second simple experiment was then carried out, in which the apparatus previously used was modified by the addition of a tube filled with liquid and placed over the opening of the central cylinder (◘ Fig. 5.2).

When the pressure exerted by the blood in the reservoir was greater than that exerted by the liquid in the tube (liquid level below blood level) the cement continued to be displaced upwards, out of the tube (■ Fig. 5.3a). When the pressure exerted by the blood in the reservoir was less than that exerted by the liquid in the tube (liquid level above blood level) the cement was displaced from the tube, through the holes and into the blood (■ Fig. 5.3b).

These simple experiments demonstrated that the time of pressurisation needed to be extended considerably (to at least 6 minutes after the start of mixing for Simplex bone cement at room temperature) to prevent a lamination of blood forming between the cement and the bone. Pressurisation of cement into bone requires the use of seals and pressurisers, many such instruments have been developed over the years. Lee and Ling [14] describe an acetabular pressuriser that was first used in 1972 and is still in use today. Use of the acetabular pressuriser was

shown to be able to maintain raised pressure for several minutes and significantly increase the penetration of cement into bone. Continuous monitoring of arterial blood pressure while using the pressuriser produced no evidence of any unusual effects due to its use [4]. Other pressurisers have been assessed for effectiveness and are reported in Dunne et al. [6].

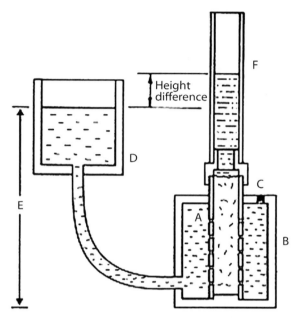

A   Cylinder, containing bone cement
B   Annulus around cylinder
C   Vent
D   Blood reservoir
E   Variable height, setting blood pressure
F   Tube, containing water

■ **Fig. 5.2.** Bleeding apparatus, modified

A   Cylinder, containing bone cement
B   Annulus around cylinder
C   Vent
D   Blood reservoir
E   Variable height, setting blood pressure

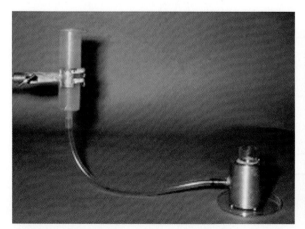
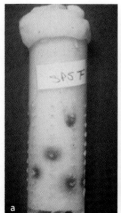
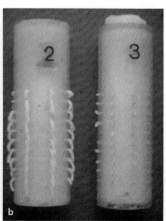

■ **Fig. 5.1.** Diagram and picture of bleeding apparatus

■ **Fig. 5.3. a** Bone cement displaced out of tube by blood. **b** Bone cement displaced through holes in tube by pressure on cement

Pressurisation of Cement in the Femur

A simple cement pressuriser has been in use in Exeter and elsewhere for a number of years (Stryker Cement Gun Mk.II, Primary Cement Syringe, Proximal Cement Seal).

The prepared femoral medullary cavity is filled with cement using the cement gun and syringe, the seal is fitted over the syringe nozzle and the nozzle cut to be flush with the end of the seal. The seal is pressed into the cut end of the femur, forming a closed cavity that is full of cement. More cement is injected into the cavity, putting the cement under pressure and forcing it into the bony spaces of the inside of the femoral medullary cavity. As the cement is forced into the bone, so fat is forced out and through the bone, visibly oozing out of the exposed surface of the femur. Pressure is maintained on the cement by periodically injecting more cement into the cavity, until sufficient time has passed for the cement to remain where it is placed. Pressures generated at the proximal end, the mid-diaphysis and the distal end of a Sawbones femur were measured in the laboratory using miniature pressure transducers. ◳ Figure 5.4a shows pressures generated dur-

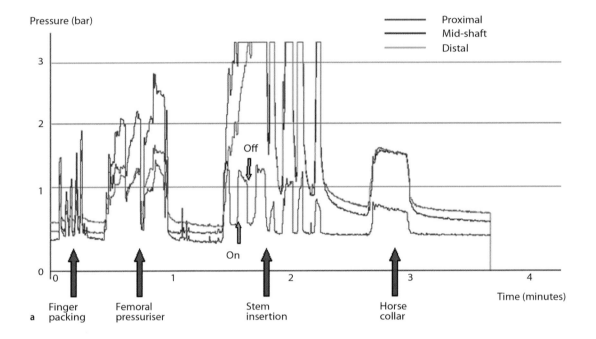

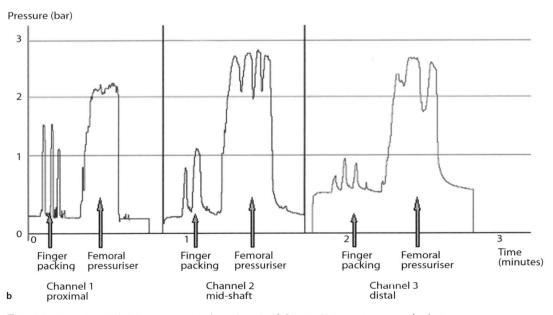

◳ **Fig. 5.4. a** Pressurisation during cementation and stem insertion. **b** Pressure in cement at measured points

ing the whole pressurisation to implant insertion cycle; ☐ Fig. 5.4b shows pressures generated at the three measuring points during cement pressurisation. It can be seen that pressures exceeding 2 bar (202,65 kPa) can be obtained using the pressuriser, ensuring excellent penetration of bone by cement. Pressures generated during stem insertion are even higher, but this is primarily caused by the cement being very viscous, leading to high pressures; the cement is stable within the bone spaces following pressurisation.

The way in which cement is mixed has changed over the years, currently most modern cementing techniques recommend the use of a vacuum mixing system – in the 1st Annual Report of the National Joint Register for England and Wales, 89.5% of cases used vacuum mixing for the femoral cement and 88.8% of cases used vacuum mixing for the acetabular cement [18]. Vacuum mixing of cement decreases the porosity of the cement but also increases the shrinkage of the cement on polymerisation (the effects of vacuum mixing and porosity in cement are also discussed elsewhere in this book: ▶ chapters 3.6, 4.1, 4.2). Gilbert et al. [7] showed that Simplex shrinks by 5.09% when hand mixed and by 6.67% when vacuum mixed; Endurance cement shrinks by 6.50% when vacuum mixed. The shrinkage typically occured between 400 and 600 seconds after start of mixing – this is after pressurisation of cement had been completed, therefore pressurisation should have little effect on countering shrinkage. Haas et al. [8] report different results – they report cement shrinkage of 2.3% with a specimen of 9.0% porosity, and 5.3% shrinkage and 0.8% porosity with a specimen polymerised in a mould at constant pressure. They state the theoretical shrinkage of cement as a result of polymerisation of the monomer to be between 7.6 and 8%.

It is also becoming more common to heat the femoral stem before insertion. Li et al. [15] showed that heating the stem changes the direction of polymerisation of the cement – with a pre-heated stem the cement polymerises first around the stem and the wave of polymerisation progresses from the stem to the bone. The effect of the pre-heating is stated to be unlikely to produce significant thermal necrosis of the bone. Iesaka et al. [12] showed that heating a stem to 37 °C decreased the porosity of the cement at the stem-cement interface by 99%, decreased the setting time by 12% and increased the bone-cement interface temperature by 6 °C. Similar effects were observed when heating a stem to 44 °C and 50 °C. Bishop et al. [3] showed that porosity was dramatically reduced at the stem cement interface when a stem was heated above 44 °C. Heating of the stem caused a negligible increase in the temperature generated in the bone. Shrinkage of the bone cement caused it to try to pull away from the cement-bone interface (it polymerises around the stem first) but shrinkage displacements were reported to be small compared with the macro interlock into bone – the load bearing capacity of this interface was unlikely to be compromised. Bone cement shrinkage and porosity around a pre-heated implant is easily seen in a

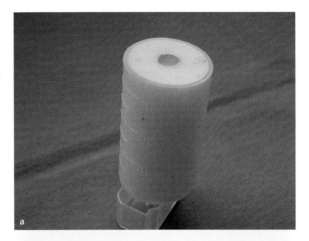

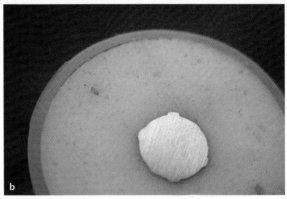

☐ **Fig. 5.5. a** Implant and cement in syringe. **b** Shrinkage gap between cement and syringe; porosity in cement forced away from implant towards syringe

simple laboratory experiment as described by Draenert [5] (▶ chapter 3.6) and repeated by the author for this chapter. ☐ Fig. 5.5a shows a specimen of cement.

Take Home Messages

- The interface between cement and bone must be as strong as possible.
- The strongest interface is formed by forcing cement into the spaces in trabecular bone and holding it there until the cement polymerises, forming a composite of bone and cement.
- A number of factors can affect the interface, including cleaning and haemostasis, cement mixing, pressurisation and component heating.
- The surgeon must be aware of the effect of all these variables in order that the strongest possible cement-bone interface is obtained at the primary procedure.
- It is the duty of the surgeon at the time of the initial operation to ensure that the mechanical interlock between cement and bone is as good as it is possible to achieve.

References

1. Askew MJ, Steege JW, Lewis JL, Ranieri JR, Wixson RL (1984) Effect of cement pressure and bone strength on polymethylmethacrylate fixation. J Orthop Res, 1(4): 412–420

2. Benjamin JB, Volz RG, Gie GA, Ling RSM, Lee AJC (1987) Cementing technique and the effects of bleeding. J Bone Joint Surg 69-B:620–624

3. Bishop NE, Ferguson S, Tepic S (1966) Porosity reduction in bone cement at the cement-stem interface. J Bone Joint Surg 78-B:349–356

4. Cadle D, James M, Ling RSM, Piper RF, Pryer DL, Wilmshurst CC (1972) Cardiovascular responses after methylmethacrylate cement. BMJ 4:107

5. Draenert K. Histomorphology of the bone-to-cement contact. In: Draenert K, Draenert Y, Garde U, Ulrich Ch (eds) Manual of cementing technology. Springer, Berlin Heidelberg New York Tokyo, pp 4–18

6. Dunne NJ, Orr JF, Beverland DE (2004) Assessment of cement introduction and pressurization techniques. Proc Inst Mech Engrs Vol.218, Part H, Eng in Med H1:11–25

7. Gilbert JL, Hasenwinkel JM, Wixson RL, Lautenschlager EP (2000) A theoretical and experimental analysis of polymerisation shrinkage of bone cement: a potential major source of porosity. J Biomed Mater Res 52:210–218

8. Haas SS, Brauer GM, Dickson G (1975) Characterization of polymethylmethacrylate bone cement. J Bone Joint Surg 57-A:380–391

9. Halawa M, Lee AJC, Ling RSM, Vangala SS (1978) The shear strength of trabecular bone from the femur, and some factors affecting the shear strength of the cement-bone interface. Arch Orthop Traum Surg 92:19–30

10. Hankin FM, Campbell SE, Goldstein SA, Matthews LS (1984) Hydrogen peroxide as a topical hemostatic agent. Clin Orthop Rel Res 186:244–248

11. Heyse-Moore GH, Ling RSM (1983) Current cement techniques. In: Marti RK (ed) Progress in cemented total hip surgery and revision. Exerpta Medica, Amsterdam

12. Iesaka K, Jaffe WL, Kummer FJ (2003) Effects of preheating of hip prostheses on the stem-cement interface. J Bone Joint Surg 85-A:421–427

13. Iwaki H, Scott G, Freeman MAR (2002) The natural history and significance of radiolucent lines at a cemented femoral interface. J Bone Joint Surg 84-B:550–555

14. Lee AJC, Ling RSM (1974) A device to improve the extrusion of bone cement into the bone of the acetabulum in the replacement of the hip joint. Biomedical Engineering 9:522–524

15. Li C, Schmid S, Mason J (2003) Effects of pre-cooling and pre-heating procedures on cement polymerisation and thermal necrosis in cemented hip replacements. Med Eng Phys 25:559–564

16. Ling RSM (1986) Observations on the fixation of implants to the bony skeleton. Clin Orthop Rel Res 210:80–96

17. Malchau H et al. (2002) Prognosis of total hip replacement – update of results and risk-ratio analysis for revision and re-revision from the Swedish National Hip Arthroplasty Register 1979–2000. 69th Annual Meeting of the AAOS, February 13–17, 2002, Dallas, USA

18. National Joint Registry for England and Wales – Summary Report to the 1st Annual Report (2004). National Joint Registry (NJR) Centre, Harwell, Oxfordshire OX11 0QJ, England

Bone Preparation: Femur

Steffen J. Breusch

Summary

The aim during cement application is to establish a durable interface between cement and cancellous bone and furthermore an even, non-deficient cement mantle. Preservation of strong cancellous bone and meticulous cleansing using pulsatile lavage are of utmost importance. A minimum cement mantle thickness of 2–3 mm is regarded essential to minimise the risk of osteolysis and loosening. Cement mantle thickness depends on femoral anatomy, femoral bone/canal preparation, stem size and design and centralizer usage. Critical zones of cement mantle thickness exist in Gruen zones 8/9 and 12, which can only be assessed on lateral radiographs. By recognising these factors, the surgeon can minimize the risk of typical modes of failure.

5.2.1 Femoral Preparation and Pulsatile Lavage

Introduction

In this chapter the rationale and technique for preparing the cancellous bone bed to establish a durable cement-bone interface are discussed.

Why Should We Preserve Cancellous Bone?

To achieve adequate cement interdigitation and a viable interlock, preservation of cancellous bone stock is of great importance. Although Charnley initially believed from his experience in fracture healing, that cancellous bone cannot carry the load [21], he later advocated preservation of cancellous bone for cemented anchorage[22]: »… The cancellous structure can be regarded as a system of springs; the superficial layer of the cancellous bone in contact with the surface of the cement will *move as one* with the cement surface when load is applied; the deflection of the cancellous structure will take place inside the bulk of cancellous bone. In this way, we can explain the paradox of the transmission of load from a hard to a soft substance without relative motion taking place between the surfaces in contact. It is on these grounds that I believe it is an advantage to have a layer of cancellous bone interposed between a cement surface and cortical bone.« Based on his further clinical experience he later recommended preservation of 2–3 mm strong cancellous bone adjacent to the endosteal surface [23]. Draenert confirmed this view (▶ chapter 3.6) with his light- and electronmicroscopy findings in meticulous animal and post-mortem studies [10, 29]. Preserved cancellous bone filled and stiffened with cement forms a viable construct/composite which is resistant to deformation and is capable to carry the load [29]. Numerous in-vitro experiments have shown a strong correlation between improved cement penetration and increased shear strength of the cement-bone interface [2, 5, 38, 47, 57, 63, 66, 74, 81] (▶ chapter 5.1). The interface strength is not only affected by the degree of cement penetration but also by the quality of the supporting cancellous framework [2, 13, 57].

This concept of creating a sound cement-bone construct is also supported by clinical and radiological experience. In a long-term radiographic study, Ebramzadeh et al. [30] discovered inferior outcome in cases where proximal cancellous bone had not been filled with cement. In conclusion, they advocated removal of all medial cancellous bone. In contrast, Beckenbaugh and Ilstrup [7] had already pointed out that poorer outcome is not determined by preservation of bone, but due to failure to adequately »pack« the cement into proximal cancellous bone. In cases with poor proximal cement penetration a twofold increase in loosening rates had been observed [7].

Based on a 3-dimensional finite element model, Ayers and Mann [3] recommended removal of weak proximal medial cancellous bone to increase the cement mantle thickness. The rigorous removal of cancellous bone was also suspected by Pellicci et al. [83] as a cause for failure. Less aggressive removal of cancellous bone has been associated with minimal femoral loosening rates after more then ten years [78] and Schulte et al. [86]. In this context, the poorer outcome of cemented femoral revisions [67] with deficient cancellous bone stock are of note and contradict the recommendation of removal of cancellous bone. Furthermore, cadaver studies [27] on the stability of the cement-bone interface in the revision scenario have provided convincing evidence supporting the concept of preservation of cancellous bone. After the first revision the interface shear strength was reduced dramatically to 20.6%, and decreased further to as little as 6.8% after the second revision compared to the primary situation.

It is therefore on these grounds that preservation of strong cancellous bone (◘ Fig. 5.6) should be regarded of great importance.

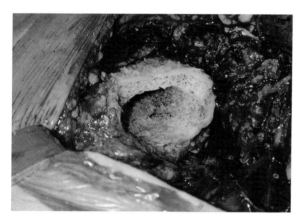

◘ **Fig. 5.6.** Intraoperative photograph of proximal end of the femur after bone preparation. Note that anteriorly and medially strong cancellous bone has been preserved for cement interdigitation

Femoral Bone Preparation

To preserve cancellous bone stock, careful femoral bone preparation is essential. Controversy exists regarding the optimal method of bone preparation for a cemented femoral stem [26]. DiGiannini [26] et al. reviewed the limited literature available on this subject and challenged the rationale and concept of the popular »ream and broach« preparation. It is indeed difficult to understand why destructive reamers should be inserted until the endosteal surface is hit. This intriguing manoeuvre removes cancellous bone thus creating a poor distal bone stock which is more similar to the revision situation. Reaming to cortex also increases the risk of bleeding by disrupting the arterial supply thus jeopardising the establishment of a sound interface. Some laboratory studies have confirmed the detrimental effect of reamers on the shear strength of the cement-bone interface [4, 73] when compared with »broach only« techniques. Impaction of bone debris, which seems to be beneficial for cementless fixation [35], may contribute to primary stability in vitro [14, 20]. But this »concept« contradicts the proven advantages of lavaged bone with improved cement penetration and shear strength [5, 13, 15, 16, 38, 57, 66].

A previous study [14] has shown, that significant destruction of the adjacent trabeculae [29] can occur when blunt chipped tooth broaches of maximum size were inserted. Fortunately, removal of cancellous bone in the curved femur is almost never complete, which may offer an explanation why the published clinical results do not reveal a distinct difference between »ream and broach« and »broach only« techniques. A less traumatic method of bone preparation and preservation can be achieved using diamond wet-grinders [29], but no clinical results are available to support the theoretical advantage of this technique. If pulsatile lavage is strictly implemented, cement penetration does not seem to depend on broach surface design, when comparing »chipped tooth« with »diamond tooth« broaches (◘ Fig. 5.7) [14].

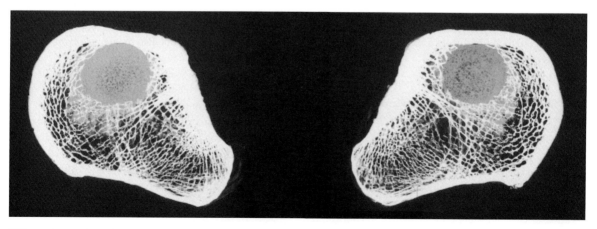

◘ **Fig. 5.7.** Microradiographic evaluation of cement penetration for matched femoral pairs broached using either a chipped or diamond tooth broach taken at the level of the lesser trochanter. There was no significant difference between broach type with regard to cement penetration

In summary, »broach only« techniques seem preferable and may be regarded as the »gold standard«, but careful bone sparing techniques should be implemented whichever technique or instruments are used.

Pulsatile Lavage is Mandatory!

In the late 1970s, Halawa et al. [38] had already demonstrated the significance of bone quality and bone lavage prior to cementation with regard to improved mechanical shear strength. Krause et al. [57] observed in human tibias that the depth of bone cleaning using lavage had a tendency to limit the depth of cement penetration. Bannister and Miles [5] had also found improved cement penetration and increased interface strength when bone lavage was used.

To our knowledge, it is common practice to use some form of lavage prior to cement application. However, only a few studies have concentrated on the effectiveness of the lavage type. Krause et al. [57] reported improved cement penetration and shear strength when high intensity lavage was used. Majkowski et al. [66] evaluated the effect of bone surface preparation upon cement penetration using slices of bovine bone. They found no difference between continuous and pulsed pressurized lavage and no further beneficial effect of brushing.

Although the benefit of pulsatile lavage has been documented both experimentally [15, 16, 38, 66] and clinically [67], national surveys in the United Kingdom [43] and Germany [12] have elucidated a low prevalence of pressurised jet-lavage in cemented THA. Syringe-lavage is often used as an alternative. Maistrelli et al. [65] compared jet-lavage versus syringe-lavage in human tibial specimens obtained at total knee arthroplasty and found significantly better penetration in the jet-lavage group. However, the authors only commented on the time of lavage but not on the amount of irrigation used. Therefore it remained unclear whether volume or lavage quality is the more important factor.

Jet-Lavage Versus Syringe Lavage

It is important to distinguish between various lavage types and volumes. In a novel model, using entire paired human femora and not bone slices to allow assessment of the entire femoral architecture, the effect of irrigation type rather than total volume upon cement penetration in the proximal femur was studied [15]. Sixteen-paired human cadaver femora were prepared using conventional broaches. Cancellous bone was irrigated with 1 litre pulsed lavage in one femur and with 1 litre syringe-lavage in the contralateral femur. The specimens were imbedded in specially designed pots (Fig. 5.8) and vacuum-mixed bone cements were applied in a retrograde manner. After application of a standardised pressure, the femora were removed, radiographed and horizontal sections were ob-

tained and analysed to assess cement penetration. These in vitro results showed that in equal quality bone, the use of jet-lavage yields significantly (p < 0.0001) improved rates of cement penetration compared to syringe-lavage specimens (Figs. 5.9 and 5.10).

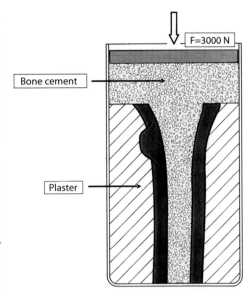

 Fig. 5.8. Experimental configuration of a femur embedded in a canister using plaster of Paris. Bone cement was applied in retrograde manner in the femoral canal and up to the top of the canister. A 3000 N load was applied to the canister lid pressurising the femoral canal in a controlled manner allowing for standardised cement pressurisation

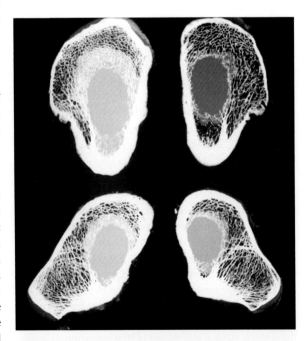

 Fig. 5.9. Microradiographs. Cement penetration for jet-lavage and syringe lavage sections taken at the level of the lesser trochanter. Cement penetration was significantly (p>0,0001) increased (see Fig. 5.10) in all specimens with jet-lavage (*left*) compared to the syringe-lavage specimens (*right*)

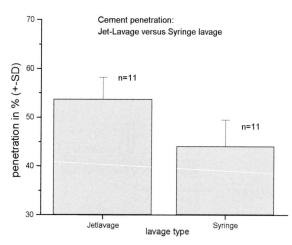

Fig. 5.10. Jet-lavage versus syringe lavage: Statistical outcome of cement penetration of paired femora (see ▣ Fig. 5.9)

To directly compare the effectiveness of both pulsatile jet- and syringe-lavage with regard to cement penetration in vivo under bleeding conditions, a new sheep model allowing for standardised bilateral, simultaneous cement pressurisation was created [16]. After femoral neck osteotomies, both femoral cavities of 10 sheep were prepared for retrograde cement application. After randomisation, one side was lavaged with 250 ml irrigation using a bladder syringe, the contralateral femur with the identical volume but using a pulsatile lavage. A specially designed apparatus was used to allow for bilateral simultaneous cement pressurisation. Microradiographs were taken and analysed using image analysis to assess cement penetration into cancellous bone. The results confirmed the superiority of jet-lavage bone surface preparation (p=0.002) compared to syringe-lavage also under in-vivo conditions.

Impact of Lavage and Pressurisation

The impact and relationship of pulsatile lavage and pressurisation (▶ chapter 5.1) had further been studied using 60 human cadaver femora [13]. Bone lavage was carried out either using jet-lavage or manual syringe lavage, cement application differed with regard to the amount of pressurisation used. Five different stem designs were implanted. Both jet-lavage and cement pressurisation significantly improved the penetration of cement into cancellous bone (p=0.027 and p=0.003, respectively). Stem insertion alone (without additional pressurisation during retrograde gun application and proximal seal) resulted in inferior rates of cement penetration. An influence of the stem type upon outcome (penetration) was not observed, confirming that the femoral stem, a sole means of pressurization, is inadequate. In correlation to the statistical clinical evidence from the Swedish hip register [67] (▶ chapter 11), the positive effect of pulsatile lavage in this study also proved at least as important as sustained pressurisation. In the presence

of strong, dense cancellous bone these findings were more pronounced [13]. High pressurising techniques are an effective means, but must be combined with jet-lavage to also reduce the risk of thrombo-embolic complications.

In summary, not only an improved cement-bone interface and longer implant survival, but also a reduced risk of fat embolism (▶ chapter 15) support the concept of pulsatile lavage. It seems justified to conclude from all experimental and clinical available, that the use of high-volume pressurised jet-lavage for cleaning of the intra-medullary cavity prior to cement application should be regarded mandatory in cemented total hip arthroplasty.

> **Take Home Messages**
>
> - When preparing the proximal femur a layer of at least 2–3 mm strong cancellous bone should be preserved for cement interdigitation and establishment of a durable cement-bone interface.
> - Clinical and experimental evidence have proven that pulsatile lavage is at least equally important for cement interdigitation when compared with pressurisation.
> - Pulsatile lavage not only improves cement penetration, but also significantly reduces the risk of embolic complications to be encountered with cement pressurisation.
> - The use of pulsatile lavage is considered mandatory for cleansing of the bone bed in cemented THA; manual bone lavage is less/not effective.

5.2.2 The Optimal Cement Mantle

Introduction

In this chapter the importance of a non-deficient cement mantle is highlighted and all aspects of how to achieve this are discussed.

Optimal Cement Mantle Thickness

Although no clear definition exists for the »ideal« cement mantle thickness, there is little doubt that a deficient cement mantle may be detrimental with regard to long-term implant survival. Thin layers of cement have less potential for energy absorption and may crack and fail [45, 59], in particular in the proximal and distal portions of the cement mantle [54]. Cement mantle fractures, localised osteolysis [19, 44, 68] and granuloma formation at the interface [1, 82] or failure [7, 79] may result as a consequence of direct implant to bone contact or very thin cement mantles around the stem tip [33, 79, 79]. Furthermore, deficient cement mantles create a pathway for particulate wear debris to migrate along the stem-cement interface down to the cement-bone interface thus initiating or accelerating particle induced osteolysis and loosening [46, 49]. In contrast, complete cement mantles with a minimum thickness of 2–3 mm have been reported to be associated with better long-term radiographic outcome [30, 52, 53].

Radiographic evaluation remains the basis for assessment of the cement mantle, the quality of cementing technique and the diagnosis of aseptic loosening. Various classifications and criteria for radiographic loosening have been proposed [6, 40, 51, 53, 70, 87, 88] including radiolucent lines, implant migration and cement mantle defects. Radiolucent lines at the cement-bone interface on the immediate postoperative film are clear evidence for inadequate cement interdigitation and poor surgical technique [36]. However, the significance of radiolucent lines [50, 60, 70] depends on stem surface (debonding), length of implantation and serial radiographic comparison. Furthermore, the adequacy of radiographic interpretation is subject to debate. Poor inter- and intraobserver reproducibility of radiographic cement mantle assessment have been reported [42, 55, 56, 64]. Cement mantle defects and the prevalence of thin cement mantles may be underestimated on routine radiographic assessment [17, 48, 79, 90]. Cadaver studies have shown a poor correlation between radiographic and microradiographic assessment of the cement-bone interface [48, 84]. Also, a clear distinction between pure cement mantles and cement mantles containing interdigitated cancellous bone has not been made and is difficult to attempt using plain radiographs.

In any case, a simple grading of postoperative cement filling of the femur is not only a useful clinical tool, but also has been shown to correlate with outcome [6].

Classification of Barrack et al. [6]:

- A = »white-out« at the cement bone interface (in which no distinction could be made between femoral cortex and cement in the diaphysis)
- B = slight radioluceny at the cement-bone interface
- C = defective or incomplete cement mantle (voids, defects, radiolucency >50%)
- D = poor cementing with failure to fill the canal, no cement below tip or 100% radiolucency

There is a high correlation between low cement grading and loosening of the femoral stem [33]. Gruen et al. [36] have described 4 modes of failure, which are all based on poor cementing: »incomplete cement encapsulation«, »poor (calcar) proximal-medial or distal (or combined) acrylic support«, and emphasising the importance of adequate cement mantle thickness. Although it is not justified to define an ideal cement mantle thickness, a minimum cement mantle thickness of 2 mm is widely accepted based on experimental, clinical and radiographic experience [2, 9, 30, 45, 53, 59, 61, 71, 83, 90]. The »optimal« cement mantle will invariably be uneven, as an inevitable mismatch between femoral stem

and intramedullary cavity exists. As a consequence, the cement mantle will be commonly asymmetric, but should not get thinner than 1–3 mm in mid and lower Gruen Zones (a.p.: 2–6, lateral: 9–13), to avoid metal-to-bone contact at all cost. In the proximal areas, where most of the load will be transmitted and in particular at the level of the medial calcar (corresponding to Gruen zone 7) probably at least 4–7 mm thickness should be achieved [3, 36, 71].

Factors Influencing Cement Mantle Quality and Thickness

The thickness and quality of a cement mantle are influenced by several factors:

- Quality of cementing technique
- Femoral anatomy (shape and bone architecture)
- Surgical technique (canal preparation and broaching)
- Stem design and instrumentation
- Centralizer usage
- Stem size

Quality of Cementing Technique

Several clinical studies have emphasised the fundamental influence of modern cementing techniques on improved outcome in cemented total hip arthroplasty [18, 40, 41, 67, 72, 85]. Modern cementing techniques aim to improve the mechanical interlock between bone and cement in order to establish a durable interface. With increased depth of cement penetration the strength of the cement-bone interface is enhanced [2, 38, 57, 81]. Thus, also the quality of the cement mantle, which comprises a layer of cement-cancellous bone composite and a pure layer of cement is improved. Thorough cleansing of the bone bed by the use of jet-lavage, of a distal intramedullary plug and a proximal seal (representing femoral pressurisation) reduce the risk for revision approximately 20% each [67]. These important aspects are covered in depth in the following chapters (▶ chapters 2.2, 3.6, 5.1, 6.1)

Femoral Anatomy

It is particularly intriguing that the hip joint is frequently visualised only in one plane in contrast to all other joints in orthopaedics! This is both true for the preoperative and the postoperative assessment of hip arthroplasty. The variation of anatomic shape of the proximal femur is an under-recognised variable affecting both stem alignment and also the cement mantle.

Several morphological bone indices have been introduced to classify different femoral geometry: Bone types A–C according to Dorr [28], the cortical index (CI) [37] and the canal flare index (CFI) [75] are the most commonly known classifications (◘ Figs. 5.11 and 5.12). Probably the most useful clinical classification (easy to use) is the one according to Dorr [28, 37], which assesses the

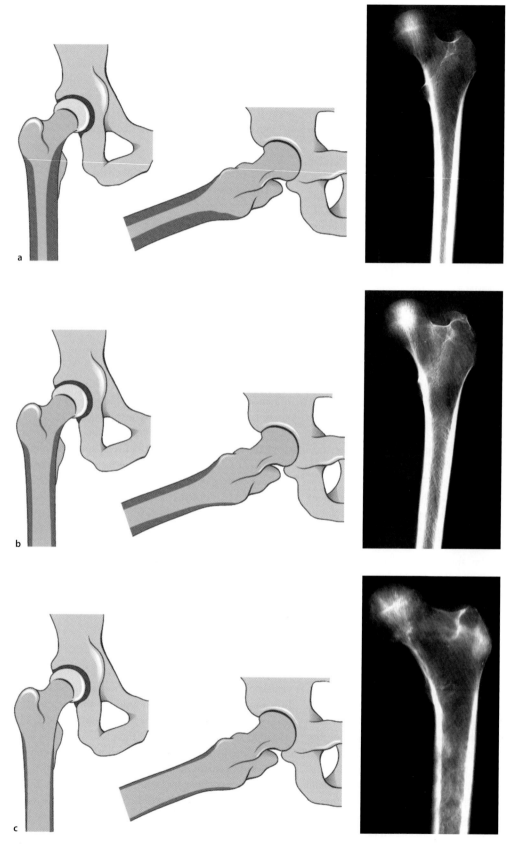

Fig. 5.11a–c. Dorr type A (**a**) with a »champagne flute« canal configuration and thick cortices. **b** Type B is the most common and normally shaped femur with moderate proximal flare. **c** With ageing and/or osteoporotic bone loss thinning of the cortices with widening of the canal leads to Type C, which is also called »stove pipe« femur

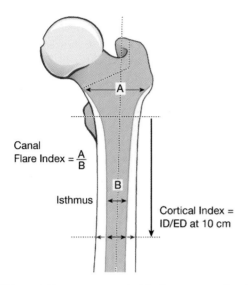

Metaphyseal width (A): _____ mm
Diaphyseal width at isthmus (B): _____ mm

Canal flare index: A/B = _____
stovepipe: < 3.0
━ normal: 3.0-4.7
━ champagne-fluted: 4.7-6.5

Internal femoral diameter (ID) at 10 cm :___ mm
External femoral diameter (ED) at 10 cm :___ mm

Cortical Index: ID/ED

◨ **Fig. 5.12.** Measurements required for determination of useful bone indices for preoperative planning: Canal flare index and cortical index

intramedullary femoral shape (◨ Fig. 5.11). Type B represents the most common canal configuration with normal thickness of the diaphyseal cortices and a mildly proximally fluted metaphysis (flare). If the inner canal narrows in the diaphysis (a), this is referred to as type A (or »champagne flute«) [75]. This is commonly the case in the younger male patient and often associated with a large femoral offset. Noble et al. [76] emphasised the effect of ageing on the shape of the proximal femur. Type-C bone with thinning of the cortices associated with osteoporosis is more common in the elderly and also called »stove pipe«.

It is obvious to say that in a wider canal a lower risk will exist for thin (<2 mm) cement mantles. Indeed, a cadaver study confirmed this correlation, but also revealed a higher risk of producing thin cement mantles in the lateral plane [17], even when preoperatively bone indices were determined [28, 37, 75] only on plain AP films. There seems to be an increased risk to produce thin cement mantles in type A femora, particularly when straight stems without centralizer are used or centralizers fail. Femoral bone indices may be useful in assessing the risk of thin cement mantles preoperatively (◨ Fig. 5.12).

Berger et al. [8] postulated that the distal anterior mid-shaft bowing of the femur predisposes anterior cement mantle deficiencies when centralizers are not used. In contrast, we could find no evidence for this mechanism and our results suggested that it is the proximal anatomy (and bowing) of the S-shaped femur which affects stem alignment in the sagittal plane most [17]. Furthermore, the tip of cemented stems with standard length do not usually extend beyond the isthmus of the distal femoral bow.

It is well worth re-visiting the lateral femoral geometry of the femur (◨ Fig. 5.13) to appreciate the proximal anatomy [25]. Crawford et al. [25] gave an anatomical explanation for incomplete cement mantles in the sagittal

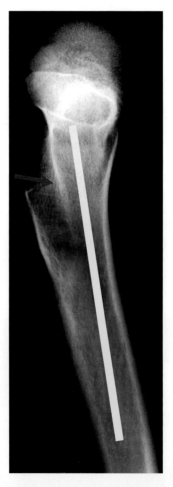

◨ **Fig. 5.13.** This lateral radiograph of the proximal femur emphasizes two important issues. Firstly, a straight stem (*yellow line*) does not follow the proximal femoral bowing. Secondly, the posterior extension of the neck, i.e. the true calcar femorale (*red arrow*) comprises a dense cortical structure (◨ Fig. 5.14), which tends to push all femoral instruments and the femoral stem anteriorly

femoral plane (see above). On the lateral radiograph the anterior proximal curve becomes evident as the femoral neck flows into the metaphysis. By simply drawing a straight line, mimicking a straight femoral stem within the canal (■ Fig. 5.13), a dilemma becomes evident: the femur is curved, but a straight femoral stem is not. Furthermore, the extension of the posterior femoral neck into the metapyhsis, the so-called calcar femorale (■ Fig. 5.14) divides the proximal femur into a posterior and an anterior compartment, with the latter accommodating the femoral stem.

Surgical Technique (Canal Preparation and Broaching)

Crawford et al. [25] emphasised the importance of operative technique necessary to minimise the risk of thin cement mantles in the sagittal plane. The assessment of the cement mantle and stem alignment is commonly done concentrating on standard anterior-posterior (AP) radiographs [6, 30, 34, 44, 56, 64]. As a topographical reference for comparison the Gruen zones 1–7 [36] are the accepted standard for evaluation of standard (AP) radiographs (■ Fig. 5.14). However, far less is known about the cement mantle thickness and stem alignment (and their clinical significance) as visualised on the lateral projection [8, 39, 42, 51, 53].

Lateral radiographs are essential to detect inadequate cement mantle thickness, which typically seem to occur antero-proximally in Gruen zones 8/9, particularly when straight stems are used and posterior-distally in Gruen zone 12 (■ Fig. 5.15) without centralizer [17, 33, 90]. If the true lateral projection is not used, than the frequency of cement mantle defects is underestimated [80].

It is impossible to always avoid posterior angulation so long as straight stems are used in a curved femur [80].

Östgaard et al. [80] found well over 1/3 of all straight stems investigated associated with a »broken« cement mantle, i.e. stem to bone contact either in Zone 12 or 8/9. To minimise this pattern of oblique stem malalignment in the lateral plane, it is important to enter the proximal femur in the piriformis fossa, similar to intramedullary nailing. During subsequent broaching the broach must be kept in contact with the posterior cortex and intraoperatively a layer of anterior cancellous bone (see ■ Fig. 5.6) must be preserved (► chapter 2.2.). Similarly, to prevent unfavourable varus stem alignment [7, 8, 36, 79] and a thin cement mantle in Gruen Zone 7, lateral canal preparation is essential.

In a cadaver study [17], posterior canal entry through the piriformis fossa and removal of a prominent posterior calcar were implemented and a »normal« femoral neck cut (1.5–2 cm above the lesser trochanter) without complete destruction of the proximal anatomy was used. Despite this technique the observed pattern of oblique (straight) stem alignment in the lateral projection associated with thin cement mantles in Gruen zones 8/9 could not always be prevented (■ Fig. 5.16).

Lower femoral neck osteotomies and more aggressive removal [91] of the posterior anatomical calcar femorale [29] have been advocated to allow a more posterior canal entry and as a consequence better alignment of a straight stem is possible. However, sacrificing the femoral neck should jeopardise rotational stability thus increasing the risk of posterior stem migration, loosening and late dislocation.

Stem Design

Garellick et al. [33] and Östgaard et al. [80] observed this identical pattern of malalignment of Charnley stems in the lateral projection in a series implanted without trochanteric

Calcar femorale

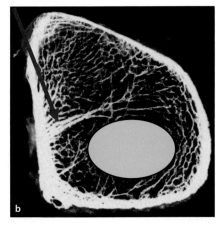

■ **Fig. 5.14a,b.** Horizontal microradiographs. The anatomical calcar femorale extends down to the lesser trochanter (**b**), thus dividing the femur into an anterior and a posterior compartment. It is in the anterior portion, where the femoral stem will be seated

osteotomies. Garellick et al. [33] compared stem alignment of Spectron (n=204) and Charnley stems (n=204) in the lateral projection and observed stem-bone contact in Gruen zone 8 (20% Charnley and 13% Spectron) and zone 12 (42% Charnley and 19% Spectron). This anatomical phenomenon may also offer an explanation, why in the initial Charnley series with trochanteric osteotomy better stem alignment (in the sagittal plane) and hence a lower risk of thin cement mantles were possible [80].

Similarly, in a standardised cadaver study [17] with radiographic and microradiographic analysis of 48 left femora, implanting four different stem designs (1 anatomic, 3 straight), the same phenomenon was found. In the frontal (AP) plane overall 88% of stems were aligned within one degree of neutral. In total 24 thin cement mantles (less than 2 mm) were determined in 19 specimens in Gruen zones 1 through 7 with no correlation to stem design or zone. In the sagittal plane typical areas of

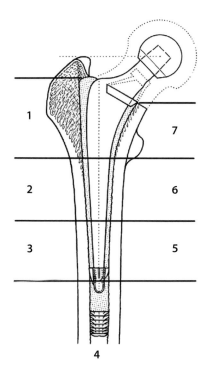

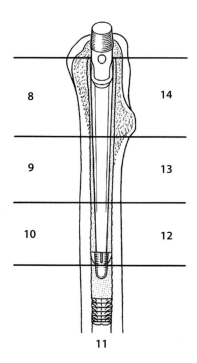

Fig. 5.15. Assessment of stem alignment and cement mantle thickness with reference to Gruen zones 1–7 in the AP plane [36] and 8–14 in the lateral plane [51]

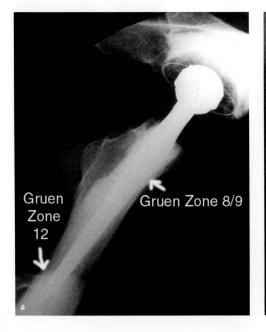

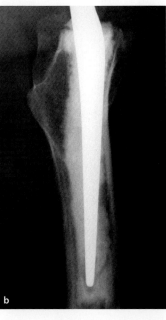

Fig. 5.16a,b. Postoperative cross-table lateral radiographs reveal a typical pattern of oblique stem alignment, particularly observed with straight stem designs. Due to the femoral geometry, naturally a risk for thin cement mantle exists antero-proximally in Gruen Zones 8/9 and if no centralizer is used in Zone 12

thin cement mantles were identified (◘ Fig. 5.17) in Gruen zones 8 and 9 (n=39) and 12 (n=21). The anatomic stem design carried the lowest risk of producing a thin cement mantle proximally in Gruen zones 8/9 (◘ Figs. 5.18 and 5.19). The risk for straight stem designs was more than 90%. Straight stems without a centralizer showed the highest risk of thin cement mantles in Gruen zone 12 (93%).

Valdivia et al. [90] compared 6 different stem designs, implanted in cadaveric femora, using plain radiography and computer tomography. The results confirmed that insertion of a straight stem will bring the implant close to the anterior and anteromedial aspects of the femur at the level of the lesser trochanter, making this region prone to deficient cement mantles and leaving little room for

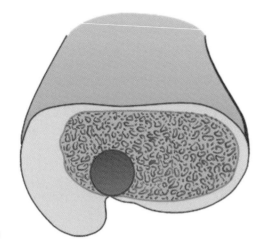
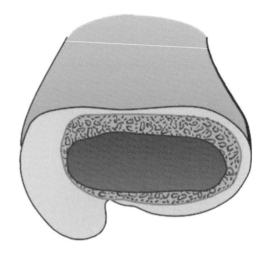

◘ **Fig. 5.17a,b.** To minimise the risk of stem malalignment and thin cement mantles, posterior canal entry in the fossa piriformis (**a**) and strict postero-lateral broaching are essential. A preserved layer of anterior-medial cancellous bone (see also ◘ Fig. 5.6) is a good intraoperative guide for correct canal preparation and reassures the surgeon

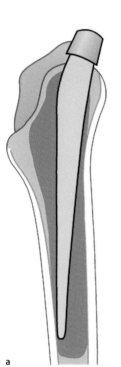
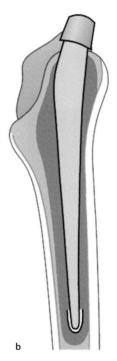
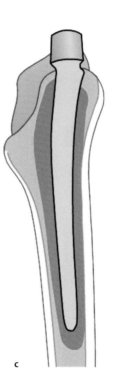
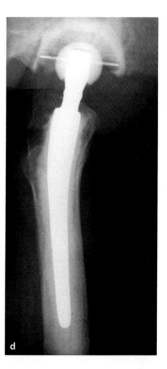

◘ **Fig. 5.18a–d.** Diagram of stem alignment in the lateral plane. A straight stem used without centralizer carries the highest risk of producing a thin cement mantle in Gruen Zone 8/9 and Zone 12 around the posterior stem tip, which typically can touch the posterior femoral cortex (◘ Fig. 5.20). In contrast, the use of a distal centralizer (**b**) eliminates the risk in Zone 12, but has no effect on the proximal cement mantle. An anatomic stem (**c,d**) respects the proximal anatomy and is associated with a lower risk of thin cement mantles technical errors. The authors [90] concluded that, »these results also should prompt manufacturers and investigators to consider the sagittal anatomy of the femur in design of the implant, instrumentation, and study of the cement mantle. A good stem design should reliably and reproducibly yield an adequate cement mantle under most conditions if implanted with reasonable skill.«

Centralizer Usage

Distal stem tip centralizers did reduce the risk of thin cement mantles in zone 12 (◘ Fig. 5.20a) but did not affect lateral stemmal alignment and thin cement mantles in zones 8/9 [17]. If anything, they seemed to increase the risk of thin cement mantles in zones 8/9, possibly by pushing the stem more anteriorly. When straight stems

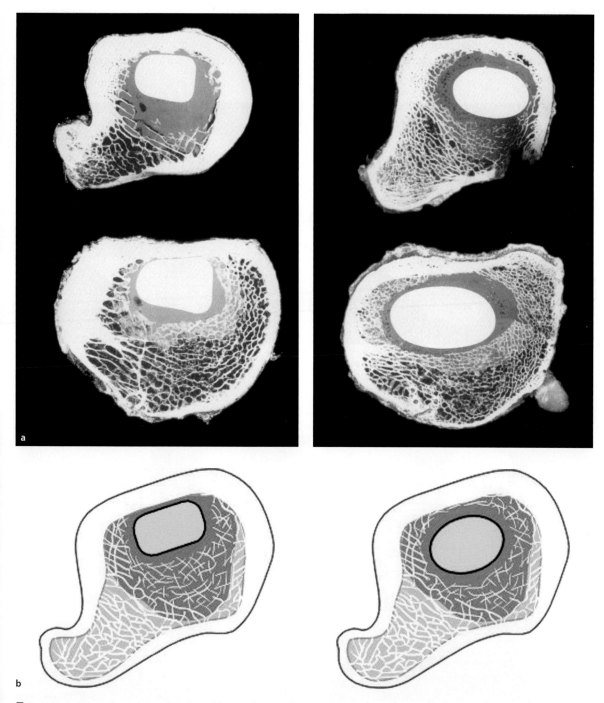

◘ **Fig. 5.19a,b.** Microradiographic analysis (**a**, *top*) from cadaver study [17] reveal the areas of thin cement mantles in Gruen zones 8 and 9 in correlation with the plain lateral radiographic appearance. In the femur with marked proximal bowing (see ◘ Fig. 5.13) the antero-proximal cement mantle may be very thin (<1–2 mm), in particular when straight stem designs are used (*left pictures*). This risk is significantly smaller with anatomic stem designs, which follow the proximal curve (◘ Fig. 5.18c). This becomes clearer on the schematic diagrams below (**b**, *bottom*)

without centralizer are used or centralizers fail, there seems to be an increased risk to produce thin cement mantles in Gruen zone 12 particularly in type A femora.

Small centralizers may fail to centralize the stem tip but were efficient to prevent direct bone-metal contact. Direct contact to bone of stem tip (◘ Fig. 5.20b) may be a starting point for osteolysis (◘ Fig. 5.21) but can also be seen in stable femoral components [19].

Similar to these findings Berger et al. [8] found centralizers only to have a significant effect in the distal zones with regard to fewer cement mantle deficiencies. Thus, it would appear that a distal centralizer fails to prevent prox-imal cement mantle deficiencies. The benefit of centralizers with regard to improved long-term outcome remains subject to debate [89]. Centralizers may adversely affect the peak strains around the stem tip [31]. Complications associated with the use of centralizers include dislodgement from the stem tip, void accumulation and fracture [8, 34, 39, 77]. However, there is increasing evidence that distal centralizers are useful to achieve a neutral stem alignment thus preventing an unfavourable varus position [7, 8, 36, 79], although stem varus/valgus malalignment in the frontal plane in our study did not correlate with the use of a centralizer or with stem or centralizer design.

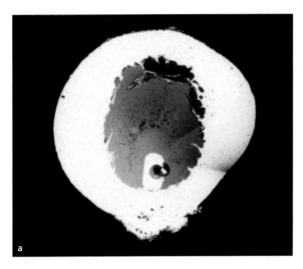
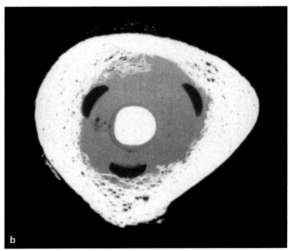

◘ **Fig. 5.20a,b.** Microradiographic images reveal direct contact between the stem tip and the posterior cortex in correlation to Gruen zone 12, when no centralizer is used (**a**). In contrast a well designed and sized centralizer is effective to assure adequate stem tip alignment and prevent cement mantle deficiencies

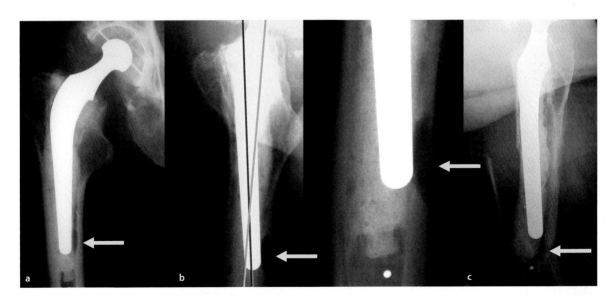

◘ **Fig. 5.21a–c.** Patchy distal osteolysis 5 years postoperatively (**a**). The lateral view reveals the typical oblique stem malalignment and shows posterior stem tip to bone contact in Gruen Zone 12 (**b**) with localized osteolysis (*yellow arrow*), which becomes more obvious at higher magnification (**c**). At 8 years the patient presented with pathological periprosthetic fracture through the distal osteolysis at the stem tip

Stem Size

Anatomy and stem shape are beyond the surgeons control, but stem size and stem design selection are the surgeon's responsibility. Large stem sizes implanted as »cemented press-fit« stems carry the risk of cement mantle deficiencies [11, 29] and may be associated with increased loosening rates [58, 69]. Krismer et al. [58] reported a revision rate of 1.9% after 6 to 8 years for Müller straight (cemented press-fit) stems, but considered another 20.1% radiographically at risk. Oversizing of the stem resulting in incomplete cement mantles has been suggested to account for early femoral component loosening also in Chinese patients with small femora [24]. This observation is supported by the finite-element model of Lee et al. [62] and the biomechanical testing of Fisher et al. [32]. Similar to Huddleston [44] they concluded that smaller stem sizes and not overbroaching are desirable to accomplish a favourable cement mantle thickness.

Results with Müller straight stems implanted using modern cementing techniques, where smaller stem sizes have probably been used to respect a minimum cement mantle thickness, are not dissimilar from results with other stem designs (Charnley, Exeter, Stanmore) [67]. Interestingly, excellent results have been achieved using the anatomically adapted prosthesis (▶ chapter 7.3, 11), e.g. SPII, [67], which carry a low risk of thin cement mantles [11, 17].

Consequences of Thin Cement Mantles

Thin layers of cement have less potential for energy absorption and may crack and fail [45, 59], in particular in the proximal and distal portions of the cement mantle [54]. Localised osteolysis [19, 44, 68] or failure [7, 79] may result as a consequence of direct bone contact or very thin cement mantles around the stem tip [76, 79, 80] – as observed in a significant number of straight stems without centralizer [33]. Radiographic scalloping has been reported to start about the proximal third of the stem [19] which would correlate to the thin cement mantles in zones 8/9 in our study which cannot be detected on AP films.

In the presence of wear, typically in straight stems without centralizer in association with the pattern of lateral stem malalignment with distal posterior stem-bone contact in Gruen zone 12, osteolysis with the risk of distal periprosthetic fracture can be observed (▣ Fig. 5.21).

Similarly, in correlation to the described thin cement mantles in Gruen zones 8/9, a late periprosthetic pathological fracture can occur through an area of antero-proximal osteolysis (▣ Fig. 5.22).

Typical modes of failure have been described in the late 1970s [36]. Varus positioning of the stem with insufficient medial calcar cement mantle can be detrimental, but as outlined above a lateral stem malalignment leading to thin cement mantles must be avoided to reduce the risk for osteolysis induced (late) periprosthetic fracture.

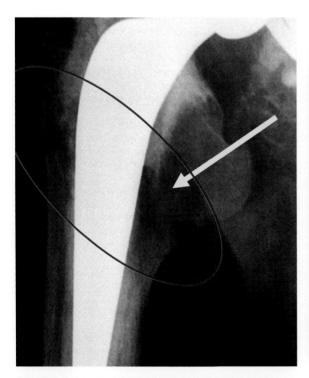 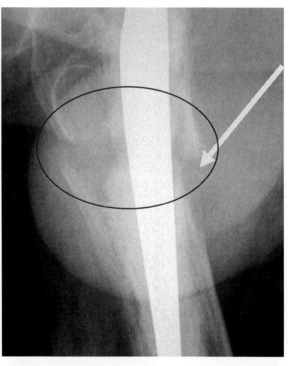

▣ **Fig. 5.22.** In correlation to the described area of thin cement mantles in Gruen zones 8/9, a late periprosthetic pathological fracture occurred 11 years postoperatively through an area of antero-proximal osteolysis

Take Home Messages

- Deficient cement mantles may be detrimental with regard to long-term outcome of cemented femoral stems.
- Optimal cementing technique and bone preparation contribute to avoid primary cement mantle deficiencies.
- Cement mantle thickness depends on cement technique, femoral anatomy, canal preparation, stem design and size, as well as centralizer usage.
- Critical zones of cement mantle thickness exist in Gruen zones 8/9 and 12, which can only be assessed on lateral radiographs.
- Posterior and lateral canal entry and preparation are essential to prevent stem malalignment and to minimise the risk of thin cement mantles.
- Straight stems without distal centralizers carry the highest risk of thin cement mantles.
- Anatatomical stem designs respect the proximal femoral geometry and reduce the risk of thin cement mantles in Gruen zones 8 and 9.
- Centralizers are effective to prevent stem tip-bone contact, but fail to minimize the risk of proximal thin cement mantles.
- The long term consequences of thin cement mantles include loosening and osteoylsis, which may act as a stress riser for periprosthetic fracture.
- It is surgical technique, as well as implant choice (design and size) which determine the long term outcome of a cemented femoral stem.

References

1. Anthony PP, Gie GA, Howie CR, Ling RSM. Localised endosteal bone lysis in relation to the femoral components of cemented total hip arthroplasties. J Bone Joint Surg 1990; 72-B: 971–9
2. Askew MJ, Steege JW, Lewis JL, Ranieri JR, Wixson RL. Effect of cement pressure and bone strength on polymethylmethacrylate fixation. J Orthop Res 1984; 1: 412–20
3. Ayers D, Mann K. The importance of proximal cement filling of the calcar region: a biomechanical justification. J Arthroplasty 2003; 18(7 Suppl 1):103–9
4. Balu GR, Noble PC, Alexander JW, Vela VL. The effect of intramedullary reaming on the strength of the cement/bone interface. Trans Orthop Res Soc 1994;19: 79
5. Bannister GC, Miles AW. The influence of cementing technique and blood on the strength of the bone-cement interface. Eng Med 1988; 17:131–3
6. Barrack RL, Mulroy RD, Harris WH. Improved cementing techniques and femoral component loosening in young patients with hip arthroplasty. J Bone Joint Surg 1992; 74-B:385–9
7. Beckenbaugh RD, Ilstrup DM. Total hip arthroplasty. A review of three hundred and thirty-three cases with long follow-up. J Bone Joint Surg 1978; 60-A:306–13
8. Berger RA, Seel MJ, Wood K, Evans RN, D'Antonio J, Rubash HE. Effect of a centralizing device on cement mantle deficiencies and initial prosthetic alignment in total hip arthroplasty. J Arthroplasty 1997; 12/4:434–43
9. Bocco F, Langan P, Charnley J. Changes in the calcar femoris in relation to cement technology in total hip replacement. Clin Orthop 1977;128: 287–95
10. Breusch SJ, Draenert K. Vacuum application of bone cement in total hip arthroplasty. Hip International 1997;7/4:1–16
11. Breusch SJ, Draenert Y, Draenert K. Anatomic basis of the cemented femur shaft. A comparative study of straight and anatomic design. Z Orthop 1998; 136:554–9
12. Breusch SJ, Berghof R, Schneider U, Weiß G, Simank H-G., Lukoschek M, Ewerbeck V. Status of cementation technique in total hip endoprostheses in Germany. Z Orthop 1999; 137:101–7
13. Breusch SJ, Schneider U, Kreutzer J, Ewerbeck V, Lukoschek M. Effects of the cementing technique on cementing results concerning the coxal end of the femur. Orthopäde 2000; 29:260–270
14. Breusch SJ, Norman TL, Revie IC, Lehner B, Caillouette JT, Schneider U, Blaha JD, Lukoschek M. Cement penetration in the proximal femur does not depend on broach surface. Acta Orthop Scand 2001; 72:29–35
15. Breusch SJ, Norman TL, Schneider U, Reitzel T, Blaha JD, Lukoschek M. Lavage technique in THA: Jet-lavage produces better cement penetration than syringe-lavage in the proximal femur. J Arthroplasty 2000; 15/7:921–927
16. Breusch SJ, Schneider U, Reitzel T, Kreutzer J, Ewerbeck V, Lukoschek M. Significance of jet lavage for in vitro and in vivo cement penetration.Z Orthop Ihre Grenzgeb. 2001;139(1):52–63
17. Breusch SJ, Lukoschek M, Kreutzer J, Brocai DRC, Gruen T. Dependency of cement mantle thickness on femoral stem design and centralizer. J Arthroplasty 2001; 16/5:648–57
18. Britton AR, Murray DW, Bulstrode CJ, McPherson K, Denham RA. Long-term comparison of Charnley and Stanmore design total hip replacements. J Bone Joint Surg 1996;78-B:802–8
19. Carlsson ÅS, Gentz C-F, Linder L. Localized bone resorption in the femur in mechanical failure of cemented total hip arthroplasties. Acta Orthop Scand 1983; 54:396–402
20. Chareancholvanich K, Bourgeault C, Loch D, Greer N, Lew W, Bechtold JE, Gustilo RB. Stability of primary cemented femoral implants with compaction of autogenous cancellous bone. 65th AAOS, New Orleans, March 1998
21. Charnley J. The closed treatment of common fractures 1957. E&S Livingstone, Edinburgh London
22. Charnley J. Acrylic cement in orthopaedic surgery 1970. E&S Livingstone, Edinburgh, London
23. Charnley J. Low friction arthroplasty of the hip: Theory and practice 1979. Springer, Berlin Heidelberg New York Tokyo
24. Chiu KH, Shen WY, Tsui HF, Chan KM. Experience with primary Exeter total hip arthroplasty in patients with small femurs. J Arthroplasty 1997; 12/3:267–72
25. Crawford RW, Psychoyios V, Gie G, Ling R, Murray D. Incomplete cement mantles in the sagittal femoral plane: an anatomical explanation. Acta Orthop Scand 1999; 70(6):596–8
26. DiGiovanni CW, Garvin KL, Pellicci PM. Femoral preparation in cemented total hip arthroplasty: Reaming or broaching? JAAOS 1999;7(6):349–357
27. Dohmae Y, Bechtold JE, Sherman RE, Puno RM, Gustilo RB. Reduction in cement-bone interface shear strength between primary and revision arthroplasty. Clin Orthop 1988;236:214–220
28. Dorr L. Total hip replacement using APR system. Techniques in Orthopedics 1986; 1(3):22–34
29. Draenert K, Draenert Y, Garde U, Ulrich Ch. Manual of cementing technique 1999. Springer, Berlin Heidelberg New York Tokyo
30. Ebramzadeh E, Sarmiento A, McKellop HA, LLinas A, Gogan W. The cement mantle in total hip arthroplasty. Analysis of long-term radiographic results. J Bone Joint Surg 1994; 76-A:77–87

31. Estok DM, Orr TE, Harris WH. Factors affecting cement strains near the tip of a cemented femoral component. J Arthroplasty 1997; 12/1:40–8

32. Fisher DA, Tsang AC, Paydar N, Milionis S, Turner CH. Cement-mantle thickness affects cement strains in total hip replacement. J Biomechanics 1997; 30:1173–7

33. Garellick G, Malchau H, Regner H, Herberts P. The Charnley versus the Spectron hip prosthesis: radiographic evaluation of a randomized, prospective study of 2 different hip implants. J Arthroplasty. 1999;14(4):414–25

34. Goldberg BA, AL-Habbal G, Noble PC, Paravic M, Liebs TR, Tullos HS. Proximal and distal femoral centralizers in modern cemented hip arthroplasty. Clin Orthop 1998, 349:163–73

35. Green JR, Nemzek DVM, Arnoczky SP, Johnson LL, Balas MS. The effect of bone compaction on early fixation on porous-coated implants. J Arthroplasty 1999, 14/1:91–7

36. Gruen TA, McNeice GM, Amstutz HC. »Modes of failure« of cemented stem-type femoral components. A radiographic analysis of loosening. Clin Orthop 1979; 141:17–27

37. Gruen T. A simple assessment of bone quality prior to hip arthroplasty: cortical index revisited. Acta Orthop Belg 1997; 63(Suppl. I):20–7

38. Halawa M, Lee AJC, Ling RSM, Vangala SS. The shear strength of trabecular bone from the femur, and some factors affecting the shear strength of the cement-bone interface. Arch Orthop Trauma Surg 1978; 92:19–30

39. Hanson PB, Walker RH. Total hip arthroplasty cemented femoral component distal stem centralizer. J Arthroplasty 1995; 10/5:683–8

40. Harris WH, McCarthy JC, O'Neill DA. Femoral component loosening using contemporary techniques of femoral cement fixation. J Bone Joint Surg 1982; 64-A:1063–67

41. Harris WH, McGann WA. Loosening of the femoral component after the use of the medullary-plug cementing technique. Follow-up note with a minimum five-year follow-up. J Bone Joint Surg 1986; 68-A:1064–66

42. Harvey EJ, Tanzer M, Bobyn JD. Femoral cement grading in total hip arthroplasty. J Arthroplasty 1998;13(4):396–401

43. Hashemi-Nejad A, Goddard NJ, Birch NC. Current attitudes to cementing techniques in British hip surgery. Ann R Coll Surg Engl 1994;76:396–400

44. Huddleston HD. Femoral lysis after cemented hip arthroplasty. J Arthroplasty 1988; 3(4):285–97.

45. Huiskes R. Some fundamental aspects of human joint replacement. Analyses of stresses and heat conduction in bone-prosthesis structures. Acta Orthop Scand 1980; Suppl. 185:109–200

46. Howie DW, Vernon-Roberts B, Oakshott R, Manthey B. A rat model of resorption of bone at the cement-bone interface in the presence of polyethylene wear particles. J Bone Joint Surg 1988; 70-A: 257–63

47. Indong Oh, Carlson CE, Tomford WW, Harris WH. Improved fixation of the femoral component after total hip replacement using a methacrylate intramedullary plug. J Bone Joint Surg 1978; 60-A:608–13

48. Jacobs ME, Koeweiden EMJ, Sloof TJJH, Huiskes R, van Horn JR. Plain radiographs inadaequate for evaluation of the cement-bone interface in the hip prosthesis. Acta Orthop Scand 1989;60(5): 541–3

49. Jasty MJ, Floyd WE, Schiller AL, Goldring SR, Harris WH. Localized osteolysis in stable, non-septic total hip arthroplasty. J Bone Joint Surg 1986; 68-A: 912–9

50. Jasty M, Maloney WJ, Bragdon CR, Haire T, Harris WH. Histomorphololgical studies of the long-term skeletal responses to well fixed cemented femoral components. J Bone Joint Surg 1990; 72-A: 1220–9

51. Johnston RC, Fitzgerald RH, Harris WH, Poss R, Müller ME, Sledge CB. Clinical and radiographic evaluation of total hip replacement. J Bone Joint Surg 1990; 72-A: 161–8

52. Joshi AB, Porter ML, Trail IA et al. Long-term results of Charnley low friction arthroplasty in young patients. J Bone Joint Surg 1993;75-B:616–623

53. Joshi RP, Eftekhar NS, McMahon DJ, Nercessian OA. Osteolysis after Charnley primary low-friction arthroplasty. A comparison of two matched paired groups. J Bone Joint Surg 1998; 80-B:585–90

54. Kawate K, Maloney WJ, Bragdon CR, Biggs SA, Jasty M, Harris WH. Importance of a thin cement mantle. Autopsy studies of eight hips. Clin Orthop 1998;(355):70–6

55. Kelly AJ, Lee MB, Wong NS, Smith EJ, Learmonth ID. Poor reproducibility in radiographic grading of femoral cementing technique in total hip arthroplasty. J Arthroplasty 1996;11:525–8

56. Kramhoft M, Gehrchen PM, Bodther S, Wagner A, Jensen F. Inter- and intraobserver study of radiographic assessment of cemented total hip arthroplasties. J. Arthroplasty 11: 272–276, 1996

57. Krause W, Krug W. Miller JE. Strength of the cement-bone interface. Clin Orthop 1982; 163:290–9

58. Krismer M, Klar M, Klestil T, Frischhut B. Aseptic loosening of straight- and curved-stem Müller femoral prostheses. Arch Orthop Trauma Surg 1991;110:190–4

59. Kwak BM, Lim OK, Kim YY, Rim K. An investigation of the effect of cement thickness on an implant by finite element analysis. Inter Orthop (SICOT) 1979; 2: 315–9

60. Kwong LM, Jasty M, Mulroy RD, Maloney WJ, Bragdon CR, Harris WH. The histology of the radiolucent line. J Bone Joint Surg 1992; 74-B:76–73

61. Lee AJC, Ling RSM. Improved cementing techniques. Am Acad Orthop Surg Instr Course Lect 1981; 30:407–13

62. Lee IY, Skinner HB, Keyak JH. Effects of variation of prosthesis size on cement stress at the tip of a femoral implant. J Biomed Mat Res 1994; 28:1055–60

63. MacDonald W, Swarts E, Beaver R. Penetration and shear strength of cement-bone interfaces in vivo. Clin Orthop 1993; 286: 283–8

64. McCaskie AW, Brown AR, Thompson JR, Gregg PJ. Radiological evaluation of the interfaces after cemented total hip replacement. Interobserver and intraobserver agreement. J Bone Joint Surg 1996;78-B:191–4

65. Maistrelli GL, Antonelli L, Fornasier V, Mahomed N. Cement penetration with pulsed lavage versus syringe lavage in total knee arthroplasty. Clin Orthop 1995; 312:261–5

66. Majkowski RS, Miles AW, Bannister GC, Perkins J, Taylor GJS. Bone surface preparation in cemented joint replacement. J Bone Joint Surg 1993; 75-B:459–63

67. Malchau H, Herberts P: Prognosis of total hip replacement in Sweden: Revision and re-revision rate in THR. Presented at the 65th Annual Meeting of the American Academy of Orthopaedic Surgeons, New Orleans, LA, February 1998

68. Maloney WJ, Jasty M, Rosenberg A, Harris WH. Bone lysis in well-fixed cemented femoral components. J Bone Joint Surg 1990; 72-B:966–70

69. Massoud SN, Hunter JB, Holdsworth BJ, Wallace WA, Juliusson R. Early femoral loosening in one design of cemented hip replacement. J Bone Joint Surg 1997;79-B:603–

70. Mjöberg B. The theory of early loosening of hip prostheses. Orthopedics 1997; 20(12):1169–1175

71. Morscher EW, Wirz D. Current state of cement fixation in THR. Acta Orthop Belg 2002;68:1–12

72. Mulroy RD, Harris WH. The effect of improved cementing techniques on component loosening in total hip replacement. An 11-year radiographic review. J Bone Joint Surg 1990; 72-B: 757–60

73. Newman MA, Bargar WL, Hayes DEJr, Taylor JK. Femoral canal preparation for cemented stems: reamers versus broaches. 60th Annual Meeting of the American Academy of Orthopaedic Surgeons, San Francisco, USA, February 1993

5

74. Noble PC, Espley AJ. Examination of the influence of surgical technique upon the adequacy of cement fixation in the femur. J Bone Joint Surg 1982; 64-B:120–1

75. Noble PC, Alexander JW, Lindahl LJ, Yew DT, Granberry WM, Tullos HS. The anatomic basis of femoral component design. Clin Orthop 1988; 235:148–165

76. Noble PC, Box GG, Kamaric E, Fink MJ, Alexander JW, Tullos HS. The effect of aging on the shape of the proximal femur. Clin Orthop 1995; 316:31–44

77. Noble PC, Collier MB, Maltry JA, Kamaric E, Tullos HS. Pressurization and centralization enhance the quality and reproducibility of cement mantles. Clin Orthop 1998; 355: 77–89

78. Older J. Low friction arthroplasty of the hip, a 10–12-year follow-up study. Clin Orthop 1986; 211: 36–42

79. Olsson SS, Jernberger A, Tryggö D. Clinical and radiological long-term results after Charnley-Müller total hip replacement. Acta Orthop Scand 1981; 52:531–42

80. Ostgaard HC, Helger L, Regner H, Garellick G. Femoral alignment of the Charnley stem: a randomized trial comparing the original with the new instrumentation in 123 hips. Acta Orthop Scand. 2001 Jun;72(3):228–32

81. Panjabi MM, Cimino WR, Drinker H. Effect of pressure on bone cement stiffness. Acta Orthop Scand 1986; 57:106–10

82. Pazzaglia UE. Pathology of the bone-cement interface in loosening of total hip replacement. Arch Orthop Trauma Surg 1990; 109:83–8

83. Pellicci PM, Salvati EA, Robinson HJ. Mechanical failures in total hip replacement requiring reoperation. J Bone Joint Surg 1979; 61-A:28–36

84. Reading AD, McCaskie AW, Gregg PJ. The inadaequacy of standard radiographs in detecting flaws in the cement mantle. J Bone Joint Surg 1999; 81-B:167–170

85. Roberts DW, Poss R, Kelley K. Radiographic comparison of cementing techniques in total hip arthroplasty. J Arthroplasty 1986; 1:241

86. Schulte KR, Callaghan JJ, Kelley SS, Johnston RC. The outcome of Charnley total hip arthroplasty with cement after a minimum twenty-year follow-up. The results of one surgeon. J Bone Joint Surg 1993; 75-A:961–75

87. Stauffer RN Ten year follow-up study of total hip replacement: With particular reference to roentgenographic loosening of the components. J Bone Joint Surg 1982; 64-A:983–90

88. Sutherland CJ, Wilde AH, Borden LS, Marks KE. A ten-year follow-up of one hundred consecutive Müller curved-stem total hip replacement arthroplasties. J Bone Joint Surg 1982; 64-A:970–982

89. Tolo ET, Wright JM, Bostrom MP-G, Pellicci P, Salvati EA. The effect of two different types of distal centralizers on the cement mantle thickness and stem alignment in total hip arthroplasty. AAOS Annual Meeting, New Orleans, March 1998, SE053

90. Valdivia GG, Dunbar MJ, Parker DA, Woolfrey MR, MacDonald SJ, McCalden RW, Rorabeck CH, Bourne RB. The John Charnley Award: Three-dimensional analysis of the cement mantle in total hip arthroplasty. CORR 2001;(393):38–51

91. Wroblewski BM, Siney PD, Fleming PA, Bobak P. The calcar femorale in cemented stem fixation in total hip arthroplasty. J Bone Joint Surg Br. 2000; 82(6):842–5

Bone Preparation: Acetabulum

Dominik Parsch, Steffen J. Breusch

Summary

In this chapter the importance of meticulous bone preparation of the acetabulum and the optimal cement mantle in the socket are outlined with a discussion of all relevant literature. It is recommended to partially preserve the subchondral bone plate of the acetabular roof, but to open the cancellous spaces for cement interdigitation with a combination of reaming, multiple drill holes and copious pulsatile lavage. The cement mantle should be a least 2–3 mm with further cement interdigitation into the roof (Zone I) to prevent radiolucent lines, which are associated with a higher risk of failure.

5.3.1 Bone Bed Preparation

Since the seventies cement anchorage holes drilled into the acetabulum have been recommended to improve fixation of cemented acetabular cups. The drilling of holes apparently increased torsional resistance at the cement-bone interface, though initially little attempt was made to further investigate this systematically.

In-vitro studies have documented the benefit of anchorage holes evaluating the optimum size and depth: Using finite element method Mootanah et al. [11] demonstrated that chamfered anchorage holes perpendicular to the surface of the acetabulum improve the mechanical stability of the implant. Based on studies with beechwood blocks, Mburu et al. [10] recommended keyholes with a diameter of 12 mm and a depth of 6 mm at each of the pubic, iliac and ischial sites, where in vivo the bone stock is greatest. However, clinical series showed that three large anchorage holes through a mainly intact subchondral plate may be inadequate to provide sufficient cement penetration increasing the risk for radiolucencies [1, 3, 17]. Nevertheless,

long-term survivorship of the acetabular component at 25 years using this technique has been reported to be 89.9% using revision for aseptic loosening as an endpoint [2].

Until today, sufficient evidence has been provided, that cement penetration and the mechanical interlock of cement and cancellous bone are the key factors for a stable bone-cement interface in vivo. If cancellous bone is not exposed adaequately, radiolucencies and loosening at the cement-bone interface may result as a consequence even in the presence of multiple anchoring holes (◻ Fig. 5.23).

Several studies have addressed the relationship between cementing technique, cement penetration and prevention of radiolucencies in cemented acetabular components [7, 12–15].

As a consequence, it has been suggested to completely remove the subchondral plate in order to provide maximum penetration of cement into the cancellous pores.

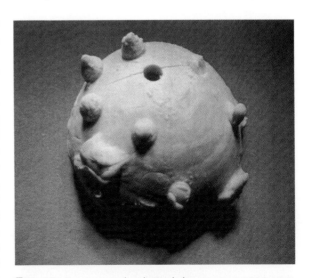

◻ **Fig. 5.23.** Despite several anchoring holes, note poor cement penetration into cancellous bone leading to subsequent loosening

However, experimental analyses showed that the bone plate within the acetabulum transmits most of the bearing load from the hip joint to the acetabular rim so that the cancellous bone within the pelvis is stressed to a much lower level [8, 16]. When the subchondral plate is removed, stresses in the cancellous bone immediately superior to the socket are remarkably increased [16]. Subsequently, fatigue failure or collapse of the cancellous bone may cause migration of the socket.

In accordance with these experimental results, clinical studies demonstrated the benefits of partial preservation of the subchondral plate penetrated only by multiple 5 or 6 mm drill holes especially in zone I in order to get optimum cement penetration [4, 6, 9]. A 77% survivorship for the acetabular component at 21 years using revision or definite loosening as a endpoint has been reported [5].

Our current practice includes partial removal of the subchondral plate to provide sufficient stability of the acetabular bone bed. Multiple (6 to 8) 4,5 to 6 mm penetration holes are drilled mostly in zone I (◘ Figs. 5.24 and 5.25).

The number of holes varies depending on the size of the acetabulum and the surface area of the remaining subchondral plate. Large cysts are grafted and routinely a bone graft taken from the last reaming is used to achieve cement interdigitation at the sclerotic medial floor.

Take Home Messages

- Bone bed preparation should be meticulous with removal of all soft tissue, cysts and opening of cancellous honeycombs.
- Partial preservation of the subchondral plate increases the mechanical stability of the acetabular bone bed.
- Multiple anchorage holes in the acetabular roof allow adequate cement penetration into the subchondral cancellous bone.
- The use of pulsatile lavage is considered mandatory.

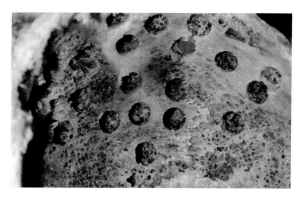

◘ **Fig. 5.24.** Partial removal of subchondral plate with multiple small drill holes in cadaver specimen. Please note exposed cancellous bone despite partial preservation of bone plate

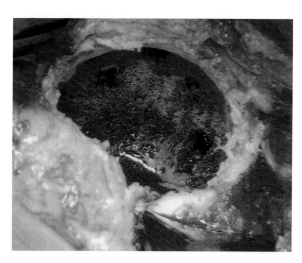

◘ **Fig. 5.25.** Intraoperative photograph demonstrating adaequate bone preparation after cyst removal and multiple drill holes (*top* = roof)

References

1. Andersson GB et al. (1972) Loosening of the cemented acetabular cup in total hip replacement. J Bone Joint Surg [Br] 54:590–599
2. Berry DJ et al. (2002) Twenty-five year survivorship of two thousand consecutive primary Charnley total hip replacements. J Bone Joint Surg [Am] 84-A:171–177
3. Charnley J (1979) Low-friction arthroplasty of the hip. Theory and practice. Springer, Berlin Heidelberg New York Tokyo
4. DeLee JG, Charnley J (1976) Radiological demarcation of cemented sokets in total hip replacement. Clin Orthop 121:20–32
5. Della Valle CJ et al. (2004) Primary total hip arthroplasty with a flanged, cemented all-polyethylene acetabular component. J Arthroplasty 19:23–26
6. Eftekhar NS, Nercessian O (1988) Incidence and mechanism of failure of cemented acetablar components in total hip arthroplasty. Orthop Clin North Am 19:557
7. Garcia-Cimbrelo E et al. (1997) Progression of radiolucent lines adjacent to the acetabular component and factors influencing migration after Charnley low-friction total hip arthroplasty. J Bone Joint Surg [Am] 79:1373–1380
8. Jacob HA et al. (1976) Mechanical function of subchondral bone as experimentally determined on the acetabulum of the human pelvis. J Biomech 9:625
9. Kobayashi S et al. (1994) Risk factors affecting radiological failure of the socket in primary Charnley low friction arthroplasty. Clin Orthop 306:84–96
10. Mburu G et al. (1999) Optimizing the configuration of cement keyholes for acetabular fixation in total hip replacement using Taguchi experimental design. Proc Instn mech Engrs 213:485–491
11. Mootanah R et al. (2000) Fixation of the acetabular cup in cemented total hip replacement: Improving the anchorage hole profile using finite element method. Technology Health Care 8:343–355
12. Ranawat CS et al. (1988) Effect of modern cement technique on acetabular fixation total hip arthroplasty. Orthop Clin North Am 19:599–603
13. Ranawat CS et al. (1995) Prediction of the long-term durability of all-polyethylene cemented sockets. Clin Orthop 317:89–105

14. Ranawat CS et al. (1997) Fixation of the acetabular component. Clin Orthop 344:207–215

15. Ritter MA et al. (1999) Radiological factors influencing femoral and acetabular failure in cemented Charnley total hip arthroplasty. J Bone Joint Surg [Br] 81-B:982–986

16. Vasu R et al. (1982) Stress distribution in the acetabular region before and after total joint replacement. J Biomech 31:133

17. Welch RB, Charnley J (1970) Low-friction arthroplasty of the hip in rheumatoid arthritis and ankylosing spondylitis. Clin Orthop 72:22–32

5.3.2 Optimal Cement Mantle?

The improvement of long-term results with cemented acetabular components compared with those of Charnley's first series has been attributed to the use of modern cementing technique with improved cement penetration creating a better cement mantle [5, 8, 9, 12, 14]. In general, 2 to 5 mm depth of cement penetration is believed to be optimal [1, 3, 7, 10, 15]. Thin layers and interruptions of the cement mantle have disadvantageous effects on the durability of the acetabular component as they result in cement fractures and increased polyethylene wear: Cement fractures have been observed to start in regions with a thin or incomplete cement mantle [4]. External wear of the polyethylene socket was associated with lack of acrylic cement in those areas [16]. Rapid polyethylene wear correlated with a thin cement mantle in the weight-bearing area [6].

Cement penetration and the mechanical interlock of cement and cancellous bone is the key factor for a stable bone-cement interface. Several studies have addressed the relationship between cement penetration and evidence of radiolucencies on postoperative radiographs and the risk of early loosening of cemented acetabular components. They showed that the most important prognostic factor for long-term survival of the acetabular component is the absence of radiolucency in DeLee-Charnley zone I on the radiograph obtained after surgery [2, 11 ,12, 13] (◙ Fig. 5.26). They found a correlation between early radiolucency, acetabular wear and loosening. In the presence of radiolucency, an increase in wear will promote the likelihood of loosening of the acetabular component.

It has been emphasised that it is possible to reduce the risk of acetabular radiolucency in zone I by careful cementing, which includes removal of eburnated bone, drilling of penetration holes, cleansing of the bone bed of marrow and debris by jet-lavage (◙ Fig. 5.27), minimisation of blood flow by means of hypotensive anaesthesia, haemostasis with hydrogen peroxide solution and sustained pressurisation (preferably with the use of a pressuriser, ► chapter 7.4) of the cement before cup insertion.

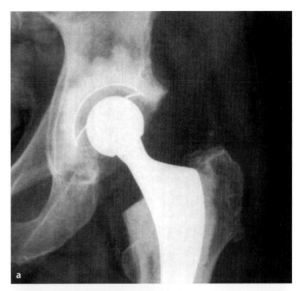

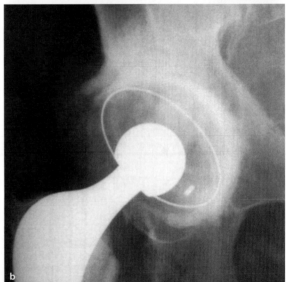

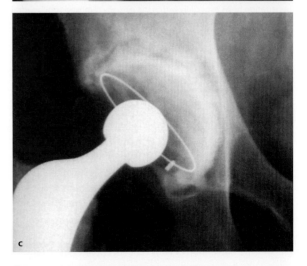

◙ **Fig. 5.26. a** Well-cemented acetabular component with an even cement mantle (*top*). **b,c** Inadequate cementing technique. Evidence of radiolucency in DeLee-Charnley zone I on early postoperative films (**b** *middle*) and progression at 5 years follow-up (**c** *bottom*)

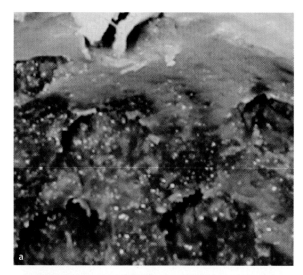

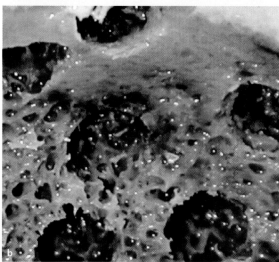

□ Fig. 5.27a,b. Prepared human acetabulum before and after jet-lavage performed to clean the cancellous bone bed. Note multiple penetration holes especially within the partially removed subchondral plate in DeLee-Charnley zone I

References

1. Askew MJ et al. (1984) Effect of cement pressure and bone strength on PMMA fixation. J Orthop Res 1:412–420
2. Garcia-Cimbrelo E et al. (1997) Progression of radiolucent lines adjacent to the acetabular component and factors influencing migration after Charnley low-friction total hip arthroplasty. J Bone Joint Surg [Am] 79:1373–1380
3. Huiskes R, Sloof TJ (1981) Thermal injuriy of cancellous bone following pressurized penetration of acrylic cement. Trans Orthop Res Soc 6:134
4. Jasty M et al. (1991) The initiation of failure in cemented femoral components of hip arthroplasties. J Bone Joint Surg [Br] 73:551–557
5. Joshi RP et al. (1998) Osteolysis after Charnley primary low-friction arthroplasty. J Bone Joint Surg [Br] 80:585
6. Kobayashi S et al. (1994) Risk factors affecting radiological failure of the socket in primary Charnley low friction arthroplasty. Clin Orthop 306:84–96
7. Krause WR et al. (1982) Strength of the cement-bone interface. Clin Orthop 163:290
8. Malchau H, Herberts P (1998) Prognosis of total hip replacement in Sweden. Presented at the 65th Annual Meeting of the American Academy of Orthopaedic Surgeons, New Orleans, USA
9. Noble PC, Swarts E (1983) Penetration of acrylic bone cements into cancellous bone. Acta Orthop Scand 54:566
10. Ranawat CS et al. (1988) Effect of modern cement technique on acetabular fixation total hip arthroplasty. Orthop Clin North Am 19:599–603
11. Ranawat CS et al. (1995) Prediction of the long-term durability of all-polyethylene cemented sockets. Clin Orthop 317:89–105
12. Ranawat CS et al. (1997) Fixation of the acetabular component. Clin Orthop 344:207–215
13. Ritter MA et al. (1999) Radiological factors influencing femoral and acetabular failure in cemented Charnley total hip arthroplasty. J Bone Joint Surg [Br] 81-B:982–986
14. Schulte KR et al. (1993) The outcome of Charnley total hip arthroplasty with cement after a minimum twenty-year follow-up. The results of one surgeon. J Bone Joint Surg [Am] 75-A:961–975
15. Walker PS et al. (1984) Control of cement penetration in total knee arthroplasty. Clin Orthop 185:155
16. Wroblewski BM et al. External wear of the polyethylene socket in cemented THA. J Bone Joint Surg [Br] 69:61–63

Take Home Messages

- A minimal cement mantle thickness of at least 2 mm should be achieved in all areas of the acetabulum.
- Commonly, much thicker layers (including the bone and cement composite) will be obtained in the acetabular roof, which are considered beneficial.
- Cement thinning or fractures may lead to increased polyethylene wear and early component loosening.
- The prevention of early radiolucent lines by means of adequate cement penetration is of utmost importance.

Part III Modern Cementing Technique

Chapter 6 Optimal Cementing Technique – The Evidence – 146

Chapter 6.1 What Is Modern Cementing Technique? – 146
S.J. Breusch, H. Malchau

Chapter 6.2 The Important Role and Choice
of Cement Restrictor – 150
C. Heisel, S.J. Breusch

Chapter 6.3 Cement Gun Performance Matters – 155
P. Simpson, S.J. Breusch

Chapter 6.4 Femoral Pressurisation – 160
A.W. McCaskie

Chapter 6.5 Acetabular Pressurisation – 164
D. Parsch, A. New, S.J. Breusch

Chapter 7 Implant Choice

Chapter 7.1 Stem Design Philosophies – 168
N. Verdonschot

Chapter 7.2 Stem Design – The Surgeon's Perspective – 180
J.R. Howell, M.J.W. Hubble, R.S.M. Ling

Chapter 7.3 Migration Pattern and Outcome of Cemented Stems
in Sweden – 190
J. Geller, H. Malchau, J. Kärrholm

Chapter 7.4 In-vitro Rotational Stability
of Cemented Stem Designs – 196
M. Thomsen, C. Lee

Chapter 7.5 Flanged or Unflanged Sockets? – 206
D. Parsch, S.J. Breusch

Chapter 7.6 Rationale for a Flanged Socket – 208
A.J. Timperley, J.R. Howell, G.A. Gie

Optimal Cementing Technique – The Evidence: What Is Modern Cementing Technique?

Steffen J. Breusch, Henrik Malchau

Summary

This chapter gives an overview of cementing technique evolution and defines the current status of modern cementing techniques. Modern cementing techniques aim to improve the mechanical interlock between bone and cement in order to establish a durable interface. The use of distal plug, cement gun, pulsatile lavage and cement pressurising devices have been shown to significantly improve long-term outcomes.

Introduction

The pioneer of cemented total hip arthroplasty (THA) Sir John Charnley created an amazingly high operative standard based on dedication and thorough basic research. His concept »low friction arthroplasty« still enjoys long term success with Kaplan-Meier survival rates of 85–90% after 20 years [24, 36, 39, 44]. Other cemented stem designs showed a wide range between poor [2, 7, 41, 45, 46] and good results [12, 15, 21, 29, 30, 47] both clinically and radiographically. However, it soon became obvious that not only stem design but, in particular, operative and cementing technique had to be considered important factors influencing the outcome of cemented THA. Beckenbaugh and Ilstrup [7] found a strong correlation between poor packing of cement and radiographic loosening [45]. Other studies have also shown higher rates of loosening when cement filling of the medullary canal was incomplete [26, 43, 45]. In this context, several authors postulated a poor prognostic bearing flaws and deficiencies in the cement mantle, manufactured by the surgeon, on the immediate postoperative radiograph [22, 42].

Evolution of Cementing Techniques

Cement Application

In the first decade of cemented THA, cementing techniques were fairly crude (◘ Table 6.1). Femoral canal preparation was done by curetting out cancellous bone. Irrigation – if used at all – was limited, and high viscosity cement was mixed and applied manually. However, it is important to note that even back then, the first form of pressurised cement application was already done by »thumbing« down the cement from proximal to distal. Charnley [13] had already emphasised the importance of achieving adequate cement pressure: »… The cement is forced down the track of the medullary canal as a stiff dough and the insertion of the point of the tapered stem of the prosthesis expands the stiff dough and injects it into the cancellous lining of the marrow space….«. This fact may offer an explanation why excellent long-term results have been achieved with so-called first-generation cementing techniques [24, 36, 39, 44].

Cement Containment and Gun Application

The introduction of a distal intramedullary cement restrictor allowed for cement containment and better pressurisation, which resulted both in improved cement penetration [23, 31] and better clinical outcome [18, 19, 34]. Retrograde cement application via cement gun [18, 19] generated higher cement pressures distally than proximally, a pattern reversed by finger packing [32]. »Sustained cement pressurisation« [27] further improved cement interdigitation [6] and provided a method able to resist the bleeding pressure, necessary to prevent blood

Table 6.1. Evolution of cementing techniques

First-Generation	Second-Generation	Third-Generation
Limited bone-bed preparation	Bone-bed preparation (bulb syringe irrigation/drying)	Thorough bone-bed preparation (pulsatile lavage)
Unplugged femur	Distal cement restrictor (bone/plastic)	Improved distal cement restrictor
Stiff, doughy cement introduced by hand	Retrograde cement application via cement gun	Retrograde cement application via cement gun
Digital pressurisation	Femoral and acetabular cement pressurisation	Femoral pressuriser Acetabular pressuriser
Hand mixing of cement	Open atmosphere cement mixing by hand	Vacuum mixing/(centrifugation of bone cement) Stem centralizers/cement spacers

entrapment and to obtain a satisfactory cementing result [1, 8] (▶ chapter 5.1, 6.4).

Bone Lavage

A further significant step towards improved cementing technique was the observation that bone lavage prior to cementation aided cement penetration [17, 25]. Both bone lavage and cancellous bone quality [17] were found to be significant factors with regard to improved mechanical shear strength [4].

The combination of distal plug, retrograde cement application via gun and bone lavage constitute the main factors of the improved second generation cementing techniques (see Table 6.1).

Cement Pressurisation and Pulsatile Lavage

A further distinction into third generation techniques (see Table 6.1) is probably more of academic and didactic interest, but a further and important evolution of cementing technique was certainly seen with the introduction of pulsatile bone lavage (▶ chapter 5.2) and pressurising devices, which facilitated a more reproducible pressurising technique [11, 27]. Also, standardised vacuum cement mixing and the use of stem centralising devices are considered third-generation techniques. Vaccum mixing of cement has been shown to contribute to the risk reduction for revision in the long term [30]. However, this may not be the case for all cement types (▶ chapter 4). Distal stem centralizers on the whole seem to have clear benefits, as the risk for stem tip to bone contact is reduced, which has been identified as a late failure mechanism due to osteolysis induced periprosthetic fracture (▶ chapter 5.2).

There may be dispute as to whether the use of pulsatile lavage and pressurising devices (▶ chapters 2.1, 2.2) should be labelled second- or third-generation techniques. However, more thorough cleansing of the bone bed by the use of pulsatile jet-lavage has been shown to be significantly more effective than manual lavage [11]. Furthermore, the use of pressurising devices to seal and contain cement at the femur and acetabulum, are proven steps to further improve cement pressurisation and hence interdigitation. The consequent use of pulsatile lavage and the pressurising devices should be considered mandatory parts of modern cementing techniques.

Impact of Modern Cementing Techniques

Modern cementing techniques aim to improve the mechanical interlock between bone and cement in order to establish a durable interface. Cement interdigitation not only depends on bone preparation, but also on lavage and mode of cement application. Good interdigitation is a product of adequate cement penetration and resistance to bleeding. Another elegant method has been advocated, where bone cement is applied under vacuum suction and femoral drainage [14], to reduce interface bleeding without the downside of intramedullary pressure increase (▶ chapter 15). However, so far no long-term data utilising this technique has been published.

In contrast, both pressurisation and lavage of cancellous bone have been identified to be the most significant factors with regard to improved cement interdigitation [1, 4, 10, 11, 17, 25, 28, 31, 38, 40] and been shown to be also clinically highly effective. Several clinical studies comparing patients before and after the introduction of modern cementing techniques have confirmed the benefit of improved cement application techniques [7, 12, 29, 30, 34, 42, 43, 45]; with the same benefit being found also in young patients [3, 5, 35]. Furthermore, if the risk for revision is taken as the measured outcome, the Swedish Hip Registry has provided important evidence

Observed survival with different cementing techniques

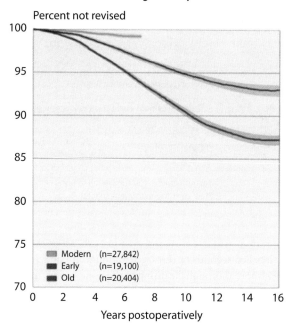

□ Fig. 6.1. Observed implant survival with different cementing techniques. Note significant improvement of implant survival with better cementing techniques in 3 cohorts. *Green*; modern (n=27,842), *red*: *early* (n=19,100), *blue*: old (n=20,404).

to support this relationship [29, 30]. Probably one of the most significant findings was, that the use of a distal intramedullary plug, pulsatile lavage, cement gun and a proximal seal (representing modern generation cement techniques) reduce the risk for revision by approximately 20% each [29]. This is highlighted by a continuous improvement of implant survival in Sweden (□ Fig. 6.1). Currently, these techniques have to be considered as »gold standard« [9, 20, 29, 32], in particular if used with a well documented bone cement [16, 21, 30, 37]. Excellent outcomes with cements of medium of higher viscosity [21], which seem more forgiving (▶ chapter 3.7), have been reported.

Take Home Messages

Modern cementing techniques are the key to long-term success.
Improved outcome has been proven for:
- Meticulous bone preparation and preservation.
- Distal femoral plug (cement restrictor).
- Pulsatile lavage.
- Retrograde cement application via gun.
- Sustained cement pressurisation (pressuriser).
Evidence exists for better outcome for:
- Vaccum-mixing of bone cement.
- Distal femoral stem centralizer.

References

1. Askew MJ, Steege JW, Lewis JL, Ranieri JR, Wixson RL. Effect of cement pressure and bone strength on polymethylmethacrylate fixation. J Orthop Res 1984; 1:412–20
2. August AC, Aldam CH, Pynsent PB. The McKee-Farrar hip arthroplasty: A long term study. J Bone Joint Surg 1986; 68-B:520–7
3. Ballard WT, Callaghan JJ, Sullivan PM, Johnston RC. The results of improved cementing techniques for total hip arthroplasty in patients less than fifty years old. J Bone Joint Surg 1994; 76-A: 959–64
4. Bannister GC, Miles AW. The influence of cementing technique and blood on the strength of the bone-cement interface. Eng Med 1988; 17:131–3
5. Barrack RL, Mulroy RD, Harris WH. Improved cementing techniques and femoral component loosening in young patients with hip arthroplasty. A 12-year radiographic review J Bone Joint Surg 1992; 74-B:385–9
6. Bean DJ, Hollis JM, Woo SL-Y, Convery FR. Sustained pressurization of polymethylmethacrylate: a comparison of low- and moderate viscosity bone cements. J Orthop Res 1988; 6:580–4
7. Beckenbaugh RD, Ilstrup DM. Total hip arthroplasty. A review of three hundred and thirty-three cases with long follow-up. J Bone Joint Surg 1978; 60-A:306–13
8. Benjamin JB, Gie GA, Lee AJC, Ling RSM, Volz RG. Cementing technique and the effect of bleeding. J Bone Joint Surg 1987; 69-B:620–4
9. Breusch SJ, Berghof R, Schneider U, Weiß G, Simank H-G., Lukoschek M, Ewerbeck V. Der Stand der Zementiertechnik bei Hüft-totalendoprothesen in Deutschland. Z Orthop 1999;137:101–7
10. Breusch SJ, Schneider U, Kreutzer J, Ewerbeck V, Lukoschek M. Einfluß der Zementiertechnik auf das Zementierergebnis am koxalen Femurende. Orthopäde 2000; 29:260–270
11. Breusch SJ, Norman TL, Schneider U, Reitzel T, Blaha JD, Lukoschek M. Lavage technique in THA: jet-lavage produces better cement penetration than syringe-lavage in the proximal femur. J Arthroplasty 2000; 15/7:921–927
12. Britton AR, Murray DW, Bulstrode CJ, McPherson K, Denham RA. Long-term comparison of Charnley and Stanmore design total hip replacements. J Bone Joint Surg 1996; 78-B:802–8
13. Charnley J. Acrylic cement in orthopaedic surgery 1970. Edinburgh, London. E&S Livingstone.
14. Draenert K, Draenert Y, Garde U, Ulrich Ch. Manual of cementing technique. Berlin, Heidelberg, New York, Tokyo: Springer, 1999
15. Fowler JL, Gie G, Lee AJC, Ling RSM. Experience with the Exeter total hip replacement since 1970. Orthop Clin North Am 1988; 19:477–89
16. Furnes O, Lie SA, Havelin LI, Vollset SE, Engesaeter LB. Exeter and charnley arthroplasties with Boneloc or high viscosity cement. Comparison of 1,127 arthroplasties followed for 5 years in the Norwegian Arthroplasty Register. Acta Orthop Scand 1997;68(6):515–20
17. Halawa M, Lee AJC, Ling RSM, Vangala SS. The shear strength of trabecular bone from the femur, and some factors affecting the shear strength of the cement-bone interface. Arch Orthop Trauma Surg 1978; 92:19–30
18. Harris WH, McCarthy JC, O'Neill DA. Femoral component loosening using contemporary techniques of femoral cement fixation. J Bone Joint Surg 1982; 64-A:1063–67
19. Harris WH, McGann WA. Loosening of the femoral component after the use of the medullary-plug cementing technique. Follow-up note with a minimum five-year follow-up. J Bone Joint Surg 1986; 68-A:1064–66
20. Hashemi-Nejad A, Goddard NJ, Birch NC. Current attitudes to cementing techniques in British hip surgery. Ann R Coll Surg Engl 1994;76:396–400

149   6

Chapter 6.1 · Optimal Cementing Technique – The Evidence: What Is Modern Cementing Technique?

21. Havelin LI, Espehaug B, Lie SA, Engesæter LB, Furnes O, Vollset SE. Prospective studies of hip prostheses and cements. A presentation of the Norwegian Arthroplasty Register 1987–1999. 67th Annual Meeting of the American Academy of Orthopaedic Surgeons, Orlando, USA, March 15–19, 2000

22. Ianotti JP, Balderston RA, Booth RE, Rothman RH, Cohn JC, Pikens GT: Aseptic loosening after total hip arthroplasty. Incidence, clinical significance, and etiology. J Arthroplasty 1986; 1:99–107

23. Indong Oh, Carlson CE, Tomford WW, Harris WH. Improved fixation of the femoral component after total hip replacement using a methacrylate intramedullary plug. J Bone Joint Surg 1978; 60-A:608–13

24. Joshi RP, Eftekhar NS, McMahon DJ, Nercession OA. Osteolysis after Charnley primary low-friction arthroplasty. A comparison of two matched paired groups. J Bone Joint Surg 1998; 80-B:585–90

25. Krause W, Krug W. Miller JE. Strength of the cement-bone interface. Clin Orthop 1982; 163:290–9

26. Kristiansen B, JensenJ.S. Biomachenical factors in loosening of the Stanmore hip. Acta Orthop Scand 1985;56:21–24

27. Lee AJC, Ling RSM. Improved cementing techniques. Am Acad Orthop Surg Instr Course Lect 1981; 30:407–13

28. Majkowski RS, Miles AW, Bannister GC, Perkins J, Taylor GJS. Bone surface preparation in cemented joint replacement. J Bone Joint Surg 1993; 75-B:459–63

29. Malchau H, Herberts P: Prognosis of total hip replacement in Sweden: Revision and re-revision rate in THR. Presented at the 65th Annual Meeting of the American Academy of Orthopaedic Surgeons, New Orleans, LA, February 1998

30. Malchau H, Herberts P, Söderman P, Odén A. Prognosis of total hip replacement: Update and validation of results from the Swedish National Hip Arthroplasty Registry. 67th Annual Meeting of the American Academy of Orthopaedic Surgeons,, Orlando, USA, March 15–19, 2000

31. Markolf KL, Amstutz HC. In vitro measurement of bone-acrylic interface pressure during femoral component insertion. Clin Orthop 1976; 121:60–6

32. McCaskie AW, Gregg PJ. Femoral cementing technique: current trends and future developments. J Bone Joint Surg 1994;76B:176–177

33. McCaskie AW, Barnes MR, Lin E, Harper WM, Gregg PJ. Cement pressurisation during hip replacement. J Bone Joint Surg 1997; 79-B:379–84

34. Mulroy RD, Harris WH. The effect of improved cementing techniques on component loosening in total hip replacement. An 11-year radiographic review. J Bone Joint Surg 1990; 72-B: 757–60

35. Mulroy RD, Harris WH: Acetabular and femoral fixation 15 years after cemented total hip surgery. Clin Orthop 1997; 337:118–28

36. Neumann L, Freund KG, Sorensen KH. Long-term results of Charnley total hip replacement. Review of 92 patients at 15 to 20 years. J Bone Joint Surg 1994;76-B:245–51

37. Nilsen AR, Wiig M. Total hip arthroplasty with Boneloc: loosening in 102/157 cases after 0.5–3 years. Acta Orthop Scand 1996 Feb;67(1):57–9

38. Noble PC, Espley AJ. Examination of the influence of surgical technique upon the adequacy of cement fixation in the femur. J Bone Joint Surg 1982; 64-B:120–1

39. Older J, Butorac R. Charnley low friction arthroplasty (LFA): a 17–21 year follow-up study. J Bone Joint Surg 1992; 74-B Supppl III:251

40. Panjabi MM, Cimino WR, Drinker H. Effect of pressure on bone cement stiffness. Acta Orthop Scand 1986; 57:106–10

41. Pavlov PW. A 15 year follow-up study of 512 consecutive Charnley-Müller total hip replacements. J Arthroplasty 1987; 2:151

42. Roberts DW, Poss R, Kelley K. Radiographic comparison of cementing techniques in total hip arthroplasty. J Arthroplasty 1986; 1:241

43. Russotti GM, Coventry MB, Stauffer RN. Cemented total hip arthroplasty with contemporary techniques. A five-year follow-up study. Clin Orthop 1988; 235:141–47

44. Schulte KR, Callaghan JJ, Kelley SS, Johnston RC. The outcome of Charnley total hip arthroplasty with cement after a minimum twenty-year follow-up. The results of one surgeon. J Bone Joint Surg 1993; 75-A:961–75

45. Stauffer RN Ten year follow-up study of total hip replacement: With particular reference to roentgenographic loosening of the components. J Bone Joint Surg 1982; 64-A:983–90

46. Sutherland CJ, Wilde AH, Borden LS, Marks KE. A ten-year follow-up of one hundred consecutive Müller curved-stem total hip replacement arthroplasties. J Bone Joint Surg 1982; 64-A:970–982

47. Van der Schaaf DB, Deutman R, Mulder TJ. Stanmore total hip replacement: A 9–10 year follow-up. J Bone Joint Surg 1988; 70-B:45

Optimal Cementing Technique – The Evidence: The Important Role and Choice of Cement Restrictor

Christian Heisel, Steffen J. Breusch

Summary

Modern cementing techniques rely on occluding and sealing of the intramedullary canal in order to generate sufficient pressure to enhance cement penetration. Each plug design should be able to withstand intramedullary pressure levels which can be expected with contemporary cementing procedures and should occlude the canal sufficiently to prevent leakage. Artificial cement restrictors have different abilities to meet these recommendations and the surgeon should carefully choose the right product.

Introduction

Since the introduction of cemented total hip arthroplasty by Sir John Charnley over forty years ago, the technique of femoral cement application has significantly changed [5, 6, 18, 26, 28, 40]. Initially, a manual antegrade technique was performed [9]:

»… The cement is forced down the track of the medullary canal as a stiff dough and the insertion of the point of the tapered stem of the prosthesis expands the stiff dough and injects it into the cancellous lining of the marrow space …«.

Although Charnley had already recognised and emphasised the importance of achieving adequate cement pressure, a more reproducible method became available with the introduction of an intramedullary cement restrictor [23, 28] and retrograde cement delivery via cement gun [13].

Why Do We Need a Cement Restrictor?

Only a distal intramedullary plug will allow for cement containment and hence pressurised cement application

[5, 24]. Plugging of the canal, cement pressurisation (proximal seal) and thorough pulsatile lavage play an integral part of modern cementing techniques [18, 32]. Improved cement penetration [2, 28], shear strength [1, 4, 22] and better clinical outcome [26, 32, 37, 40] have been demonstrated as a consequence.

Danter et al. [11] concluded from their study that cement leakage and restrictor migration might compromise the magnitude of cement penetration. Sufficient and sustained pressure levels, which are also important to withstand the potentially detrimental effect of intramedullary bleeding pressure [4, 19], can only be generated if the cement restrictor is not displaced and distal cement bypass/leakage is minimal [12]. Maximum peak pressures during cemented total hip arthroplasty in current studies vary between 122 kPa and more than 1500 kPa [10, 12, 33, 36, 41]. Yee et al. [41] and Churchill et al. [10] reported these high peak pressures which are mostly seen distally, just above the plug, during insertion of the stem [10, 36, 41]. Each intramedullary plug should be able to withstand these pressure levels which can be expected with contemporary cementing procedures and should occlude the canal sufficiently to prevent leakage.

Are the »Bone Plug« or the »Cement Plug« Sufficient?

In the 1980s, occlusion of the distal intramedullary canal was done with a bone plug [40] or by sealing with bone cement [28]. Some studies which compared bone plugs to artificial plugs suggested that sufficient stability with the bone plug was not always achieved [3, 20, 38]. The technique may achieve good results in the hands of an experienced surgeon but it is less reliable than an artificial plug and dependent on the bone quality of the patient.

Another concern is the growing number of revision surgeries. Many hospitals run their own bone bank where they store the retrieved femoral heads from primary total hip arthroplasty patients. Using this bone as a cement restrictor would waste precious bone material which otherwise could be used for revision cases.

Another option for the femoral canal occlusion is the use of bone cement [3, 28] or the use of bone cement in combination with an artificial plug [25, 30]. This seems to yield good stability but an additional batch of cement and more time is needed to perform this technique.

Artificial Cement Restrictors – Which One is the Right One?

Today, with the evolution of biomaterials in orthopaedic surgery, numerous plug designs and materials (non-resorbable, resorbable) are available. Regardless of design, however, intramedullary cement leakage and plug migration during cement and stem insertion should not occur to ensure adequate intramedullary pressures [24, 36]. Various studies have been published about the efficacy of intramedullary plugs, but they often investigated only one

[18, 28, 41] or two [8, 31, 38] plug designs or they did not include a sufficient statistical evaluation [3, 21].

Johnson et al. [16] compared five different models using a rigid wooden pipe with an absolute cylindrical diameter to simulate the canal. They found statistical differences in the stability of the different plugs dependent on varying canal diameters but not in the different designs.

Another study compared various different cement restrictor designs in artificial bones (same set-up for all tests) and in fresh-frozen femora (intraoperative situation) [15]. The results of this study are shown in ▢ Table 6.2.

There are three different design principles used to achieve intramedullary locking of cement restrictors:

Some plugs have to be inserted oversized to occlude the intramedullary canal press-fit (e.g. Biostop G/IMSET, Plugin´Tech, Buck, Universal Cement Restrictor; ▢ Fig. 6.2). The designs are made of flexible materials like gelatine (resorbable) or polyethylene. Plugs made of polyethylene remain in the canal after surgery and with these plugs a foreign body reaction to PE particles is possible, but there are no existing studies which prove this assumption. They also have to be removed in the situation of a failure of the prosthesis when revision surgery is required.

▢ **Table 6.2.** Results of pressure measurements with various designs in artificial bones and fresh frozen femora. Columns at the right show the relationship between failure and migration of the plugs at three different selected levels. The difference between these two values represents failure due to cement leakage

Cement Restrictor	Sawbones (max. Pressure in kPa)					Fresh-frozen Femora (max. Pressure in kPa)				Fresh-frozen Femora Number of Plugs which Failed at Defined Pressure Level (X/) and Number of Plugs Migrated at that Level (/X)			
	n	Min	Max	Median	No. of Cement Leakages	n	Min	Max	Median	n	350 kPa	700 kPa	1000 kPa
REX Cement Stop (a-one medica, Netherland)	10	180	970	466	0	11		1290	1121	11	0/0	1/1	1/1
BIOSTOP G (Depuy) IMSET (Aesculap)	10	355	598	423	0	11	757	1283	1129	11	0/0	0/0	4/4
Plugin´Tech (implantcast, Germany)	10	170	614	302	4	10	372	1201	1027	10	0/0	3/2	4/3
EXETER plug (Srtyker Howmedica)	–	–	–	–	–	10	860	1253	1157	10	0/0	0/0	1/0
Palacos-Plug (Biomet Merck)	–	–	–	–	–	10	634	1042	991	10	0/0	1/0	7/0
Universal-Cem.-Restr. (aap, Germany)	9	162	350	260	6	9	821	1217	1037	9	0/0	0/0	3/0
BUCK (Smith & Nephew)	10	71	216	121	4	10	294	1080	690	10	1/1	5/5	8/7

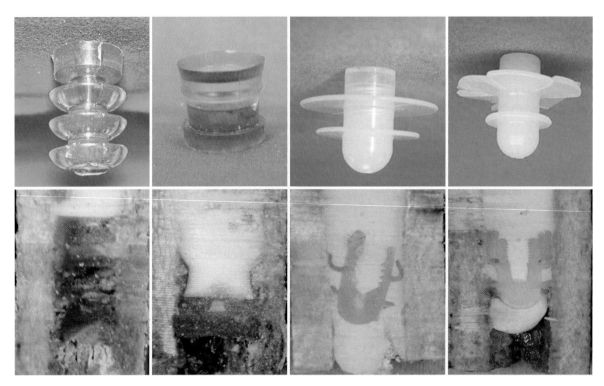

Fig. 6.2. *Upper row from left*: BIOSTOP G (DePuy)/IMSET (Aesculap), Plugin Tech (implantcast, Germany), BUCK Cement Restrictor (Smith&Nephew), Universal-Cement-Restrictor (aap, Germany). Cross-sections of the fresh frozen femora show typical modes of failure: gelatine plugs occlude the canal, but migrate with high pressures; polyethylene plugs show cement leakage and additional migration

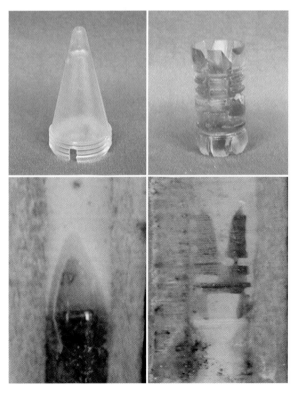

Fig. 6.3. EXETER plug (left, Stryker Howmedica), Palacos-Plug (right, Biomet Merck). Good occlusion and stability with the design on the left, good stability but severe leakage on the right

Some plugs are made of Polymethylmethacrylate (PMMA) (e.g. Exeter Plug, Palacos Plug; Fig. 6.3) and are implanted in a slightly larger size than the true canal diameter, as they are rigid and designed to lock in the conical intramedullary cavity above the femoral isthmus. In stove pipe femora this may be difficult to achieve. The other difficult anatomical situation one can be confronted with is the short femur or the high isthmus. The anatomical analysis of fresh frozen femora showed that the isthmus is located about 86 to 131 mm below the lesser trochanter [15]. In the case of a very proximal isthmus, these PMMA plugs have to be placed below the isthmus where they cannot be locked safely because the canal width is opening in the distal direction. They also have their disadvantages in revision total hip arthroplasty where often a longer stem has to be used which shifts the area where the plug has to be placed further distally. These disadvantages also apply to the gelatine and PE plugs but because of their flexible material they seem to be more forgiving. The significant difference between the two PMMA plugs shown in Fig. 6.3 is due to the design of the cement restrictors. The Exeter Plug has a conical shape with a thin PMMA wall, which allows the plug to adapt to the oval cross-section of the canal. The Palacos Plug on the other hand is a solid, round cylindrical PMMA plug, which allows no deformation and, therefore, cement leakage is often the consequence.

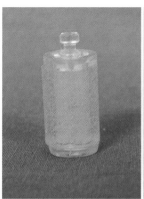
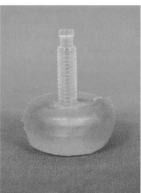
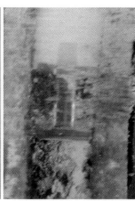

Fig. 6.4. Rex Cement Stop before insertion and expanded (A-one medical, Netherland). Cross-section shows good stability and occlusion

The third available design is different and works by an expandable mechanism (REX Cement Stop; Fig. 6.4). The PMMA parts of the plug are in direct contact to the inserted cement, which makes a removal in a revision case possible. The advantage of this plug design is the possibility to use this plug distal to the femoral isthmus. This design principle reduces the risk of fat embolism [6], which can occur if an oversized plug is implanted and fat and bone marrow are forced distally in the intramedullary canal [6, 14, 17, 24, 29, 39]. For this reason, pulsatile jet-lavage should be used prior to implantation and in fact also prior to templating for an occlusive plug design [14]. It also prevents an intraoperative split fracture of the proximal femur which can happen if an oversized plug is introduced [35]. Sakkers et al. [34] reported that a human femur can withstand pressures of at least 2000 kPa, but if an oversized plug is inserted forcefully into a weak bone (e.g. osteoporotic bone) to achieve good occlusion, this complication can occur even at lower pressure levels. The intrafemoral expanding mechanism should in theory minimise this complication.

The Right Choice

Artificial cement restrictors can be used to occlude the femoral canal to prevent cement leaking and to allow for high intramedullary pressures [6, 15, 16, 21, 31]. Most studies are based on experimental data but all these results need to be evaluated in the clinical situation. In a recent study with our own patients, we could identify a significant number of migrated plugs in the clinical setting with an oversized gelatine plug. Soft-gelatine cement restrictors can occlude the canal sufficiently if they are implanted oversized. They can migrate if high intramedullary pressures are generated. Soft polyethylene plugs can be used but if the polyethylene is rigid cement leakage occurs and soft polyethylene restrictors do not withstand the pressure with modern cementing techniques. If PMMA plugs are used, the Exeter Plug design shows high

stability and occlusion because its thin wall can adapt to the oval shaped femoral canal. Rigid PMMA plugs cannot be recommended due to the high rate of cement leaking around the plug. The design which allows handling of all intraoperative situations is the expandable design. This plug allows good stability in primary total hip arthroplasty cases, revision cases and difficult anatomical situations. It can be placed below the isthmus and reduces the risk of fat embolism in the elderly and the risk for femoral fracture in osteoporotic bone with the use of oversized plugs.

The surgeon should be aware of the different design features of artificial cement restrictors. Appropriate plug selection is important [3] to minimise the risk of failure due to migration or cement leakage.

Take Home Messages

- The use of a distal plug is mandatory in cemented THA to ensure adequate cement pressurisation.
- All plug designs have their intrinsic weaknesses and failure mechanisms.
- For routine practice a well designed artificial plug seems preferable.
- The intramedullary canal should be thoroughly cleansed using pulsatile lavage prior to templating and plug insertion to prevent fat embolism.
- In cases where plug stability is in question (stove pipe femur, high isthmus, long stem in revision), an expandable plug design should be used.

References

1. Bannister GC, Miles AW. The influence of cementing technique and blood on the strength of the bone-cement interface. Engl Med 1988; 17(3):131–3
2. Bean DJ, Hollis JM, Woo SL, Convery FR. Sustained pressurization of polymethylmethacrylate: a comparison of low- and moderate-viscosity bone cements. J Orthop Res 1988; 6(4):580–584
3. Beim GM, Lavernia C, Convery FR. Intramedullary plugs in cemented hip arthroplasty. J Arthroplasty 1989; 4(2):139–41

4. Benjamin JB, Gie GA, Lee AJ, Ling RS, Volz RG. Cementing technique and the effects of bleeding. J Bone Joint Surg Br 1987; 69-B(4):620–624

5. Breusch SJ. Cementing technique in total hip arthroplasty – factors influencing survival of femoral stems. *In:* Walenkamp GHIM, Murray DW (eds): Bone cements and cementing technique, Springer Verlag, Heidelberg 2001, 53–80

6. Breusch SJ, Heisel C. Insertion of an expandable cement restrictor reduces intramedullary fat displacement. J Arthroplasty. 2004;19(6):739–44

7. Breusch SJ, Berghof R, Schneider U, Weiss G, Simank HG, Lukoschek M, Ewerbeck V. Status of cementation technique in total hip endoprostheses in Germany. Z Orthop Ihre Grenzgeb 1999; 137(2):101–7

8. Bulstra SK, Geesink RG, Bakker D, Bulstra TH, Bouwmeester SJ, van der Linden AJ. Femoral canal occlusion in total hip replacement using a resorbable and flexible cement restrictor. J Bone Joint Surg Br 1996; 78(6):892–8

9. Charnley J. Acrylic cement in orthopaedic surgery. Edinburgh, London: E&S Livingstone, 1970

10. Churchill DL, Incavo SJ, Uroskie JA, Beynnon BD. Femoral stem insertion generates high bone cement pressurization. Clin Orthop 2001; 393:335–344

11. Danter MR, King GJ, Chess DG, Johnson JA, Faber KJ. The effect of cement restrictors on the occlusion of the humeral canal: an in vitro comparative study of 2 devices. J Arthroplasty 2000; 15(1):113–9

12. Dozier JK, Harrigan T, Kurtz WH, Hawkins C, Hill R. Does increased cement pressure produce superior femoral component fixation? J Arthroplasty 2000; 15(4):488–95

13. Harris WH. A new approach to total hip replacement without osteotomy of the greater trochanter. Clin Orthop 1975;(106):19–26

14. Heisel C, Mau H, Borchers T, Muller J, Breusch SJ. [Fat embolism during total hip arthroplasty. Cementless versus cemented--a quantitative in vivo comparison in an animal model]. Orthopäde. 2003;32(3):247–52

15. Heisel C, Norman T, Rupp R, Pritsch M, Ewerbeck V, Breusch SJ. In vitro performance of intramedullary cement restrictors in total hip arthroplasty. J Biomech 2003; 36(6):835–843

16. Johnson JA, Johnston D, el Hawary R, Tan SR, Wong LA, Gross M. Occlusion and stability of synthetic femoral canal plugs used in cemented hip arthroplasty. J Appl Biomater 1995; 6(3):213–8

17. Kallos T, Enis JE, Gollan F, Davis JH. Intramedullary pressure and pulmonary embolism of femoral medullary contents in dogs during insertion of bone cement and a prosthesis. J Bone Joint Surg Am 1974; 56(7):1363–7

18. Lee AJ, Ling RS. Improved cementing techniques. Instr Course Lect 1981; 30:407–413

19. Majkowski RS, Bannister GC, Miles AW. The effect of bleeding on the cement-bone interface. An experimental study. Clin Orthop 1994; 299:293–297

20. Mallory TH. A plastic intermedullary plug for total hip arthroplasty. Clin Orthop 1981;(155):37–40

21. Maltry JA, Noble PC, Kamaric E, Tullos HS. Factors influencing pressurization of the femoral canal during cemented total hip arthroplasty. J Arthroplasty 1995; 10(4):492–7

22. Markolf KL, Amstutz HC. In vitro measurement of bone-acrylic interface pressure during femoral component insertion. Clin Orthop 1976; 121:60–66

23. Markolf KL, Amstutz HC. Penetration and flow of acrylic bone cement. Clin Orthop 1976; 121:99–102

24. McCaskie AW, Barnes MR, Lin E, Harper WM, Gregg PJ. Cement pressurisation during hip replacement. J Bone Joint Surg Br 1997; 79(3):379–84

25. McLaughlin JR, Harris WH. A composite plug for occluding the femoral canal prior to cementing a total hip femoral component. Orthop Rev 1994; 23(4):344–6

26. Mulroy RD, Jr., Harris WH. The effect of improved cementing techniques on component loosening in total hip replacement. An 11-year radiographic review. J Bone Joint Surg Br 1990; 72-B(5):757–760

27. Noble PC, Collier MB, Maltry JA, Kamaric E, Tullos HS. Pressurization and centralization enhance the quality and reproducibility of cement mantles. Clin Orthop 1998;(355):77–89

28. Oh I, Carlson CE, Tomford WW, Harris WH. Improved fixation of the femoral component after total hip replacement using a methacrylate intramedullary plug. J Bone Joint Surg Am 1978; 60(5):608–13

29. Orsini EC, Byrick RJ, Mullen JB, Kay JC, Waddell JP. Cardiopulmonary function and pulmonary microemboli during arthroplasty using cemented or non-cemented components. The role of intramedullary pressure. J Bone Joint Surg Am 1987; 69(6):822–32

30. Owens P, Lavernia CJ. Technique for a composite femoral intramedullary plug in cemented hip arthroplasty. J Arthroplasty 1999; 14(3):369–71

31. Prendergast PJ, Birthistle P, Waide DV, Kumar NV. An investigation of the performance of Biostop G and Hardinge bone plugs. Proc Inst Mech Eng [H] 1999; 213(4):361–5

32. Prognosis of total hip replacement: Update and validation of results from the Swedish national hip arthroplasty registry. AAOS, Orlando, FL, 2000

33. Reading AD, McCaskie AW, Barnes MR, Gregg PJ. A comparison of 2 modern femoral cementing techniques: analysis by cement-bone interface pressure measurements, computerized image analysis, and static mechanical testing. J Arthroplasty 2000; 15(4):479–87

34. Sakkers RJ, Valkema R, de Wijn JR, Lentjes EG, van Blitterswijk CA, Rozing PM. The intramedullary hydraulic pressure tolerance of the human femur. Clin Orthop 1995;(311):183–9

35. Schneider M, Heisel C, Breusch SJ. [Femoral fissure after cement restrictor implantation]. Z Orthop Ihre Grenzgeb 2003; 141(5):554–556

36. Song Y, Goodman SB, Jaffe RA. An in vitro study of femoral intramedullary pressures during hip replacement using modern cement technique. Clin Orthop 1994;(302):297–304

37. Suominen S, Antti-Poika I, Tallroth K, Santavirta S, Voutilainen P, Lindholm TS. Femoral component fixation with and without intramedullary plug. A 6-year follow-up. Arch Orthop Trauma Surg 1996; 115(5):276–9

38. Thomsen NO, Jensen TT, Uhrbrand B, Mossing NB. Intramedullary plugs in total hip arthroplasty. A comparative study. J Arthroplasty 1992; 7(Suppl):415–8

39. Tronzo RG, Kallos T, Wyche MQ. Elevation of intramedullary pressure when methylmethacrylate is inserted in total hip arthroplasty. J Bone Joint Surg Am 1974; 56(4):714–8

40. Wroblewski BM, van der Rijt A. Intramedullary cancellous bone block to improve femoral stem fixation in Charnley low-friction arthroplasty. J Bone Joint Surg Br 1984; 66(5):639–44

41. Yee AJ, Binnington AG, Hearn T, Protzner K, Fornasier VL, Davey JR. Use of a polyglycolide lactide cement plug restrictor in total hip arthroplasty. Clin Orthop 1999; 364:254–66

Optimal Cementing Technique – The Evidence: Cement Gun Performance Matters

Phil Simpson, Steffen J. Breusch

Summary

In this chapter, the handling characteristics and performance of eight different cement guns/mixing systems in terms of efficient cement delivery are compared. No ideal system exists on the market, which offers both excellent vacuum-mixing and a well-designed, efficient cement gun.

Introduction

Survival of stems in cemented total hip replacement has been improved by modern generation cementing techniques in both primary and revision surgery [1, 6, 7]. During cementing of the femoral component, back-bleeding from the intramedullary canal can prevent adequate cement penetration into the cancellous bone [2, 4] and can cause laminations in the cement mantle which can weaken its biomechanical properties. Rapid retrograde filling of the femoral canal with cement and early pressurisation are therefore very important components of modern cementing technique and are largely dependent upon surgical technique and the performance of the cement gun used. Many different commercial cement guns and mixing systems exist to serve this purpose.

Surprisingly, to date very little is known about the performance [3] and efficacy of cement guns used most commonly in routine practice. More sophisticated mixing systems have been developed over the years, but very little knowledge exists on the functioning of the cement guns, which are commonly simple mechanical devices.

Material and Methods

The performance of a cement delivery system depends both on the operator and the type/viscosity of cement used. In this experiment five cements of known different viscosities were used (◻ Table 6.3) to test eight different cement mixing and delivery systems commercially available in Europe (◻ Fig. 6.5, ◻ Table 6.4). To test the efficacy of the systems with regards to cement extrusion, all evaluations were carried out in a controlled operating-room environment. The mixing of cements was performed by a single person who was trained to competency on each system by the manufacturer. At a standardised time-point, the gun was handed to a blinded researcher who proceeded to extrude the cement as quickly as possible from the delivery system. The nozzles of all systems had been cut to equal lengths. The time taken to completely empty a double mix of cement (i.e. 80 g) from the cement cartridge/gun and the weight of cement extruded were then recorded so that the speed of extrusion could be documented in grams per second. The process was then repeated three times for each type of cement and mean values were calculated.

◻ **Table 6.3.** Bone cements used

Cement	Supplier
Simplex P	Stryker
CMW 1	DePuy, Blackpool, UK
Palamed	Biomet, UK
Smartset HV	DePuy, Blackpool, UK
Palacos R	Schering-Plough, UK

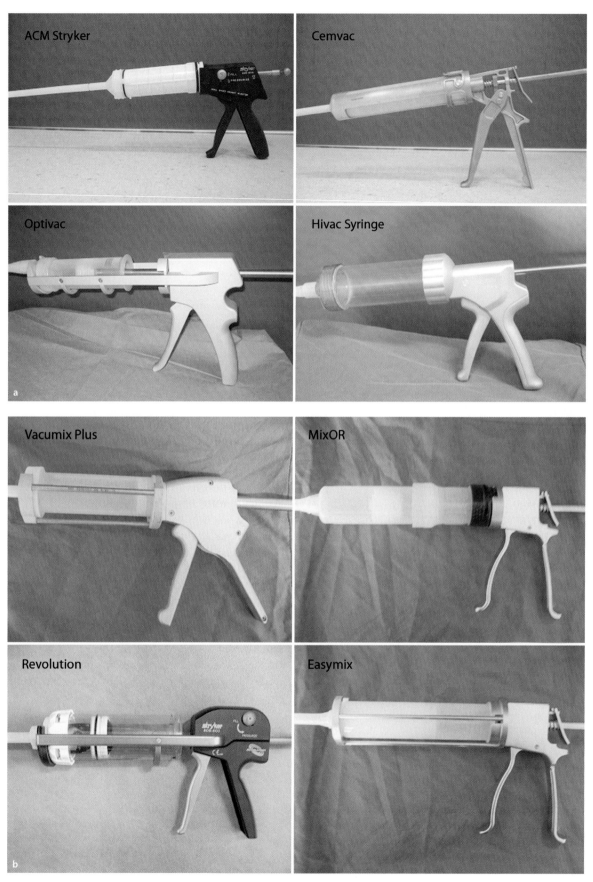

☐ **Fig. 6.5a,b.** Cement guns

Table 6.4. Advantages and disadvantages of cement mixing systems and guns

Cementing System	Manufacturer	Ratchet/ Non-ratchet	Advantages	Disadvantages	Mean Microporosity [7] (%)
Revolution	Stryker	Ratchet	Excellent mixing of all cements. Powered mixing. Easy to use. Dual ratchet for filling and pressurisation	Slow cement delivery	Not tested
ACM system	Stryker	Ratchet	Dual ratchet for filling and pressurisation. Good consistent gun performance with all cements.	Mixing system only works well with Simplex. Large cement wastage with mixing system.	Not tested
Easymix	Coripharm	Non-ratchet	Fast cement extrusion from gun.	Cannot deliver double mix of Simplex. Mixing system not particularly robust, separating occasionally during mixing.	Not tested
MixOR	Coripharm	Non-ratchet	Good consistent quality of cement mixing with all brands.	Extension section used to allow double mixes can unscrew during cement extrusion. Gun/cartridge interlock is not very stable.	1.9
Optivac	Biomet	Ratchet	Gun extrudes cement reasonably quickly. Produces a consistent quality of cement mix.	Cartridge can fracture during cement extrusion. Screw at end of cartridge can be expelled with cement if not tightened properly.	0.7
Hivac Syringe	Summit Medical	Ratchet	Fast cement extrusion from gun. Syringe can take a triple mix of cement.	Mixing system wastes cement	3.6
Cemvac	DePuy	Non-ratchet	Excellent mixing of all cements with easy to use system.	Slow cement delivery	0.7
Vacumix	DePuy	Ratchet	Fast cement extrusion	Mixing system wasted cement and was not very user-friendly.	2.2

Results

All of the systems tested used vacuum-mixing of the cement and all but one system mixed the cement in the container which was to be inserted into the gun. The guns themselves were either ratcheted or non-ratcheted (■ Fig. 6.5). The different gun mechanisms both seemed to work well when brand new (as tested), but it is our clinical experience that with repetitive use and wear the non-ratcheted devices can fail intra-operatively by slipping of the feeding rod. This may lead to potential problems with retrograde filling or loss of pressurisation when cementing the femur. With regards to the ease of use and

quality of cement mixing, each system appeared to have its strong and weak points (■ Table 6.4).

The performance of each cement gun varied with the cement used (■ Fig. 6.6). Cements of lower viscosity at the time of cement extrusion yielded faster delivery speeds. Looking at all individual combinations of cement and cement gun, the Vacumix system from DePuy delivered the fastest cement extrusion when used in combination with pre-chilled Palacos R cement (15.3 g/sec). This finding was in agreement with the only other piece of work published on this subject [3]. Ironically, this gun is no longer being manufactured and serves to highlight the continuing deficiencies in the development of cementing

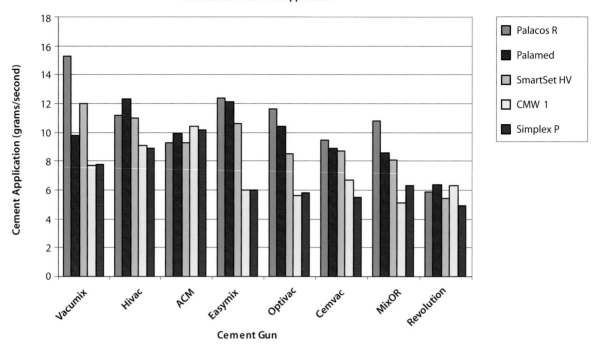

□ Fig. 6.6. Graph displaying the mean rates of cement extrusion achieved by each cement gun with different cements

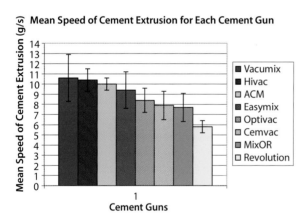

□ Fig. 6.7. Graph displaying the mean speed of cement extrusion for each cement gun taking into account all cements. 99% confidence intervals are included

systems for the femoral component. If the extrusion times for each cement are combined together to give an overall mean extrusion time for each cement gun (□ Fig. 6.7), it can be seen, that some systems are statistically superior to others. The Vacumix, Hivac Syringe, ACM and Easymix systems achieved the highest mean cement extrusion values but their performance was not necessarily consistent with all cements. In this respect, the ACM and Revolution systems were the most consistent devices as was evidenced by their smaller confidence intervals. The Revolution system had the lowest mean cement extrusion

value, however, and was statistically worse than all the other systems except MixOR. This was probably related to the width of the cement cartridge which resulted in a high ratio of nozzle to plunger diameter.

The speed of cement extrusion is only one of the important factors when considering the performance of a cement gun and many of the guns that expelled the cement quickly did not have reliable or easy to use mixing systems (□ Table 6.4). Two systems on the market – Cemvac and Revolution – appear to have concentrated very much on addressing this issue. However, this appears to have been at the expense of cement gun performance, which was significantly inferior in the case of Revolution, to a previous model of a gun produced by the same company. Although they did not test all the systems used in this study, another research group [5] previously tested the quality of cement produced and found significant differences in the porosity of the cement produced by different systems. In their series, Cemvac and Optivac performed best and produced the lowest microporosity values.

None of the guns/mixing systems reviewed here fulfilled all the attributes we believe are necessary for good cementing of the femur, but the Cemvac system seems to come closest.

Future testing of cement guns, in addition to the tests on speed of extrusion, should include a mechanical analysis of the maximum cementation pressures achievable with each gun or a system failure pressure. This would tell a potential user that a gun could not only achieve rapid retrograde filling but could also achieve adequate pressures for good cement interdigitation. Fatigue testing would help delineate if non-ratcheted devices were indeed more prone to rod slippage as they wear, confirming our clinical experience. The clinical advantages of rapid retrograde filling of the femoral canal will always be difficult to prove, but there is little doubt regarding the efficacy of modern generation cementing techniques. Hence, intraoperative failure of cement delivery (by cement gun failure) must be avoided at all cost. The theory behind the improved clinical success of the technique appears clear and it therefore seems appropriate that we should attempt to refine each part of it as best possible.

In this respect, we still believe that no ideal cement gun is offered currently on the market and that there is significant room for improvement from all manufacturers.

Take Home Messages

- The handling characteristics of cement guns have shown a significant difference in performance.
- Performance does not appear to be dependent on the mechanism of cement delivery (ratchet vs. non-ratchet), but clinical experience suggests a ratchet mechanism to be superior.
- Newly available (mixing) systems appear to have concentrated on the quality and consistency of cement mixing at the expense of cement gun performance.
- Although no ideal system exists, the surgeon must choose a combination of mixing system, gun and cement, which provides acceptable performance.

References

1. Barrack RL, Mulroy RG Jr, Harris WH (1992) Improved cementing techniques and femoral component loosening in young patients with hip arthroplasty: a twelve year radiographic review. J Bone Joint Surg Br 74:385–389
2. Benjamin JB, Gie GA, Lee AJC, Ling RSM, Volz RG (1987) Cementing technique and the effects of bleeding. J Bone Joint Surg Br 69:620–624
3. Heisel C, Schelling K, Thomsen M, Schneider U, Breusch SJ (2003) Cement delivery depends on cement gun performance and cement viscosity. Z Orthop 141:99–104
4. Majkowski RS, Bannister GC, Miles AW (1994) The effect of bleeding on the cement bone interface. Clin Orthop 299:293–297
5. Mau H, Schelling K, Heisel C, Wang J-S, Breusch SJ (2004) Comparison of various mixing systems and bone cements as regards reliability, porosity and bending strength. Acta Orthop Scand; 75(2):160–172
6. Mulroy WF, Harris WH (1996) Revision total hip arthroplasty with use of so-called second-generation cementing techniques for aseptic loosening of the femoral component. A fifteen-year-average follow-up study. J Bone Joint Surg Am. 78:325–30
7. Neumann L, Freund KG et al. (1994) Long-term results of Charnley total hip replacement. J Bone Joint Surg Br 76:245–251

Optimal Cementing Technique – The Evidence: Femoral Pressurisation

Andrew W. McCaskie

Summary

This chapter focuses on cement pressurisation during femoral fixation. It includes theoretical concepts and a description of the supporting evidence in the literature. It then utilises the concepts to describe the surgical technique in a practical »how to do« style. This step-by-step account concentrates on femoral preparation, cement introduction and pressurisation and finally component insertion.

Introduction

Pressurisation is pivotal to optimal cemented femoral fixation. During arthroplasty, a composite structure is created with a central metal prosthesis, an outer cylinder of cortical bone, and between them a layer of bone cement and cancellous bone. This produces two critical interfaces: the cement-bone and prosthesis-cement. The durability of the implant depends on the integrity of the interfaces. These simple facts are clinically important because the operating surgeon is responsible for interface »manufacture«.

Micro-Interlock

The main technical objective is to drive cement into the trabecular structure of cancellous bone, and create micro-interlock. Any material that occupies the trabeculae during pressurisation will prevent the flow of cement. This explains why the quality of surface preparation is so important (▸ chapter 5.1). A further impediment exists, namely the bleeding surface of bone. This is a problem not only in a physical sense but also a dynamic one.

The blood flows in the opposite direction to the desired flow of cement, leading to a potential disruption of the cement-bone interface [3, 18]. The pressure generated by bleeding has been measured at 36 cm of water [15] which, when the cement is at a low viscosity, could be sufficient to displace cement from trabeculae [16] or cause laminations [5].

Applying pressure to cement can overcome such problems. Firstly, during pressurisation the cement is made to flow in the desired direction, along the pressure gradient. Secondly, a sustained pressure, above the bleeding pressure, will overcome the effects of bleeding bone.

Pressure, Fluid Flow, and Viscosity

The fluid velocity of an incompressible substance (moving into a porous structure) upon pressure application is determined by the Darcy Law [2]. The flow is proportional to the pressure gradient and inversely proportional to the viscosity. In simple terms a greater flow will be achieved as cement viscosity decreases and as the pressure gradient increases. Bone cement changes viscosity throughout its use and the change varies not only with formulation but also with other factors such as the environmental temperature and humidity. This complex relationship has been clarified by research but remains at the heart of the technical challenge faced by the surgeon using cement during surgery.

Understanding the Effects of Pressurisation

In terms of cement penetration under applied pressure, Markolf and Amstutz evaluated cement flow through holes of differing diameter in an aluminium disc [20]. Penetration depth increased with increasing pore size and applied pressure. Halawa et al. demonstrated the benefit of an applied pressure of 300 KPa, when compared with 150 KPa [13]. Panjabi used a canine model to compare insertion pressures of between 110 and 1230 KPa with a constant pressure of 35 KPa [23]. Relative penetration (percentage of available cancellous bone occupied by cement) increased with insertion pressure. Analysis concluded that 520 KPa was high enough to achieve adequate penetration of cement but sufficiently low to avoid complications.

A further question arises over whether an increase in cement penetration produces an improved biomechanical performance of the cement-bone interface. Convery and Malcolm reported that 700 KPa achieved 80% more penetration and a 388% increase in shear strength [10]. Askew et al. evaluated the cement penetration and interface strength with different pressures and duration of application [1]. Although both penetration and interface strength increased with increasing pressure, there was no further improvement with longer application times.

From the clinical standpoint, various viscosity options exist. Bean compared standard viscosity cement with low viscosity cement in a human femoral model [4] in which the applied pressure varied. The shear strength increased significantly with pressure until the pressure reached 410 KPa. There was no difference between cements in this respect. A canine model has been used to demonstrate that shear strength at the cement-bone interface is linearly dependent upon depth of cement penetration [17]. An 82% increase in shear strength and 74% increase in penetration were observed with distal bone plugging and pressurised cement insertion, with lower viscosity cement giving a further increase. In a human femoral model, a retrograde gun technique achieves both improved penetration and interface strength at proximal levels with reduced viscosity cement rather than high viscosity cement [24].

The pressure generated on stem insertion and the flow of cement that results, is another interesting question. Continuous pressure measurement throughout cementation has demonstrated that stem insertion achieves the highest pressures and it has been suggested that prior impaction of the cement was probably unnecessary [25]. Furthermore, the pressure generated during stem insertion has been measured in a cadaveric femur fitted with pressure transducers [6]. Greater pressures were generated distally (758 KPa for large prostheses and 359 KPa for small) when compared with proximal pressures (200 KPa for large and 131 KPa for small). The timing of prosthesis insertion can affect the pressure generated [9]. Late insertion of a stem creates both increased pressure and intrusion factor compared with early introduction, an effect

enhanced by a tapered design. In addition, a cadaver model has demonstrated less cement-bone radiolucencies (significant in zones 2 and 6) with late stem insertion [11].

There are two common ways to generate pressure in clinical practice. First, pressure can be generated before prosthesis insertion using a gun and seal. This utilises a medium or reduced viscosity phase of the cement. This phase is regarded the most crucial and ideally full cement interlock should be achieved at this stage before prosthesis insertion. Second, (distal) pressure can be generated by the prosthesis during insertion. This utilises a relatively higher cement viscosity. An evaluation of pressure generated at all stages has demonstrated the ability of a proximal seal to sustain pressure and also that a component design (Exeter and custom) can generate pressure throughout the length of a cavity model [12].

Clinical Technique and Pressurisation

Over the past 40 years, the debate about cement and how to use it has developed with lack of consensus and variation in practice [14, 21]. Charnley described kneading the cement followed by pressurised insertion with the two-thumb technique [8]. Pressurisation was completed during prosthesis insertion.

The gradual refinement of cementation technique has taken place and there are now higher levels of agreement particularly in terms of gun insertion and pressurisation [22]. The foundation of interlock is the preparation. The following account is clearly a summary of key steps to achieve pressurisation, not a comprehensive account of a modern cementing technique. ◘ Figure 6.8 shows schematically how the phases of the technique are related to pressure generation.

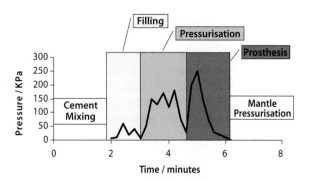

◘ **Fig. 6.8.** This schematic representation shows the phases of femoral cementation in time order and gives an indication of the relative pressures produced. The timings and pressures shown are hypothetical and are for illustration only. They do not represent a timing guide for clinical usage (see text)

Preparation

- Where possible, bleeding from the bone surface should be reduced by control of the blood pressure e.g. hypotensive anaesthesia/epidural.
- The production of an even mantle is related to stem position. Therefore, particular care is required to ensure the canal entry point is sufficiently lateral and posterior to minimise both stem malalignment and cement mantle deficiencies (▶ chapter 5.1).
- The reaming and broaching processes should aim to preserve a healthy/sound layer of cancellous bone, with blood supply minimally disrupted. The size of stem and mantle thickness should be planned preoperatively with templates.
- The bone surface should then be cleared of debris by meticulous and copious high-pressure pulsatile lavage (usually 1 liter of irrigation fluid is necessary).
- A cement restrictor is inserted 1.5–2 cm distal to the expected tip of the prosthesis. This creates a proximal clean compartment ready for pressure application.
- Lavage is repeated and the canal is packed with 3–5% H_2O_2 or saline soaked ribbon gauze.

Cement Mixing, Introduction and Pressurisation

- The author prefers a caulking gun in-syringe mixing system. The technique will require at least 2 mixes (80 g), with more required for capacious canals.
- A vent tube placed at the restrictor will remove trapped air and blood as cement is extruded.
- Cement insertion begins with canal filling. The modern technique utilises retrograde insertion.
- The timing of introduction will depend on the formulation and environment but the author prefers a medium viscosity. It is clearly important to avoid introduction with the cement at such a low viscosity that it cannot be controlled or contained.
- Pressurisation (sustained) begins when the canal has been filled. The author's preferred method is to utilise the cement gun. After retrograde filling the surgeon's thumb generates pressure, whilst the nozzle is shortened and a deformable seal positioned around it. The seal is positioned on the femoral neck at the osteotomy site to create a closed compartment (▶ chapter 2.2). Slow cement intrusion is achieved by slow steady trigger pulls. A sustained pressure can be generated by this technique that encourages cement flow and resists the bleeding pressure. Fat will be seen being displaced from the bone at this point.

Stem Insertion

- The stem is inserted immediately after the release of the seal and pressure, at a time when the cement is at a high viscosity. The timing of insertion will depend on the formulation and environment. It is clearly important to avoid too low a viscosity such that the cement is extruded as the prosthesis is inserted. It is equally important that the viscosity is not so high that the cement cures during insertion before the prosthesis reaches its final position.
- The author prefers to maintain a partial seal over the medial neck cut (corresponding to Gruen zone 7) using a thumb, which also guides the implant during insertion. The prosthesis should be inserted with careful regard to position. It is usually possible to use the insertion of the first two thirds of the stem to assess resistance. The final third of stem insertion can therefore be optimised to correspond with maximal working viscosity. No hammering is required.
- After reaching the desired position it is important to maintain position until final polymerisation (some surgeons maintain a pressure seal during this period). Particularly rotation of leg and stem relative to each other should be avoided.

The postoperative radiographic appearance after using this kind of approach is shown in ◘ Fig. 6.9.

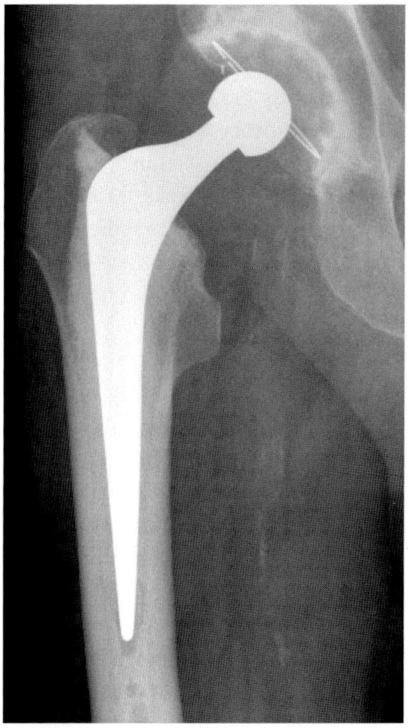

◘ **Fig. 6.9.** Postoperative radiograph after cemented total hip replacement. Note particularly the femoral cement mantle and the optimal cement penetration

Clinical Outcome with Pressurisation

The change has been supported by clinical evidence. UK joint registers have been used to evaluate patients with loosening at 5 years. Outcome was based on the grade of postoperative cementation derived from radiographs. Failure was associated with significantly poorer grades of cementation when compared to the non-failure group [7]. A very useful guide to practice is found in the Swedish arthroplasty register [19]. The change to modern cementing technique has been associated with an increase in rates of survival. Moreover, pulsatile lavage, a proximal femoral seal and the use of a distal plug are associated with a reduced risk of revision.

Conclusion

This chapter has reviewed the link between pressure and bone cement, in terms of both theory and practice. Such knowledge when put into practice as part of modern cementation techniques can reduce the risk of revision and increase the survival of the femoral stem. In this way, the surgeon becomes critical in the final »manufacturing« process of a hip replacement.

Take Home Messages

- Pressure applied to bone cement will direct flow.
- Pressure applied to cement, when sustained and of sufficient magnitude can overcome the bleeding pressure.
- Flow of cement increases with an increase in applied pressure and a decrease in cement viscosity.
- Pressurisation is key to cement intrusion and the creation of micro-interlock.
- From a clinical perspective the surgeon makes use of:
  - the medium viscosity phase by applying pressure with a sealed sustained technique,
  - the high viscosity phase, by applying pressure with prosthesis insertion.
- Pressurisation, as a part of modern cementing, has improved the long-term performance of the cemented stem.

References

1. Askew MJ, Steege JW, Lewis JL, Ranieri JR, Wixson RL (1984) Effect of cement pressure and bone strength on polymethylmethacrylate fixation. J Orth Res 1:412–420
2. Baeudoin AJ, Mihalko WM, Krause WR (1991) Finite element modeling of polymethylmethacrylate flow through cancellous bone. J Biomechanics 24(2):127–136
3. Bannister GC, Miles AW (1988) The influence of cementing technique and blood on the strength of the bone-cement interface. Engineering in Medicine 17(3):131–133
4. Bean DJ, Hollis JM, Woo SLY, Convery FR (1988) Sustained pressurization of polymethylmethacrylate: A comparison of low- and moderate- viscosity bone cements. J Orth Res 6:580–584
5. Benjamin JB, Gie GA, Lee AJC, Ling RSM, Volz RG (1987) Cementing techniques and the effect of bleeding. J Bone Joint Surg 69-B:620–624
6. Bourne RB, Oh I, Harris WH (1984) Femoral cement pressurization during total hip replacement. The role of different femoral stems with reference to stem size and shape. Clin Orthop 183:12–16
7. Chambers IR, Fender D, McCaskie AW, Reeves BC, Gregg PJ (2001) Radiological features predictive of aseptic loosening in cemented Charnley femoral stems. J Bone Joint Surg [Br]; 83-B: 838–42
8. Charnley J (1979) Low Friction Arthroplasty of the Hip. Theory and Practice. Springer, Berlin Heidelberg
9. Churchill DI, Incavo SJ, Uroskie JA, Beynnon BD (2001) Femoral stem insertion generates high bone cement pressurization. Clin Orthop Rel Res 393:335–344
10. Convery FR, Malcolm LL (1980) Prosthetic fixation with controlled pressurized polymerisation of polymethylmethacrylate. Trans Orthop Res Soc 4(2):205
11. Dayton MR, SJ Incavo, DL Churchill, JA Uroskie, BD Beynnon (2002) Effects of Early and Late Stage Cement Intrusion Into Cancellous Bone. Clinical orthopaedics and related research 405:39–45
12. Dunne NJ, Orr JF, Beverland DE (2004) Assessment of cement introduction and pressurisation techniques. Proc Instn Mech Engrs Part H J Engin Med 218(12):11–25
13. Halawa M, Lee AJC, Ling RSM, Vangala SS (1978) The shear strength of trabecular bone from the femur, and some factors affecting the shear strength of the cement-bone interface. Arch Orthop Traumat Surg 92:19–30
14. Hashemi-Nejad A, Birch NC, Goddard NJ (1994) Current attitudes to cementing techniques in British hip surgery. Ann R Coll Surg Engl 76:396–400
15. Heys-Moore GH, Ling RSM (1982) Current cementing techniques. In: Marti R (ed) Progress in cemented total hip surgery and revision: Proceedings of a symposium held in Amsterdam. Amsterdam, Geneva, Hong Kong, Princeton, Tokyo: Excerpta Medica, p 71
16. Lee AJC, Ling RSM (1984) Loosening. In: Ling RSM (ed) Complications of total hip replacement. Churchill-Livingstone, Edinburgh
17. Macdonald W, Swarts E, Beaver R (1993) Penetration and shear strength of cement-bone interfaces in vivo. Clin Orthop 286:283–288
18. Majkowski RS, Miles AW, Bannister GC, Perkins J, Taylor GJS (1993) Bone surface preparation in cemented joint replacement. J Bone Joint Surg 75-B:459–463
19. Malchau H, Herberts P, Soderman P, Oden A (2000) Prognosis of total hip replacement-update and validation of results from the Swedish National Hip Arthroplasty Register 1979–1998. Scientific Exhibition 67th AAOS Meeting, March 15–19, Orlando, USA
20. Markolf KL, Amstutz HC (1976) Penetration and flow of acrylic bone cement. Clin Orthop 121:99–102
21. McCaskie AW, Gregg PJ (1994) Femoral cementing technique: trends and future developments. J Bone Joint Surg 76-B:176–177
22. National Joint Registry (2004) National Joint Registry for England and Wales. 1st Annual Report, Crown Copyright
23. Panjabi MM, Goel VK, Drinker H, Wong J, Kamire G, Walter SD (1983) Effect of pressurization on methylmethacrylate-bone interdigitation: an in vitro study of canine femora. J Biomechanics 16(7):473–480
24. Reading AD, McCaskie AW, Barnes M, Roberts M, Gregg PJ (1997) Comparison of two modern femoral cementing techniques: in vitro study using cement-bone interface pressure and computerised image analysis. J Bone Joint Surg 79-B:Supp IV:468–469
25. Song Y, Goodman S, Jaffe R (1994) An in-vitro study of femoral intramedullary pressures during hip replacement using modern cement techniques. Clin Orthop 302:297–304

Optimal Cementing Technique – The Evidence: Acetabular Pressurisation

Dominik Parsch, Andrew New, Steffen J. Breusch

Summary

In this chapter the rationale and technique of acetabular cementing technique with particular emphasis on cement pressurisation are discussed and different pressuriser models are compared.

Introduction

The goal of modern cementing technique in general is to improve both the long-term properties of cement and cement-bone interface. Cleansing of the cancellous bone bed of marrow and debris by jet lavage [9, 16], the minimisation of blood flow by means of hypotensive anaesthesia [2, 24] and hemostasis with hydrogen peroxide solution [13] are all important steps to enhance the degree of intrusion and interlock. However, apart from pulsatile lavage, pressurisation of the cement is considered the most decisive factor. Elevated pressure during cement application and curing may help to reduce porosity of cement improving its mechanical properties [5, 11]. In addition, higher strengths at the cement-bone interface can be achieved by intrusion of cement into cancellous bone [3, 6, 14, 20]. The magnitude and duration of the applied pressure required to achieve adequate penetration and to prevent displacement by bleeding depend on cement properties, bone bed quality and preparation as well as bleeding pressure [7, 14, 17, 27].

In analogy to these findings mostly derived from studies performed at the proximal femur, different acetabular cement pressurisers have been designed with the idea of sealing off the acetabular margins before cup insertion, thus creating a closed space and allowing pressure to be applied to create cement intrusion into bone.

Experimental Evidence

Experimentally, pressures of 35–50 kPa for 30–60 seconds were found to produce near-optimal cement penetration into cleaned cancellous bone [19]. In addition, sustained pressures greater than 5–20 kPa seem to be sufficient to prevent cement displacement by intraosseous blood pressure [7, 26], thus preventing blood lamination, which has been shown to be associated with a significant reduction of the mechanical interface strength [4] (◘ Fig. 6.10).

Different acetabular pressurisers and pressurising techniques have been promoted in the past [1, 8, 12, 15, 18, 21, 22] ranging from the previously removed femoral head, sponge-filled sterile gloves, standard and more sophisticated instruments (◘ Figs. 6.11, 6.12 and 6.13). More recently, a sequential cementation procedure with individual anchoring hole cement injection with subsequent filling of the rest of the acetabulum through a standard pressuriser has been shown to improve cement penetration [12].

In-vitro studies with the Exeter pressuriser revealed peak pressures of 110 kPa at the acetabular wall [15]. Similar pressures were found with the use of a »cement compactor« [22]. Both studies used human acetabula without simulation of intraosseous bleeding. No sustained pressures were reported, cement penetration was stated to be improved, though not quantified [15, 22]. Bernoski presented a newly designed pressuriser creating peak pressures of 180 kPa and maintained pressures in the range of 80–90 kPa [8]. However, model pelvices without simulation of intraosseous bleeding were used in their study. New et al. [18] designed an instrumented pressuriser to allow the intraoperative measurement of acetabular cement pressurization. They found average pressures were close to 50 kPa and peak pressures in the range of 75–90 kPa. Cement penetration measurements were not performed.

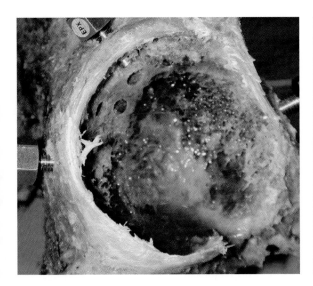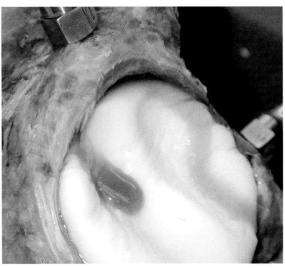

Fig. 6.10. Immediate and adequate pressurisation in the acetabulum cannot be overemphasised. Even after only 10 seconds after cement insertion, without pressurisation the bleeding pressure may cause blood laminations at the interface (*right*)

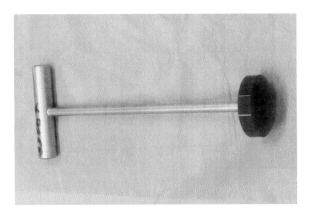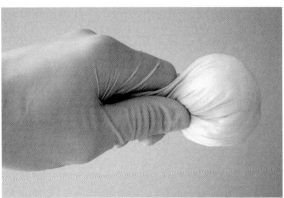

Fig. 6.11. Standard acetabular pressuriser

Fig. 6.12. Provisional pressuriser – sponge-filled sterile glove inserted by hand

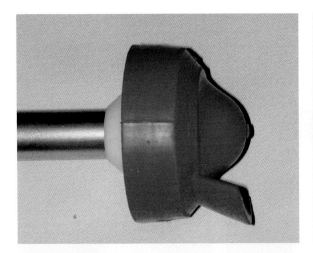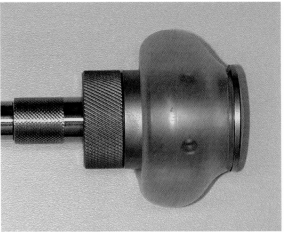

Fig. 6.13. Acetabular cement pressuriser used in our study: The Bernoski pressuriser (*left*, DePuy, Germany) has a silicone rubber head to occlude the acetabulum, with a flap to cover the cotyloid notch. A central plunger is advanced with a handle to bulge the central diaphragm of the head. The Exeter pressuriser (*rigth*, Howmedica, Germany) consists of an expandable balloon, which is filled with fluid and expanded as an attached handle is pulled. (Permitted reprint from [23])

In a recent study, we installed a new model with human cadaver pelvices simulating the intraosseous blood pressure [23]. Intraacetabular pressures and cement penetration as the key outcome of cement pressurisation were quantified. Using paired specimens two different designs of pressurisers (Bernoski and Exeter) were compared with each other (□ Fig. 6.13)

Both pressurisers tested appear to fulfil the minimum requirements for optimal cement pressurisation (□ Fig. 6.14): We found similar peak pressures with both pressurisers in the range of 68–86 kPa. The clinically more relevant sustained pressures tended to be higher using the Exeter pressuriser (45–52 kPa) compared to the Bernoski pressuriser (21–28 kPa). This is confirmed by measurements of the resulting cement penetration, which showed improvements in percentages of penetrated areas as well as absolute depths of penetration with the use of the Exeter pressuriser, though statistically not significant. AP radiographs revealed no radiolucency in either group in DeLee-Charnley zone I, where postoperative radiolucent lines have been shown to be predictors of early failure [25] (□ Fig. 6.15).

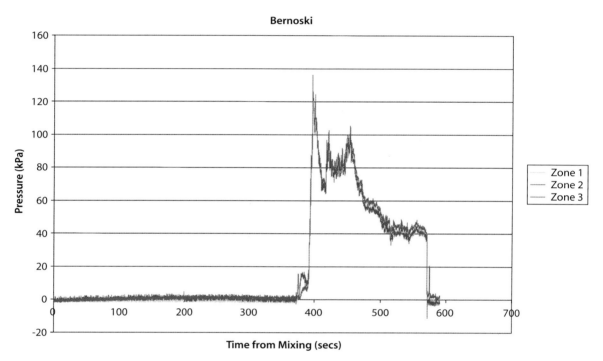

□ **Fig. 6.14.** Typical pressure curve achieved with acetabular pressuriser. Note sustained pressurisation over several minutes without pressure drop below 40 kPA in all three zones

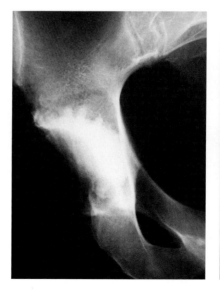
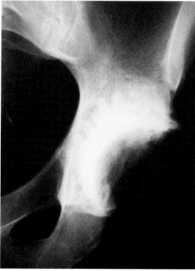

□ **Fig. 6.15.** AP radiographs of paired hemipelvices after cement pressurisation with the Bernoski pressuriser (right acetabulum) and the Exeter pressuriser (left acetabulum). (Permitted reprint from [23])

To our knowledge, there are no clinical studies documenting the effectiveness of pressurisers alone. However, pressurisation has been part of the »second generation« cementing technique, which also included perforation of the subchondral bone, jet lavage and drying of the bone bed. The combination of those factors were found to be essential for the long-term success of cemented acetabular components [10].

Our current practice includes pressurisation of the bone cement using a standard pressuriser (▶ chapter 2.1, ◘ Fig. 6.11) until the cement is almost cured. The acetabular component is then inserted late into the well penetrated cement bed.

Take Home Messages

▬ Pressurisation of the cement is a key element of modern cementing technique.
▬ Cement penetration can be obtained by various pressurisers.
▬ Adequate cement penetration should be achieved before cup insertion.

References

1. Altchek M. A readily available improvised acetabular cement pressurizer. Clin Orthop 1983; 174:164–165
2. An HS, Mikhail WE, Jackson WT, Tolin B, Dodd GA. Effects of hypotensive anesthesia, nonsteroidal antiinflammatory drugs and PMMA on bleeding in THA patients. J Arthroplasty 1991;6:245–250
3. Askew MJ, Steege JW, Lewis JL, Ranier JR, Wixson RL. Effect of cement pressure and bone strength on PMMA fixation. J Orthop Res 1984;1:412–42
4. Bannister GC, Miles AW. The influence of cementing technique and blood on the strength of the cement-bone interface. Eng Med 1988;17:131–133
5. Bayne SC, Lautenschlager EP, Compere CL, Wildes R. Degree of polymerization of acrylic bone cement. J Biomed Mater Res 1995;9:27
6. Bean DJ, Hollis JM, Woo SLY, Convery FR. Sustained pressurization of PMMA: A comparison of low- and moderate-viscosity bone cement. J Orthop Res 1988;6:580–584
7. Benjamin JB, Gie GA, Lee AJC, Ling RSM, Volz RG. Cementing technique and the effects of bleeding. J Bone Joint Surg [Br] 1987;69-B:620–624
8. Bernoski FP, New AM, Scott RA, Northmore-Ball MD. An in vitro study of a new design of acetabular cement pressurizer. J Arthroplasty 1998;13:200
9. Breusch SJ, Norman TL, Schneider U, Reitzel T, Blaha JD, Lukoschek M. Lavage technique in THA: Jet-Lavage produces better cement penetration than syringe-lavage in the proximal femur. J Arthroplasty 2000;15:921–7
10. Crites BM, Berend ME, Ritter MA. Technical considerations of cemented acetabular components. Clin Orthop 2000;381:114–119
11. Davies JP, Jasty M, O'Connor DO et al. The effect of centrifuging bone cement. J Bone Joint Surg Br 1989;71:30
12. Flivik G, Wulff K, Sanfridsson J, Ryd L. Improved acetabular pressurization gives better cement penetration. J Arthroplasty 2004;19:911–918
13. Hankin FM, Campbell SE, Goldstein SA, Matthews LS. Hydrogen peroxide as a topical haemostatic agent. Clin Orthop 1984;186:244
14. Krause WR, Krug W, Miller J. Strength of the cement-bone interface. Clin Orthop 1982;163:290
15. Lee AJ, Ling RS. A device to improve the extrusion of bone cement into the bone of the acetabulum in the replacement of the hip joint. Biomed Eng 1974;9:522
16. Majkowski RS, Bannsiter GC, Miles AW. The effect of bleeding on the cement-bone interface. Clin Orthop 1994;299:293–297
17. Markolf KL, Kabo JM, Stoller DW, Zager SA, Amstutz HC. Flow characteristics of acrylic bone cements. Clin Orthop 1984;183:246–254
18. New AM, Northmore-Ball MD, Tanner KE, Cheah SK. In vivo measurement of acetabular cement pressurization using a simple new design of cement pressurizer. J Arthroplasty 1999;14:854
19. Noble PC, Swarts E. Penetration of acrylic bone cements into cancellous bone. Acta Orthop Scand 1983;54:566
20. Oates KM, Barrera DL, Tucker WN, Chau CCH, Bugbee WD, Convery FR. In vivo effect of pressurization of PMMA bone cement. J Arthroplasty 1995;10:373–381
21. Oh I, Harris WH. A cement fixation system for total hip arthroplasty. Clin Orthop 1982;164:221–229
22. Oh I, Merckx DB, Harris WH. Acetabular cement compactor. Clin Orthop 1983;177:289–293
23. Parsch D, Diehm C, New A, Schneider S, Breusch SJ. A new bleeding model of the human acetabulum and a pilot comparison of two different cement pressurizers. J Arthroplasty 2004; 19:381–386
24. Ritter MA, Zhou H, Keating CM, Keating EM, Faris PM, Meding JB, Berend ME. Radiological factors influencing femoral and acetabular failure in cemented Charnley total hip arthroplasty. J Bone Joint Surg [Br] 1999;81-B:982–986
25. Ranawat CS, Rawlins BA, Harju VT. Effect of modern cement technique on acetabular fixation total hip arthroplasty. Orthop Clin North Am 1988;19:599–603
26. Shelley P, Wroblewski BM. Socket design and cement pressurization in the Charnley low-friction arthroplasty. J Bone Joint Surg [Br] 1988;70-B:358–363
27. Walker PS, Soudry M, Ewald FC, McVickar H. Control of cement penetration in total knee arthroplasty. Clin Orthop 1984;185:155

Implant Choice: Stem Design Philosophies

Nico Verdonschot

Summary

In this chapter various aspects of cemented stem designs such as shape, surface roughness and material properties are discussed. An attempt is made to provide some guidelines of design features, or combinations of them, that are known to lead to early failure. A design philosophy can be regarded as a good (or optimal) combination of design features. It will be shown that various design philosophies work equally well, but that an inferior design can result if their features are mixed. This will be illustrated by analysing the design philosophies of successful and unsuccessful cemented femoral hip stems.

Introduction

A large variety in cemented stem design is available on the orthopaedic market. Most of the current designs perform very well with survival rates over 90% after 10 years. For the younger patients, however, the survival rates are less positive with survival rates of 72–85% after 10 years [10, 11, 27]. The Scandinavian Registers effectively show that we have succeeded in continuous improvement of this medical service. However, the ultimate goal should be to create a generation of THA designs that last a lifetime, in particular for the younger patient. Hence, there is still a need to improve the performance of THA.

To be able to improve current designs, it is important to understand the failure mechanisms involved in aseptic loosening of hip prostheses and to be able to separate good and bad prosthetic design features. Huiskes provided a basis to discriminate between different failure scenarios of THA reconstructions [13]. Application of these failure scenarios allows one to analyse and test designs in a more systematic way. However, they do not provide direct guidelines that can be used in the design process of THA systems. The purpose of this paper is to provide some general guidelines on prosthetic design features of cemented stems such as prosthetic shape, surface roughness and stem material. More specifically it will be discussed how these features affect the mechanical failure process of cemented stems in terms of stem-cement debonding, cement abrasion and stem burnishing (□ Fig. 7.1), and failure of the cement mantle. In addition, different design philosophies of cemented stems that have proven to either work or fail are discussed. These views may then serve as a basis for new designs or at least act as discussion document for individuals that work in this field.

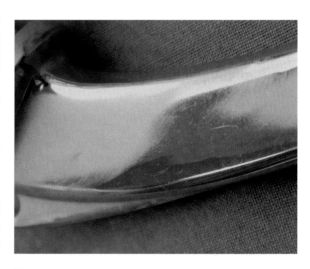

□ **Fig. 7.1.** Photograph of retrieved stem at revision for infection. Note burnishing and self-polishing at the (matt) stem surface

Design Features

Surface Roughness

Migration studies suggest that all stems do migrate within their cement mantle [18]. Hence, one could pose the hypothesis that all current stem designs do debond from the cement within a limited time period. In the past, it has been postulated that debonding could be prevented by increasing the surface roughness [3, 5] or by using stems that had been pre-coated with PMMA in the factory [6]. There is currently little to no evidence that these surface treatments create a long lasting bond between the stem and the cement. One of the reasons that the interfacial strength is not adequate with rough surfaces is the fact that rough stems usually have an incomplete attachment to the cement mantle resulting in substantial pores at the stem-cement interface and weakening of the interfacial bond [28, 35]. If we adopt the hypothesis that all stems do debond from the cement mantle, we must consider the consequences after stem-cement debonding; most importantly the abrasive behaviour of the debonded stem. We analysed this in an in-vitro experiment (❑ Fig. 7.2) whereby we implanted metal tapers with three different surface roughness values (Ra's were 0.02, 1.1 and 11 µm,

respectively) and exposed the tapers to a cyclic load. We measured the migration and determined the amount of damage at the interface (abrasion) and in the cement (cracks) in sections using scanning electron microscopy (SEM). It was very clear that, although the migration was less for the rough tapers, the amount of (abrasive) damage was larger for these components (❑ Fig. 7.3) [35]. This phenomenon was also demonstrated by Crowninshield et al. [5] who applied a cyclic displacement on a rough piece of metal that was compressed against bone cement. They also found, that cement abrasion increased with surface roughness. However, one could argue that the application of a cyclic *displacement* is not what happens clinically. In the in-vivo situation, a cyclic *force* is applied and it may be that a rougher surface would increase the friction coefficient at the stem-cement surface and would therefore reduce the cyclic motions and potentially its abrasive potential. We have analysed this mechanism with finite element micro-models [34] (❑ Fig. 7.4) and established first a relationship of surface roughness and cyclic micro-motions. Obviously, the micro-motions reduced with increasing surface roughness. Subsequently, we applied these micro-motions to a micro-model that simulated the asperities of the surface of the stem and calculated the peak stresses in the cement around the asperities of the roughness profile. It appeared

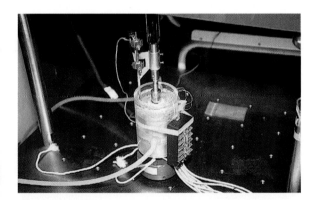

❑ **Fig. 7.2.** Experimental set-up of a taper in a cement mantle. The specimen was put in saline solution (temperature was 38 °C). The taper was cyclically loaded and the migration was measured. (Adapted from [35])

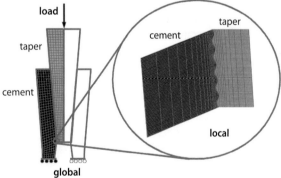

❑ **Fig. 7.4.** Finite element analysis of the local effects of surface roughness. The displacement field calculated in the global model were applied to the local (micro) model

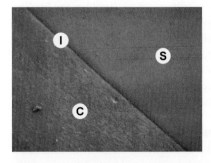
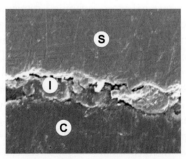
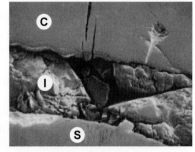

❑ **Fig. 7.3.** SEM details of the taper-cement interface around a taper with a different surface roughness (*from left to right:* Ra=0.02, 1.1, 11 µm).

I interface; *S* stem; *C* cement. Cement and interface damage increased with surface roughness. (Adapted from [35])

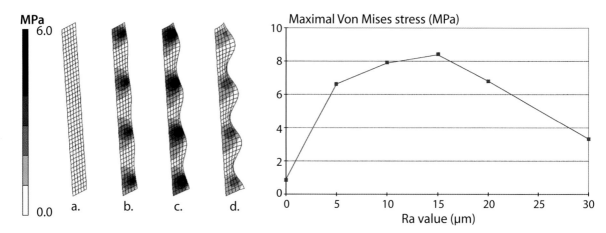

🔲 **Fig. 7.5.** Results from a finite element micro-analysis of the surface roughness of a straight tapered unbonded stem. *Left*: Shown is the Von Mises stress distribution in the cement around the asperities of the roughness profile of the stem surface. Surface roughness values (Ra) are: 0.0, 5.0, 15.0 and 30.0 μm (*from left to right*). *Right*: The local stresses around the asperities of the stem surface did show a maximum at 15 microns; beyond that value the local stresses reduced with surface roughness indicating a lower abrasive potential. (Adapted from [34])

that although the cyclic micro-motions were maximal for a surface roughness of 0 microns (theoretical case), the local cement stresses remained low due to the absence of asperities on the metal surface (🔲 Fig. 7.5). At a roughness value of Ra=15 μm, the local cement stresses were very high indicating a high abrasive mechanism. Interestingly, when the surface roughness was further increased, local cement stresses reduced again because of reduced cyclic motions caused by the better 'grip' of the metal surface on the cement (🔲 Fig. 7.5). Obviously, this is only an example that shows the complexity of stem-cement interface mechanics and cement abrasion. The surface roughness beyond which the abrasive potential diminishes depends on many other factors such as the prosthetic design, loading conditions, location, etc. Likewise, it is also difficult to state which surface finish can be considered to generate negligible cement abrasion. After reviewing the literature one could come to the conclusion that in some cases roughened stems have shown to fail earlier than polished versions of the same implant. Examples of these are the Exeter stem (rough versus matt; Swedish Register) and the Iowa Stem [4]. In addition, Muller et al. [22] analysed the in-vivo failure behaviour of a stem with a surface roughness of Ra=2.0 μm. They concluded that the stem was not stable, and generated excessive osteolysis, particularly around defects in the cement mantle. On the other hand, Von Knoch et al. [37] analysed 11 retrieved femoral CoCr stems which had a surface roughness of Ra=1 μm. They found no marks of burnishing on the stem surfaces, suggesting that the stem had been very stable and had not produced any cement abrasion. In addition, the Spectron prosthesis has a roughness of Ra=2.8 μm [18] and has an excellent survival record [11]. These clinical findings show the complex interactions of design features of femoral stem designs that cannot be judged on an individual parametric basis.

Nevertheless, the question 'what is rough and what is polished?' is often posed and I believe that it is possible to define a classification of abrasive potential in relation to the surface roughness of cemented femoral stems. Be reminded that the term 'polished' does not reflect how it looks, but what its abrasive capacity is:

- *polished*: Ra <1.0 μm usually cause little to no cement abrasion;
- *matt*: Ra <2.0 μm; no excessive abrasion, but if the stems are designed such that they create large micro-motions, cement abrasion and surface burnishing may occur;
- *rough*: Ra >2.0 μm; this surface finish can only be applied at locations where micromotions are expected to be minimal, with most designs this is at the proximal level and in combination with a bulky proximal part, sometimes in combination with geometrical features that further stabilise the implant.

Shape

To facilitate the discussion about the shape of cemented femoral stems, it is convenient to consider the loading modes that are applied to the reconstruction. These are axial forces, bending forces and rotational forces. The mechanism of load-transfer of the axial and bending forces is primarily affected by the mid-frontal plane shape of the stem, whereas the cross-sectional shape primarily determines the rotational stability of the design.

Mid-Frontal Shape

Axial forces can by transferred from stem to cement by different mechanisms. As discussed by Huiskes et al. [14], designs can be separated into a so called 'force-closed' or a 'shape-closed' system. The 'force-closed' type of design relies on a taper that transfers the load to the cement at the stem-cement interface. The external load is in mechanical equilibrium with the (frictional) forces at the stem-cement interface. As the cement creeps or micro-cracks accumulate in the cement, the circumferential stresses reduce and, with those, the frictional forces. Therefore, the stem will migrate to increase the fictional forces to balance the external forces. Examples of such a type of design are the Exeter stem (Stryker-Howmedica), the Collarless Polished Taper (Zimmer), and the C-stem (DePuy) (◘ Table 7.1). A 'shape-closed' design type has features that transfer a relatively large portion of the axial load to the cement. These features can be collars, ridges, profiles and also an anatomic design can be considered as 'shape-closed' design feature. These features all contribute to the mechanical stability of the implant, even after debonding of the stem-cement interface.

The way bending forces are transferred to the cement depends on the bending stiffness of the stem relative to the cement/bone construct. If one performs stress calculations, almost all designs have stress concentrations at the proximal and distal region. By changing the stiffness, the areas with high stresses can be adapted. A relatively stiff stem will transfer more load distally, whereas a flexible stem will generate higher stresses in the proximal region. Particularly when a flexible material such as Titanium is used, one should be careful not to have a proximal section with a small proximal M-L dimension. In that case the stem will behave too flexible resulting in early debonding and relatively high micromotions at the stem-cement interface.

Cross-Sectional Shape

The first designs of the cemented hip prostheses were primarily designed to withstand loads in the frontal plane i.e. they had to withstand the axial and bending forces. Only over the last decade has it become more apparent that the design also needs to withstand the rotational (A-P) forces that are exerted on the reconstruction. Particularly, during activities such as rising from a chair or stair climbing the A-P forces can be quite substantial [1] and it can be suspected that not all cemented stems are equally suited to withstand these forces. Migration studies have also demonstrated the rotational movement of some implants [8, 18]. Hence, the rotational resistance has become an important parameter of the design. Stems with a circular cross-sectional shape have a smaller rotational stability by definition. The cross-sectional shape should therefore be far from circular and could be rectangular or irregular to improve the rotational stability. Stems with proximal-distal profiles along the surface also have an improved rotational stability. However, a downside of these non-circular shapes is that the irregular cross-sectional shape may create stress intensities at the stem-cement interface and

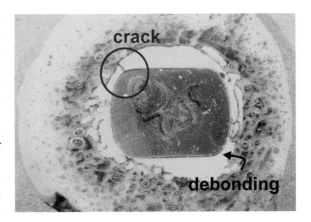

◘ **Fig. 7.6.** A cross section of an example of a retrieved specimen showing stem-cement debonding and cement cracking at the corner of the stem

in the cement. This may create stem-cement debonding and cement cracks (◘ Fig. 7.6). Rotational stability also depends on the cross-sectional size of the implant. The high failure rates with the rough surfaced pre-coated stem analysed by Sylvain and co-workers showed a clear trend with the smaller sizes [32]. This suggests that because of its small size the rotational stability of the stem was not adequate resulting in rotational migration and subsequent failure of the reconstruction. This indicates that, particularly for heavy patients with a large offset, one should be critical to the rotational stability of the stem and certainly not implant a very small stem size.

Hence, in terms of rotational stability, the cross sectional shape should be far from circular but should also not include any sharp corners. Definite limitations to the fillet radius of the corners of the stem are difficult to provide, but should at least be 2 mm and preferably over 3 mm. Most current designs that perform well clinically fulfil these requirements.

Stem Material

Basically there are three types of materials that are commonly used for cemented femoral stems. These are cobalt-chromium alloys, stainless steels, and titanium alloys. The use of titanium seemed attractive because its stiffness is closer to that of bone and bone cement than the other materials, which are relatively stiff. In addition, some companies offer titanium implants with modular heads whereas the stainless steel versions are of the monoblock type. Hence, titanium implants have also been selected for use because of their modularity and subsequent intra-operative flexibility.

The designs made of titanium alloy have gradually received a reputation to fail earlier than the CoCr or stainless steel designs [7, 17, 19]. On the other hand, there are

▣ Table 7.1.

Manufacturer	Type	Material (Alloy)	Surface Roughness (Micons)	Design Features
Stryker Howmedica	Exeter	Stainless Steel	<0.05	Symmetric design. No collar to allow for cement creep. Double tapered design to produce compressive stresses at the stem-cement and cement-bone interfaces.
	Omnifit	CoCr	0.9	Symmetric design with a collar. Proximal profiles to produce compressive stresses rather than shear stresses at the stem-cement interface.
	Definition	CoCr	>2.5 (grit blasted regions)	Symmetric design with a collar. Proximal and distal integrated PMMA centralizers/pre-cement mantles. Proximal and distal grit blasted surfaces to enhance stem-cement bonding in these areas.
	Accolade-C	CoCr	0.9	Symmetric design. Collar and profiles together with satin surface finish provide for mechanical stability
Zimmer	Muller Straight Stem	CoCr	0.5–1.5	Symmetric design with a small collar. Proximal to distal profiles create extra stability. Rotational stability is obtained by a distinct rectangular cross sectional shape. Medial/lateral stem-bone contact possible.
	VerSys precoat Plus	CoCr	1.5–2.5	Symmetric design. Proximal and distal centralizers to optimize cement mantle thickness. Collared to improve prosthetic stability
	MS30	Stainless Steel	<0.22	Symmetric, tapered design. Tri-tapered design with rounded corners to optimize cement stresses and stem stability
	CPT		0.025–0.05	Symmetric design. Collarless to allow for cement creep. Double tapered design to produce compressive stresses at the stem-cement and cement-bone interfaces
Smith & Nephew	Spectron EF	CoCr	2.8 proximally 0.7 distally	Straight design, with a collar. Proximally roughened for extra proximal fixation.
DePuy J&J	Charnley	CoCr	0.75 (Race et al)	Flanged prosthesis with a mini-internal collar. First introduced in the 1960's.
	C-stem	Stainless Steel	Polished	Symmetric design. No collar to allow for accommodation of cement creep. Triple tapered design to increase proximal load-transfer
	G2	CoCrMo	Polished	Double tapered design. No collar. Designed for optimal continuous cement mantle
Biomet	Stanmore	CoCr	0.5	Symmetric design with a collar. No additional ridges or profiles.
	Olympia	Stainless Steel	0.01	Anatomical design to promote an intact cement mantle. Smooth cross sections to prevent stress intensities.
	SHP (old version)	CoCr	3.8 proximally 2.0 distally	Designed to provide a thick proximal and distal cement mantle
Aesculap	Bicontact	CoCr	1.5–2.5	Straight stem, no collar, flanges for rotational stability
	Centega	CoCr	1.5–2.5	Anatomical design for equal cement mantle thickness, no collar, anterior flange for rotational stability
	Centrament	CoCr	1.5–2.5	Straight design, no collar, 3-D taper, proximal centralizer
Waldemar-Link	Lubinus SPII	CoCr	1.5	Anatomical design for equal cement thickness. Proximal to distal profile for extra stability
Wright Medical Technology	Perfecta-IMC	CoCr	5–6 proximally 2 distally	Proximal fixation by stepped collars to reduce circumferential hoop stresses
	Extend	CoCr	5	Proximal load transfer by a tri-polar wedge

reports, which show satisfactory results with titanium stems [2]. The use of titanium alloy as implant material can have two disadvantages.

First of all the material has a stiffness of about 50% relative to CoCr or stainless steel. The result is that a Titanium implant behaves more flexible in the cement mantle increasing the potential of stem-cement debonding. This is comparable to the iso-elastic cementless stems that were implanted in the 1980s, which failed in large quantities because they were too flexible [16, 23]. In addition, the higher flexibility of the stem will increase proximal cement stresses. In some designs, with a bulky proximal shape, these stresses may be within an acceptable range, but for designs that have small proximal dimensions, particularly in the M-L direction, cement stresses may become too high resulting in cement failure.

The second disadvantage of the titanium designs is the susceptibility of the material to crevice corrosion. This type of corrosion is driven by the generation of a gap (the crevice) between the stem and the cement. Willert et al. [38] were the first to report on this, but occasional reports have appeared since that time [9, 33]. In contrast, there are no reports about this type of corrosion for designs made of stainless steel or CoCr. It is not yet fully clear how high the impact of crevice corrosion is on clinical failure rates, but it is evident that it is a negative aspect of cemented titanium implants.

Based on the above stated considerations it seems fair to conclude that there are concerns when using titanium material for a cemented stem. The flexibility of the implant may become a particular problem in heavy patients with small femurs.

Design Philosophies

Because there is a clinical database representing over three decades survival data one would expect that it should not be such a problem to distill the optimal design parameters. However, as already discussed above, survival of THAs is a complex matter. Even from a clinical point of view, the failure criteria are unclear (revision, migration, or radiographic loosening). In large studies such as the national registers, survival of the cup and stem are sometimes not separated, prosthetic parameters may have changed over time, or the same prosthetic system sometimes performs well in one study, but insufficient in another. This illustrates that there is no such thing as 'the survival' of a particular hip system. Despite these restrictions in the interpretation of clinical data, it has become clear that a design feature can have a negative effect for a particular design, whereas it has none or even a beneficial effect for another prosthetic design. As an example one can consider the surface finish as a prosthetic design parameter. The Swedish Register tells us that the Exeter matt

stem with a surface finish of about Ra=1.0 μm, produced significantly worse results than the polished version (with a roughness of Ra=0.02 μm). This would suggest that a rough surface finish would lead to inferior survival. However, in the same register, there are stems with rough stem surfaces that perform clinically very well.

Hence, it certainly is a combination of inferior design features that result in a bad implant. In this respect, one must rather think in a certain design philosophy rather than in individual design features. When a certain design philosophy is adopted all design features can be chosen as to match the philosophy and optimise clinical performance.

⬛ Table 7.1 shows the result of a query to the major manufacturers to provide a list of their most important cemented hip systems. The data illustrates that there is a wide range of designs on the marked with variations in material, surface roughness and design features. The most interesting design may be the Muller Straight stem. This hip system does not prescribe the aim of a complete cement mantle. Although this may be in contradiction with current thoughts about cementing techniques, the clinical results are favourable for this design [11]. This may be due to a rather flat cross sectional shape of the stem, which provides for an excellent inherent (rotational) stability.

The table also indicates that companies are refraining from selling cemented titanium stems in large quantities. With regard to the surface finish, it appears that most stems are either rough or polished. All rough stems have a collar. Moreover, all collarless designs are highly-polished. Hence, these combinations fit nicely within the design philosophies as discussed above.

Mixing Design Philosophies

To demonstrate the importance of the paradigm of design philosophies one could consider two totally different design philosophies of prosthetic stems that perform clinically very well and mix the design features and discuss the potential consequences. As an example we will discuss the Exeter stem and the Lubinus SPII stem designs (⬛ Fig. 7.7).

The Exeter stem is double tapered, has no collar, has a highly-polished surface, is symmetric, and is made of stainless steel. The philosophy behind the design is that it anticipates on stem-cement debonding, distributes the stresses evenly in the cement mantle (no collar or ridges) and accommodates creep and stress relaxation in the cement mantle. It therefore can migrate (subside) without any cement damage. We have analysed this in an in-vitro study in which we cemented 10 Exeter stems in composite femora and applied a cyclic load to them (⬛ Fig. 7.8) [36]. Five of them were exposed to a continuous dynamic load; five of them were loaded for only 2.5 hours per day

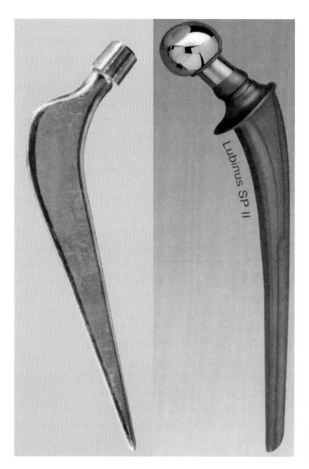

⊡ Fig. 7.7. *Left:* the Exeter stem with a tapered shape and a polished surface; *right:* the Lubinus SPII stem with an anatomical shape a collar, stem profiles and a matt surface finish

(the remaining 21.5 hours were regarded as 'resting time' during which the cement could relax, ► chapter 3.2). All 10 stems migrated and the stems that were exposed to a discontinuous load migrated in a stepwise fashion (⊡ Fig. 7.9). The cases with the highest migration were sectioned and carefully examined using SEM. We could not detect any cement damage, which indicates that the migration must have been accompanied with stress relaxation and cement creep.

The design philosophy of the Lubinus SPII is completely different. The stem has an anatomical shape, has longitudinal profiles, a matt surface finish, and has a collar. These features of the Lubinus SPII stem are design parameters that promote the philosophy of maximal mechanical stability of the stem in the cement mantle, even if the stem would debond from the cement mantle. This correlates also very well with the relatively small migration rates of this stem [18]. For the Exeter stem, higher migration values are reported. Hence, this is a 'migrating' stem with a so called force-closed load transfer mechanism [14]. With such kind of stem a polished surface finish, a tapered shape and no collar is beneficial. If the Exeter stem would be provided with a collar the migration would decrease, but a major part of the load would be transferred at the proximal level and in some cases this would probably lead to more cement damage in this region. If the surface roughness of the Exeter stem would be increased, the stem might debond from the cement at a later stage, but once debonded the prosthesis would produce more cement (and stem) abrasion leading to an imperfect fit of the stem in the cement mantle,

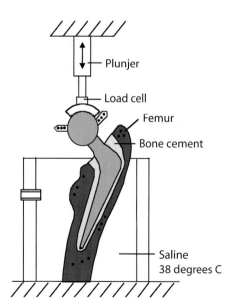
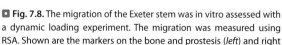

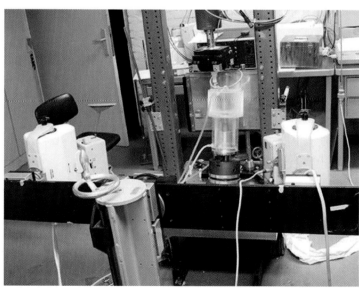

⊡ Fig. 7.8. The migration of the Exeter stem was in vitro assessed with a dynamic loading experiment. The migration was measured using RSA. Shown are the markers on the bone and prostesis (*left*) and right the stereo-X-ray set-up in the laboratory. The reconstruction was tested in saline of 38 °C. (Adapted from [36])

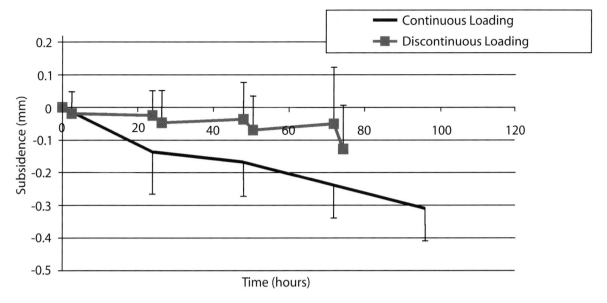

Fig. 7.9. Averaged migration pattern of 10 Exeter stems: 5 continuously loaded; 5 loaded with a discontinuous cyclic load. The latter group showed a step-wise subsidence pattern

pathways for wear debris transportation and higher local cement stresses. If the Exeter stem would be changed from a straight tapered design into an anatomic design such as the Lubinus SPII shape, migration would be reduced, but due to the polished surface finish and the absence of a collar the stem may still migrate more than the Lubinus SPII design and create gaps between the stem and the cement. This may lead to wear particle pathways and an uneven stress distribution in the cement mantle leading to earlier failure of the reconstruction.

In a clinical experimental study performed by Kärrholm et al. [18] the design philosophies are mixed on purpose. The study included 3 types of Lubinus stems: a polished version without a collar, a pre-coated stem with a collar and the standard. Logically, the polished stem without a collar subsided more than the other two components, which subsided a comparable amount. However, the polished Lubinus stem migrated much less than the values reported for the Exeter stem (0.3 mm versus 1.0 mm after one year [18]. This is understandable when one realises that the polished Lubinus stem has an anatomical shape and has surface profiles. These two features limit the migration of the stem. The collarless polished Lubinus SPII stem, which is only used in this clinical experiment, has a clear mixture of features from the 'force-closed' and 'shape-closed' design philosophies. It therefore is very valuable to follow this study to determine what the clinical consequences are of these design modifications.

In the paper from Huiskes et al. [14] the SHP stem was taken as an example of 'shape-closed' (□ Fig. 7.10). This stem has been designed in the mid 1980s with the assumption that the stem would remain bonded to the cement. Subsequently, a finite element computer simula-

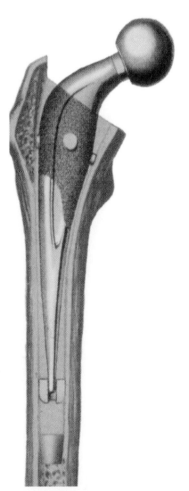

Fig. 7.10. The scientific hip prosthesis had a small M-L dimension at the resection level and in the tip region; a few centimetres under the resection level the M-L dimension is relatively large

tion calculated the optimal shape in order to minimise cement stresses [12]. The stem had a relatively small A-P dimension at the proximal and distal region (■ Fig. 7.10). That this shape works in terms of more global cement stresses has been recently confirmed with experimental work [25]. However, current migration data suggest that (almost) all stems debond from the cement and that the assumption of a bonded interface is incorrect. For the SHP prosthesis this has become evident by migration data reported by Nivbrand et al. [24]. A debonded SHP stem has only a limited number of features that represent a 'shape closed' design. Hence, in retrospect, the SHP design was designed with a mixed design philosophy. If the computer assumptions would have been changed from a bonded to an unbonded stem-cement interface, the shape of the SHP as optimised by the computer would certainly have been different.

The Capital Hip – Absence of a Design Philosophy

The choice of a good design philosophy is more difficult than it seems. The best way to design a stem that prob-

ably works adequately well as clinically good performing implants is to learn from earlier mistakes. An example of erroneous design considerations is the Capital hip design marketed in the 1990s by 3M Health Care Ltd., particularly in the UK. In 1997 it was taken off the market as reports of high failure rates appeared in the media and literature [20, 29]. It is often stated that the Capital design is a copy of the Charnley design. However, when one looks carefully to the designs, the surface roughness is higher than the Charnley design, and it appears that the Capital hip in fact represents four different types. The 3M company made two geometries (the round back and the flanged design (■ Fig. 7.11) and both components were made of two materials (Stainless Steel, SS, or Titanium, Ti). There seems to be little, not to say none, scientific consideration behind these design variations and certainly does not show any prove of a scientific design philosophy other than the argument that the stems looked like a Charnley and that the modifications were presumed to have minor effects. The reality is that these design variations did affect the clinical survival rates as is shown in ■ Table 7.2. The surfaces of the Capital hip stems were all treated with the same shot-blasted procedure to give it some roughness. Given the fact that titanium is softer

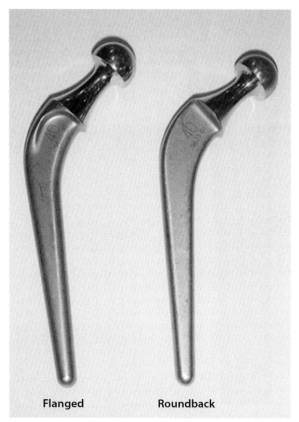 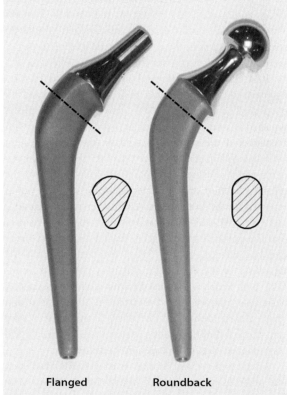

■ **Fig. 7.11.** The Charnley hip system (*left*) and the Capital hip system (*right*). Note that the flanged Capital hip really differs from the flanged Charnley stem

as compared to stainless steel, it is not surprising that the titanium stems were rougher than the stainless steel designs [31]. In addition, the flanged design did not replicate the Charnley flanged design because of patent restrictions. Therefore, the flange on the Capital hip was much less pronounced as compared to the Charnley flanged design.

The failure mechanism of the Capital Ti design (primarily of the flanged type) was described by McGrath et al. [21]. It started with lateral/proximal debonding, cement abrasion, migration and osteolysis. From a mechanical point of view these observations are quite logical. The Ti stems, in combination with the relatively slim design, are rather flexible as compared to the SS versions. The flexibility promotes early debonding of the stem. After debonding of the Capital Ti stem, cement (and stem) abrasion is promoted because of the high surface roughness in combination with high micro-motions caused, again, by the high flexibility of the implant. Due to the higher flexibility of the Ti stems, they also created higher cement stresses as compared to the SS designs. As a consequence, more cement damage can accumulate resulting in an increased likelihood of cement crack formation. This mechanism has been demonstrated by

Janssen et al. [15], who simulated the mechanical failure mechanism around the Capital hip stems using finite element techniques. They found considerably more cement cracks around the Ti stems as compared to the SS stems (■ Fig. 7.12a).

The fact that the round back stems performed clinically better than the flanged designs may be due to the better rotation stability of the round back as compared with the flanged design. This has been reported by Ramamohan et al. [29] and became apparent in the finite element simulations of Janssen et al. [15], where the roundback stem was much more susceptible for out-of-plane loading (stair climbing) than the round back design (■ Fig. 7.12b).

As stated earlier, not all Capital hip designs failed in large numbers. The stem that was most similar to the Charnley was the stainless steel roundback Capital hip. The failure rate is indeed quite low (■ Table 7.2). For the patients and the 3M company it is just bad luck that about 50% of the Capital hips were of the Titanium, flanged design type (see ■ Table 7.2). If the majority of the Capital hips would have been of the roundback stainless steel type, the high failure rate of the flanged titanium design might not have surfaced.

■ **Table 7.2.** Details of the Capital hip system. Source: Royal College of Surgeons of England, 2001.a; 001.b.

Stem Design	Stem Material	Loosening Rate [%]*	Distribution [%]
Flanged	Titanium	9.1	48.2
Roundback	Titanium	6.1	20.5
Flanged	Stainless Steel	4.4	22.0
Roundback	Stainless Steel	1.5	9.4

*Loosening rate until issue Hazard Notice in 1997.

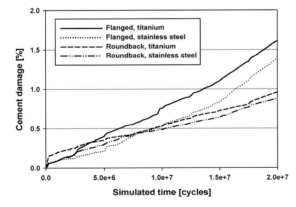

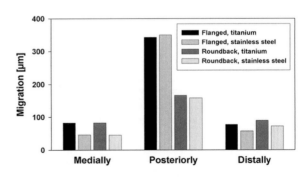

■ **Fig. 7.12.** Results of computer finite element simulation of the four Capital hip stems. *Left:* Shown is the accumulation of damage in the complete cement mantle. Note that the flanged design produced more damage than the roundback and that the Titanium implants produced more damage than the stainless steel ones. *Right:* Shown is the migration of the femoral head relative to the bone in the model after the damage and creep simulation. Note that the migration in posterior direction of the head of the flanged design was considerably more than the roundback types, indicating the inferior rotational stability of the flanged types

Conclusion

The clinical survival of cemented femoral components depends on many design factors, but is obviously also largely affected by patient and surgeon factors. It is this complex interaction of factors that makes it difficult to identify the design parameters that will lead to a successful implant. The examples of failed implants included in this paper highlight this complex interaction and illustrate, once again, the urgent need of reliable pre-clinical test methods, careful introduction of new implants to the orthopaedic community, and rigid post marketing surveillance of these new devices [13].

The principle attitude towards novel designs should be to establish a design philosophy and check whether all design features contribute to optimise the design philosophy and decrease the sensitivity of the design to patient and surgeon related factors. In this way, we can learn from previous mistakes and improve the performance of cemented THA components further, particularly for the younger patient.

Take Home Messages

- In the cross sectional plane, avoid sharp corners and a circular outer geometry.
- If the stem is made of Titanium alloy, be aware that the stem should be relatively bulky in order to avoid that the stem is too flexible at the proximal level.
- When designing new cemented THA stems, think in design philosophies rather than in individual design parameters. Be aware that an optimal factor (such as a rough surface finish) for one design may be inferior for another design.
- Most implants currently on the market are based on a design philosophy. Seemingly small deviations have led to dramatically high failure rates. Hence, there is no such thing as a 'small change to the design'; it can have a severe impact on prosthetic survival.

References

1. Bergmann G, Deuretzbacher G, Heller M, Graichen F, Rohlmann A, Strauss J, Duda GN. Hip contact forces and gait patterns from routine activities. J Biomech 2001; 34(7):859–71
2. Bowditch M, Villar R. Is titanium so bad? Medium-term outcome of cemented titanium stems. J Bone Joint Surg Br 2001; 83(5):680–5
3. Chen CQ, Scott W, Barker TM Effect of metal surface topography on mechanical bonding at simulated total hip stem-cement interfaces. J Biomed Mater Res 1999; 48(4):440–6
4. Collis DK, Mohler CG. Comparison of clinical outcomes in total hip arthroplasty using rough and polished cemented stems with essentially the same geometry. J Bone Joint Surg Am 2002; 84-A(4):586–92
5. Crowninshield RD, Jennings JD, Laurent ML, Maloney WJ. Cemented femoral component surface finish mechanics. Clin Orthop 1998; (355):90–102
6. Davies JP, Harris WH. Strength of cement-metal interfaces in fatigue: comparison of smooth, porous and precoated specimens. Clin Mater 1993; 12(2):121–6
7. Ebramzadeh E, Normand PL, Sangiorgio SN, Llinas A, Gruen TA, McKellop HA, Sarmiento A. Long-term radiographic changes in cemented total hip arthroplasty with six designs of femoral components. Biomaterials 2000; 24(19):3351–63
8. Gill HS, Alfaro-Adrian J, Alfaro-Adrian C, McLardy-Smith P, Murray DW. The effect of anteversion on femoral component stability assessed by radiostereometric analysis. J Arthroplasty 2002; 17(8):997–1005
9. Hallam P, Haddad F, Cobb J. Pain in the well-fixed, aseptic titanium hip replacement. The role of corrosion. J Bone Joint Surg Br. 2004; 86(1):27–30
10. Havelin LI, Engesaeter LB, Espehaug B, Furnes O, Lie SA, Vollset SE. The Norwegian Arthroplasty Register: 11 years and 73,000 arthroplasties. Acta Orthop Scand 2000; 71(4):337–53
11. Herberts P, Malchau H, Garellinck G. Annual report 2003, The Swedish National Hip Arthroplasty Register. 2004
12. Huiskes R, Boeklagen R. Mathematical shape optimization of hip prosthesis design. J Biomech. 1989; 22(8–9):793–804
13. Huiskes R: Failed innovation in total hip replacement. Diagnosis and proposals for a cure. Acta Orthop Scand 64(6):699–716, 1996
14. Huiskes R, Verdonschot N, Nivbrant B. Migration, stem shape, and surface finish in cemented total hip arthroplasty. Clin Orthop 1998; (355):103–12
15. Janssen DW, Aquarius R, Stolk J, Verdonschot N. Inferior design characteristics of the Captital Hip can be detected by numerical analysis. ORS, 2005
16. Jacobsson SA, Djerf K, Gillquist J, Hammerby S, Ivarsson I. A prospective comparison of Butel and PCA hip arthroplasty. J Bone Joint Surg Br 1993; 75(4):624–9
17. Jergesen HE, Karlen JW. Clinical outcome in total hip arthroplasty using a cemented titanium femoral prosthesis. J Arthroplasty. 2002; 17(5):592–9
18. Kärrholm J, Nivbrant B, Thanner J, Anderberg C, Börlin N, Herberts P, Malchau H. Radiossstereometric evaluation of hip implant design and surface finish. Scientific Exhibition, AAOS, Orlando, USA, 2000
19. Lichtinger TK, Schurmann N, Muller RT. Early loosening of a cemented hip endoprosthesis stem of titanium. Unfallchirurg 2000; 103(11):956–60
20. Massoud SN, Hunter JB, Holdsworth BJ, Wallace WA, Juliusson R. Early femoral loosening in one design of cemented hip replacement. J Bone Joint Surg Br 1997; 79(4):603–8
21. McGrath LR, Shardlow DL, Ingham E, Andrews M, Ivory J, Stone MH, Fisher J. A retrieval study of capital hip prostheses with titanium alloy femoral stems. J Bone Joint Surg Br 2001; 83(8):1195–201
22. Muller RT, Heger I, Oldenburg M The mechanism of loosening in cemented hip prostheses determined from long-term results. Arch Orthop Trauma Surg. 1997; 116(1–2):41–5
23. Niinimaki T, Puranen J, Jalovaara P. Total hip arthroplasty using isoelastic femoral stems. A seven- to nine-year follow-up in 108 patients. J Bone Joint Surg Br. 1994; 76(3):413–8
24. Nivbrant B, Karrholm J, Soderlund P. Increased migration of the SHP prosthesis: radiostereometric comparison with the Lubinus SP2 design in 40 cases. Acta Orthop Scand 1999; 70(6):569–77
25. Peters CL, Bachus KN, Craig MA, Higginbotham TO. The effect of femoral prosthesis design on cement strain in cemented total hip arthroplasty. J Arthroplasty. 2001; 16(2):216–24
26. Thomas SR, Shukla D, Latham PD. Corrosion of cemented titanium femoral stems. J Bone Joint Surg Br 2004; 86(7):974–8

27. Puolakka TJ, Pajamaki KJ, Halonen PJ, Pulkkinen PO, Paavolainen P, Nevalainen JK. The Finnish Arthroplasty Register: report of the hip register. Acta Orthop Scand. 2001; 72(5):433–41

28. Race A, Miller MA, Ayers DC, Cleary RJ, Mann KA. The influence of surface roughness on stem-cement gaps. J Bone Joint Surg Br. 2002; 84(8):1199–204

29. Ramamohan N, Grigoris P, Schmolz W, Chappell AM, Hamblen DL. Early failure of stainless steel 3M Captial femoral stem. J Bone Joint Surg Br. 2000 82-B suppl-1 p. 71

30. Royal College of Surgeons of England. 3M Capital Hip System: The lessons learned from an investigation, 2001a

31. Royal College of Surgeons of England. An Investigation of the Performance of the 3M Capital Hip System, 2001b

32. Sylvain GM, Kassab S, Coutts R, Santore R. Early failure of a roughened surface, precoated femoral component in total hip arthroplasty. J Arthroplasty. 2001; 16(2):141–8

33. Thomas SR, Shukla D, Latham PD. Corrosion of cemented titanium femoral stems. J Bone Joint Surg Br 2004; 86(7):974–8

34. Verdonschot N, Tanck E, Huiskes R. Effects of prosthesis surface roughness on the failure process of cemented hip implants after stem-cement debonding. J Biomed Mater Res 1998 15; 42(4):554–9

35. Verdonschot N, Huiskes R. Surface roughness of debonded straight-tapered stems in cemented THA reduces subsidence but not cement damage. Biomaterials. 1998; 19(19):1773–9

36. Verdonschot N, Barink M, Stolk J, Gardeniers JW, Schreurs BW. Do unloading periods affect migration characteristics of cemented femoral components? An in vitro evaluation with the Exeter stem. Acta Orthop Belg. 2002; 68(4):348–55

37. von Knoch M, Bluhm A, Morlock M, von Foerster G. Absence of surface roughness changes after insertion of one type of matte cemented femoral component during 2 to 15 years. J Arthroplasty. 2003 Jun;18(4):471–7.

38. Willert HG, Broback LG, Buchhorn GH, Jensen PH, Koster G, Lang I, Ochsner P, Schenk R. Crevice corrosion of cemented titanium alloy stems in total hip replacements. Clin Orthop 1996; (333):51–75

Implant Choice:
Stem Design – The Surgeon's Perspective

Jonathan R. Howell, Mathew J.W. Hubble, Robin S.M. Ling

Summary

This chapter considers the principles behind the design of cemented femoral stems and concentrates on the issues that are important to the surgeon when selecting a stem for use in clinical practice. Two main issues are central to a surgeon's choice of implant in hip replacement surgery: long-term function of the prosthesis and the versatility of the hip replacement system. The first part of the chapter examines how stem design may affect fixation of the stem within the femur and the long-term performance of a hip replacement. The second part of the chapter considers the needs of the surgeon in the operating room and how design of a cemented stem system may help the surgeon recreate each patient's anatomy and thereby achieve the optimum outcome.

Introduction

In 1960, Sir John Charnley revolutionised hip-replacement surgery when he described the use of acrylic cement to fix the femoral prosthesis inside the shaft of the femur [16]. During the initial experience with cemented hip replacements, relatively crude techniques were used to introduce the cement by hand and then insertion of the prosthesis was relied upon to achieve extrusion of the cement into the inner surface of the bone. Using these techniques, variable results were seen, with failure rates at 10 years ranging between 1.5% and 40% [42, 62].

Over the past 40 years, concerted efforts have been made to improve the results of cemented hip replacement and to achieve more reliable results. These efforts have included engineering and laboratory research and clinical studies, which have led to greater understanding of

the properties and use of bone cement and the influence of stem design on the longevity of hip replacements. In addition, advances in the design of implants and surgical instruments have helped the surgeon to achieve a more reliable result for patients with widely varying anatomy, and for both primary and revision procedures.

In choosing a cemented stem system for use in clinical practice, a surgeon is faced with two main areas for consideration. The first of these is the influence that the stem design has on the long-term clinical performance of the prosthesis, and thus the success of the operation. The second pertains to practical issues of use including instrumentation, and the versatility of the system in meeting the requirements posed by a wide range of clinical scenarios. In this chapter we shall examine how stem design may influence events at the interfaces of a cemented hip replacement, how it may affect the cement itself, and how, ultimately it may determine the long-term result of the operation. We shall then consider some of the practical issues of use that a surgeon will need to bear in mind when choosing a cemented stem.

Stem Design, Fixation and Survivorship

Materials and Interfaces of a Cemented Hip Replacement

The femoral component of a cemented total hip replacement has been described as a rod inside two tubes [60], the inner tube of which is the polymethylmethacrylate cement and the outer tube of which is the femur. This model illustrates that there are three materials present in a cemented hip replacement: the metal of the stem, the cement and the bone; and they are separated by two interfaces: the stem/

cement interface and the cement/bone interface. Gruen described the modes of failure of total hip replacements [32], illustrating that failure may occur within any of these materials or at either of the interfaces. Stem fracture was a common mode of failure in early designs of hip replacement [29], but the use of strengthened alloys in modern designs has almost abolished this form of failure [45], and when failure occurs in the modern cemented femoral stem it does so most commonly through loosening at the cement/bone interface [65], which is associated with loss of bone stock. However, the initiator of this loosening can occur at either of the interfaces or within the cement itself [38] and two major pathways are thought to contribute to the loosening of THR components [65]. The first is accumulated damage within the materials and at the interfaces leading to mechanical loosening of the implant. The second is the biological reactions made by the host in response to the presence of wear particles [4, 41, 53] and changes in fluid pressure around the femoral stem [5, 7]. These biological reactions ultimately lead to bone resorption and the loss of fixation at the cement/bone interface. In the following sections we consider fixation of the femoral stem and how this may fail, and how both of these issues may be affected by stem design.

Philosophy of Femoral Stem Fixation

The design of a cemented femoral stem has fundamental influence over its ability to attain stable and durable fixation but there has been considerable debate about how this can best be achieved. In the last few years, scientific opinion has become increasingly divided into two design philosophies highlighted in 1998 by Huiskes et al. [15] who reintroduced the concept of shape-closed fixation versus force-closed modes of fixation for cemented femoral stems.

A shape-closed fixation design is one in which the stem achieves fixation at the stem/cement interface through a match in the shapes of the surfaces of the stem and the cement with the cement gripping the surface of the stem. These designs have matt or textured surfaces into which it is intended the cement will penetrate, thus achieving a solid bond of the stem to the cement. Conversely, a force-closed system is one in which the fixation of the stem within the cement is achieved through the balance of forces without the need for the existence of a bond between the stem and the cement.

Shen [60] has argued along similar lines and has suggested that a cemented stem may act either as a composite beam or as a loaded taper. For a stem to act as a composite beam there must be perfect bonding at all times between the stem and cement. These two materials have markedly different Young's modulus, indicating that the stiffness of the two materials differs widely. For this type of fixation to

succeed, the strains in the stem and cement must be equal at the interface at all times, and for all loading conditions, but the strain in the material is dependent upon the stiffness. This means that for any given load the strain in the cement is likely to be greater than that in the metal of the stem surface and there is likely to be micro-motion and hence debonding at the stem/cement interface.

Alternatively, a stem may act as a taper within the cement, in which case fixation is achieved through the balance of forces across the interface and bonding between the stem and cement is neither necessary nor desirable. The balance of forces arises from the ability of a polished tapered stem to subside over short distances within the cement mantle. As the stem subsides it applies a radial compression force to the cement and the greater the load that is applied to the stem, the tighter its fit becomes across the stem/cement interface through its action as a taper.

Composite Beam Stem Fixation

In attempts to achieve shape-closed fixation, several authors have investigated the relationship between stem surface roughness and the shear strength achieved at the interface [6, 13, 17, 23]. In push out tests [6, 17, 23] and in torsional testing [13] it has been shown that increasing the stem roughness leads to increased strength of the stem/cement interface, although in many cases the testing methods have been unrealistic and have disregarded the effects of cyclical loading [6, 17]. These experimental data have led to the belief that a rough surface finish is beneficial [35] and to the development of a number of femoral prostheses with roughened surfaces. In addition, attempts have been made to improve the bonding between stem and cement by pre-coating the stem surface with cement applied onto the surface during manufacture of the stem [35]. The pre-coated stem is then inserted into the cement in the femoral canal, which binds with the pre-coated surface. Barb et al. [8] examined the interfacial strengths of pre-coated stems in an animal model and found that interfacial strengths were significantly higher in pre-coated stems. Raab et al. [56] showed that pre-coated metal/cement interfaces exhibited fracture toughness in excess of the acrylic cement, a finding that contrasted with their studies of uncoated metal surfaces [55]. Fatigue testing studies [25, 56] have suggested that pre-coating significantly increased the fatigue life of the stem/cement interface and initial clinical trials suggested that the use of pre-coated stems was associated with favourable short to medium term survival in some studies [9, 31, 59]. However, Callaghan et al. [14, 15] have found that the use of a pre-coated stem was associated with poor survival, with a loosening rate of 24% at an average of only 8 years follow-up and this poor survival of pre-coated femoral stems has been confirmed by several other clinical studies [18, 27,

30, 52, 70]. Therefore, it appears that, despite theoretical advantages, the use of pre-coating is detrimental to the long-term survival of femoral implants.

Several authors have suggested that attempts to strengthen the stem/cement interface using pre-coated stems or roughened stems causes failure at the cement/bone interface [30, 45, 57] and finite element analysis studies [47, 63] has suggested that a firm bond at the stem/cement interface may have harmful effects at the cement/bone interface.

Polished Tapered Stem Fixation

The original design of the Exeter stem was a collarless taper and its original surface finish was polished because the industry standards at the time of its introduction in 1970 demanded such a surface finish. The tapered geometry was chosen for its ability to compress the cement into the endosteal surface of the bone during stem insertion [29] and the collar was removed because of clinical observations of calcar resorption underneath the collars of other stems in use at the time. This loss of calcar height occurs even in cases in which there was intimate initial contact between the collar and calcar [58] and indicates that the collar is not an effective method of load transfer to the proximal femur.

Early experience with the collarless polished taper demonstrated several features that suggested that this stem may transmit loads to the endosteal surface of the bone in a different way to that of conventional stems. The most striking finding was that of distal migration of the stem, usually over distances of 2 mm or less, and without cement fracture or disruption of the cement/bone interface [29]. Subsequent retrieval analysis and laboratory experiments have shown that this subsidence is accommodated by cement creep. Indeed the subsidence of the polished taper within the cement means that this type of stem can maintain satisfactory fixation despite changes in the cement mantle over time, a phenomenon that will not be seen with stems that utilise shape-closed fixation. This ability to subside may allow the loading of the stem to be distributed evenly, especially in the proximal femur where remarkable preservation of calcar bone was seen with this stem [29].

The taper action of stems utilising force-closed fixation means that the cement and bone are loaded principally in compression and shear forces are reduced. This is likely to be protective for both the cement and bone. The effect of stem surface finish on cement stresses has been investigated by Miles et al. [50] who have shown that for polished stems the major load component was radial compression but for textured stems there was significant shear. There has been much research into the physical properties of acrylic cement [44] and this has shown that cement is sig-

nificantly stronger when loaded in compression compared to loading in tension or shear. A 3-D numerical stress analysis [22] has concluded that loading in compression may be the only reliable mechanism of loading in vivo. Certainly, clinical experience with polished tapered stems has shown that this design is associated with exceptional long-term performance despite the appearance of debonding at the stem/cement interface [29, 49, 69].

Stem Migration and Wear

For a stem to achieve shape-closed fixation there must be a perfect bond between the cement and the stem, and this bond must be durable to provide long-term success of the hip replacement. There is evidence in the literature that such a bond does not exist even immediately after stem insertion [11, 12, 67] and that a gap exists between stem and cement that allows fluid migration [20] and the formation of a membrane at this interface [28]. Such a gap may exist due to thermal shrinkage of the cement or due to imperfect cement interdigitation into the stem surface features [1, 21, 28, 44, 46, 67]. Additionally, both experimental [55, 26, 34, 64] and in-vivo [40, 52] studies have shown that during the service lifetime of a hip replacement the stem further debonds from the cement, opening up a gap between the stem and cement and many believe that this is an inevitable occurrence that cannot be prevented, at least in a proportion of hip replacements [15, 22, 49, 65].

There is increasing evidence from radiostereometric analysis (RSA) that femoral stems of all designs undergo migration [43], although the pattern of migration is dependent upon the stem design. In a comparison of the Exeter (force-closed fixation) and the Charnley Elite (shape-closed fixation) stems, Alfaro-Adrian et al. [3] have shown fundamental differences exist in the patterns of migration of the two systems. The Exeter stems tended to migrate distally at a higher initial rate than the Charnley Elite, but they had a slower posterior migration of the femoral head. The pattern of movement of the Charnley Elite was one of rapid initial posterior head migration and slower distal migration. The migration of both stems slowed after the first year. The difference in the direction of stem movement has important consequences for the long-term survival of hip replacements. Traditionally, it has been believed that distal migration of cemented stems is predictive of failure, but it is important to distinguish at which interface movement is occurring. The distal subsidence of the Exeter stem has been shown to occur at the stem/cement interface [2] and not at the cement/bone interface, and as the Exeter subsides distally it loads the cement in compression and the cement/bone interface is protected. In contrast, the Charnley Elite stem loads the cement in shear and distal migration occurs at both the stem/cement and cement/bone interfaces.

The posterior migration of the Charnley Elite stem is of particular importance. During activities such as stair-climbing and rising from a chair the femoral head is subjected to a large posteriorly-directed component of the joint reaction force [10], which tends to displace the femoral stem posteriorly within the cement, which may lead to early failure of the hip [51]. Alfaro-Adrian et al. [3] found that there was a subset of Charnley Elite stems that exhibited abnormally rapid posterior migration in the first year, which continued in the second year of service, and these stems are likely to fail. In contrast, none of the Exeter stems in their study exhibited rapid posterior migration, probably because the distal migration of the tapered stem and the rectangular cross-sectional geometry make the Exeter particularly resistant to torsional forces.

Debonding of the stem/cement interface may allow micro-movement of the stem within its cement mantle [28, 39, 40, 43] leading to abrasion of the two surfaces, the loss of stem fixation and the generation of wear debris that can produce three body wear [23, 33, 65, 66]. The present authors have undertaken a systematic analysis of stem wear [36] on the surface of 172 femoral stems of 23 different designs. Wear was analysed using three different methods: visual inspection and light microscopy; interference microscopy, and scanning electron microscopy. This study demonstrated that wear changes affected 93% of stems in the study and this included 74 stems that were stated as being well fixed by the revising surgeon. However, these wear changes were often difficult to see with the naked eye and in 30 cases they would have been missed altogether without specialised techniques. The wear was often very localised and was concentrated along the anterolateral and posteromedial borders of the stems. These are the areas of the stem that Berme and Paul [10] demonstrated were subjected to the highest torsional forces as a result of the posteriorly-directed component of the joint reaction force, that also causes the posterior migration of the femoral head seen in RSA studies.

One of the most striking findings of this study was the fundamental difference in wear morphology found on matt and polished stems, summarised in ◘ Table 7.3. Matt stems were found to wear through abrasive polishing of the surface (◘ Fig. 7.13) and debris from the wear process was removed from the stem surface. Removal of debris

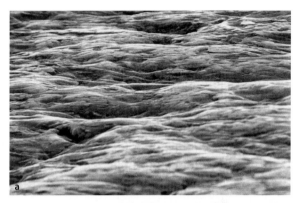
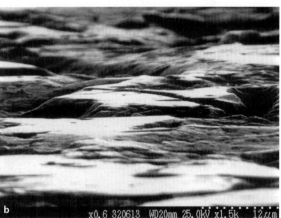

◘ **Fig. 7.13a,b.** Scanning electron micrograph showing typical wear of matt stems. **a** An unworn area of stem showing well-defined surface asperities. **b** Localised abrasive wear of a matt stem. Note how the tips of the asperities have been removed at a uniform height (Reprinted from [36] with permission from Elsevier)

◘ **Table 7.3.** The morphology and distribution of wear changes found on matt and polished stems

	Matt Stems	Polished Stems
Wear morphology	*Polishing* wear 92% (122/132)	*Pitting* wear 94% (44/47)
Debris retention	3% of stems showed retention of debris on surface	86% of stems showed retention of debris on surface
Wear distribution (areas of highest wear)	Anterolateral border Posteromedial border Collar under surfaces	Anterolateral border Posteromedial border
Other phenomena	Slurry Wear Release of Alumina	Not Seen Not Seen

is likely to be brought about by fluid in the stem/cement interface and in our electron microscopy studies we found evidence of slurry wear of the matt stem surfaces, caused by high pressure fluid containing hard particles (■ Fig. 7.14). In contrast, the wear morphology of polished stems was typical of fretting wear and we found the stem surface surrounding the areas of wear were unaffected by the wear process (■ Fig. 7.15). This has important implications as it implies that the stem/cement interface surrounding the localised wear on polished stems is not disturbed and we believe it explains why debris was found locked into the boundaries of the wear pits.

Several authors [15, 23, 66] have suggested that the long-term success of a hip replacement depends on minimising the effects of micro-motion at the stem cement interface. In our wear studies, we found fundamental differences between the action of matt and polished stems in this respect. The abrasive polishing of a matt surface is likely to be mirrored by abrasive wear of the cement mantle, which may have several important effects. Firstly, it generates large numbers of particles that may contribute to three body effects both at the stem/cement interface and at the articulation if they can gain access to it through fluid flow. In this regard, it is interesting to note that a universal finding during the electron microscopy of matt stems was the exposure and release of alumina particles from the stem surface (■ Fig. 7.16). Alumina is used to shot blast the stem surface in the production of a matt finish, and some of the grains appear to become embedded within the surface, only to be uncovered by subsequent stem wear. The release of hard ceramic particles from the surface of matt stems is likely to add to the three body effects caused by metal and cement particles.

The second important effect of abrasive wear of the cement mantle is enlargement of the internal dimensions, which means that cyclical movements of the stem are likely to increase leading to further cement wear. The effect is to destabilise the stem within its cement mantle and to enlarge the space available for fluid flow along the interface. As the amplitude of stem micromotion increases, significant hydrostatic effects may be generated that may lead to slurry wear, and which may contribute to the development of lysis. The fretting wear of polished stems occurs below the level of the original stem surface and as ■ Fig. 7.15 shows the surrounding stem is unaffected. It is therefore likely that the surrounding cement is also unaffected and that polished stem wear represents a more benign process. Furthermore, a stem with a polished surface and the correct geometry may function as a taper within the cement [29, 54, 60], allowing subsidence of the stem within the cement mantle, thus closing the stem/cement interface and so prevent fluid migration and the dispersal of particulate debris.

In view of the differences between polished and matt stems in their wear morphology and their propensity for

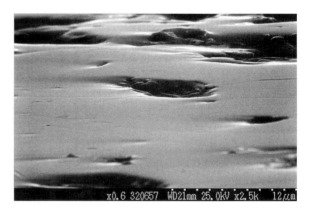

■ **Fig. 7.14.** Scanning electron micrograph of erosion or »slurry wear« seen on the surface of a matt stem. A comet tail appearance is seen on one side of each surface depression, a typical appearance of slurry wear caused by high pressure fluid containing hard particles (Reprinted from [36] with permission from Elsevier)

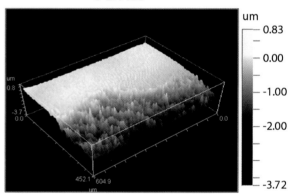

■ **Fig. 7.15.** Interference microscopy appearance of fretting wear of a polished stem. The edge of a fretting pit is shown and illustrates that the wear occurs below the level of the original stem surface. Note how the surrounding stem surface is unaffected by the localised wear pit and therefore the stem/cement interface surrounding the pit is unlikely to be disturbed (Reprinted from [36] with permission from Elsevier)

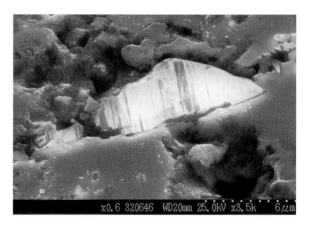

■ **Fig. 7.16.** Scanning electron micrograph showing an alumina particle that had been embedded on the surface of a matt stem, and that was uncovered by the abrasive wear process (Reprinted from [36] with permission from Elsevier)

◩ **Table 7.4.** Clinical outcomes of stems that have existed with different surface finishes during their histories

Reference	Stem	Alloy	Ra [µm]	Follow-up [Years]	Loosening [%]	Focal Lysis [%]	Revision for ASL [%]
Dall et al. 1993 [24]	Charnley Flat back	EN58J	0.03	3–17	3.1		
	Subsequent Charnleys	316L	0.6	3–17	11.4		
Crawford et al. 1998 [19]	Polished Exeter Monoblock	REX734 –'Orthinox'	0.01–0.03	8–10		0	
	Matt Exeter Monoblock	REX734 –'Orthinox'	0.8–1.2	8–10		21.7	
Howie et al. 1998 [37]	Polished Exeter Monoblock	REX734 –'Orthinox'	0.01–0.03	8–10			0
	Matt Exeter Monoblock	REX734 –'Orthinox'	0.8–1.2	8–10			20
Collis et al. 1998 [18]	T28	316L	0.03	11.04		0	
	TR28	CoCrMb	0.9–1.2	10.48		4.9	
Collis et al. 1998 [18]	Iowa (bb*)	CoCrMb	0.75	10.46			***
	Iowa (gb**)	CoCrMb	2.0	7.21			***
Sporer et al. 1999 [61]	Iowa (bb*)	CoCrMb	0.8	11.3			6
	Iowa (gb**) + pre-coat	CoCrMb	2.1	8.2			18
Meding et al. 2000 [48]	T28	316L	0.03	17–21	11.1		
	TR28	CoCrMb	0.9–11.2	17–21	15.8		

* bead blasted, ** grit blasted, *** in the first 5 years, revision rate was 5 times higher for the grit-blasted and pre-coated stems than for the bead blasted. stems

damage of the cement mantle, it could be expected that patterns of behaviour should have emerged in the orthopaedic literature regarding stems, like the Exeter, that have existed over time with identical geometry but with different surface finishes. In ◩ Table 7.4, the literature on this subject is summarised, and it shows that in no instance has a stem exhibited better long-term results with a rougher surface finish. Thus it appears that stem and cement wear may be of fundamental importance to the long-term survivorship of a cemented total hip replacement.

Stem Design, Versatility and Practical Use

Reproducing the Anatomy

In order to achieve a successful result for a wide range of patients and clinical situations, a surgeon must have available a system that allows considerable tailoring to the needs of the individual. The anatomical considerations that will need to be addressed at the time of the operation include femoral offset, leg length, femoral neck anteversion and the canal size, and the ideal femoral stem system will allow a surgeon to address each issue independently.

Femoral offset is the horizontal distance between the centre of the femoral head and a line drawn vertically down the midline of the femur. The offset affects tension within the soft-tissue envelope of the hip as well as the lever arm of the abductors. Decreasing a patient's femoral offset will tend to reduce tissue tension around the hip and will risk dislocation of the hip. In addition, it will shorten the lever arm of the abductors, meaning that the abductors will need to increase the force of their contraction in order to stabilise the pelvis. This in turn increases the joint reaction force to which the hip is subjected, which will predispose to aseptic loosening of the hip-replacement components. On the other hand, increasing a patient's offset is also poorly tolerated, as it tends to increase tension within the fascia lata, and predisposes to the development of trochanteric bursitis. It is therefore essential for the surgeon to reproduce the patient's own offset as closely as possible at the time of the operation. To achieve this will require a femoral stem system that offers a range of offsets independent of other variables. In addition, modularity of the head with a range of head offsets is desirable, as it will allow fine-tuning after insertion of the main components.

Leg-length discrepancy is a significant source of dissatisfaction and a major cause of litigation following total hip-replacement surgery. It is therefore essential that a surgeon should take the utmost care to achieve equality of leg length through control of the depth of insertion of the femoral stem. The design of the femoral stem can help in this regard in that a collarless stem may be seated at a variable depth, unconstrained by the presence of a collar, which will limit further insertion of the stem once contract is made with the calcar. The surgical instrumentation can also help the surgeon achieve equal leg lengths if a trial reduction can be performed using the stem broaches, particularly if the broaches bear markings that correspond to insertion depth guides on the femoral stem (☐ Fig. 7.17). During preparation of the femur, the broach is inserted to the depth that the surgeon believes is correct to restore leg length. A trial reduction is then carried out and the depth of broach insertion is adjusted as necessary. Having achieved the correct leg length, the surgeon marks the femur at the point opposite the insertion depth guide on the broach, and during final stem insertion the surgeon places the stem so that the corresponding mark on the prosthesis lies opposite the same mark, thus restoring the patient's anatomy.

During the operation it is important for a surgeon to be able to insert the femoral stem in the correct anteversion to optimise the range of movement and to minimise the risk of post-operative dislocation. The anteversion that is required will differ between surgeons, according to their individual surgical technique, and even for each surgeon subtle variations in femoral stem placement will be required depending on the position of the acetabular component so that a balanced hip is achieved. Therefore,

the design of the femoral stem should allow placement of the stem in variable anteversion independent of offset, leg length and stem size. In some patients, particularly in dysplastic cases, the patient's natural offset will need to be significantly modified and this may require a derotation osteotomy, often performed in association with a shortening osteotomy to allow restoration of the correct centre of hip rotation. The ideal stem design will allow such significant modification of anteversion without loss of stem fixation.

The last aspect of anatomy that requires replication is the stem size, which should be matched to the patient's femoral canal to ensure that an adequate cement mantle is achieved in every case. Use of a stem that is too large risks creating a cement mantle defect, and it may also be a cause of post-operative thigh pain, particularly if used in the ectatic osteopenic femur. Use of a stem that is too small risks stem fracture, particularly in the young, active and heavily built male patient. Therefore, the design of a femoral stem range should include the availability of a range of femoral stem sizes, independent of other factors such as offset. Ideally, the range of sizes should include stem sizes for patients with very narrow femora, such as encountered in the dysplastic femur and in cases of juvenile rheumatoid arthritis. In addition, smaller stem sizes will be required for some ethnic groups, particularly patients from Asia and the Far East, and the stem design should allow for this so that a surgeon is able to accommodate any eventuality that he or she encounters intra-operatively.

The development of navigation and computer-assisted surgery may mean that in the future surgeons have a further tool available to them to assist in the restoration of correct femoral offset, leg length and stem version, although the efficacy of this technology in this regard is as yet unproven. If navigation is shown to be effective, then in the future surgeons may wish to choose a femoral stem system for which appropriate software has been developed.

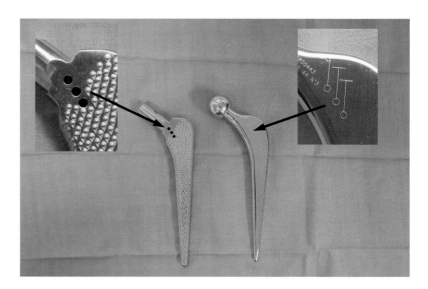

☐ **Fig. 7.17.** Depth markers on the broaches corresponding to markings on the prosthesis help a surgeon carry out an accurate trial reduction and assist with the restoration of correct leg length

Stem System Versatility

When selecting a design of stem system for use, surgeons look for a system that is versatile and that allows its use in a wide range of clinical situations. It is, for instance, useful for a surgeon to be able to use the same system for both primary and revision total hip replacement, and ideally for hemiarthroplasty as well. This allows the surgeon to gain familiarity and confidence with the system during easier primary cases, in preparation for its use in the more complex primary and revision cases. However, in order for the system to be effective in the revision setting, a number of stem options will be needed including the availability of a range longer stems, so that the surgeon is able to bypass cortical defects and periprosthetic fractures. The additional availability of instruments for impaction grafting allows the surgeon to deal with femoral bone stock loss, particularly in the younger patient and enhances the versatility of the stem system.

In many instances revision of a socket is required when femoral bone stock and fixation are well preserved. In order to facilitate socket exposure the femoral stem often needs to be removed, but with a composite beam type of stem such removal will often be difficult because of the bonding between stem and cement, and removal will of course destroy the fixation of this type of stem. This is not the case for a polished tapered stem, which can be removed with ease after the surgeon has cleared the cement over the top of the stem shoulder with a burr. The stem is tapped out, which does not affect the cement mantle, and at the end of the case the stem is reinserted into the old cement mantle. The authors tend to cement in a slightly smaller stem using a liquid mix of cement, which chemically binds to the old cement mantle. This technique of cement-in-cement revision has been used at the authors' institution for several years and a review of the results has just been completed. There were 189 patients with minimum five years follow-up after cement-in-cement revision, and there have been no revisions for aseptic loosening of the stem following this procedure. These results have demonstrated that the unique fixation and loading properties of the polished tapered stem allow its removal and reinsertion without deleterious effects on the survivorship of the implant, and the stem and cement can be considered as a truly modular system. The success of this technique has led to the development recently of a stem designed specifically for cement-in-cement revision (Fig. 7.18). This is a slightly shorter stem than the standard, but the offset is the same and it allows the surgeon to revise almost all designs of cemented stems without the need for cement removal. Instruments have been designed to prepare the distal cement for insertion of a hollow centralizer so that the stem continues to function as a taper.

Incorporation of a hemiarthroplasty option into the stem range adds to the versatility of the system, particu-

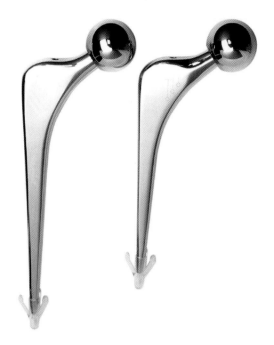

 Fig. 7.18. A short stem prosthesis developed for use in cement-in-cement revision

larly if it allows cement-in-cement revision. One of the major complications following hemiarthroplasty for intracapsular femoral neck fractures is acetabular erosion and the development of late post-operative pain, which may necessitate revision. The revision of a hemiarthroplasty may be a difficult operation and the documented rates of major intra-operative and post-operative complications are as high as 50% [68]. Intra-operative complications include femoral perforation and fracture, which are particular problems during the revision of curved cemented stems because the cement mantle must be removed before the revision stem can be inserted. The curved direction of the cement mantle tends to push instruments towards the weak cortices of the femur risking fracture and perforation. These problems can be overcome by using a straight stem for hemiarthroplasty that has the same geometry as the surgeon's usual primary stem, particularly if a polished tapered system is utilised as this will allow a cement-in-cement revision without compromising stem fixation.

Finally, the versatility of a hip-stem system will be enhanced through the capacity to use alternative bearings, tailored to the needs of the individual patient. Many surgeons now favour the use of a hard-on-hard bearing in the younger patient, in the hope that the reduced wear characteristics of these bearings will help reduce rates of loosening and lysis in the longer term. In addition, many of the hard bearing allow the use of large diameter heads, which may reduce dislocation rates. For these reasons modular stems and heads are of great benefit to surgeons, particularly if the stem spigot has been designed for use with different bearing options.

Take Home Messages

- In selecting an appropriate stem for use, surgeons take into account two main facets of design: the effect of the design on the long-term clinical result, and the practical issues of using a stem and its instrumentation.

- The philosophy of stem fixation has become increasingly polarised into two schools of thought: composite beam versus polished taper fixation.

- Composite beam fixation relies on perfect bonding between the stem and cement at all times and for all loading conditions.

- Polished taper fixation achieves stability through a balance of forces that result from the ability of the stem to subside within the cement mantle. Bonding is neither necessary or desirable.

- Perfect bonding between stem and cement may not be present, even immediately after the operation, and attempts to improve bonding have been clinically unsuccessful.

- RSA studies have shown micro-movement in all designs of stem examined, calling into question the whole issue of bonding at the stem/cement interface

- Not all migration is associated with a poor outcome. The distal migration of a polished tapered stem within the cement mantle is an essential feature of stem function and does not predict failure. Early posterior migration of a stem is predictive of early failure.

- Wear studies have shown that stem surface wear is almost a universal finding, again suggesting that micro-motion at the stem/cement interface is inevitable.

- Fundamental differences are seen in the wear morphology of matt and polished stems, with the abrasive wear of matt stems more likely to damage the cement, thus destabilising the stem and opening a gap for dispersal of debris through fluid flow.

- The clinical literature supports the hypothesis that differences in the pattern of stem wear may be of fundamental importance to the long-term success of a total hip replacement.

- Stem design should help the surgeon restore a patient's individual anatomy, and this should include the ability to tailor the offset, leg length, neck anteversion and stem size independent of each other.

- Stem versatility is enhanced through the availability of stems for hemiarthroplasty, primary total hip replacement and revision surgery. This will include the availability of a range of stem lengths and impaction grafting instruments. The ability to carry out cement-in-cement revision vastly increases the ease of use of a stem system, and the availability of a range of bearing options is also of great benefit.

References

1. Ahmed AM et al. (1982) Transient and residual stresses and displacements in self curing bone cement – Part I: Characterization of relevant behaviour of bone cement. J Biomech Eng 104: 21–7
2. Alfaro-Adrian J et al. (1999) Cement migration after THR: a comparison of Charnley Elite and Exeter femoral stems using RSA. J Bone Joint Surg Br 81:130–4
3. Alfaro-Adrián J et al. (2001) Should total hip arthroplasty femoral components be designed to subside? A radiosterometric analysis study of the Charnley Elite and Exeter stems. J Arthroplasty 16(5):598–606
4. Amstutz HC et al. (1992) Mechanism and clinical significance of wear debris-induced osteolysis. Clin Orthop 276:7–18
5. Anthony PP et al. (1990) Localised endosteal bone lysis in relation to the femoral components of cemented total hip arthroplasties. J Bone Joint Surg Br 72(6):971–9
6. Arroyo NA, Stark CF (1987) The effects of textures, surface finish and precoating on the strength of bone cement/stem interfaces. Proceedings 13th Society for Biomaterials, New York: 218
7. Aspenberg P, Van der Vis H (1998) Migration, particles and fluid pressure. A discussion of causes of prosthetic loosening. Clin Orthop 352:75–80
8. Barb W et al. (1982) Intramedullary fixation of artificial hip joints with bone cement- precoated implants. I. Interfacial strengths. J Biomed Mater Res 16(4):447–58
9. Berger RA et al. (1996) Hybrid total hip arthroplasty: Seven to ten year results. Clin Orthop 333:134–46
10. Berme N, Paul JP (1979) Load actions transmitted by implants. J Biomed Eng 1:268–72
11. Brumby SA (1997) Migration, micromotion and debonding: The effect of the femoral stem surface finish and a collar. Transactions of Orthopaedic Research Society 22:353
12. Brumby SA (1998) Radiographic and histologic analysis of cemented double tapered femoral stems. 335: 229–37
13. Bundy KJ, Penn RW (1987) The effect of surface preparation on metal/bone cement interfacial strength. J Biomed Mater Res 21(6):773–805
14. Callaghan JJ et al. (1996) Primary hybrid total hip arthroplasty: An interim follow-up. Clin Orthop 333:118–25
15. Callaghan JJ et al. (1997) Total hip arthroplasty in the young adult. Clin Orthop 1997 344:257–62
16. Charnley J (1960) Anchorage of the femoral head prosthesis to the shaft of the femur. J Bone Joint Surg Br 42:28–30
17. Chen CQ et al. (1999) Effect of metal surface topography on mechanical bonding at simulated total hip stem-cement interfaces. J Biomed Mater Res 48(4):440–6
18. Collis DK, Mohler CG (1998) Loosening rates and bone lysis with rough finished and polished stems. Clin Orthop 355:113–22
19. Crawford RW et al. (1998) An 8–10 year clinical review comparing matt and polished Exeter stems. Orthop Trans 22(1):40
20. Crawford RW et al. (1999) Fluid migration around model cemented femoral components. J Bone Joint Surg Br 81 SUPP I:82
21. Crawford RW et al. (1999) Fluid flow around model femoral components of differing surface finishes – In vitro investigations. Acta Orthop Scand 70(6):589–95
22. Crowninshield RD et al. (1980) The effect of femoral stem cross-sectional geometry on cement stresses in total hip reconstruction. Clin Orthop 28;(146):71–7
23. Crowninshield RD et al. (1998) Cemented femoral component surface finish mechanics. Clin Orthop 355:90–102
24. Dall DM et al. (1993) Fracture and loosening of Charnley femoral stems: comparison between first-generation and subsequent designs. J Bone Joint Surg Br 75:259–65

7

25. Davies JP, Harris WH (1993) Strength of cement-metal interfaces in fatigue: comparison of smooth, porous and precoated specimens. Clin Mater 12(2):121–6

26. Davies JP et al. (1996) Monitoring the integrity of the cement-metal interface of total joint components in vitro using acoustic emission and ultrasound. J Arthroplasty 11(5):594–601

27. Dowd JE (1998) Failure of total hip arthroplasty with a precoated prosthesis: 4-toll-year results. Clin Orthop 355:123–36

28. Fornasier VL, Cameron HU (1976) The femoral stem/cement interface in total hip replacement. Clin Orthop 116:248–52

29. Fowler J et al. (1988) Experience with Exeter Hip since 1970. Orthop Clinics N America 19:477–89

30. Gardiner RC, Hozack WJ (1994) Failure of the cement-bone interface. A consequence of strengthening the cement-prosthesis interface? J Bone Joint Surg Br 76(1):49–52

31. Goldberg VM et al. (1996) Hybrid total hip arthroplasty: A 7- to 11-year follow-up. Clin Orthop 333:147–54.

32. Gruen TA et al. (1979) 'Modes of Failure' of cemented stem-type femoral components. Clin Orth 141:17–27

33. Harrigan TP, Harris WH (1991) A three-dimensional non-linear finite element study of the effect of cement-prosthesis debonding in cemented femoral total hip components. J Biomech 24(11): 1047–58

34. Harrigan TP et al. (1992) A finite element study of the initiation of failure of fixation in cemented femoral total hip components. J Orthop Res 10(1):134–44

35. Harris WH (1992) Is it advantageous to strengthen the cement-metal interface and use a collar for cemented femoral components of total hip replacements? Clin Orthop Dec 285:67–72

36. Howell JR et al. (2004) In vivo surface wear mechanisms of femoral components of cemented total hip arthroplasties: the influence of wear mechanism on clinical outcome. J Arthroplasty 19(1):88–101

37. Howie DW et al. Loosening of matt and polished cemented femoral stems. J Bone Joint Surg Br 80(4):573–6

38. Huiskes R (1993) Failed innovation in total hip replacement. Acta Orthop Scand 64:699–716

39. Huiskes R et al. (1998) Migration, stem shape, and surface finish in cemented total hip arthroplasty. Clin Orthop 355:103–12

40. Jasty M et al. (1991) The initiation of failure in cemented femoral components of hip arthroplasties. J Bone Joint Surg Br 73(4):551–8

41. Jasty M et al. (1992) Acrylic fragmentation in total hip replacements and its biological consequences. Clin Orthop 1992;116–28

42. Johnstone RC, Crowninshield RD (1983) Roentgenologic results of total hip arthroplasty. Clin Orth 181:92

43. Karrholm J et al. (2000) Radiosteriometric evaluation of hip implant design and surface finish. Scientific exhibit 67th Annual Meeting of the AAOS, March 15–19, Orlando, USA

44. Lewis G (1997) Properties of acrylic bone cement: state of the art review. J Biomed Mater Res 38(2):155–82

45. Ling R (1992) The use of a collar and pre-coating on cemented femoral stems is unnecessary and detrimental. Clin Orth 285: 73–83

46. Ling RS, Lee AJ (1998) Porosity reduction in acrylic cement is clinically irrelevant. Clin Orthop 1998 355:249–53

47. Mann KA et al. (1992) The effect of using a plasma-sprayed stem-cement interface on stresses in a cemented femoral hip component. Trans Orthop Res Soc 17:317

48. Meding JB (2000) Long-term survival of the T-28 versus the TR-28 cemented total hip arthroplasties. 15(7): 928–33

49. Middleton RG et al. (1998). Effects of design changes on cemented tapered femoral stem fixation. Clin Orthop 1998 355:47–56

50. Miles AW et al. (1990) The effect of the surface finish of the femoral component on load transmission in total hip replacement. J Bone Joint Surg Br (Suppl) 72:736

51. Mjoberg B et al. (1984) Instability of total hip prostheses at rotational stress: a roentgen stereophotogrammetric study. Acta Orthop Scand 55:504–6

52. Mohler CG et al. (1995) Early loosening of the femoral component at the cement-prosthesis interface after total hip replacement. J Bone Joint Surg Am 77(9):1315–22

53. Muller RT et al. (1997) The mechanism of loosening in cemented hip prostheses determined from long-term results. Arch Orthop Trauma Surg 116:41–5

54. Norman TL et al. (1996) Axisymmetric finite element analysis of a debonded total hip stem with an unsupported distal tip. J Biomech Eng 118:399–404

55. Raab S et al. (1982) The quasistic and fatigue performance of the implant/bone-cement interface. J Biomed Mat Res 15:159

56. Raab S et al. (1982) Thin film PMMA precoating for improved implant bone-cement fixation. J Biomed Mat Res 16:679

57. Ramaniraka NA et al. (2000) The fixation of the cemented femoral component. Effects of stem stiffness, cement thickness and roughness of the cement-bone surface. J Bone Joint Surg Br 82(2):297–303

58. Rickards R, Duncan CP (1986). The collar-calcar contact controversy. J Bone Joint Surg Br 68:851

59. Schmalzried TP, Harris WH (1993) Hybrid total hip replacement: A 6.5 year follow-up study. J Bone Joint Surg Br 75:608–15

60. Shen G (1998) Femoral stem fixation: An engineering interpretation of the long-term outcome of Charnley and Exeter stems. J Bone Joint Surgery Br 80:754–56

61. Sporer SM et al. (1999) The effects of surface roughness and polymethylmethacrylate precoating on the radiographic and clinical results of the Iowa hip prosthesis. J Bone Joint Surg Am 81:481–92

62. Sutherland CJ et al. (1982) A ten-year follow-up of 100 consecutive Muller curved-stem total hip replacement arthroplasties. J Bone Joint Surg Am 64:970–82

63. Verdonschot N, Huiskes R (1996) Mechanical effects of stem cement interface characteristics in total hip replacement. Clin Orthop 329:326–36

64. Verdonschot N, Huiskes R (1997). Cement debonding process of total hip arthroplasty stems. Clin Orthop 336:297–307

65. Verdonschot N, Huiskes R (1998) Surface roughness of debonded straight-tapered stems in cemented THA reduces subsidence but not cement damage. Biomaterials 19:1773–9

66. Verdonschot N et al. (1998) Effects of prosthesis surface roughness on the failure process of cemented hip implants after stem-cement debonding. J Biomed Mater Res 42(4):554–9

67. Wang JS (1999) Interface gap after implantation of a cemented femoral stem in pigs. Acta Orthop Scand 1999 70(3):234–9

68. Warwick D et al. (1998) Revision of failed hemiarthroplasty for fractures at the hip. Int Orthop 22(3):165–8

69. Williams HD et al. (2002) The Exeter universal cemented femoral component at 8 to 12 years. A study of the first 325 hips. J Bone Joint Surg Br 2002 84(3):324–34

70. Woolfson ST, Haber DF (1996) Primary total hip replacement with insertion of an acetabular component without cement and a femoral component with cement. Follow-up study at an average of six years. J Bone Joint Surg Am 78:698–705

Implant Choice:
Migration Pattern and Outcome
of Cemented Stems in Sweden

Jeffrey Geller, Henrik Malchau, Johan Kärrholm

Summary

In this chapter we will focus on the femoral side of cemented hip implants and review the outcome in the Swedish Hip Registry. We will also describe the migration pattern of different stem designs over their lifespan and how this information contributes to the long-term outcomes of some of the more commonly used prostheses. Much of this data has been collected through studies using Radio Stereometric Analysis (RSA) data and will continue to provide further insight as these patients are tracked to obtain long term data. Presently, this data has shown that femoral stems that subside more than 0.1 mm in the first 2 years are at a significantly higher risk of failure than stems that exhibit less subsidence.

Introduction

An enormous number of cemented femoral stem designs are available to the orthopaedic surgeon. The minority of femoral implants has a published long-term track record and can be regarded as well-documented designs. Very different design rationales have produced similar excellent outcomes after 10 years [11] but the detailed function of each design »philosophy« is often not fully understood. The rationale for different stem geometries will be covered in a different chapter (▶ chapter 7.1), but in the context of the current discussion, stem geometry has an important effect on the pattern of migration. Among other factors such as grade of cement mantle, bone quality, and surface finish, stem geometry most closely correlates with migration pattern. For example, a stem with a tapered geometry behaves different than a straight stem.

For some designs the mechanism of failure has been identified, such as the roughened finish on the Centralign

hip in combination with its narrow, rounded geometry, or the extraordinarily high rate of stem-cement debonding in the 3M Capital hip [18]. Controversy still exists whether there is an ideal stem surface [10], but clinical experience has shown that both polished and matt stem designs can work. Each type of stem relies on a different force profile for solid fixation. A roughened femoral stem, most often accompanied by a collar, is maintained in position by »shape closed« fixation; stability is achieved in the original implanted position by the stem architecture and surface finish in the cement mantle. A smooth femoral stem, by contrast achieves stability by »force closed« fixation. In this scenario, the stem gains stability when the smooth stem, most often in a tapered shape, is supported by the surrounding cement mantle. The tapered shape can tolerate subsequent cement creep and still maintain good rotational stability [12, 24]. In a laboratory study examining the microscopic integration and adherence to roughened stems, the authors showed that the cement did not flow into the macro-texturing completely. This led to the formation of hollow spaces termed »volcanoes« and when these constructs were tested in vitro, the volcanoes were noted to be areas of early debonding of cement from the stem. This initiated the sequence of particle generation from debonding and subsequent loosening [7].

Several studies have supported roughened stems, both biomechanically as well as clinically. Most biomechanical models comparing femoral stems with different surface finishes report that the initial stability of a roughened, cemented, straight femoral stem with a collar is the most stable configuration when subjected to simulated walking and stair climbing forces compared to smooth stems. The testing regimens used in these investigations are often designed to only simulate activity within the first month of implantation only, and do not address longer term stability (and cement creep) and their value is thus limited [6, 8].

Some clinical studies have also supported the use of femoral stems with a roughened finish with published survival rates of 95–99% after ten to fifteen years [5, 14, 19].

Other investigations have shown no difference between surface finishes. Rasquinha and associates showed no difference between smooth and roughened surface finish in a short-term prospective trial [20]. This may be misleading, as other longer-term data show that after 8–11 years, these results deteriorate for the roughened femoral stems with markedly higher failure rates and resultant bony destruction. As a result of this experience, the use of stems with roughened finish was abandoned by the investigators and led them to advocate the routine use of polished stems when cementing the femoral side of a total hip replacement [21].

Finally, several published reports have demonstrated excellent long term results using smooth, tapered cemented femoral stems [3, 13, 26]. These stems have shown excellent results between 7 and 16 years with a revision rate of 0–7% for aseptic loosening, respectively. All stems had a similar stem geometry including a tapered geometry with a relatively flat back design, as introduced by Charnley. As of the time of this writing, there have been no such dramatic failures reported of smooth cemented stems. It is of significant value to continuously evaluate existing stem designs by monitoring long-term performance, but it is equally important to evaluate newer stem designs.

Evaluation of Stem Design Performance in Sweden

Outcome of cemented femoral stems can be evaluated with several methods. The vast majority of knowledge has historically been via reports in the literature. The limitation to solely relying on this medium for all of our information is the inherent risk for bias in these investigations. Many of these reports are of small series with limited numbers of surgeons performed in a retrospective manner. Nonetheless, they do provide a type of documentation about implants that might not ever else be published. Another important, yet fairly crude way is to report implant survival or revision rates without any clinical or radiographic data input (i.e. implant registries). Several countries have established national implant registries which are beneficial in several ways. There is tremendous variation in the implants used in different regions of the world and a national registry provides both local feedback to surgeons as well as comparative information versus global trends. The model often used in establishing national implant registries is the Swedish Hip Register. The large number of total hip arthroplasties included in the Swedish Hip Register allows measuring statistical outcomes and comparing various stem designs, implanted by a multitude of surgeons. The outcome figures therefore are much more realistic and

representative compared to a single surgeon or specialty hospital centre report. For this reason, even manufacturers have used information gleaned from the Swedish Hip Register to support use of their respective prostheses when appropriate. Some of the most successful implants such as the Charnley stem, the Exeter stem, the Spectron, and the Lubinus stem have excellent results after 10 to 20 years according to the Register. By the latest reports, the femoral stem in the original Charnley low-friction arthroplasty have enjoyed 20–30 year success rates between 85–90% [2, 4] and this benchmark is still considered the golden standard among stem designs.

Examples of Implants with Poor Track Records

Although it seems at times that almost everyone has designed a stem at one time or another, most of these designs are rapidly and quietly eliminated from the marketplace when signs of failure occur. Few of these clinical results are ever reported in the literature. A few popular examples of femoral stems with poor results are the Centralign hip prosthesis, the Iowa precoat hip prosthesis, the 3M hip prosthesis, and the Cenator stem.

The Centralign stem had a very high failure rate when used in large statured patients due to the shorter diameter of the femoral stem. This led to stem fracture or loosening with lysis after a very short term follow-up. The Iowa Hip prosthesis also showed a 3% failure rate within 3 years. This was a result of early debonding with subsequent aggressive bony lysis. The Cenator femoral stem is another stem with a tenuous record. The failure rate of this stem increased markedly between 5 and 10 years post-operatively, going from a success rate of 94.2% to 83.7%, respectively, as documented in the Swedish Hip Register [11]. The 3M Capital hip prosthesis was shown by Massoud et al. [18] to have a very high rate of cement-stem debonding by 26 months with 16% of stems definitely loose and another 10% probably loose. The authors postulated that this was largely due to the instrumentation accompanying the prosthesis that lead the surgeon to implant the prosthesis with a thin cement mantle and large amount of cancellous bone in the calcar region, thus leading to a high rate of early aseptic loosening [18].

Results of Currently Used Stems

As evidenced in the Swedish Hip Registry, several cemented femoral stems have shown excellent long term survival rates [11]. The revision rates for aseptic loosening of these stems have been exceptional. Based on this evidence, these stems should strongly be considered for routine use in the cemented femoral component. In contrast, some components have shown dramatic failure rates between 5 and 10

☐ **Table 7.5.** Femoral stem survival rates from the Swedish Hip Registry, 2003

Stem	5 Years [%]	10 Years [%]	15 Years [%]
Bi-Metric	97.4	91.4	90.6
Cenator	94.2	**83.7**	
Charnley	97.8	93.6	91.7
Exeter (Polished)	99.2	96.0	93.3
Lubinus SP II	99.6	97.9	97.0
Muller (straight)	99.6	98.0	98.0
Scan Hip Collar	98.8	93.4	89.9
Spectron EF	99.4	97.2	95.9
Stanmore	97.6	91.3	

years from the index procedure (☐ Table 7.5). Both scenarios have been clearly demonstrated in a timely manner using the Swedish Hip Register and the power demonstrated by the large number of implants tracked by the Register.

The two stems most commonly used today in Sweden are the (anatomic) Lubinus II and the (straight) Spectron EF stems. This is in large part due to their respective outstanding long-term clinical performance. Both stems show similar geometries, notably smooth surfaces, tapered flat back designs with excellent rotational stability. These stems have shown very low revision rates for aseptic loosening starting at five years and continuing consistently out to fifteen years.

Migration Pattern of Cemented Femoral Stems

Another method to evaluate femoral stem behaviour and performance is to study the movement pattern of each individual design using RadioStereometric analysis (RSA). RSA is a radiographic method of evaluating the position of components in total hip arthroplasty. Briefly, it begins with the implantation of small tantalum marker beads at the time of the index total hip operation. Approximately 7–9 beads are inserted into the pelvis and proximal femur. In the follow up period, the patient undergoes radiographic evaluation using a dual X-ray tube technique. The patient is placed on a calibration tube and radiographic images are generated. The dual X-ray tubes generate oblique radiographic views of the hip and pelvis clearly visualising the tantalum markers. These images are then scanned into a computer model to calculate relationships between the tantalum markers and the patient's native anatomy. Based on these measurements, very precise changes in component position can be detected. RSA has been shown to be an extremely sensitive means to measure femoral implant subsidence, polyethylene wear, or acetabular component loosening [15].

On the femoral side, it has been shown that micro-movement and migration can precede clinical loosening

and failure in some stem designs [9, 16, 17, 25]. Any movement at any interface can initiate a special failure mechanism. The most common site of femoral loosening occurs between the cement and the bone interface, however early movement (»loosening«) often occurs between the stem and the cement. RSA studies have shown that within the first 6 months after implantation, femoral stems subside within the cement mantle. This subsidence varies based on the type of stem implanted. Micro-motion at the stem-cement interface can be associated with abrasive wear, in particular when the stem surface is rough, and ultimately particularly in association with thin cement mantle and sharp implant corners cement mantle fracture can occur. Abrasive wear particles and hydraulic pressure at the interface generated from pumping of joint fluid can contribute to a cascade of wear induced osteolysis and loosening. Some stem design philosophies (► chapter 7.2) accept that the stem will debond from the interface and polish the stem surface to minimise abrasive wear [1].

However, there is evidence from the RSA studies that debonding occurs with all implant designs which may ultimately initiate a failure mechanism [22, 23]. It has also been postulated that the critical interface is the cement-stem interface [10], but this only seems true for very rough stem surfaces. To minimise the risk of stem debonding, as a consequence many stem designs have addressed this phenomenon by texturing or precoating the stem surface or by adding a collar in the attempt to increase implant bonding and stability within the cement mantle over time. Experimental work has been used to support these concepts [24]. However, ultimately only clinical studies on the migration and movement pattern of each individual stem will allow a full assessment of whether the postulate holds true that migration (subsidence and retroversion) can be stopped or at least significantly limited by these measures.

Radiostereometric Analysis Data of Popular Stem Designs

In a study [15] presented at the American Academy of Orthopaedic Surgeons in 2000, investigators demonstrated the stem subsidence characteristics of several of the more commonly implanted prostheses used in the Swedish Hip Register (☐ Table 7.6).

- *Lubinus SP groups:* This stem design is made of CoCr-alloy and showed a small early subsidence with only minimum increase after 6 months. The higher values for the stems made of titanium alloy could be an effect of a smoother surface finish and a lower elastic modulus (☐ Fig. 7.19).
- *The Spectron EF groups:* These stems showed no or almost no subsidence until after the 6 months follow-up. There was a levelling of the curve after 2 years, suggesting a period of deformation of the cement or

debonding in only a few of the cases followed by secondary stabilization (◘ Fig. 7.19).

— *The Anatomic-Option and the Tifit groups:* Both designs tended to show increasing subsidence after the 6 months follow up, but the distal migration was faster. The Tifit stems, followed for 5 years, migrated more slowly after the 2 years follow-up (◘ Fig. 7.20).

— *The SHP and Exeter groups:* The collarless stems and Exeter designs showed early and fast subsidence. The migration rate tended to decrease somewhat after 1 year.

— *Experimental variations of Lubinus design* (original SP II, polished, CPC stem). These 3 groups constitute the first cases in a prospective and randomised study aimed to study the influence of surface finish. 76 cases have been operated and 40 have been followed for 1 year. The stem designs are based on the original Lubinus SP II. Group 8a is the original one (see Group 1). In Group 8b the collar has been removed and the stem has been polished (not commercially available). In Group 8c the original SP II design is coated with a thin layer PMMA (not commercially available).

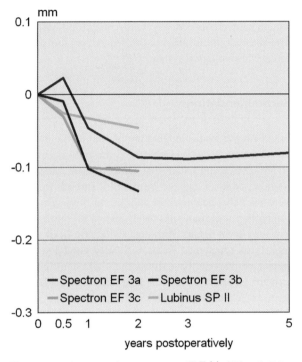

◘ **Fig. 7.19.** Subsidence of Spectron stems (◘ Table 7.5) with SPII as reference

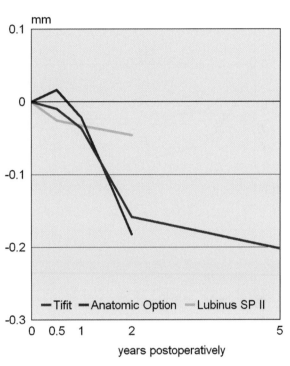

◘ **Fig. 7.20.** Subsidence of groups 4 and 5 (◘ Table 7.6) with SPII as reference

◘ **Table 7.6.** The different stem designs and patient materials

Gro	Name	Material	Surface Finish [μm]		Male/Female	Mean Age	Original Study
			Proximally	Distally			
1	Lubinus SP II	CoCr alloy	1.5	1.5	8/12	67 (52–78)	RS against 5
2	Lubinus SP II	TiA/V alloy	1.0	1.0	9/14	65 (51–76)	Control group in RS
3a	Spectron EF	CoCr alloy	2.8	0.7	6/10	70 (65–76)	Control group in RS
3b	Spectron EF	CoCr alloy	2.8	0.7	10/11	58 (42–70)	Consecutive study
3c	Spectron EF	CoCr alloy	2.8	0.7	4/13	71 (61–81)	Control group in RS
4	Anatomic Op	CoCr alloy	1.5	1.5	15/29	58 (32–69)	Control group in RS
5	Tifit	TiA/V alloy	1.3	1.3	12/8	52 (38–66)	Control group in RS
6	SHP	CoCr alloy	3.8	2.0	8/12	67 (55–78)	RS against 1
7	Exeter	Stainless	<0.5	<0.5	11/5	71 (63–81)	Consecutive study
8a	Lubinus SP II	CoCr alloy	1.5	1.5	5/7	66 (53–77)	RS against 8b/c
8b	Lubinus pol	CoCr alloy	<0.5	<0.5	8/8	66 (46–77)	RS against 8a/c
8c	Lubinus pre	CoCr alloy	1.5	1.5	5/7	65 (55–78)	RS against 8a/b

The data from the RSA study [15] revealed that after 2 years most cemented stem designs had migrated into retroversion and that surprisingly all stem designs regardless of the surface finish, macrostructure or collar had subsided. The stems that had mechanically failed and had been revised after 3–5.5 years all had failed by the same pattern, subsidence and retroversion. Subsidence of the stem had occurred more frequently than subsidence of the entire bulk of the cement mantle (■ Table 7.7).

The amount of tolerable stem migration will be intrinsic to and dependent on the design of the stem [12]. Hence, a degree of subsidence may be detrimental to one stem design, but not as relevant in another. But clearly the most important result from this comprehensive RSA study was the finding that all designs migrate, hence must debond at the stem cement interface. Those stems that migrate/subside excessively in the early post-operative period are significantly more likely to go onto clinical failure and thus need revision surgery.

All interfaces in a cemented THA are important. If the cement bone interface is poor than mechanical loosening can result irrespective which stem design is used. Hence the establishment of this interface remains the most critical. However, the stem-cement interface and any migration pattern within also play an important role in this complex interaction between stem, cement and host bone. The ultimate performance will depend on the weakest link in this biological system.

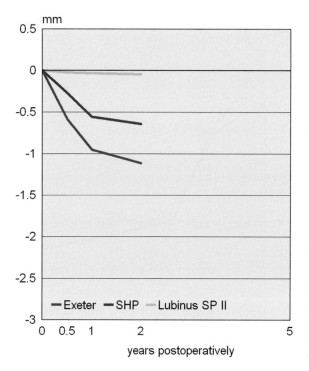

■ **Fig. 7.21.** Subsidence of groups 6 and 7 (■ Table 7.6) with SPII as reference

Recommendations

Based on the available literature as well as the data observed in the Swedish Hip Registry, the authors currently recommend using a stem that has a flat back design with rounded edges, a tapered stem and a smooth finish. A stem with this geometry in addition to third generation cementing technique has been shown to have excellent long-term results. Although there have been several reports of roughened stems with very good long-term results, many series have shown that these stems perform well in the short to intermediate term, but in the long term, as they tend to debond and incite a viscous cycle of debris formation and subsequent bone lysis with dramatic bony destruction. The stems which have performed well based on information from the Swedish Hip Registry include the Spectron, the Exeter, and the Lubinus stems. Additionally, RSA data has shown that all cemented femo-

	Implant	Total	Significant Subsidence (p <0.01)*	Cement mantle		Stem Inside Mantle	
				Subsiding > Significant Value	Values (Range)	Subsiding >Significant Value	Values (Range)
1	Lubinus SP II	4	0.11	0		4	–0.20 to –
2	Lubinus SP II	13	0.18	2	–0.32 to –0.20	10	–0.46 to –
3a	Spectron EF	11	0.18	0		4	–0.25 to –
3b	Spectron EF	16	0.20	3	–0.30 to –0.23	4	–0.46 to –
3c	Spectron EF	12	0.11	4	–0.25 to –0.17	5	–0.28 to –
6	SHP	14	0.11	2	–0.42 to –0.32	14	–1.10 to –
7	Exeter	16	0.20	0		16	–1.94 to –
8a**	Lubinus SP II	7	0.11	2	–0.45 to –0.11	2	–0.16 to –
8b**	Lubinus	8	0.11	0		7	–0.89 to –
8c**	Lubinus	7	0.11	0		1	–0.15

■ **Table 7.7.** Stem subsidence inside the cement mantle in mm. Groups 1–7: 2-year results. Group 8: 1-year results

ral stems subside within the first two years after implantation. The most common failure pattern is that of subsidence with accompanying retroversion of the stem. Those stems that subside greater than 0.1 mm in the first two years, regardless of stem geometry, are at significantly higher risk for loosening and subsequent failure.

Take Home Messages

- Based on RSA data all cemented femoral stems exhibit subsidence and retroversion in the first 6 months after implantation.
- All stem designs migrate, hence must debond at the stem cement interface.
- Those stems that subside greater than 0.1 mm within two years after implantation show a significantly higher revision rate compared to stems with less subsidence.
- Few joint implants have documented long term clinical data, however various outcome studies in addition to the Swedish Hip Register have been able to show extensive results for many such hip implants.

References

1. Anthony PP, Gie GA, Howie CR et al. Localised endosteal bone lysis in relation to the femoral components of cemented total hip arthroplasties. J Bone Joint Surg Br 72:971, 1990
2. Berry DJ, Harmsen WS, Cabanela ME, et al. Twenty-five-year survivorship of two thousand consecutive primary Charnley total hip replacements: factors affecting survivorship of acetabular and femoral components. J Bone Joint Surg Am 84-A:171, 2002
3. Britton AR, Murray DW, Bulstrode CJ, et al. Long-term comparison of Charnley and Stanmore design total hip replacements. J Bone Joint Surg Br 78:802, 1996
4. Callaghan JJ, Templeton JE, Liu SS, et al. Results of Charnley total hip arthroplasty at a minimum of thirty years. A concise follow-up of a previous report. J Bone Joint Surg Am 86-A:690, 2004
5. Clohisy JC, Harris WH: Primary hybrid total hip replacement, performed with insertion of the acetabular component without cement and a precoat femoral component with cement. An average ten-year follow-up study. J Bone Joint Surg Am 81:247, 1999
6. Crowninshield RD, Jennings JD, Laurent ML, et al. Cemented femoral component surface finish mechanics. Clin Orthop:90, 1998
7. Duffy GP, Muratoglu OK, Biggs SA, et al. A critical assessment of proximal macrotexturing on cemented femoral components. J Arthroplasty 16:42, 2001
8. Ebramzadeh E, Sangiorgio SN, Longjohn DB, et al. Initial stability of cemented femoral stems as a function of surface finish, collar, and stem size. J Bone Joint Surg Am 86-A:106, 2004
9. Freeman MA, Plante-Bordeneuve P: Early migration and late aseptic failure of proximal femoral prostheses. J Bone Joint Surg Br 76:432, 1994
10. Harris WH: Is it advantageous to strengthen the cement-metal interface and use a collar for cemented femoral components of total hip replacements? Clin Orthop Relat Res:67, 1992
11. Herberts P MH, Garellick G: Annual Report 2003. The Swedish National Hip Arthroplasty Register, in www.jru.orthop.gu.se, 2003
12. Huiskes R, Verdonschot N, Nivbrant B: Migration, stem shape, and surface finish in cemented total hip arthroplasty. Clin Orthop:103, 1998
13. Issack PS, Botero HG, Hiebert RN, et al. Sixteen-year follow-up of the cemented spectron femoral stem for hip arthroplasty. J Arthroplasty 18:925, 2003
14. Jaffe WL, Hawkins CA: Normalized and proportionalized cemented femoral stem survivorship at 15 years. J Arthroplasty 14:708, 1999
15. Kärrholm J, Nivbrant B, Thanner J, Anderberg C, Börlin N, Herberts P, Malchau H. Radiosstereometric evaluation of hip implant design and surface finish. Scientific Exhibition, AAOS, Orlando, USA, 2000.
16. Kärrholm J, Borssen B, Lowenhielm G, et al. Does early micromotion of femoral stem prostheses matter? 4–7-year stereoradiographic follow-up of 84 cemented prostheses. J Bone Joint Surg Br 76:912, 1994
17. Krismer M, Biedermann R, Stockl B, et al. The prediction of failure of the stem in THR by measurement of early migration using EBRA-FCA. Einzel-Bild-Roentgen-Analyse-femoral component analysis. J Bone Joint Surg Br 81:273, 1999
18. Massoud SN, Hunter JB, Holdsworth BJ, et al. Early femoral loosening in one design of cemented hip replacement. J Bone Joint Surg Br 79:603, 1997
19. Meneghini RM, Feinberg JR, Capello WN: Primary hybrid total hip arthroplasty with a roughened femoral stem: integrity of the stem-cement interface. J Arthroplasty 18:299, 2003
20. Rasquinha VJ, Ranawat CS, Dua V, et al. A prospective, randomized, double-blind study of smooth versus rough stems using cement fixation: minimum 5-year follow-up. J Arthroplasty 19:2, 2004
21. Sporer SM, Callaghan JJ, Olejniczak JP, et al. The effects of surface roughness and polymethylmethacrylate precoating on the radiographic and clinical results of the Iowa hip prosthesis. A study of patients less than fifty years old. J Bone Joint Surg Am 81:481, 1999
22. Thanner J, Freij-Larsson C, Karrholm J, et al. Evaluation of Boneloc. Chemical and mechanical properties, and a randomized clinical study of 30 total hip arthroplasties. Acta Orthop Scand 66:207, 1995
23. Verdonschot N, Huiskes R: The effects of cement-stem debonding in THA on the long-term failure probability of cement. J Biomech 30:795, 1997
24. Verdonschot N, Tanck E, Huiskes R: Effects of prosthesis surface roughness on the failure process of cemented hip implants after stem-cement debonding. J Biomed Mater Res 42:554, 1998
25. Walker PS, Mai SF, Cobb AG, et al. Prediction of clinical outcome of THR from migration measurements on standard radiographs. A study of cemented Charnley and Stanmore femoral stems. J Bone Joint Surg Br 77:705, 1995
26. Wroblewski BM, Siney PD, Fleming PA: Triple taper polished cemented stem in total hip arthroplasty: rationale for the design, surgical technique, and 7 years of clinical experience. J Arthroplasty 16:37, 2001

Implant Choice: In-vitro Rotational Stability of Cemented Stem Designs

Marc Thomsen, Christoph Lee

Summary

This chapter describes the primary rotational stability of cemented stems. The 6-DOF measurement system type Heidelberg-Göttingen, which can track the complex spatial movement of stems, has characterised the anchoring stability of more than 50 uncemented stem designs. Different polished cemented hip stems have shown an overall tight fixation and excellent torsional stability using this system. Measurements have been repeated after debonding of the stems.

Introduction

The success of any type of femoral prosthesis is influenced by the design and the mode of fixation [1, 12, 14, 16, 39, 44]. The incorporation of femoral stems fixed without cement depends on tight anchoring of the implant to the femur via frictional connection at several points. The extent of micro-movement at the implant-bone interface, i.e. the slip between stem and bone, represents a quantitative measure for initial anchoring stability. Initial torsional stability may serve as a valuable predictor for successful incorporation and function of femoral stems [19, 23, 38, 43, 44]. It has been well documented, that a femoral stem is subjected to large axial torsional loads which occur during regular walking, stair climbing, and getting up from a chair [4, 10, 30]. A standardised in-vitro comparison of the initial (torsional) stability of different types of prostheses is possible with the 6-degrees of freedom (DOF) measurement system type Heidelberg-Göttingen. This method allowed to track the complex spatial movements with high precision and also to characterise the typical modes of fixation (and movement in space) of more than 50 different uncemented stem designs [21, 31, 40, 41].

When cementing a femoral stem, the space between prosthesis and inner surface of the bone is completely filled, thus creating a form fit with a frictional connection. At the stem-cement interface micromotion and subsidence of the stem have been shown to be unavoidable [2, 28]. This movement will eventually lead to debonding at the stem-cement interface, which in some stem designs (with rough surfaces) may lead to secondary problems at/within the cement mantle [17, 24, 26]. The possible abrasion of the two surfaces, the loss of stem fixation and the generation of wear debris can further provoke three body wear [22, 27]. It is important to also understand the pattern of fixation and the mode of implant motion in cemented stem designs.

Hence, we tested different polished designs of cemented hips to compare the initial rotational anchoring stability, the location of torque transfer from the stem within the cement mantle to the bone, and the twist of the stem. Debonding was simulated to register potential micromovement of the stem within its cement mantle.

Experimental Measurement of Stem Movement

Measurement of complex spatial movement is difficult. In most previous studies [9, 19, 23, 38, 43], micro-movements in uncemented prostheses were measured in one dimension at maximally two locations on the prosthesis. Gilbert et al. reported on spatial movements of the prosthesis [20]. However, because the stem was modelled as a rigid body, its bending and twisting was not taken into account. Schneider et al. used a four-degrees-of-freedom apparatus, which was unsuitable for determining spatial movements [37]. The method reported by Dürselen et al. [13] used six-degrees-of-freedom. However, its 20 μm resolution was too small to reach the required reliability.

None of these studies examined the specific aspects of torsional loading, which are highly effective at producing micro-movements.

The method reported here relies on three main features:

- The testings including the implantations are done under uniform conditions following an established protocol.
- The application of a pure torque, which is free from counter-action.
- The measurement tracked the complete spatial micro-movements of the stem and bone at defined sites.

Standardised Experimental Model

A standardised protocol had been established for the measurement of uncemented implant designs. One particular type of synthetic femur (composite bone 2nd generation (#3106), Sawbones Europe AB, Malmö, Sweden) was used to ensure for consistency and comparability [7]. It closely resembles the human femur in mechanical properties and dimensions. Cortical structures are mimicked by longitudinally laminated fibres bound by epoxy, and the cancellous bone is simulated by rigid polyurethane foam. For consistency, all implantations were done by the same surgeon in cooperation with a manufacturer bioengineer or product manager of the prosthesis. Bones were osteotomised just below the tip of the greater trochanter to avoid cortical contact of spongiosa-anchored prostheses. The bones were hollowed out by rasping, aligned parallel with the direction of the torque vector applied in the experiment, and rigidly supported at their condyles.

Using a materials testing machine (Frank-Universalprüfmaschine 81816/B, Karl Frank GmbH, Weinheim-Birkenau, Germany), the uncemented stems were pressed into the composite bone in a stepwise manner by 25 cycles of 2000 N followed by 25 cycles of 4000 N. This was 500 N more than what is typically achieved by a metal hammer during surgery [36], but represents loads that occur during daily activities of life [9].

Applied to a newly developed prosthesis, the testing provides characteristics in the implanted state in-vitro and may help to predict the clinical performance. The results of three uncemented prostheses are presented for reference of typical patterns of fixation.

For the measurement of the cemented stems, the same protocol was adapted. The cemented stems were implanted by an experienced surgeon. A minimum of 2 mm cement mantle was ensured by overbroaching and undersizing the stem. Preoperative templating guaranteed equal or near equal stem sizes in medial to lateral dimensions of the different designs. The Palacos bone cement used and the polyurethane foam formed a tight unit simulating highest cementing quality in order to focus on

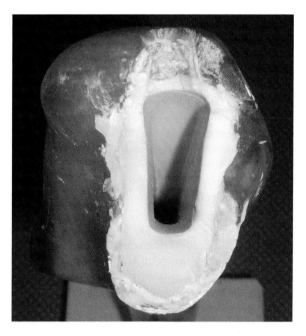

Fig. 7.22. Sawbone with a homogenous cement mantle after prosthesis explantation

the stem/cement interface (**Fig. 7.22**). Radiographs in two planes were taken to ensure neutral stem alignment, an overall good fit and a minimal cement mantle thickness >2 mm. The axial rotational micro-movements in these experimental models were studied using one of our devices as published 2002 by our lab [21]. Measurements were repeated after debonding of the implant.

Tested Uncemented Prostheses

The Alloclassic Stem (Zimmer/SULZER Orthopedics Ltd, Winterthur, CH, formerly Zweymüller stem) relies on distal fixation. For the implantations, size-7 stems were used to achieve distal cortical press-fit fixation. The broaches touched the cortical structures distally.

The CLS femoral prosthesis (Zimmer/ SULZER Orthopedics Ltd.) has been designed as a three-dimensional taper for press-fit implantation. It is tapered in the frontal, sagittal, and transverse planes. Its distal part is made so small that it cannot fill the intramedullary canal in the proximal diaphysis. The four ribs on the proximal part of the stem have been reported to minimize rotational migration [5]. This stem has been used for implantation since 1984 at the authors' institution [1].

The Standard Range of Motion (S-ROM) prosthesis (DePuy/Johnson & Johnson) is an uncemented modular femoral component. The surgical technique involved a three-step reaming process: distal cylindrical reaming to establish the diameter of the distal prosthesis, followed by proximal conical reaming, and placement of the characteristic modular metaphyseal sleeve. The distal slit of this circular stem is designed to reduce the bending stiffness.

Tested Cemented Prostheses

The Exeter cemented stem (Stryker/Howmedica) has a more than 30 year track record [18, 46]. It features a polished, rectangular, double tapered steel design to create radial compressive loading. The double taper should promote cement engagement and provide rotational stability. The surface is highly-polished in order to reduce friction between the cement and the implant and therefore significantly reducing the potential for third body wear. A hollow centralizer made from polymethylmethacrylate (PMMA) allows the stem to engage distally within the cement mantle during subsidence [2] and avoids end bearing of the stem directly onto the cement.

The G2 Hip System (DePuy/Johnson & Johnson) has uncemented and cemented fixation options, with a single set of instruments for both techniques. The cemented stem is made of CoCr and polished to reduce wear. Tapered in the longitudinal and posterior to anterior direction, proximal load transfer and rotational stability are maximised. A light lateral flare is said to limit subsidence. The shape and well-rounded corners are intended to lead to a consistent cement mantle of 2 mm thickness avoiding peak loading of parts of the cement. A distal centralizer is designed to sit 10 to 30 mm from the tip.

The OLYMPIA cemented anatomic femoral stem (Biomet) is made from high nitrogen stainless steel and is highly-polished. It has an oval metaphyseal part, which follows the natural femoral torque, thus providing intrinsic rotational locking and stability without the need for sharp corners. A reduced tri-taper limits subsidence and increases rotational stability. The anatomic shape requires a different prosthesis for the left and the right side (14 sizes in total) but improves centralisation of the stem and allows a thick (>2 mm) and more homogeneous cement mantle also in the lateral plane. The diaphyseal extremity is round, double tapered and symmetrical. The smooth sections help to distribute stresses evenly avoiding local stress concentrations, which may lead to cement mantle fracture. A range of PMMA distal centralizers have been designed to sit 5–10 mm from the tip of the stem.

Torque and Preload Application

Axial torques are produced by two counterbalanced weights 1 and 2 (◨ Fig. 7.23). The axially aligned preload is generated by weights 3 and 4 [21]. The forces are transferred onto the prosthesis neck via ropes and a rod. First, by adjusting the positions of the weights 1 and 2, the line of action of the forces F1 and F2 are set to coincide. The

weights are then shifted by stepper motors in an anti-parallel fashion. A force couple is formed [31] which produces an axially acting torque T_z. Since F1 = F2 = F, it holds:

$$T_z = a \cdot F.$$

a is the distance between the application lines of F1 und F2. The weights 1 and 2 are shifted step-by-step producing a stepped triangular time-dependent torque function T(t) with the amplitude of 6 Nm, a period of 2 min, and a step increment of +/-0.16 Nm.

This method of applying a pure torque ensures that the axes of rotation of stem and bone at their measured sites are not affected by the way of torque transfer to the neck of the stem: The axes are determined by the subjects themselves. Furthermore, the experimental setup ensures that $T_z(t)$ remains independent of the motion of the prosthesis, hence keeping the torque transfer free of counter action. The applied torsional loads (± 6 Nm) are comparatively small and do not exceed physiological limits since Bergmann et al. reported that approximately 35 Nm axial load are exerted to the femoral prosthesis during walking [4].

Measurement of Spatial Movement

The axial torque twists the stem and the bone and produces differential movements between them. In order to track the relative micro-motions and deformations, the displacements of more than one site on each subject has to be measured. The lesser trochanter is used as the reference system. Measurements are carried out at five different locations, two of which are at the implanted stem (# 1: shoulder, # 2: stem apex) and the remaining three on the synthetic bone (# 3: 2 cm or 8 cm below the lesser trochanter, # 4: at the same level as # 2, # 5: 20 cm below the lesser trochanter). To measure the spatial movement at a particular location, a cube (edge length: 3.1cm) is rigidly attached to the site via a metal rod. To reach the apex of the stem, a hole of greater diameter than the rod is drilled through the bone. The position of the cube is recorded by six displacement transducers (LVDT #1300, Fa. Mahr, Göttingen, Germany), which in turn are attached to the lesser trochanter in a three-two-one configuration, as depicted in ◨ Fig. 7.24. This arrangement makes it possible to track the spatial movement (translation and rotation) of the selected sites relative to the lesser trochanter, as a function of the applied axial torque $T_z(t)$.

Data Analysis

In the initial position, three planes of the cube determine a Cartesian co-ordinate system which is fixed to the lesser trochanter and serves as the reference system. When movement of the respective site takes place, the same

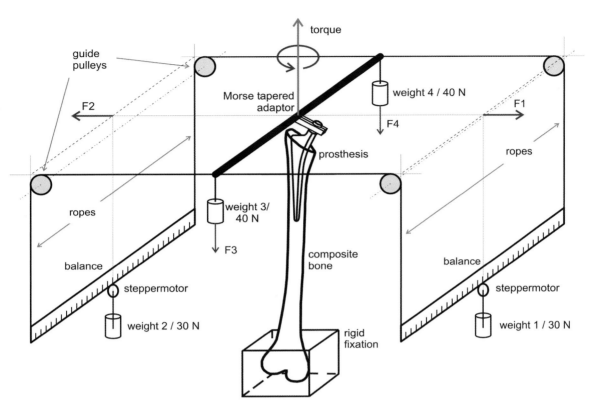

Fig. 7.23. Sketch of the device used to study the axial rotational micro-movements. The axial torque was produced by weights 1 (30 N) and 2 (30 N). The horizontal distance between the weights was adjusted by two computer-controlled stepper motors. The role of weight 3 and 4 was to generate the axial preload of 80 N

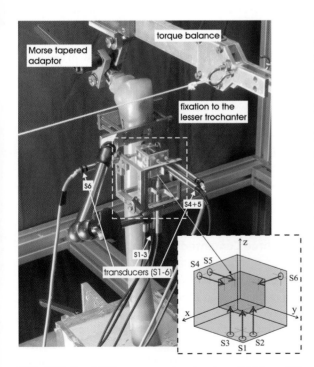

Fig. 7.24. The 6-DOF measurement system type Heidelberg-Göttingen. Six linear variable differential transducers in a three (S1, S2, S3) – two (S4, S5) – one (S6) setting were used to measure the spatial position of the movable cube. In this view, the cube was rigidly tied to site #3 (8 cm below the lesser trochanter)

three planes of the cube define a displaced co-ordinate system. The position of the displaced co-ordinate system is calculated using the S_i position vectors of the contact points of the six transducers S_i.

Due to the high precision and resolution of the six displacement transducers the translation vector d (resolution <0.1 μm) and rotational vector α (resolution <0.5 millidegrees) of stem or bone at the selected sites can be determined with high accuracy.

In order to correlate the measured movements with the geometrical structures of the subjects the helical axes of the diverse movements are calculated. The parameters of a helical axis (HA) are: the unit polar vector $e = \alpha/|\alpha|$ (direction of the HA), the normal vector $n = \frac{\alpha \times d}{\alpha^2}$ (distance of the HA from the origin of the reference system), and the helical shift $\Delta z = e \cdot d$. For detailed proofs of these formulae see Beatty and Kinzel et al. [3, 29].

The cyclic application of the axial torque yields an $\alpha = \alpha(T_z)$ characteristics with a small hysteresis. The inclination of the linear fit is taken as the normalized rotation α/T_z. The relative normalised rotation between the lesser trochanter and the respective site #1 is denoted by α_i.

Normalised rotation α_5 of the bone at site # 5 reveals the bone twist between the reference at the lesser trochanter and site # 5. Since site # 5 is lying sufficiently far below the apex of the stem, α_5 mainly depends on the location of the centre of torque transfer from the stem to the bone. Therefore, α_5 characterises the stiffening because of the prosthesis and the location of the fixation, which is lying more proximally for greater α_5 values. The rotation α_3 and α_4 of the bone at sites # 3 and # 4 depends on the location and the spatial spread of the torque transfer. The proximal rotational slip α_1 is the proximal relative rotation between stem and bone at the location of the reference. For practical reasons, site #1 at the stem is shifted proximally by a few centimetres. Since the values at the position of the reference (lesser trochanter) are of interest, they have to be interpolated.

Modes of Fixation

The measurements revealed not only differences between the types of prostheses examined in respect to their responses to torsional loading but also indicated constructive peculiarities as an explanation for clinical and radiological findings.

In all prostheses, the unit vectors e of the helical axes of stem or bone movement at the five sites were found to be parallel to the applied torque vector T_z i.e. to the corresponding anatomical femur axis within the accuracy of measurements. Because of this coincidence of the rotational directions in each prosthesis tested, the magnitudes of the respective rotational angles may be related arithmetically. Statistical analysis of the normal vectors also showed that the corresponding helical axes of the movements at the five sites intersected the centre of the respective femurs in all cases. Therefore, it was also possible to relate the corresponding rotational angles of the tested prostheses arithmetically. All helical shifts Δz were detectable, but small ($\Delta z < 0.3$ μm/Nm). The maximum translation parallel to the femoral long axis did not exceed 0.3 μm/Nm · 6 Nm = 1.8 μm.

The Three Uncemented Prostheses

Primarily, uncemented prostheses rely on a frictional connection. They wedge in and mechanical contact occurs at discrete spots of asperities in the contacting surfaces. Torque transfer occurs at these locations which differ depending on the type of anchorage. The three uncemented prostheses chosen are representatives of typical movement patterns which range from proximal to distal fixation [18].

Not listed is an example for proximal fixation. The CLS (◘ Fig. 7.25) shows a proximal 2/3 fixation. The vertical axis shows the rotational displacement in millidegrees/Nm. The horizontal axis reveals that these measurements are dependent on the location of the measurement site. Note that the lines connecting the data points do not rep-

resent the deformed shape of the objects. Their purpose is to indicate that sites # 1 and # 2 belong to the stem, while sites # 3, # 4 and # 5 are located on the bone. A proximal 2/3 fixation is in accordance with the observation that clinically the least loss on bone mineral density is found in Gruen zone 5.

The Alloclassic prosthesis has a typical distal fixation (◘ Fig. 7.26), which was very rigid: $\alpha_{2-4} = 3.0$ millidegrees/Nm. While the distal torque transfer was associated with a minimal twist of the bone between the reference (lesser trochanter) and site # 3: $\alpha_3 \approx 4.0$ millidegrees/Nm, there was considerable proximal movement. Considering the Bergmann values of 35 Nm [4] a transversal slipping shift of $\Delta s_1 = 140$ μm between stem and spongiosa must be expected to occur at the proximal sites of this prosthesis. This value is within a clinically relevant range because the proximal slip α_1 mainly is produced by the twist of a still distally fixed metallic stem. The presented measurements suggest that distally cortically fixed Alloclassic prostheses suffer from loosening along their proximal third, despite solid anchoring of the prosthesis to the femur. This hypothesis has been confirmed clinically by the work of Dohle et al. [11], who found cortical hypertrophy and trabecular condensation in the area of the distal stem and frequently observed linear radiolucencies in Gruen zone 1 and 7. In some cases, they were extended into zone 2 and 6. Nevertheless the clinical function of the implants is not impaired.

The S-ROM (◘ Fig. 7.27) prosthesis showed the so-called overall fixation. It remained in continuously close contact to the bone: $\alpha_1 = 5.0$ millidegrees/Nm, $\alpha_{2-4} = 6.5$ millidegrees/Nm, and correspondingly stem and bone were twisted over the same distance in a similar fashion. These findings are in agreement with that of Ohl et al. who reported excellent torsional fixation of the S-ROM [32]. The detected micro-movement of the proximal sleeve relative to the stem is striking. This finding is consistent with the observation by Bobyn et al. who found evidence of surface modification and fretting wear. It remains to be clarified whether this micro-movement of 3 millidegrees/Nm is ultimately responsible for stem loosening [6].

The Three Cemented Prostheses

All cemented prostheses formed a very close overall fixation in combination with the cement (◘ Figs. 7.28 to 7.30). Between 2 and 8 cm distal from the lesser trochanter there was a nearly parallel movement of the three partners (stem, cement and sawbone). Already these values were hardly reached by the uncemented systems. Looking at the level of the lesser trochanter, all three prostheses showed an even closer contact. Regarding twist of the bone, values were largest for the G2, which reached slightly less distally in comparison to the other two designs.

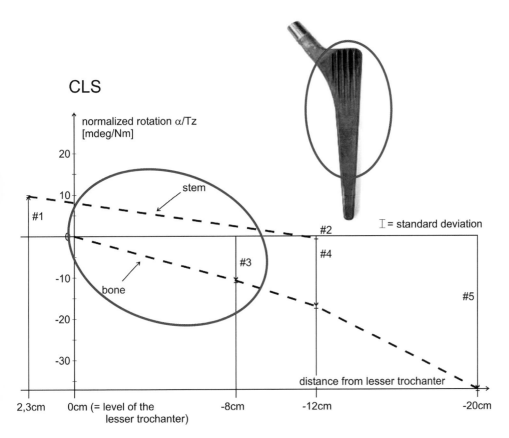

■ **Fig. 7.25.** CLS: pattern of proximal 2/3 torque transfer. The micro-motions between stem twist and bone twist are graphically indicated. The ordinate shows rotational displacement in millidegrees/Nm. The abscissa reveals these measurements are dependent on the location of the measurement site

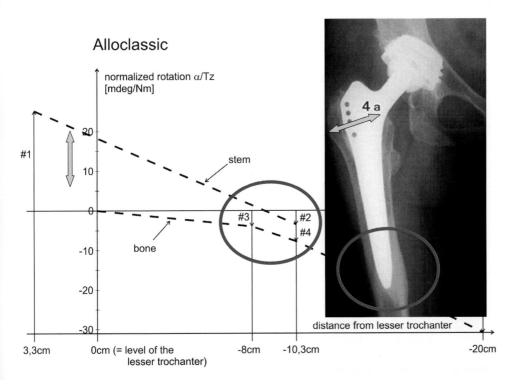

■ **Fig. 7.26.** Alloclassic: pattern of distal torque transfer. Consistent with this behaviour is the finding of proximal radiolucency and distal cortical hypertrophy in radiographic imaging

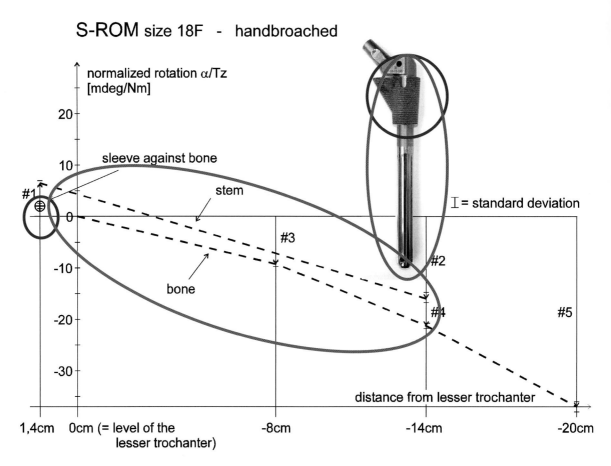

Fig. 7.27. S-ROM: pattern of overall fixation. Remarkable is the fact, that the micro-motion between sleeve and stem is larger than between sleeve and bone

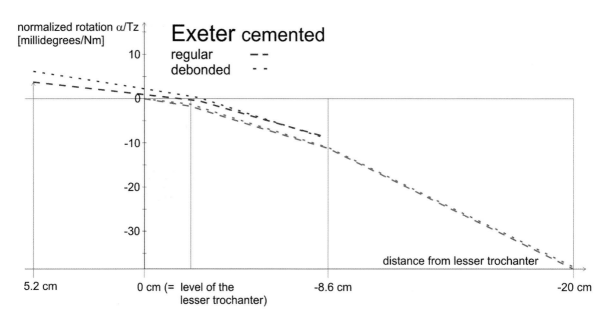

Fig. 7.28. Exeter: a collarless, polished, double tapered design. Results of two conditions have been included in one graph. The dashed curves represent a regular cemented prostheses and sawbone, the dotted lines show the changes of stem and sawbone after debonding has occurred

After debonding all three designs still had a very good fixation in the system, but compared to the cemented non-debonded data the twist between the stem and the »bone« at the lesser trochanter level doubled proximally. This made the curves of stem and bone become nearly parallel from the lesser trochanter up to 2 cm distally. Since the curves up to 8 cm distally did not change much except for a slight parallel shift of the G2 stem, all three cemented designs displayed a truly overall fixating and loading anchorage.

Discussion

Rotational stability of cemented designs has not been studied to the same extent as with uncemented designs. As expected, the results for instrinsic stability for the cemented prostheses are much better and more alike than those of the uncemented designs. With the cementing an »individual metal-PMMA implant« is created for the bone. Only a few custom-made uncemented designs offer this quality of anchorage through form fit. Com-

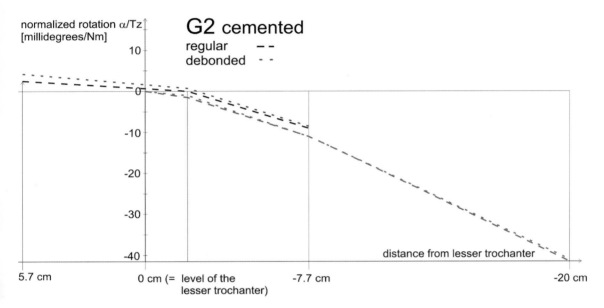

Fig. 7.29. G2: The multitapered, well-rounded and polished cemented design has been measured. The dashed curves represent the regular cemented prostheses and sawbone, the dotted lines show the changes of stem and sawbone after debonding has occurred

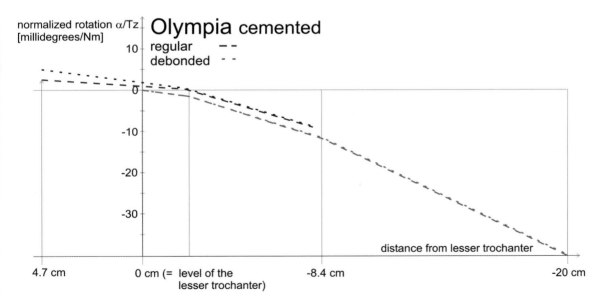

Fig. 7.30. Olympia: features an anatomic design with a polished surface. Again, results of two conditions have been included in one graph. The dashed curves represent a regular cemented prostheses and sawbone, the dotted lines show the changes of stem and sawbone after debonding has occurred

mon uncemented designs rely on mere press-fit and only with sufficient primary stability ingrowth of bone may provide a form fit which leads to excellent secondary stability.

Interesting was the debonded situation. Compared to the primary situation the relative movement nearly doubled. However, these changes were small in magnitude as visualized on the graphs (◘ Figs. 7.28 to 7.30). This may be seen as a hint for the successful polished designs, but further investigations need to be carried out. Creep of the cement plays an important role in vivo and this is a situation, which mere debonding cannot not simulate in the experimental set-up used. In real bone, interlocking of the cement bone interface will not be the same, especially because of the variation in cancellous structure and bone remodelling. In our model we »glued together« polyurethane foam and PMMA forming one tight unit, similar to the composite formed between cement and cancellous bone in vivo. Yet, with a slight modification of the measuring protocol we would expect to also measure micro-motion at the cement bone interface in cadaveric femora. This is an issue especially with stems with matt surfaces [22].

As for now, the mainly proximal effect of the »debonding« of the Olympia and Exeter relates to clinical findings of proximal debonding [15, 27] and computer simulation [25]. The G2 showed overall slightly reduced anchorage stability, but whether the increase in micro-motion seen in all three designs may further lead to increased abrasive wear remains speculative, in particular as all designs are highly-polished. However, reduced torsional stability may lead to posterior migration as shown for several stem design using Röntgen stereogrammetric analysis [28].

Further studies on cemented stem designs with matt or rougher surface structure are required to identify their patterns of movement and debonding.

Take Home Messages

- Complex spatial measurement of the anchoring stability of uncemented and cemented prosthesis designs is possible using the 6-DOF measurement system type Heidelberg Göttingen.
- Because of form fit with a frictional connection, the primary stability of the three polished cemented stems has been high with a pattern of overall fixation.
- The effects of debonding: Micro-movement of the three polished stems nearly doubled proximally in concordance with clinical and numerical results, yet remained a tight overall fixation.
- Further studies on cadaveric femora and cemented designs with matt or rougher surface structure should additionally focus on micro-movement in the interface cement and bone.

References

1. Aldinger PR, Breusch SJ, Lukoschek M, Mau H, Ewerbeck V, Thomsen M (2003) 10-15 Year Follow-up of the Cementless Spotorno Stem. J Bone Joint Surg Br Mar; 85(2):209–14
2. Alfaro-Adrian J, Gill HS, Marks B, Murray DW (1999) Cement migration after THR: A comparison of Charnley Elite and Exeter femoral stems using RSA. J Bone Joint Surg Br 81(1):130–4
3. Beatty MF (1966) Kinematics of Finite, Rigid-Body Displacements. Am J Phys 34:949–954
4. Bergmann G, Graichen F, Rohlmann A (1993) Hip loading during walking and running measured in two patients. J Biomech 26:969–990
5. Blaha JD, Spotorno L, Romagnoli S (1991) CLS press-fit total hip arthroplasty. Techniques Orthop 6:80–86
6. Bobyn JD, Dujovne AR, Krygier JJ, Young DL (1993) Surface Analysis of the Taper Junctions of Retrieved and in Vitro Tested Modular Hip Prostheses. In: Morrey BF (ed). Biological, Material and Mechanical Considerations of Joint Replacement. Raven Press Ltd., New York
7. Cristofolini L, Viceconti M, Cappello A, Toni A (1996) Mechanical validation of whole bone composite femur models. J Biomech 29:525–535,
8. Cristofolini L, Teutonico AS, Monti L, Cappello A, Toni A (2003) Comparative in vitro study on the long term performance of cemented hip stems: validation of a protocol to discriminate between »good« and »bad« designs. J Biomech Nov;36(11):1603–15
9. Callaghan JJ, Fulghum CS, Glisson RR, Stranne SK (1992) The effect of femoral stem geometry on interface motion in uncemented porous-coated total hip prostheses. J Bone Joint Surg Am 74(6):839–848
10. Davy DT, Kotzar GM, Brown RH, et al (1976) Telemetric force measurement across the hip after total hip arthroplasty. J Bone Joint Surg 58A:618–623
11. Dohle J, Becker W, Braun M (2001) Radiological analysis of osseointegration after implantation of the Zweymuller-Alloclassic total hip system. Z Orthop 139: 517–24
12. Ducheyne P, De Meester P, Aernoudt E (1977) Influence of a functional dynamic loading on bone ingrowth into surface pores of orthopedic implants. J Biomed Mater Res 11(6):811–824
13. Dürselen L, Claes L, Wilke HJ (1991) Non-contact measurement of small translations and rotations in all degrees of freedom. Biomed Tech 36: 248–252
14. Engh CA, O'Connor D, Jasty M, McGovern TF, Bobyn JD, Harris WH (1992) Quantification of implant micromotion, strain shielding, and bone resorption with porous-coated anatomic locking femoral prostheses. Clin Orthop 285:13–29
15. Ek ET, Choong PF (2005) Comparison between triple-tapered and double-tapered cemented femoral stems in total hip arthroplasty. J Arthroplasty 20(1):94–100
16. Fischer KJ, Carter DR, Maloney WJ (1992) In vitro study of initial stability of a conical collared femoral component. J Arthroplasty 7:389–395
17. Fornasier VL, Cameron HU (1976) The femoral stem/cement interface in total hip replacement. Clin Orthop 116:248–52
18. Franklin J, Robertsson O, Gestsson J, Lohmander LS, Ingvarsson T (2003) Revision and complication rates in 654 Exeter total hip replacements, with a maximum follow-up of 20 years. BMC Musculoskelet Disord. Mar 25;4(1):6
19. Gebauer D, Refior HJ, Haake M (1989) Micromotions in the primary fixation of cementless femoral stem prostheses. Arch Orthop Trauma Surg 108:300–307
20. Gilbert JL, Bloomfield RS, Lautenschläger EP, Wixson RL (1992) A computer-based biomechanical analysis of three-dimensional motion of cementless hip prosthesis. J Biomech 25:329–340

21. Görtz W, Nägerl UV, Nägerl H, Thomsen M (2002) Spatial micro-movements of uncemented femoral components after torsional loads J Biomech Eng (ASME) 124:706–713

22. Howell JR Jr, Blunt LA, Doyle C, Hooper RM, Lee AJ, Ling RS (2004) In vivo surface wear mechanisms of femoral components of cemented total hip arthroplasties: the influence of wear mechanism on clinical outcome. J Arthroplasty 19(1):88–101

23. Hua J, Walker PS (1994) Relative Motion of Hip Stems under Load. An in Vitro Study of Symmetrical, Asymmetrical, and Custom Asymmetrical Designs. J Bone Joint Surg 76-A: 95–103

24. Huiskes R, Verdonschot N, Nivbrant B (1998) Migration, stem shape, and surface finish in cemented total hip arthroplasty. Clin Orthop 355:103–12

25. Hung JP, Chen JH, Chiang HL, Wu JS (2004) Computer simulation on fatigue behavior of cemented hip prostheses: a physiological model. Comput Methods Programs Biomed 76(2):103–13

26. Jasty M, Maloney WJ, Bragdon CR, O'Connor DO, Haire T, Harris WH (1991) The initiation of failure in cemented femoral components of hip arthroplasties. J Bone Joint Surg Br 73(4):551–8

27. Jones RE, Willie BM, Hayes H, Bloebaum RD (2005) Analysis of 16 retrieved proximally cemented femoral stems. J Arthroplasty 20(1):84–93

28. Kärrholm J, Nivbrant B, Thanner J, Anderberg C, Börlin N, Herberts P, Malchau H (2000) Radiostereometric Evaluation of Hip Implant Design and Surface Finish. Scientific Exhibition presented at the 67th Annual Meeting of the American Academy of Orthopaedic Surgeons, March 15-19, Orlando, USA.

29. Kinzel GL, Hall AS, Hillberry BM (1972) Measurement of the total motion between the two body segments – I. Analytical development. J Biomech 5:93–105

30. Mjörberg B, Hansson LI, Selvik G (1984) Instability of total hip prostheses at rotational stress. Acta Orthop Scand 55:504–506

31. Nägerl H, Kubein-Meesenburg D, Schäfer W, Cotta H, Thomsen M, Strachwitz B, Fanghänel J (1996) Measuring spatial micro-movement of the femur shaft of endoprostheses in relation to the spatial force system. Z Orthop 134:99–110

32. Ohl MD, Whiteside LA, McCarthy DS, White SE (1993) Torsional fixation of a modular femoral hip component. Clin Orthop 287:135–141

33. Panjabi MM, Krag MH, Goel VK (1981) A technique for measurement and description of three-dimensional six degree-of-freedom motion of a body joint with an application to the human spine. J Biomech 14:447–460

34. Pilliar RM, Lee JM, Maniatopoulos C (1986) Observation on the effect of movement on bone ingrowth into porous-surfaced implants. Clin Orthop 208:108–113

35. Rossi P, Sibelli P, Fumero S, Crua E (1995) Short-term results of hydroxyapatite-coated primary total hip arthroplasty. Clin Orthop 310:98–102

36. Schmidbauer U, Brendel T, Kunze KG, Nietert M, Ecke H (1993) Dynamic force measurement in implantation of total endoprostheses of the hip joint. Unfallchirurgie 19:11–15

37. Schneider E, Eulenberger J, Steiner W, Wyder D, Friedman RJ, Perren SM (1989) Experimental method for the in vitro testing of the initial stability of cementless hip prostheses. J Biomech 22:735–744

38. Sugiyama H, Whiteside LA, Engh CA (1992) Torsional fixation of the femoral component in total hip arthroplasty: The effect of surgical press-fit technique. Clin Orthop 275:187–193

39. Schenk RK, Wehrli U (1989) Zur Reaktion des Knochens auf eine zementfreie SL-Femur-revisionsprothese. Orthopäde 18:454–462

40. Thomsen M (2004) Robotically milled bone cavities in comparison with hand-broaching in total hip replacement. In: Stiehl JB, Konermann WH, Haaker RGA: Navigation and Robotics in Total Joint and Spine Surgery. Springer Verlag, Berlin

41. Thomsen M, Breusch SJ, Aldinger P, Görtz W, Lahmer A, Honl M, Birke A, Nägerl H (2002) Robotically milled bone cavities. A comparison with hand broaching in different types of cementless hip stems. Acta Orth Scand, 73 (4):379 –385

42. Tonino AJ, Romanini L, Rossi P et al. (1995) Hydroxyapatite-coated hip prostheses. Early results from an international study. Clin Orthop 312:211–225

43. Vanderby Jr R, Manley PA, Kohles SS, McBeath AA (1992) Fixation stability of femoral components in a canine hip replacement model. J Orthop Res 10:300–309

44. Whiteside LA, Easley JC (1989) The effect of collar and distal stem fixation on micromotion of the femoral stem in uncemented total hip arthroplasty. Clin Orthop 239:145–153

45. Wheeler JP, Miles AW, Clift SE (1999) The influence of the time-dependent properties of bone cement on stress in the femoral cement mantle of total hip arthroplasty. J Mater Sci Mater Med Aug;10(8):497–501

46. Williams HD, Browne G, Gie GA, Ling RS, Timperley AJ, Wendover NA (2002) The Exeter universal cemented femoral component at 8 to 12 years. J Bone Joint Surg Br Apr;84(3):324–34

Implant Choice:
Flanged or Unflanged Sockets?

Dominik Parsch, Steffen J. Breusch

Summary

In this chapter, experimental and clinical evidence is presented to compare unflanged and flanged acetabular components.

The Evidence

The theoretical advantage of a flanged cup is evident. The continuous flange restricts the size of the region through which cement can escape during cup insertion, thus increasing pressure in the cement (◘ Fig. 7.31). Early in-vitro studies confirmed the efficacy of the flange and recommended its use: Oh et al. [6] used a »simulated acetabulum« allowing the cup flange to be inserted flush with the surface. They concluded that a cup with a continuous flange generated significantly higher cement pressures and greater intrusion depths when compared with other cups. Shelley et al. [8] used »acetabulum-shaped cavities with simulated cancellous bone«. They found that flanged cups produced higher peak pressures as well as higher intruded cement volumes compared to unflanged cups.

However, in a recent study we did not find a significant effect on cement penetration of a flanged compared to an unflanged cup [7] (◘ Fig. 7.32). We can only speculate on the reasons for this discrepancy. One possibility is that we used paired human acetabula, which, unlike the previous studies [6, 8], do not exclude the possible effects of the irregularities in the acetabular rim, which may have a detrimental impact on the theoretically convincing sealing effect of the flange. Secondly, we used a »realistic« insertion force of approximately 80 N and decided against a robotic insertion set-up, as previously used [6, 8]. This is because in the operative situation, the surgeon must control the posi-

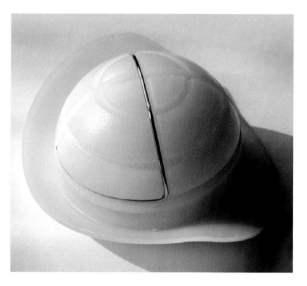

◘ **Fig. 7.31.** Flanged cup (Ogee cup, DePuy, Germany). (Permitted reprint from [7])

tion of the cup as well as the pressurisation of the cement to avoid »bottoming out«, which in some circumstances may necessitate reduction of the force applied to the cup. Bottoming-out as well as friction of the cup flange on the sides of the acetabular cavities may have an important impact on the pressure measurements [3, 8]. On the other hand, the variability of the insertion force induced by the surgeon within the above mentioned ranges, may provide a bias. Finally this is, to our knowledge, the first study simultaneously evaluating both intra-acetabular pressures and the clinically more important cement penetration. While it was confirmed that flanged cups increase the peak intra-acetabular pressure, as previously reported [6], in this more realistic simulation of surgical practice they do not improve

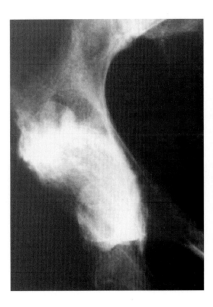
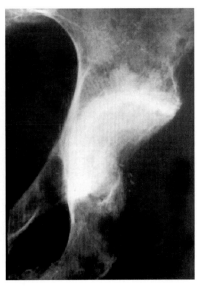

■ **Fig. 7.32.** AP radiographs of paired hemipelvices after cup implantation (right acetabulum: unflanged cup; left acetabulum: flanged cup). Note that orientation wires had been removed before insertion. (Permitted reprint from [7])

sustained pressurisation over the whole cup implantation process. Sustained pressurisation, however, has been reported to be much more effective in causing intrusion of the visco-elastic cement into the small cancellous pores [4, 5].

Based on our results, pressurisation of the cement should be completed before cup insertion i.e. using a pressuriser. The use of flanged cups as the sole means of cement pressurisation in the acetabulum cannot be recommended.

However, clinical studies have documented excellent long-term results with flanged cups [1–3]. An 11-year survival analysis, using aseptic loosening as the end point showed 100% survival of flanged cups [2]. At 21-years survivorship analysis revealed a 77% survivorship for the flanged acetabular component with revision or definite loosening as an endpoint [1].

Take Home Messages

- Excellent clinical results have been published with the use of flanged cups.
- The theoretical advantage of a flange in terms of cement pressurisation during cup insertion could not be confirmed experimentally.
- Adequate cement penetration should be achieved before cup insertion.

References

1. Della Valle CJ, Kaplan K, Jazrawi A, Ahmed S, Jaffe WL. Primary total hip arthroplasty with a flanged, cemented all-polyethylene acetabular component : evaluation at a minimum of 20 years. J Arthroplasty 2004;19:23–26.
2. Garellick G, Malchau H, Herberts P. Survival of hip replacements. A comparison of a randomized trial and a registry. Clin Orthop 2000; 375:157–167.
3. Hodgkinson JP , Maskell AP, Paul A, Wroblewski BM. Flanged acetabular components in cemented Charnley hip arthroplasty. Ten-year follow-up of 350 patients. J Bone Joint Surg 1993; 75-B: 464–467.
4. Markolf KL, Kabo JM, Stoller DW, Zager SA, Amstutz HC. Flow characteristics of acrylic bone cements. Clin Orthop 1984; 183:246–254.
5. Oh I, Merckx DB, Harris WH. Acetabular cement compactor. An experimental study of pressurization of cement in the acetabulum in total hip arthroplasty. Clin Orthop 1983; 177:289–293.
6. Oh I, Sander TW, Treharne RW. Total hip acetabular flange design and its effect on cement fixation. Clin Orthop 1985; 195:304–309.
7. Parsch D, Diehm C, Schneider S, New A, Breusch SJ. Acetabular cementing technique in THA – flanged versus unflanged cups, cadaver experiments. Acta Orthop Scand 2004; 75(3):269–75.
8. Shelley P, Wroblewski BM (1988) Socket design and cement pressurization in the Charnley low-friction arthroplasty. J Bone Joint Surg [Br] 70:358–363.

Implant Choice:
Rationale for a Flanged Socket

A. John Timperley, Jonathan R. Howell, Graham A. Gie

Summary

In clinical practice, flanged cemented sockets have been shown to give better results than simple hemispherical cemented sockets. Laboratory studies have demonstrated their efficacy in increasing the cement injection pressure and thereby improving the cement-bone interface. The flange confers other benefits – it is helpful in attaining accurate socket orientation and the correct depth of insertion in order to establish an adequate, congruent cement mantle.

Introduction

There is irrefutable evidence that the fate of a cemented socket, with regard to mechanical loosening, is determined by the quality of the surgery performed by the surgeon. In order to establish the very best cement-bone interface at the time of surgery there is data supporting the use of a flanged polyethylene socket since there is a sustained rise in cement injection pressure behind the flange at socket implantation.

History of the Flanged Polyethylene Socket and the Original Surgical Technique

A pressure-injection flanged socket made of high density polyethylene was introduced in Wrightington in 1976. The original concept was for the trimmed rim of the flange to make contact with the periphery of the acetabulum before the body of the socket touched the floor of the acetabulum. The rim would trap the cement and pressure would be induced by deflection of the semi-rigid rim when the

body of the socket was pushed to full depth. Charnley noted that this ideal situation arose only rarely since the geometry of that design of socket meant that the deepest part of the body of the socket usually made contact with the acetabulum at the same time as the flange [1]. To trim the flange, Charnley advocated making two tangential cuts to fit the antero-posterior diameter of the socket, extending this cut around the appropriate diameter inferiorly and then sequentially trimming the superior lobe so that it was ultimately left deliberately long but would sit under the roof of the acetabulum if digital pressure was applied to it. He felt that with digital pressure on the rim, the superior lobe would deflect with a lateral concavity thus pressurising the superior cement. He conceded that this type of fit could not always be achieved.

The injection-moulded Ogee socket, made of cross-linked polyethylene, became available in 1981. The name Ogee derived from the architectural term denoting the change in direction of a curved plane. The ogee part of the flange is on the posterior aspect of the cup and its purpose was to maximise the area of contact between cement and bone when the socket was inserted in neutral orientation in the acetabulum [9]. It is advocated that the Ogee flange should be trimmed relatively large to fit on the posterior acetabular rim since, as this part is more flexible than other areas of the flange, it will then bend under pressure to facilitate pressurisation.

The flanged sockets described above were both designed to be introduced through a trochanteric approach to the hip and it was a fundamental part of Charnley's teaching on the Low Friction Arthroplasty that the socket should *not* be anteverted [1]. He taught that the absence of anteversion, combined with retention of the anterior capsule, was important in preventing anterior dislocation of the hip in external rotation. Few surgeons now use the trochanteric approach to the hip and it is contemporary surgical practice to antevert the socket whether it is inserted through an anterolateral or posterior approach. The geometry of the Ogee flange is less effective at pressurising cement if the socket is positioned in significant anteversion since it often impossible to trim the flange to seat against the acetabular bone posterosuperiorly. Additionally, whilst the flange undoubtedly confers some benefits in ensuring accurate positioning of the implant, it can be seen that both of the techniques previously described rely on the deflection of one segment of the flange to pressurise the cement thus allowing the possibility of change in alignment of the face of the cup as pressurisation is attempted. For these reasons a different geometry of flange and technique of insertion may be appropriate (vide infra).

Clinical Evidence for the Use of Flanged Sockets

Hodgkinson and his colleagues [3] demonstrated a significant reduction in radiolucency on the post-operative X-rays when a flanged socket is inserted when compared with a normal hemispherical socket. At ten years it was statistically significant that more of the flanged group were free of radiolucencies compared with the unflanged group and they concluded that the improved long-term radiological result was due to the superior cement-bone interface created at the time of implantation. Kobayashi et al. [4] also studied the effect of a flange on the incidence of radiological demarcation in the medium term. Observing the 5-year radiographs, the authors demonstrated a statistical correlation between socket demarcation and socket fixation technique with *no* demarcation being evident in 80% of a group with flanged sockets compared with 33% of an earlier group in whom unflanged sockets were inserted. These two series differed in the way the acetabular bone was prepared but it is likely the flange was primarily responsible for these differences which support the observations of Hodgkinson.

Other reports in the literature have demonstrated improved results when a flanged socket is used in both primary [2, 6] and revision cases [8].

Experimental Evidence for the Use of Flanged Sockets

When introducing a socket into bone cement it is important to induce sustained pressures within the cement to achieve adequate penetration of trabecular bone and thereafter to protect the interface from the accumulation of blood (▶ chapter 6.5). Experimentally only modest cement injection pressures have been measured behind an unflanged cup and these fall when the socket »bottoms

out« [5, 9]. Conversely, much higher pressures can be induced behind a flanged implant and these pressures are maintained throughout the polymerisation cycle. In a cadaver study by Parsch et al. [7], higher peak, but not average pressures were measured in the acetabulum behind a flanged cup compared with an unflanged device and the authors suggested that the flange should not be the *sole* method of pressurising cement. In the experiment by Shelley and Wroblewski [9], the Exeter balloon pressuriser gave slightly better cement injection pressures than the flange and in practical terms the use of the Exeter pressuriser, or other proprietary pressuriser, followed by the late insertion of a flanged socket would appear to be logical.

Contemporary Surgical Technique Using a Flanged Socket

1. The socket is adequately exposed as described elsewhere.
2. The true medial wall is identified by using reamers or a long-handled gouge to remove any curtain osteophytes and expose the true medial wall of the acetabulum (▶ chapter 2.1).
3. Powered reamers may now be used, increasing in size in 2 mm increments, to remove cartilage and subchondral bone. Care is taken not to thin the walls excessively. A note is made of the largest reamer used to clear the rim of the acetabulum. Often it is useful to revert to a smaller reamer to expose further trabecular bone (▶ chapter 2.1); particular attention is paid to the rim of the acetabulum since it is important to achieve interdigitation of bone in this area.
4. A step drill is used to make multiple holes. The smaller part of the drill is used all around the rim of the socket, the larger part of the step makes multiple holes in the dome of the ilium, pubis and ischium. Care is taken not to perforate the walls. If this does occur then morcellised bone graft is packed into the hole to prevent egress of cement during cementation.
5. A socket with an outside diameter 2 mm smaller than the largest reamer used is usually the appropriate implant. A trial flange is placed on the introducer and trial socket and trimmed along the line indicating the size of the largest reamer used (◻ Fig. 7.33). A trial positioning of the cup is now carried out with further trimming of the flange until the rim of the flange lies just within the mouth of the acetabulum (◻ Fig. 7.33).
6. When satisfied with the seal achieved, the introducer is mounted on the trial flange and definitive socket and the true flange trimmed appropriately (◻ Fig. 7.34). A further rehearsal is made to ensure that the socket can be introduced through the soft tissues into the correct position without difficulty (◻ Fig. 7.34).

7. The socket is normally orientated in a position of 45 degrees abduction (the handle of the introducer will point vertically upwards) and 35 degrees flexion (the transverse handle of the introducer is rotated around the transverse axis of the patient by 35 degrees).

8. A sucker aspirator device (■ Fig. 7.35), which is placed into the acetabular roof, is turned on at this point and, to save time, the nursing staff are asked to start mixing the cement during final preparation of the bone. Thorough lavage of the socket is carried out to clean the interstices of the trabecular bone of marrow and fat. Fluid is sucked out of the wing of the ilium by the sucker aspirator. When the bone is clean, hydrogen peroxide soaked gauze swabs are packed into the socket to further clean the bone and promote haemostasis.

9. The cement may be handled approximately 3.5 minutes after the beginning of mixing (Simplex cement at 20 degrees centigrade). Immediately before it is placed in the socket, bone graft reamings may be impacted against the smooth cortical medial wall since the cement cannot adequately gain fixation against a surface of this sort. After introduction of the cement bolus excess material is removed so the surface of the cement lies with a slightly concave surface within the mouth of the socket. This step prevents escape of surplus cement into the soft tissues when the acetabular pressuriser is applied.

10. The pressuriser (■ Fig. 7.35) consists of a saline filled balloon which can be inflated from a reservoir in the handle of the device. The pressurising technique entails inflating the balloon so that it conforms perfectly within the mouth of the socket and then applying full body weight onto the device to drive the cement into the bone and, by maintaining pressure, protect the bone cement interface from back-bleeding from the host bone. The sucker aspirator also serves to suck cement into the wing of the ilium and remove blood from the interface. If there is excessive blood loss through the sucker, the level of vacuum should be reduced.

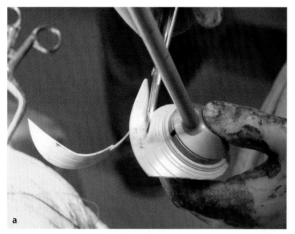

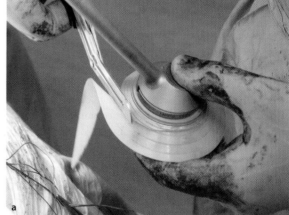

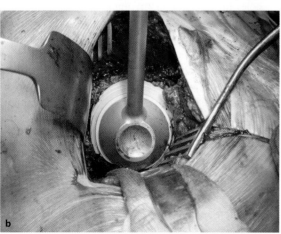

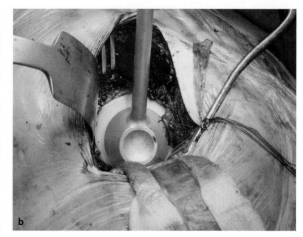

■ **Fig. 7.33a,b.** Trimming (**a**) of the trial socket flange (*blue*) and trial positioning (**b**)

■ **Fig. 7.34a,b.** Final trimming of definite implant by superimposing trail template (**a**). A final rehearsal is then done with the adjusted implant (**b**)

11. The pressuriser is applied as soon as the cement has been placed in the socket and full pressure is maintained until the cement viscosity has risen to a level suitable for socket insertion – usually about 6 minutes after the commencement of mixing (when using Simplex bone cement). In the elderly, or where it has been possible to expose a larger surface area of trabecular bone, it can happen that so much cement is pressurised into the acetabulum that a further bolus is required on top of the initial bolus of cement This will become apparent when the pressuriser is removed. If more cement is to be used, then the existing cement should be dried before it is applied.

12. The flanged socket is then inserted, as rehearsed, using the introducer and an axial pusher to drive the socket to the seated position. This exercise should require significant force and there should be a constant flow of cement around the edge of the cup. Excess cement can be removed with a small curette. The timing is perfect when the flange is delivered to the final seated position just as it is impossible to advance further the cup into the viscous cement (◘ Fig. 7.36a).

13. The post-operative radiograph should show good cement penetration and no radiolucent lines in any Zone (◘ Fig. 7.36b).

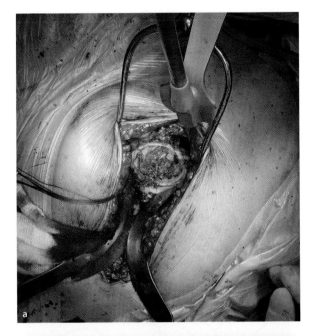

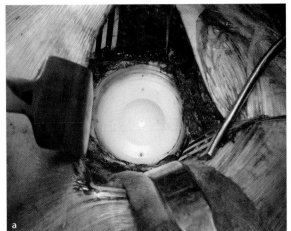

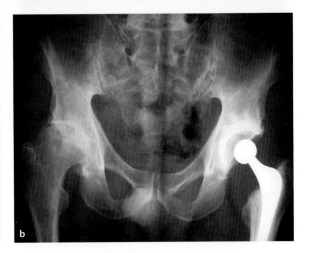

◘ **Fig. 7.35a,b.** An intraosseous, aspiration cannula is placed in the ilium to reduce bleeding (**a**). The cement is pressurises with an expandable Exeter balloon pressuriser (**b**)

◘ **Fig. 7.36a,b.** Implanted cup after cement curing (**a**) and corresponding postoperative radiograph (**b**) with no radiolucent lines

Modification of the Basic Technique – Use of the Rim-Cutter

The basic technique described above has been modified in Exeter with development of an instrument that will ensure accurate placement of a flanged cup with a congruent cement mantle into a pre-rehearsed position. This new instrument (the rim-cutter, patent pending) also facilitates exposure of trabecular bone around the periphery of the acetabulum, so potentially enhancing fixation in this important area (▶ chapter 9.1).

The principle is to cut a rim around the periphery of the acetabulum to a set depth. The flange of the socket seats into this rim thus guaranteeing the correct orientation and depth of insertion of the socket if the rim cutter has been used correctly. Accurate positioning can be ensured since the rim cutter can be navigated to the desired position. Another benefit of this technique is that it allows the possibility of carrying out a trial reduction to rehearse stability and leg length before cementation; the trimmed socket may be introduced into the acetabulum supported only by the flange resting in the rim and the hip reduced with the trial femoral component in place.

The Rim-Cutting Technique

- The acetabulum is reamed and drill holes made as described previously.
- A cup 2 mm smaller than the largest reamer used is chosen.
- The rim cutter marked with the same size as the cup is attached to a power tool (◘ Fig. 7.37a). This will cut a groove in the periphery of the acetabulum of the appropriate diameter for the flange.
- The hemispherical guide of the rim cutter centralises the cutter in the reamed socket and sets the depth of the rim and thus the position of the cup (◘ Fig. 7.37b).
- The orientation of the rim cutter is shown by the alignment rod on the device.
- Accurate inclination and flexion can be ensured by using a navigation device on the shaft of the rim cutter.
- The rim cutter is advanced to the fullest extent allowed by exerting pressure against the spring between the dome and cutting ring.
- Any debris created, including the innermost fibres of the transverse ligament, is excised.
- The flange is trimmed to the diameter defined by the chart to fit within the rim.
- A trial reduction may be carried out if chosen.
- The technique is thereafter as described above (step 7 onwards).

It will be seen from the diagram (◘ Fig. 7.38) that the cement spacers on the implant should not touch bone

with this technique, and, for all but the smallest cup size, a cement mantle of 4 mm will be guaranteed around the socket. Implantation of the cup into the rim is timed so that the flange engages the rim as the cement is becoming very viscous. Since no other part of the cup is touching bone, further pressure on the introducer will act to distort the flange and increase the cement injection pressure.

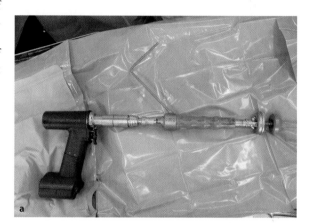

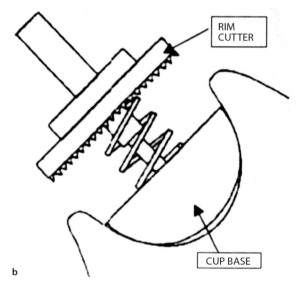

◘ **Fig. 7.37a,b.** Photograph of the rim cutter (**a**). In the diagram (**b**) the principle mechanism is outlined

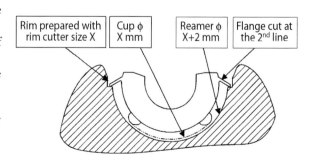

◘ **Fig. 7.38.** Diagram, showing the step in the acetabular wall created by the rim cutter and the relative cup position

> **Take Home Messages**
>
> - An accurately trimmed flange on a socket increases the cement injection pressure behind the implant.
> - There is laboratory and clinical evidence supporting the use of flanged UHMWPE sockets.
> - Modifications to the original technique are useful in ensuring correct orientation of the socket and concentricity within the mantle.

References

1. Charnley J. Low friction arthroplasty of the hip. Theory and practice. Springer Verlag, Berlin. 1979
2. Della Valle CJ, Kaplan K, Jazrawi A, Ahmed S, Jaffe WL. Primary total hip arthroplasty with a flanged, cemented all-polyethylene acetabular component: evaluation at a minimum of 20 years. J.Arthroplasty 2004;19(1):23–6
3. Hodgkinson JP, Maskell AP, Paul A, Wroblewski BM. Flanged acetabular components in Charnley hip arthroplasty. Ten year follow-up of 350 patients. J Bone Joint Surg 1993;75-B:464–7
4. Kobayashi S, Terayama K. Radiology of low-friction arthroplasty of the hip. A Comparison of Socket fixation techniques. J. Bone Joint Surg 1990; 72-B (3):439–443
5. Oh I, Sander TW, Treharne R. Total hip acetabular cup flange design and its effect on cement fixation. Clin Orthop 1985;195:304–9
6. Onsten I, Besjakov J, Carlsson AS. Improved radiographic survival of the Charnley prosthesis in rheumatoid arthritis and osteoarthritis. Results of new versus old operative techniques in 402 hips. J.Arthroplasty 1994;9(1):3–8
7. Parsch D, Diehm C, Schneider S, New A, Breusch SJ. Acetabular cementing technique in THA--flanged versus unflanged cups, cadaver experiments. Acta Orthop Scand 2004;75(3):269–75
8. Raut VV, Kay P, Siney PD, Wroblewski BM. Factors affecting socket fixation after cemented revision. Int.Orthop 1997;21(2):83–6
9. Shelley P, Wroblewski BM. Socket design and cement pressurisation in the Charnley low-friction arthroplasty. J.Bone Joint Surg 1988;70-B(3):358–63

Part IV   Clinical Outcome

Chapter 8   Femoral Components

Chapter 8.1   Cemented Stems for Everybody?   – 216
                 O. Furnes, L.I. Havelin and B. Espehaug

Chapter 8.2   Long-Term Outcome after Charnley Low Frictional Torque
                 Arthroplasty   – 221
                 B.M. Wroblewski, P.D. Siney, P.A. Fleming

Chapter 8.3   Long-Term Success with a Double Tapered Polished
                 Straight Stem   – 228
                 M.J.W. Hubble, A.J. Timperley, R.S.M. Ling

Chapter 8.4   Outcome with the MS-30 Stem   – 235
                 E.W. Morscher, M. Clauss, G. Grappiolo

Chapter 8.5   Outcome with a Tapered, Polished,
                 Anatomic Stem   – 242
                 L.J. Taylor, G. Singh, M. Schneider

Chapter 8.6   The French Paradox   – 249
                 G. Scott, M. Freeman, M. Kerboull

Chapter 8.7   Cemented Stems with Femoral Osteotomy   – 254
                 C. Howie

Chapter 9   Acetabular Components

Chapter 9.1   Is It Justified to Cement All Sockets?   – 260
                 A.J. Timperley, G.A. Gie, R.S.M. Ling

Chapter 9.2   Long-Term Success of a Well-Cemented Flanged
                 Ogee Cup   – 268
                 J. Older

Chapter 9.3   Long-Term Survival of Cemented Sockets
                 with Roof Graft   – 273
                 C. Howie

Chapter 10   What Bearing Should We Choose?   – 279
                 C. Heisel, M. Silva, T.P. Schmalzried

Chapter 11   The Evidence from the Swedish Hip Register   – 291
                 H. Malchau, G. Garellick, P. Herberts

Femoral Components:
Cemented Stems for Everybody?

Ove Furnes, Leif Ivar Havelin and Birgitte Espehaug

Summary

There is considerable evidence from our register studies, that cemented implants both in femur and acetabulum give satisfactory long-term (15 years) results. These findings apply both for young and old patients, and for all diagnostic groups. Cemented polished tapered stems have been reported with good results both in the Norwegian and Swedish hip implant registers. The Exeter and Charnley total hip implants (cup and stem) had similar results after 15 years follow up.

Introduction

During the 1980s, the use of uncemented femoral stems in total hip arthroplasty (THA) gained popularity, but still many surgeons regard the cemented metal stem with a small head articulating with a cemented all polyethylene acetabular socket as the gold standard for hip replacements. The Norwegian Arthroplasty Register started registration of hip implants in 1987 as a prospective ongoing study. The unique identification number given to each inhabitant of Norway enabled us to follow implants in many patients for extended periods of time. In several studies we have focused on the survival of different types of cemented and uncemented hip prostheses used in Norway [5]. In this paper we will present the latest update on femoral stem prostheses with up to 15 years of follow up.

Results of Cemented and Uncemented Stems

Our results indicated that both cemented and uncemented stems do well both in young and old patients (Figs. 8.1 and 8.2). Uncemented stems had marginally better results than the cemented stems in young patients (<60 years) [3], when the smooth pressfit Biofit stem was excluded (Fig. 8.3). The uncemented stem with the best result in Norway was the HA coated Corail stem with a 15 year survival of 95.1%. In patients younger than 60 years, the Corail stem had a 12-year survival of 96.2%. For several uncemented stems concern has been raised due to increased incidence of thigh pain documented. In one randomised study the uncemented implant gave 17% thigh pain and the cemented implant 3% [8]. There is also concern as to what will happen when the hydroxylapatite disappears, will there subsequent be more aseptic loosening?

The cemented stems are well documented both regarding the survival of the implant and for pain relief [1]. The polished tapered Exeter stem had the best results of the cemented stems with a 15 year survival of 97.0%. In patients younger than 60 years, the Exeter stem had a 12 year survival of 95.2%. There were differences in results among the cemented stems. The polished tapered Exeter stem had better survival than the straight vaquashined Charnley stem (Fig. 8.2, Table 8.1). These results compared well with the results of the Exeter implant in the Swedish Hip Register [9].

Results of THA System (Cup and Stem Combined)

However, it is arbitrary to look at only one of the components, as the results may change when we study the whole prosthetic system (cup and stem). Both in all patients and in patients younger than 60 years the result of the whole prosthesis was similar for Exeter and Charnley implants (Fig. 8.4). The reason was less revisions of the

Cemented and uncemented stems, 10 most common prostheses

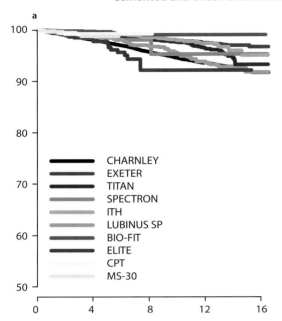

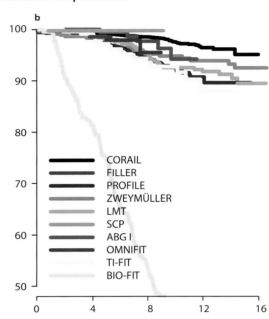

Fig. 8.1a,b. Cox-adjusted survival curves for cemented (Palacos or Simplex) and uncemented stem brands in all age groups. Adjusted for age, gender and diagnosis. **a** Cemented stems, endpoint revision of stem. **b** Uncemented stems, endpoint revision of stem. (The Norwegian Arthroplasty Register 1987–2004)

Cemented and uncemented stems in patients <60 years

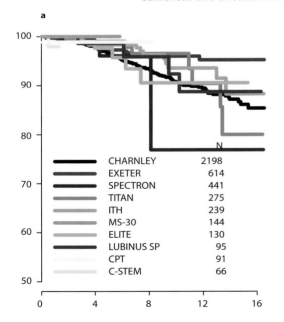

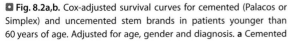

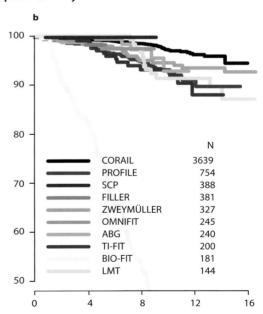

Fig. 8.2a,b. Cox-adjusted survival curves for cemented (Palacos or Simplex) and uncemented stem brands in patients younger than 60 years of age. Adjusted for age, gender and diagnosis. **a** Cemented stems, endpoint revision of stem. **b** Uncemented stems, endpoint revision of stem. (The Norwegian Arthroplasty Register 1987–2004)

Cemented and uncemented cup/stem combinations, age < 60, 10 most common prostheses

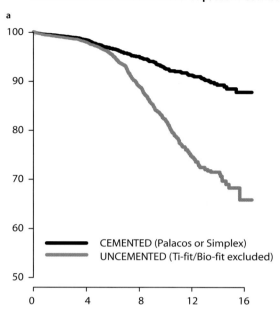

Fig. 8.3a,b. Cox-adjusted survival curves for prostheses commonly used in patients younger than 60 years of age. Adjusted for age, gender and diagnosis. **a** Cemented and uncemented cup/stem, revision of cup. **b** Cemented and uncemented cup/stem, revision of stem. (The Norwegian Arthroplasty Register 1987–2004)

Cemented and uncemented cup/stem combinations, age < 60, 10 most common prostheses

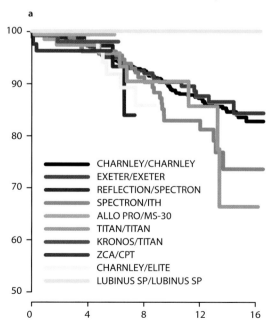

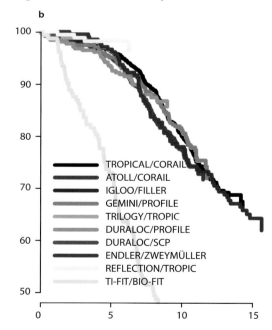

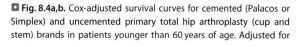

Fig. 8.4a,b. Cox-adjusted survival curves for cemented (Palacos or Simplex) and uncemented primary total hip arthroplasty (cup and stem) brands in patients younger than 60 years of age. Adjusted for age, gender and diagnosis. **a** Cemented arthroplasties, endpoint any revision. **b** Uncemented arthroplasties, endpoint any revision. (The Norwegian Arthroplasty Register 1987–2004)

Table 8.1. The 10 most commonly used cemented stems used in Norway. The revision percentage were calculated by Cox regression adjusting for age, gender and diagnosis and cement (Palacos, Simplex). The Norwegian Arthroplasty Register 1987–2004

Stem Prostheses	N	R	Median Follow-up in Years	Revision % at 10 Years	Revision % at 15 Years
Charnley	26221	976	5.8	5.5 (5.0–5.9)	7.9 (7.1–8.7)
Exeter	7567	138	5.7	2.2 (1.7–2.7)	3.0 (2.3–3.8)
Titan	7439	118	5.1	2.4 (1.9–3.0)	6.8 (4.6–8.9)
Spectron	3889	17	1.6	*	*
ITH	3533	64	7.2	2.1 (1.5–2.7)	4.9 (2.6–7.2)
Lubinus SP	1657	62	5.8	4.5 (3.1–5.9)	8.3 (5.2–11.3)
Bio-Fit	1556	10	6.8	1.0 (0.3–1.6)	*
CPT	875	6	2.8	*	*
Elite	829	24	3.4	7.9 (3.9–12)	*
MS-30	816	7	2.4	*	*

*Insufficient follow-up

Charnley acetabular components. This was probably due to the smaller head (22,2 mm) in the Charnley implant compared to the Exeter implant (28 mm and 30 mm). The smaller heads give less wear and subsequently less aseptic loosening of the acetabular component [10].

The uncemented implants had worse results than the cemented implants because of more aseptic loosening and polyethylene wear in press-fit HA coated cups, and polyethylene wear and osteolysis in press-fit hemispheric porous coated cups ▫ Fig. 8.4 [3, 6, 7].

The titanium stem prostheses (Titan and ITH) used in Norway had good 15 years results, with a 93.2% and 95.1% survival of the stem (▫ Fig. 8.2). These prostheses were mainly used in patients over 60 years of age.

The cemented anatomic Lubinus SP stem had good results in the Swedish register [5], but in the Norwegian register the Lubinus SP stem had a survival of 91.7% after 15 years (▫ Table 8.1). The results from Norway with the Lubinus SP stem were mainly based on operations from two hospitals, and the inferior results were from one hospital. The results must therefore be interpreted with caution.

Why Were Results Worse in Young Patients?

In a study of the influence of the hip diagnosis we used cemented Charnley prostheses as a control group [4]. We found that the reason for poor prognosis in some hip diseases in young patients were due to the fact that these young patients had been given a poorly performing uncemented hip implant. These implants were introduced as more promising than the established cemented implants during the 1980s. During the last 15 years these implants have failed in large numbers. The reason for failures were aseptic loosening of uncemented smooth press-fit stems, threaded cups with smooth surface, or porous coated stems without circumferential coating. If the patient had been given a cemented Charnley prosthesis using a well-documented cement (Palacos or Simplex), the survival of the implant was good both in young and old patients in all hip-diagnosis groups [4].

There is considerable evidence from our register studies that cemented implants both in femur and acetabulum give good long-term results in all age groups. At our institution, we use cemented implants (both in femur and acetabulum) with a small head (22 mm) in young patients. In older patients (>80 years) where the polyethylene wear problem is negligible and the dislocation problem is greater, we use femoral heads of 32 mm [2].

Take Home Messages

- Implant survival should not only be judged by evaluation of stem or cup in isolation, but assessed as a THA system.
- Cemented THA performs equally well in all age groups compared to the best uncemented systems.
- Uncemented acetabular components pose the increased risk of wear and osteolysis (and aseptic loosening).
- Cemented THA remains the gold standard also for the young patient until better outcome has been documented for new uncemented designs.

Acknowledgements. We thank orthopaedic surgeons at all hospitals in Norway, without whose co-operation the Norwegian Arthroplasty Register would not be possible. The work of the register is a teamwork and we thank our co-authors Lars B. Engesæter, Stein Emil Vollset and Stein Atle and our secretaries Adriana Opazo, Inger Skar and Ingunn Vindenes for their accurate registration.

References

1. Aamodt A, Nordsletten L, Havelin LI, Indrekvam K, Utvåg SE, Hviding K. Documentation of hip prostheses used in Norway. A critical review of the literature from 1996–2000. Acta Orthop Scand 2004;75 (86):663–676

2. Byström S, Espehaug B, Furnes O, Havelin LI. Femoral head size is a risk factor for total hip luxation: a study of 42,987 primary hip arthroplasties from the Norwegian Arthroplasty Register. Acta Orthop Scand. 2003;74:514–24

3. Furnes O, Espehaug B, Lie SA, Engesæter LB, Vollset SE, Hallan G, Fenstad AM, Havelin LI. Prospective studies of hip and knee prostheses. Scientific exhibition AAOS 2005, Washington, USA

4. Furnes O, Lie SA, Espehaug B, Vollset SE, Engesæter LB, Havelin LI. Hip disease and the prognosis of total hip replacements. A review of 53 698 primary total hip replacements reported to the Norwegian Arthroplasty Register 1987–1999. J Bone Joint Surg (Br) 2001;83-B:579–86

5. Havelin LI, Espehaug B, Lie SA, Engesæter LB, Furnes O, Vollset SE. The Norwegian Arthroplasty Register. 11 years and 73,000 arthroplasties. Acta Orthop Scand 2000;71:337–53

6. Havelin LI, Engesæter LB, Furnes O, Espehaug B, Vollset SE, Lie SE. 5300 uncemented acetabular cups in young patients. A comparative study with 0–13 years of follow-up in the Norwegian Arthroplasty Register. Proceedings AAOS 2002, Dallas, USA

7. Havelin LI, Espehaug B, Engesæter LB. The performance of two hydroxyapatite- coated acetabular cups compared with Charnley cups. From the Norwegian Arthroplasty Register. J Bone Joint Surg (Br) 2002;84-B:839–45

8. Kim YH. Bilateral cemented and cementless total hip arthroplasty. J Arthroplasty 2002;17 (4):434–40

9. The Swedish National Hip Arthroplasty Register. Annual Report 2003. www.jru.orthop.gu.se

10. Wroblewski BM, Siney PD, Fleming PA. Wear of the cup in the Charnley LFA in the young patient. J Bone Joint Surg Br. 2004 May;86(4):498–503

Femoral Components: Long-Term Outcome after Charnley Low Frictional Torque Arthroplasty

*B. Michael Wroblewski, Paul D. Siney, Patricia A. Fleming**

Summary

The Charnley low-friction arthroplasty has reached 42 years of clinical application: 96.5% of patients consider it a success in respect of pain relief, 74.5% have normal or near normal function and 74.3% have full or nearly full range of hip movements – with a mean follow up of 19.1 years (10–36 years).

The incidence of cup loosening and revision is exponentially related to the depth of cup penetration. Ceramic ultra high molecular weight polyethylene combination has produced results with total penetration of 0.41 mm with a follow-up to 18 years and no cup loosening.

Triple tapered polished C stem offers better load transfer from the stem to the femur avoiding strain shielding of the proximal femur.

Continuous evolution of the design, surgical technique and materials has paid dividends in the long-term success of this method of total hip arthroplasty (THA).

Introduction

The Charnley low-frictional torque arthroplasty (LFA), with a 22.225 mm diameter stainless steel head articulating with an ultra high molecular weight polyethylene (UHMWPE) cup, both components grouted with self-curing acrylic cement, has reached 42 years of successful clinical application. It has withstood the test of time when other designs made frequent changes of their basic concepts. But the Charnley LFA has not stood still. Improvements and modifications in surgical technique, design and even materials, formed an integral part of the evolutionary progress. These were brought in as a result of the study of long-term results, findings at revision surgery and examination of explanted components. Radical departure from the basic concept has not been a part of that process. It is not usually understood, let alone appreciated, that availability of long-term results has certain fundamental implications. Any patient with the longest follow-up must have been relatively young at the time of surgery. Any analysis selects ever younger patients with increasing follow-up. It is this group that can be expected to be relatively active. Such patients no longer represent »the average« for the originally selected group: they can only represent the results of the earliest application of the concept without the benefit of improvements brought in later.

It is not possible to have the benefits of long-term experience, long-term follow-up and young patients all at the same time. Furthermore, long-term problems can only be experienced after long-term success has been achieved. A suggestion is also made that any presentation of the longest follow-up results must indicate the benefits of that experience. It is no longer sufficient to claim after 42 years of the success rate of the Charnley LFA, that clinical results of a THA are good: that is the reason why this type of surgery is still practiced. This fact can almost be taken for granted.

Clinical results have become, inevitably, a measure not of the efficacy of the operation, but the skill of selecting patients for the operation. The exception will always be the group of patients with the longest follow-up: they will continue to be the measure of clinical success with an ever increasing follow-up.

Clinical assessment will remain an integral part of medical practice for we usually treat symptomatic patients. Any total hip arthroplasty, however, can be expected to offer pain relief, for it offers a neuropathic interposition spacer – provided of course the components remain well fixed.

* Research supported by the Peter Kershaw and John Charnley Trusts

For the same reason clinical results may not reflect the mechanical state of the arthroplasty: radiographic follow-up is essential. Claims of exceptional functional performance after surgery, made by an individual, can only be regarded as anecdotal and a reflection of the result for that individual. Any attempt to use that as an indicator of long-term success of the method must be considered inappropriate. We must distinguish between a successful result for an individual and a long-term success of a method.

The aim of this chapter is to remind the reader of the success, the reason for that success, and the benefits of the continuity of the evolution of the Charnley LFA spanning 42 years of clinical experience. It must be appreciated that even the earliest experience with the Charnley LFA offered 6 years and 2500 LFAs before the first revision for loose cup, loose stem or fractured stem had to be carried out [1].

No other design has ever been documented to have matched what can be called the Charnley golden standard. It can probably be argued that any method of THA should pass, even if not exceed that standard, if long-term success is to be expected.

Material and Method

Patients aged 50 years or younger, at the time of the LFA, have been selected for an indefinite follow-up. All operations had been performed at Wrightington Hospital between November 1962 and December 1990. Clean air enclosure and total body exhaust suits were used. Lateral approach with trochanteric osteotomy was the routine exposure. Both components, the UHMWPE cup and the stainless steel monoblock stem with the 22.225 mm diameter head, were implanted with cold curing acrylic cement, polymethylmethacrylate (PMMA) used as a grout.

Patients were mobilised usually within one week using elbow crutches, weight bearing, for six weeks following routine procedures. The follow-up was at 3 months then every 1–3 years or according to radiographic appearances – with free access on request.

The radiographic appearances on the acetabular side were recorded according to Hodgkinson et al. [4] and on the femoral side according to Pacheco et al. [5]. Wear measurements of the UHMWPE cup, recorded as penetration, were made on serial radiographs as documented by Griffith et al. [3].

Clinical assessment, before and after surgery, was according to d'Aubigne and Postel [2] as modified by Charnley [1].

Since clinical results do not reflect the mechanical state of the arthroplasty [9], it has been our practice to carry out revisions early, if need be, for radiographic changes only. We have taken revision, for whatever reason, as the end point. We define revision as a secondary operative intervention into cases of THA documenting reason or reasons.

Results

In the study we had 1092 patients, 1434 LFAs: 424 males and 668 females. Three hundred and forty two patients (31.3%) had had bilateral arthroplasties; 98 (9%) having had both hips replaced at a single operation. Patients mean age at surgery was 41 years (range 12–51 years). The underlying hip pathology is shown in ◘ Table 8.2 and previous hip operations (excluded were hemi- and total hip arthroplasties) in ◘ Table 8.3. Patients excluded from the continuing follow-up are shown in ◘ Table 8.4. Indications for revisions are listed in ◘ Table 8.5.

A group of 652 patients (860 LFAs) continue the follow-up and have not had a revision. They represent 59.7% of the original group of patients and 60% of the LFAs.

The mean follow-up for this group is 19.1 years (range 10–36 years). They form the basis of detailed clinical and radiographic analysis (◘ Figs. 8.5., 8.6 and 8.7).

◘ **Table 8.2.** Underlying hip pathology

Diagnosis	Number	%
Primary O.A.	298	20.8
Secondary arthritis		
▬ Congenital dislocation, dysplasia, subluxation	395	27.6
▬ Perthes disease	77	5.4
▬ Slipped upper femoral epiphysis	55	3.8
▬ Trauma (including fracture of the neck of the femur)	123	8.6
▬ Sepsis – acute	5	0.4
▬ Sepsis – chronic	37	2.6
▬ Quadrantic head necrosis	68	4.7
▬ Paget's disease	1	0.1
Rheumatoid arthritis – Still's disease	292	20.4
Ankylosing spondylitis	91	6.4
Protrusio acetabuli	47	3.3
Fusion for unspecified pathology	18	1.3
Unspecified	10	0.7

◘ **Table 8.3.** Previous operative procedures

Procedure	Number	%
None	1164	81.2
Osteotomy: femoral/pelvic	139	9.7
Open reduction and internal fixation	42	2.9
Fusion/attempted fusion	36	2.5
Cup arthroplasty	15	1.1
Pin/plate/screw fixation	4	0.3
Other (soft-tissue procedures)	78	5.4

Table 8.4. Patients excluded from the continuing follow-up

Reason	Number of Patients	% Patients	Number of Hips	% Hips
Lost to follow up	108	7.7	136	10.5
Deaths during follow up	126	12.1	174	9.1
Revised	206	15.0	264	18.4

Table 8.5. Indication for revision

Indication	Number of Revisions	Revised (%)
Infection	22	1.5
Dislocation	7	0.5
Loose cup/wear	188	13.1
Loose stem	75	5.2
Fractured stem	22	1.5
Unexplained pain	3	0.2

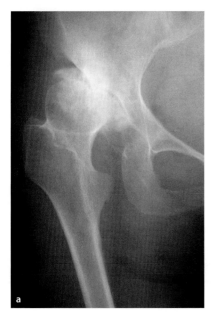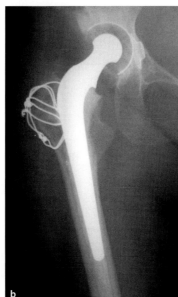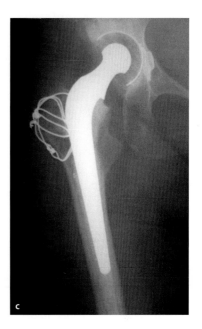

Fig. 8.5a–c. Long term follow-up. **a** Pre-operative radiograph, **b** post-operative radiograph at 1 year, **c** radiograph at 28 years post-operatively

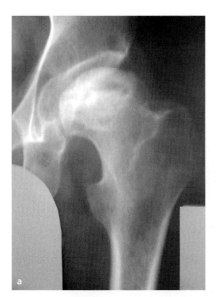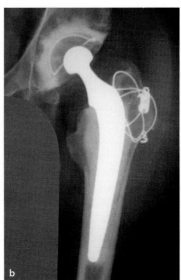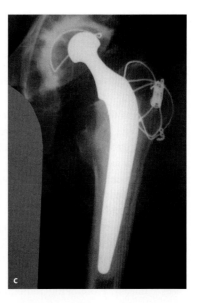

Fig. 8.6a–c. Penetration of the UHMWPE cup and no femoral cavitation. **a** Pre-operative radiograph, **b** Post-operative radiograph at 1 year, **c** radiograph at 18 years follow-up

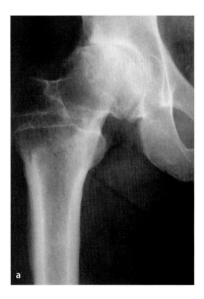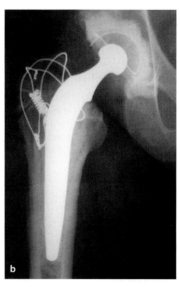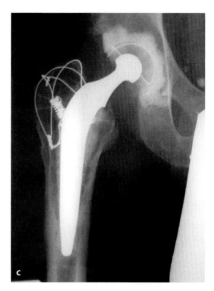

Fig. 8.7a–c. No penetration of the UHMWPE cup and femoral cavitation. **a** Pre-operative radiograph, **b** post-operative radiograph at 1 year, **c** radiograph at 20 years follow-up

Clinical Results

Clinical results remain successful:
- Pain:
  - 87.9% are pain-free (grade 6).
  - 8.6% have no more than an occasional discomfort (grade 5).
- Function:
  - 58.62% have normal or near normal function (grade 6) for age, gender and underlying hip pathology.
  - 15.9% have near normal function (grade 5).
- Movement:
  - 38.7% have full range of movement (grade 6) on the operated hip.
  - 35.6% have nearly full range of movement (grade 5).

Radiographic Assessment – Acetabulum

According to the classification of Hodgkinson et al. [4] 76 of the cups (8.8%) are radiologically loose they show change in position on serial radiographs. Further 67 cups (7.8%) show complete demarcation of 2 mm or more at the bone cement interface. Although not migrated they are classed as being loose. Thus radiologically loose cups were found in 143 (16.6%) of 860 cases which have reached 19.1 years of follow-up (range 10–36 years) and have not been revised at this stage.

The radiographic appearances have not affected clinical results to the extent as to allow identification of these cases clinically. Continuing radiographic assessment is essential.

Radiographic Assessment – Femur

Excluding the stems that have been revised (detailed in Table 8.5) before the recent review, nine stems (1.1%) are definitely loose and two further stems (0.2%) are probably loose – an overall stem loosening rate of 1.3% past 19.1 years mean follow up (10–36 years).

Cup Wear (Penetration)

The mean cup penetration was 0.08 mm/yr with a range of 0.01–0.48 mm/year and a total penetration pf 1.54 mm (range 0.1–8.0 mm). The correlation between the depth of cup penetration and the incidence of cup migration in all patients is shown in Table 8.6 and Fig. 8.8.

Survivorship Analysis

With regular follow-up, relatively low loss of patients and early intervention in cases of failure, it is probably acceptable to use survivorship analysis with revision as the end point. The survivorship for the whole group of 1092 patients, 1434 LFAs, carried out on 10th September 2004 is shown in Table 8.7 and Fig. 8.9. The survivorship was 93.7% at 10 years. 85.0% at 15 years. 75.0% at 20 years 65.7% at 25 years and 49.3% at 30 years.

What the survivorship analysis has also revealed is that once trained, the success rate for both senior trainees and the permanent staff was identical.

Table 8.6. Wear of UHMWPE cup. Cup migration and revision for aseptic cup loosening

Cup penetration [mm]	0	≤1	≤2	≤3	≤4	≤5	>5
Number of cases	47	630	291	217	116	48	27
Number migrating	0	73	75	76	58	26	16
% Migrating	0	11.6	25.8	35.0	50	54.2	59.3
Number revised	0	27	35	40	26	13	9
% Revised	0	4.3	12.0	18.4	22.4	27.1	33.3

Table 8.7. Survivorship analysis. Endpoint – revision for any reason

Follow-up [Years]	Number at Start	Withdrawn	Failure	Number at Risk	Cumulative Success Rate	Confidence Limits Higher	Confidence Limits Lower
0	1434	0	0	1434	100.00	100.00	100.00
1	1434	0	0	1434	100.00	100.00	100.00
2	1434	27	3	1420.5	99.79	100.00	99.55
3	1404	24	4	1392	99.50	99.87	99.13
4	1376	13	5	1369.5	99.14	99.62	98.65
5	1358	19	4	1348.5	98.84	99.41	98.27
6	1335	23	10	1323.5	98.08	98.82	97.35
7	1302	21	6	1291.5	97.62	98.44	96.80
8	1275	23	16	1263.5	96.35	97.37	95.34
9	1236	26	12	1223	95.37	96.52	94.22
10	1198	29	20	1183.5	93.68	95.02	92.34
11	1149	49	21	1124.5	91.81	93.35	90.28
12	1079	43	16	1057.5	90.30	92.00	88.61
13	1020	56	24	992	87.88	89.79	85.98
14	940	61	8	909.5	87.00	89.04	84.96
15	871	72	17	835	84.97	87.20	82.73
16	782	59	24	752.5	81.78	84.27	79.28
17	699	73	10	662.5	80.27	82.98	77.55
18	616	66	8	583	78.90	81.84	75.95
19	542	68	8	508	77.32	80.52	74.12
20	466	59	10	436.5	75.03	78.55	71.51
21	397	51	5	371.5	73.68	77.53	69.84
22	341	48	6	317	71.79	75.99	67.59
23	287	55	8	259.5	68.71	73.38	64.03
24	224	45	6	201.5	65.73	71.04	60.42
25	173	35	0	155.5	65.73	71.78	59.68
26	138	27	5	124.5	61.71	68.42	55.01
27	106	30	3	91	58.42	66.16	50.68
28	73	23	4	61.5	51.91	60.91	42.92
29	46	15	1	38.5	49.32	60.41	38.23
30	30	9	0	25.5	49.32	62.94	35.69
31	21	10	0	16	49.32	66.52	32.11
32	11	2	0	10	49.32	71.08	27.56
33	9	2	0	8	49.32	73.65	24.99
34	7	3	0	5.5	49.32	78.66	19.97
35	4	0	0	4	49.32	83.72	14.91
36	4	2	0	3	49.32	89.05	9.59
37	2	2	0	1	49.32	100.00	0.00

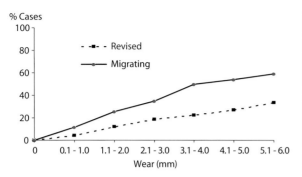

Fig. 8.8. The correlation between the depth of cup penetration and the incidence of cup migration and revision

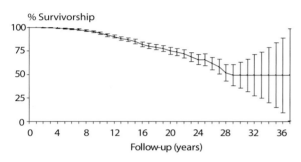

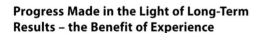

Fig. 8.9. Survivorship analysis. Endpoint – revision for any reason

Progress Made in the Light of Long-Term Results – the Benefit of Experience

Cup Wear and Loosening

These two closely related problems have been identified in 1984 as limiting the life of the arthroplasty [6].

Reduced Diameter Neck

The problem was identified as impingement of the neck on the rim of the cup, with progressive cup penetration. The diameter of the neck of the stem was reduced from 12.5 to 10 mm. This was made possible with high nitrogen stainless steel and the cold forming process in stem manufacture (ORTRON, DePuy International, Leeds U.K.).

A 20 year prospective study (in print) has shown a combined effect on reduction of aseptic cup loosening and revisions of over 50%.

Low-Wear Materials

A combination of alumina ceramic 22.225 mm diameter head articulating with chemically cross-linked polyethylene has given excellent results [9]. With the follow up

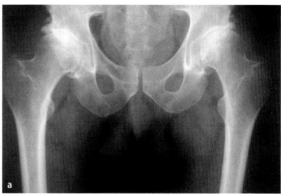

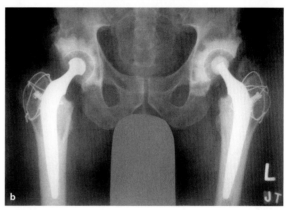

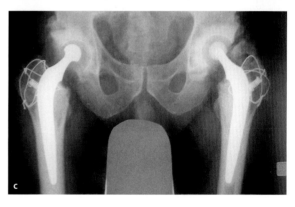

Fig. 8.10a–c. Bilateral Charnley LFA. The left side is a combination of an alumina ceramic femoral head and a cross-linked polyethylene cup and the right side a combination of a metal femoral head and a UHM-WPE cup. Both sides were operated on within one year of each other. **a** Pre-operative radiograph, **b** post-operative radiograph at 1 year, **c** radiograph at 18 years post-operatively. The left side has a total penetration of 0.41 mm and the right side has a total penetration of 4.1 mm

now to 18 years, the total penetration of the cup has not exceeded 0.41 mm (**Fig. 8.10**).

A 22.225 mm diameter zirconia head articulating with UHMWPE, with a follow-up to 9 years, has shown that 77% show no measurable wear, and in a further 10% this is less than 0.02 mm/year [12]. Clearly a ceramic polyethylene combination is the way forward. It offers the confidence of long-term information without the fear that may accompany the introduction of radically new materials.

The Stem

Stem fracture, initially the most common complication, has been totally eliminated. Two factors played a vital role; stronger stem with a better geometry and an improved method of stem fixation. By closing off the medullary canal distally with a cancellous bone block and pressurisation of the cement, the success rate was achieved in 99% at 10 years in patients with a mean age of 41 years [7].

Strain Shielding of the Proximal Femur

Stem, fracture, proximal endosteal cavitation and aseptic stem loosening have been identified as having the same basic cause: lack or loss of proximal stem support with good distal fixation. Although the early failures may have been due to surgical technique, failures after 11 years are due to defunctioning of the proximal femur [7]. The radiographic appearances indicating effects of this change present in only 5.9% of cases at a mean follow-up of 19.1 years (10–36 years), but this was 10.6% at a mean follow-up of 15.8 years (1–36 years). This apparent reduction in the incidence is due to a number of revisions of stem loosening which were carried out during the intervening period.

The introduction of the triple-tapered polished stem – the C-Stem – (DePuy International, Leeds. U.K) and the surgical technique to avoid distal stem support, have prevented the changes and even improved the radiographic changes in a large proportion of the cases [11].

Conclusions

The Charnley LFA, with 42 years of clinical application, continues to offer consistently successful clinical results. Pain relief has been offered to over 96% of patients. Improvement of function will always depend on the underlying hip pathology, patients' age and general health. Two major factors will decide the ultimate fate of the arthroplasty: wear and the effect of the implant on the function of the skeleton.

With the availability of combinations of low-wear materials, the local effects of wear products on the bone-implant interface are likely to become of academic interest only. Time and long-term follow-up will give indications of any possible systemic effects of the wear debris using metal on metal articulations.

Skeletal changes are inevitable both with increasing age and declining function. Some may and do lead to fractures, even with minor trauma. How will clinically successful THAs affect the skeletal changes ultimately is yet to be established. Will they become non-progressive or will the skeleton fail around the implant that does not?

What is clear is that with 42 years of success of the Charnley LFA we are in a position to have strong indications as to what should happen in the clinical practice rather than attempting to find out what is happening.

Take Home Messages

- The Charnley low-friction arthroplasty has reached 42 years of clinical application with pain relief in more than 95%.
- The survivorship was 93.7% at 10 years, 85.0% at 15 years, 75.0% at 20 years, 65.7% at 25 years and 49.3% at 30 years.
- The incidence of cup loosening and revision is exponentially related to the depth of cup penetration.
- Two major factors will decide the ultimate fate of the arthroplasty: wear and the effect of the implant on the function of the skeleton.
- Continuous evolution of the design, surgical technique and materials has paid dividends in the long-term success of this method of hip arthroplasty.

References

1. Charnley J (1972) The long term results of low-friction arthroplasty of the hip performed as primary interventions. J Bone Joint Surg (Br.) 54-B:61–76
2. d'Aubigne RM, Postel M (1954) Function results of hip arthroplasty with acrylic prosthesis. J Bone Joint Surg (Am.) 36-A:451–75
3. Griffith MJ, Seidenstein MK, Williams D, Charnley J (1978) Socket wear in Charnley low-friction arthroplasty of the hip. Clin Orthop 137: 37–47
4. Hodgkinson JP, Shelley P, Wroblewski BM (1989) The correlation between roentgenographic appearances and operative findings at the bone-cement junction of the socket in the Charnley low-friction arthroplasties. Clin Orthop 228:105–9
5. Pacheco V, Shelley P, Wroblewski BM (1988) Mechanical loosening of the stem in Charnley arthroplasties. J Bone Joint Surg (Br.) 70-B:596–9
6. Wroblewski BM (1985) Charnley low-friction arthroplasty in patients under the age of 40 years: In Sevastick Y, Goldie I (eds) The young patient with degenerative hip disease. Almquist and Wiksell, Stockholm, pp 197–201
7. Wroblewski BM, Fleming PA, Siney PD, Hall RM (1998) Stem fixation in the Charnley low friction arthroplasty in young patients using an intramedullary bone block. J Bone Joint Surg (Br) 80-B:273–8
8. Wroblewski BM, Siney PD, Fleming PA (1991) Charnley low-friction arthroplasty of the hip. Long term results. Clin Orthop 292:191–201
9. Wroblewski BM, Fleming PA, Siney PD (1999) Charnley low friction arthroplasty of the hip – 20 to 30 year results. J Bone Joint Surg (Br.) 81-B:427–9
10. Wroblewski BM, Siney PD, Fleming PA (1999) Low-friction arthroplasty of the hip using alumina ceramic and cross-linked polyethylene. A ten year follow-up report. J Bone Joint Surg (Br.) 81-B:54–5
11. Wroblewski BM, Siney PD, Fleming PA (2001) Triple taper polished cemented stem in total hip arthroplasty. J Arthroplasty 16(8):37–41
12. Wroblewski BM, Siney PD, Nagai H, Fleming PA (2004) Wear of ultra-high-molecular-weight polyethylene cup articulating with a 22.225 mm zirconia diameter head in cemented total hip arthroplasty. J Orthop Sci 9(3):253–5

Femoral Components: Long-Term Success with a Double Tapered Polished Straight Stem

Mathew J.W. Hubble, A. John Timperley, Robin S.M. Ling

Summary

The first double tapered, polished, collarless, straight femoral stem for cemented total hip arthroplasty (THA) to be used in clinical practice was the Exeter stem, designed in 1969 by Robin Ling and Clive Lee, in Exeter, UK. It has been in use in clinical practice since 1970 and excellent long-term results up to 33 years are now available. The Exeter is currently the most commonly used cemented stem, not only in the UK, but worldwide.

Introduction

A decision was made in Exeter in 1969 to develop a new design of total hip replacement because of the disappointing results with the McKee Farrar THA and a reluctance to perform the trochanteric osteotomy at that time advocated with the Charnley Low Friction Arthoplasty. A collar on a femoral stem was perceived to predispose to calcar lysis, and the new stem was therefore designed without a collar or proximal flare. A straight, double taper to the stem was selected to maximise the pressurisation of bone cement during insertion, and as the British standard for stainless steel orthopaedic implants at that time required them to have a polished surface, the stem was polished. Thus, largely by serendipity, a collarless, straight, double tapered polished stem was produced, which was first used in clinical practice in October 1970 (◘ Fig. 8.11).

The combination of a relatively slim prosthesis, weak (by modern standards) stainless steel, and over machining of some of the femoral stems resulted in a number of neck and stem fractures. As a result of this, in 1976 a change was made in the type of steel used. Unfortunately, it was fashionable at this time to manufacture components with a matt surface, and as the importance of a polished surface had not at that time been appreciated, the stems made from the new material were no longer polished. Although the change in material all but eliminated the problem of stem fractures, aseptic loosening and osteolysis soon

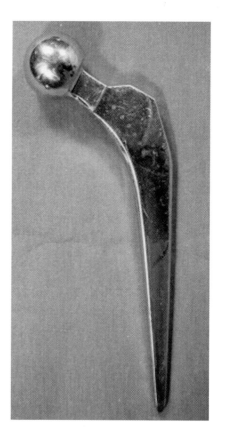

◘ **Fig. 8.11.** Photo of original Exeter stem

began to occur around the matt stems, whereas it was virtually never seen around the older polished stems. It was also noted that the polished stems routinely subsided a millimetre or two in the cement mantle, but this was not seen with the matt stems. It became clear that the polished stem was able to act as a taper, to subside and load the proximal femur, whereas the matt stem was not able to function in this manner. Therefore in 1986, a return to polished stems was made, with the introduction in 1988 of modularity. This has been mirrored by a return to the excellent result seen with the original polished stems.

The Original Series

The first Exeter stem was inserted in 1970, and between 1970 and 1975, 433 original polished stems were inserted by 16 different surgeons at the Princess Elizabeth Orthopaedic Hospital, in Exeter, using 1st generation cementing techniques (no plug, no lavage, finger packing of the canal). The stems were monoblock, with a head size of 30 mm. Of the 433 hips, 56 had had a previous procedure, and 21 were revisions (■ Table 8.8).The mean age of the patients at the time of surgery was 67 years (range 30–89 years). Follow up ranges from 28 to 33 years.

Of the 433 THAs, 6.46% had been lost to follow up by a mean of 30 years.

The survival of femoral stems for aseptic loosening, over this 30 year period was 91.4% (■ Fig. 8.12). A total of 17.8% of hips underwent a revision procedure, the most common cause being aseptic cup failure (■ Table 8.9).

By the end of 2003 there were 27 surviving patients, with 34 THAs, from the original 433. The mean length of follow up of these patients is 30 years (28–33). The average age at the time of their surgery was 56 years (now 87 years). 2 of these stems have been revised for aseptic loosening during these 30 years (at 18 and 20 years respectively). One further case is awaiting revision (91% survival for aseptic stem loosening), 12 acetabular cups have been revised, 10 for aseptic loosening, and 2 for late recurrent dislocation. The medial femoral bone stock in these patients is still well preserved (■ Table 8.10). Localised endosteal bone lysis is present in 5 cases.

■ **Table 8.8.** Pathology of 433 cases: Original series

Osteoarthritis	323
Failed osteotomy	27
Rheumatoid	22
Revision THA	17
Previous fracture	5
Revision hemiarthroplasty	4
Other	22

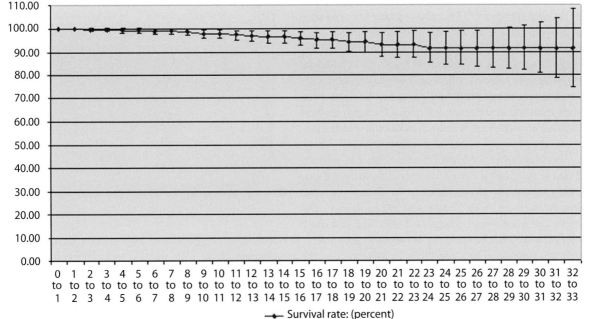

Original Exeter polished stems -
Survival rate to 33rd year with end-point revision for aseptic stemloosening: (percent)

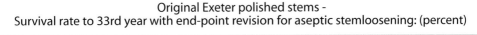

■ **Fig. 8.12.** Survival curve for original series aseptic stem loosening

Table 8.9. Indications for re-operation: All series

	Original Series (n=433)	Universal Series (n=325)	Under 50s (n=88)
Aseptic cup loosening	8.54%	2.2%	6.8%
Neck fracture	3.46%	0	0
Stem fracture	3.69%	0	0
Aseptic stem loosening	3.46%	0	1.1%
Sepsis	1.84%	1.2%	2.3%
Recurrent dislocation	0.46%	1.5%	0
Periprosthetic fracture	0.46%	0.6%	0

Table 8.10. Loss of height of medial femoral neck (mm): Original series

0	17
<1	1
1–2.9	5
3–4.9	1
5–6.9	1
7–8.9	2
>9.	1

Table 8.11. Pathology necessitating THA: Universal series

Primary osteoarthritis	245
Rheumatoid	17
Protrusio acetabuli	15
Revision hemiarthroplasty	9
Failed osteotomy	7
Previous fracture	6
Other	26

The Universal Series

In 1988, a modular version of the original double tapered polished collarless Exeter stem was introduced. This stem retained a geometry similar to the original Exeter stem (manufactured from EN58J stainless steel), but was made of stronger steel (Rex 734), had a taper that extended throughout its length, and had a morse taper at the end of the neck (■ Fig. 8.13). This allows a range of head sizes and offsets to be used with the stem. Two further offset options (35.5 and 50 mm) were added to the existing range of sizes (37.5 and 44 mm; ■ Fig. 8.14). In addition, the stem was inserted with a hollow polymethyl-methacrylate centralizer (■ Fig. 8.15), designed to prevent the stem from end bearing, and facilitating the small amount of subsidence (■ Fig. 8.16) known to be central to the mechanical behaviour of stems of this design [13].

Between March 1998 and February 1990, 325 primary THAs were performed in 309 patients at the Princes Elizabeth Orthopaedic Hospital, using the Exeter universal femoral stem. 113 were in men and 192 in women. The mean age was 67 years (range 24 to 87). The pathology necessitating THA is shown in ■ Table 8.11. The operation was performed by a consultant in 48% of cases, the remainder by fellows (9.5%) or residents (42.5%). The posterior approach was used in 248 hips, and the transgluteal (direct lateral) in 77. All acetabular components were polyethylene and cemented. 94% were metal backed, and a head size of 26 mm was used in 97%. Third-generation

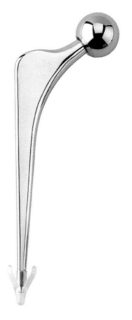

■ Fig. 8.13. Photo of modular universal Exeter stem

cementing techniques were used (plug, pulsatile lavage, retrograde filling with suction and a cement gun, and proximal pressurisation). Follow up ranged from 8 to 12 years, with a mean of 9 years. 94 patients have died, but none were lost to follow up.

Analysis of serial radiographs revealed a mean subsidence at the stem cement interface of 1.32 mm at 8 to 10

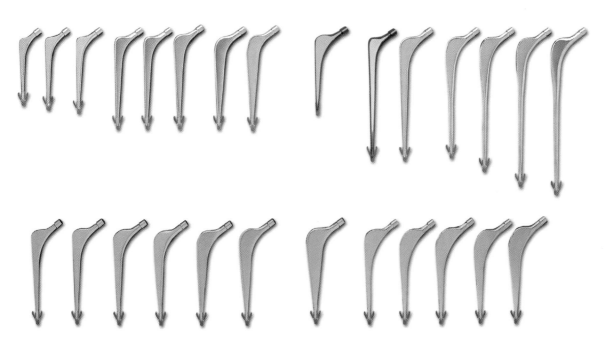

Fig. 8.14. Current range of Exeter stems

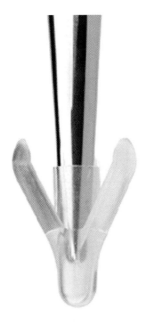

Fig. 8.15. Photo of hollow distal centralizer

years. No migration was demonstrated at the cement bone interface. Radiolucent lines were noted at the cement bone interface in 9% of hips, but only exceeded 14% of the interface in one case. Localised endosteal lysis was only seen in one case (0.5%). The medial femoral neck was preserved in the vast majority of cases (■ Table 8.12 and ■ Fig. 8.17).

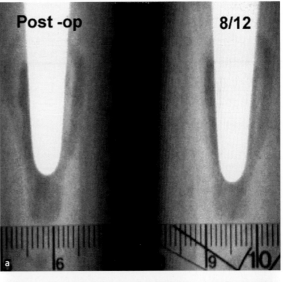

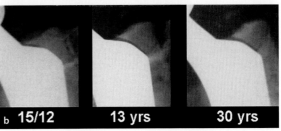

Fig. 8.16a,b. Subsidence at the tip of the Exeter stem within the cement mantle (**a**). Subsidence at the shoulder of the Exeter stem within the cement mantle (**b**)

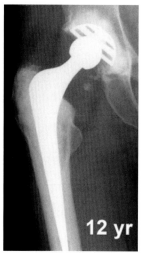

Fig. 8.17. Medial femoral neck and proximal bone stock preservation. Note the metal backed cemented acetabular component

Table 8.12. Radiological analysis: Universal series

Subsidence [mm]	
<1	51
123	
2–2.9	17
3–3.9	3
4–4.9	0
>5	2
Mean	1.32

Loss of Height of Medial Femoral Neck [mm]	
163	
<1	3
19	
6	
2	
4–4.9	2
>5	2

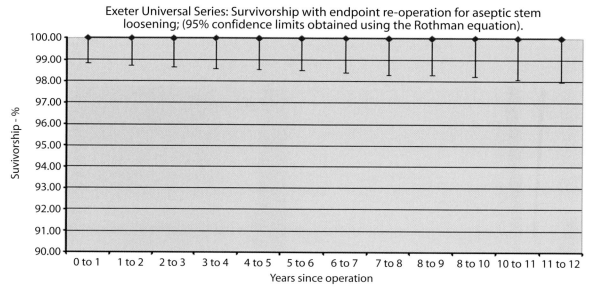

Fig. 8.18. Survival curve for Universal series aseptic stem loosening

At a follow up of 12 years, survivorship with revision of the femoral component for aseptic loosening was 100% (Fig. 8.18). There were no stem fractures. Survivorship for revision of the acetabular component for aseptic loosening was 97% and for any re-operation 92%. All the acetabular components that required revision were metal backed.

Young Patients

One of the greatest challenges facing total joint arthroplasty is the long-term survival of implants in younger, more active patients. The Universal stem series contained 31 THAs that were performed in patients from Exeter who were under the age of 50 years at the time of surgery. A wider review of patients from Exeter, North Devon and Torbay Health districts between March 1988 and June 1991 revealed a further 57 cases, making a total of 88 THAs that were performed in 71 patients with a mean age of 43 years [11]. A cemented acetabular component with a Universal Exeter stem was used in all cases. The acetabular component was metal backed in 66 cases (75%). A total of 25 different surgeons performed the procedures. 69% were consultants, 31% residents or fellows. Cementing technique varied, with a 3rd gen-

☐ Table 8.13. Pathology necessitating THA in patients under 50 years

Osteoarthritis	25
Inflammatory arthropathy	25
Acetabular dysplasia	11
Avascular necrosis	8
CDH	5
SUFE	4
Acetabular fracture	3
Other	7

eration technique in 80% of cases and orthograde finger packing of cement in 16%. Latest follow up ranged from 12 to 15 years, with a mean of 13.4 years. 7 patients died during the review period. No patients have been lost to follow up. As might be expected in such young patients, the pathology necessitating arthroplasty differed significantly from the Original and Universal series (☐ Table 8.13).

2 femoral components were revised for aseptic loosening (2.3%) by 15 years. These had both been inserted with 1st generation cementing techniques with finger packing of cement. There were 2 cases of localised femoral endosteal bone lysis, one of 28% and the other 24% of the cement/bone interface. 7 cups were revised, including one failed block graft. There were also 2 revisions for deep sepsis and 1 for recurrent dislocation. At a follow up of 15 years, survivorship with revision of the femoral component for aseptic loosening was 98%, and re-operation for any cause 85%.

Discussion

The results achieved in terms of femoral component survival, retention of proximal femoral bone stock and scarcity of femoral endosteal bone lysis in all these series are outstanding. These include femoral component survivorship in excess of 90% at 33 years and of 98% even in young and active patients at 15 years of follow up. The experience to date suggests that the universal Exeter stem, used in combination with 3rd generation cementing techniques, is capable of producing results even better than the Original stem at the same time interval (☐ Figs. 8.12 and 8.18). It is important to note that these are the results of multi-surgeon series, with surgeons of differing levels of seniority and expertise. The Exeter stem would appear to be relatively forgiving, performing well in the hands of surgeons of differing ability. The results seen in the younger, more active patients is particularly important. This is the very group where longevity of implant survival and preservation of proximal femoral bone stock is so critical, in view of the patients potential life expectancy

and the risk of the need for future revision surgery. The fact that so few (less than 10%) of the surviving patients in the Original series (who had a mean age of 56 at the time of their surgery) have required revision of their femoral component for aseptic loosening at 30 years of follow up strongly supports the selection of a prosthesis of this design for use also in young and active patients.

The acetabular components fared less well in all these series, but still had survivorship of 97% at 15 years. This fell to 87% in the under 50 year old patients, and 57% in the survivors in the Original series at 33 years. All the acetabular components that failed in the universal and young patient groups were metal backed, which despite its theoretical advantages has been shown to be clinically detrimental and was abandoned in Exeter in 1990.

Other centres have reported similarly gratifying results with the Exeter femoral component. The Swedish, Finnish and Norwegian Arthroplasty registries have all reported 10 year survival rates in excess of 95% with this prosthesis, and similar results have been reported from a variety of institutions [4, 5, 9, 12].

The Exeter polished tapered stem is functionally different from more conventional cemented stems, and challenges many of the previously accepted theories of cemented femoral stem biomechanics [6]. It has a unique migration pattern on radiosterogrametric analysis, migrating an order of magnitude more in the first 2 years at the stem cement interface than any other design of cemented stem tested. Conversely, none of the studies have shown any axial migration at the cement bone interface. These findings support the theory that the Exeter stem, due to its polished, collarless, straight, tapered design is able to function on the 'taper-slip' or 'force closed' principle (▶ chapters 7.1 and 7.2), as described by Shen and Huiskes [1, 8, 9]. Subsidence of the stem at the stem cement interface allows the taper to engage and generate a loading regime dominated by compression rather than shear (▶ chapter 3.2). This also contributes to the overall stability of the stem, especially in torsion, and minimises stress shielding of the proximal femur [1]. This perhaps explains the relative preservation of proximal femoral bone stock and limited calcar resorption seen in these series (see ☐ Tables 8.10 and 8.12, ☐ Fig. 8.16). The energy expended in this manner at the stem cement interface is not available to challenge the cement bone interface, which is thus protected in this environment. In addition, it would appear that stem subsidence helps to seal the stem cement interface, limiting the flow of fluid and debris [2, 3, 7].

The polished surface, as well as permitting subsidence, influences the mechanism and morphology of stem wear (▶ chapter 7.2). It has been shown that polished stems have a much more benign pattern of stem wear, with minimal damage of the cement mantle or release of particulate debris compared to matt surfaced stems [7]. As a consequence, arthroplasties employing a polished stem, at least in theory, are less prone to the resultant third body wear or the effects of debris and fluid flow.

Hopefully, future advances in bearing surfaces and acetabular fixation will result in further improvement in the overall survival of total hip arthroplasties, to compliment that which is already achievable with the femoral component.

Take Home Messages

- Excellent results at up to 35 years of follow up are reported with the polished double tapered Exeter femoral component.
- The fixation principle of the Exeter stem design relies on limited subsidence of the stem within the cement mantle, aided by a hollow distal centralizer (the taper-slip principle).
- A highly-polished surface is central to this principle, and also minimises stem cement abrasion and the generation of wear particles, as seen with stems with a rougher surface.
- The Exeter femoral component can be used with confidence in patients of all ages and activity level. At a follow up of 30 years, survivorship for revision of the femoral component for aseptic loosening was 91%, and even in young, active patients, 98% at 15 years.
- The polished double tapered Exeter stem is a forgiving component and performs well in the hands off surgeons of differing ability and experience, with good results reported from a variety of units.

References

1. Alfaro-Adrian J, Gill HS, Murray DW. Should total hip arthroplasty femoral components be designed to subside? A radiostereometric analysis of the Charnley elite and Exeter stems. J. Arthroplasty 2001; 16:598–606
2. Anthony PP, Gie GA, Howie CR, Ling RSM. Localised endosteal bone lysis in relation to the femoral components of cemented total hip athroplasties. J. Bone Joint Surg. Br 1990; 72B:971–9
3. Crawford RW, Evans M, Ling RS, Murray DW. Fluid flow around model femoral components of differing surface finishes: in vitro investigations. Acta Orthop Scand 1999; 70:589–95
4. Finnish Arthroplasty Registry. The 2000–2001 implant book of orthopaedic endoprostheses. http://www.nam.fi/english/publications/medical devices.html
5. Franklin J, Robertson O, Gestsson J, Lohmander LS, Ingvarsson T. Revision and complication rates in 654 Exeter total hip replacements with a maximum follow up of 20 years. BMC Musculoskelet Disord. 2003; 25:4(1):6
6. Harris WH, McCarthy JC, O'Neill DA. Femoral component loosening using contemporary techniques of femoral cement fixation. J. Bone Joint Surg Am 1982; 64A:1063–7
7. Howell JR, Blunt LA, Doyle C, Hooper RM, Lee AJC, Ling RSM. In vivo surface wear mechanisms of femoral cemented total hip arthroplasties. The influence of wear mechanism on clinical outcome. J Arthroplasty 2004; 19:88–101
8. Huiskes R, Verdonschot N, Nivbrandt B. Migration, stem shape and surface finish. Clin Orthop. 1998; 355:103–12
9. Norwegian Arthroplasty Registry. Prospective studies of Hip Prostheses and Cements 1987–1999. http://www. haukeland.no/nrl/
10. Shen G. Femoral stem fixation: an engineering interpretation of the long term outcome of Charnley and Exeter stems. J. Bone Joint Surg. Br 1998; 80B:754–6
11. Squires B, Ellis AM, Timperley AJ, Gie GA, Ling RSM, Wendover NA. The Exeter Universal Hip Replacement for the young patient. J. Bone Joint Surg. Br. 2003; 85B: Suppl 2
12. Swedish National Hip Arthroplasty Register. Annual Report 2002. http://www.jru.orthop.gu.se/
13. Williams HDW, Browne G, Gie GA, Ling RSM, Timerley AJ, Wendover NA, The Exeter cemented femoral component at 8 – 12 years. J. Bone Joint Surg B. 2002; 84B: 324–334

Femoral Components: Outcome with the MS-30 Stem

Erwin W. Morscher, Martin Clauss, G. Grappiolo

Summary

The reported follow-up studies show that excellent results with a 10-year survivorship of the MS-30 stem of 100% can be achieved. The outcome of a THR not only depends on the design of the implant but also on the conditions of its surface and the material. Last but not least the operative, and especially the cementing technique play a decisive role.

Introduction

The MS-30 femoral stem (Zimmer prior Centerpulse, Switzerland), manufactured from stainless steel (Fe-CrNiMnMoNb ISO 5832–9) and designed for cemented fixation in total hip replacement (THR), was developed by the first author (EWM) and Spotorno/Italy. The primary goal for the development of this stem was to generate an optimal cement mantle [30], which is known to be the most important factor for the longevity of a cemented femoral stem (■ Fig. 8.19). The fixation of the stem occurs according to the press-fit principle. No changes in stem design have been made since market introduction in 1990.

The quality of the cement mantle itself depends on the implant design, the implant's surface conditions and material characteristics, as well as on the operative, i.e. the cementing technique. Inadequate cementing techniques were the main cause of the high rates of aseptic loosening and, thus, of the increase in revision rates in the past [28]. Main causes of failure of cemented femoral stems are: insufficient medial support [8], an insufficient cement mantle with metal/bone contact [7], insufficient cement/ bone interdigitation [28] and an inadequate position of

the stem [12, 27, 39]. Therefore, a series of various factors, which are closely related to each other, play a decisive role for the outcome of a cemented THR.

The design of the implant determines the amount and the direction of the forces transmitted between the bone and the prosthesis through the cement. Furthermore, the design and size of the implant determine the thickness of the cement mantle. According to laboratory and clinical

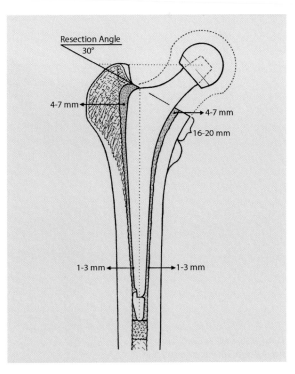

Resection Angle
30°

4-7 mm

4-7 mm

16-20 mm

1-3 mm

1-3 mm

■ **Fig. 8.19.** Schematic drawing of the MS-30 stem inserted into the proximal femur, indicating the optimum dimensions of the cement mantle and the 30° angle of the resection of the femoral neck.

experience, the optimum dimensions of a cement mantle are asymmetric and non-uniform. The cement mantle should be thicker in the region where main forces are transmitted, i.e. in Gruen zones 7, 3 and 5. Overall, the thickness of the cement mantle around the stem should be no less than 2 mm [8, 9].

The MS-30 stem is three-dimensionally tapered. Thus, the system functions according to the press-fit concept. The selected stem is undersized in comparison to the medullary canal prepared by reamers, in order to provide the necessary space for the bone cement between implant and bone. The thickness of the cement mantle must already be taken into account in the preoperative planning, which is vital for the success of a THR. The edges of the stem are rounded off, in order to minimise the creation of stress risers within the cement mantle. The flanges in the proximo-lateral part of the prosthesis increase its rotational stability. The rotational stability is further improved by a high neck resection [11, 34] of 30° in relation to the horizontal plane (◘ Fig. 8.19). An integral part of the system is the distal centralizer, which helps to position the component distally, hence avoiding metal/bone contact and malalignment [30]. A varus position of the stem, however, is first of all avoided by lateral reaming of the medullary canal.

The MS-30 has been manufactured from its introduction in clinical practice in 1990 both with a matt (Ra 0.5–1.5) as well as a polished surface (◘ Fig. 8.20). Since 2002, a lateralised version of the MS 30-stem has been available, but no other changes in stem design have been made since general market introduction in 1990.

The aim of this chapter is to summarise four follow-up studies of the MS-30 stem performed in three different orthopaedic institutions in Switzerland (Basel), Italy (Pietra Ligure) and in Germany (Heidelberg).

Patients

We report (◘ Tables 8.14 and 8.15):

1. the 10-year results of a consecutive series of 126 THRs in 123 patients with the MS-30 stem with a matt surface, which were implanted between January 1990 and December 1992 at the Orthopaedic Department of the University of Basel/Switzerland;

2. the results of a prospective study of the Orthopaedic Department of the University of Basel/Switzerland in which the outcome of 127 MS-30 stems with a matt and 128 stems with a polished surface implanted between 1994 and 1997 was compared;

3. the 10-year results of the MS-30 stem with a polished surface. The 197 stems were implanted between March 1990 and December 1992 at the Santa Corona Hospital in Pietra Ligure/Italy.

4. the mid-term multi-surgeon results of 333 consecutive MS-30 stems with a matt surface and a follow-up between 6 and 10 years from the Orthopaedic Department of the University of Heidelberg/Germany.

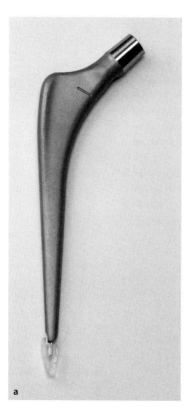 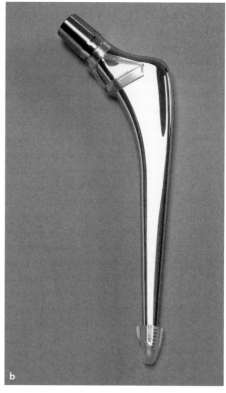

◘ **Fig. 8.20. a** MS-30 cemented femoral stem with matt surface and original (solid) centralizer. **b** MS-30 stem with polished surface and 2nd generation (hollow) distal centralizer and (optional) proximal centralizer

▢ Table 8.14. Patients data

Follow-up study No.	1	2	3	4
Surface characteristics	matt	matt/polished	polished	matt
No. of hip joints/patients	126/123	127/116 128/117	197/193	333/318
Bone cement used	Palacos-G	Palacos-G/Palacos-G	Palacos-G	Palacos
Gender male, unilateral female, unilateral	45 78	47, 55 59, 52	44 149	86 232
Bilateral, other stem	23	12, 19	5	–
Age (y) male (at surgery) female	67.3 (49–86) 67.6 (36–89)	65 (41–86) 66 (35–88) 72 (54–89) 70 (40–91)	69(51–81) 70(51–90)	70.6 (27–88) 72.4 (41–91)
Deceased until 12/2001	27	16, 15	35	73/70 pts.
Unable to come to FU	9	2, 5	58	48
Lost to FU	0	0, 0	5 (2.6%)	5 (0.9%)
No. of clin. + radiol. FU	90	109, 108	95	195
Observation time (y)	10.2 (8.3–12.1)	6.6 (5.5–7.3)	10,2 (8,5–11,9)	6.5 (7d–10.8)

▢ Table 8.15. Diagnoses (percentage)

Follow-up study No.	1	2	3	4
Surface characteristics	matt	matt/polished	polished	matt
No. of hip joints/patients	126/123	127/116 128/117	197/193	333/318
Osteoarthritis	80	82.7, 72.7	80,9	76.8
Fracture	3	3.1, 3.9	1,5	9.4
CDH	5	5.5, 7.8	2,9	4.2
Rheumatoid arthritis	2	1.6, 3.9	2,2	3.6
Avascular necrosis	10	7.1, 11.7	2,2	3.6
Others	0	0, 0	10,3	2.7

As an acetabular component, the first author's press-fit cup (Zimmer prior Centerpulse, Switzerland) was used for all patients of the follow-up studies of the Department of Orthopaedic Surgery of the University of Basel (Nr. 1 and 2) and 166 Spotorno's expansion cups + 14 standard cups (Zimmer-Centerpulse) + 17 Harris-Galante cups (Zimmer) in the Orthopaedic Hospital in Liguria/Italy (Nr. 3). In study Nr. 4 in 95% (316) of the cases cemented all-polyethylene cups (Aeskulap, Germany) were inserted.

The patients were operated in supine position, and THRs were inserted in a lateral approach in the study 1, 2, and 4, and in lateral position with a posterior approach in study 3. No trochanteric osteotomy was done in any of the cohorts.

So-called modern cementing technique was used to anchor the femoral stem in studies 1, 2 and 3, whereas in study 4 (Germany) this was not routinely the case. In modern cementing technique the medullary canal is irrigated and packed with sponges until immediately prior to the introduction of the bone cement. Furthermore, the cementing technique included the use of a cement gun, plugging of the distal femoral canal and pressurisation. For all cases Palacos bone cement – in the great majority with Gentamicin – was used to anchor the MS-30 stem.

In studies 3 and 4 the number of female patients outweighed by far the number of males. The age distribution in both female and male patients in all 4 studies was about the same (▢ Table 8.14).

The total number of hips that were available for a complete clinical and radiographic follow-up was 597. The mean follow-up times were 10.2, 6.6, 10.2 and 6.5 years, respectively.

Methods

Clinical assessment was in accordance with the International Documentation and Evaluation System (IDES) forms from the Institute of Documentation of the M.E. Müller Foundation in Berne/Switzerland [18]. The clinical evaluation was additionally done using the Harris hip score system [10]. Whereas the studies 1, 2 and 3 were prospective, study 4 was retrospective and, therefore, preoperative clinical data were not available.

In the radiological evaluation, osteolysis was defined as a newly developed, cystic lesion with endosteal scalloping and/or migration, which had not been noticed on the 6-week postoperative radiograph [19]. The radiograph of the latest follow-up was also examined for radiolucent lines at the cement/bone interface. The films were rated according to the Gruen zone system. The sites of radiolucent lines (>2 mm) at the cement/bone interface and osteolysis were recorded as being present in one or more of the 7 Gruen zones [12]. The stem was checked for varus/valgus position. A varus/valgus malalignment of the stem was defined as a deviation from the longitudinal axis of 3 or more degrees [17]. The cement mantle was examined for cement fractures. Subsidence of the stem within the cement mantle was measured as the difference of the distance between the upper circumference of the prosthesis shoulder and the sclerotic line above the shoulder (◘ Fig. 8.21) [1, 10], in other words by measuring the expansion of the radiolucency between the two.

Heterotopic ossification was assessed using the method of Brooker et al. [6].

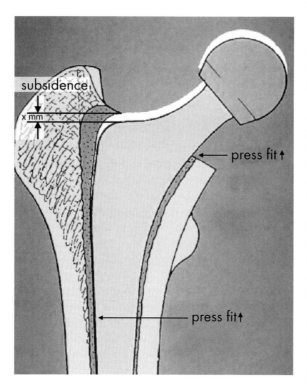

◘ **Fig. 8.21.** Measurement of subsidence. Through subsidence of a tapered femoral stem (within the cement mantle) press-fit, and therefore stability, in the metal-cement interface increases (»second line of defence«)

Results (◘ Tables 8.16 to 8.18)

The distribution of the diagnoses within the four cohorts was not significantly different and, therefore the cohorts were comparable for overall analysis.

With the exception of the 6 infections (1.8%) in study 4, the overall rate of complications was low. Taking into account that in study 4 modern cementing techniques were not used yet, even a revision rate for aseptic loosening of 0.9% after 6.5 years can be regarded as acceptable, especially in light of the fact that the authors of study Nr. 4 found a thin cement mantle around the MS-30 stem in about two thirds of the cases. The rate of osteolysis was low. The rate of radiolucencies varied between 16 and 26%.

The incidence of subsidence varies between 4.2% and 22.5% depending, of course, on the amount of migration. In studies 1 and 2 no stem had migrated more than 5 mm, an amount that would have been considered as definitive loosening.

Discussion

According to the NIH (National Institute of Health, Great Britain) a survival rate of 95% regarding aseptic loosening justifies or even recommends further clinical use of the respective endoprosthesis system [32]. Two of our studies revealed survival rates for aseptic loosening of 100% after 10 years, one cohort 99.6% and one 98.8%. The latter one was the multisurgeon study, which was not performed at one of the author's clinics. This also was the only one where modern cementing techniques had not been formally implemented. Both the rate of infection and the rate of overall revisions by far outnumbered those in the other studies. On the other hand, the three other studies were performed in the departments of the designing surgeons of the MS-30 stem and therefore a potential bias can not be excluded [26]. There is, however, no doubt that the results of large multi-surgeon studies do not match the results of experts using modern cementing techniques [31].

Past experience with the Exeter stem, reported by Ling [23], Howie [16] and the Swedish Implant Register [24], documents a statistically significant difference in the outcome between stems with a matt and a polished surface. A significantly higher rate of revisions with cemented titanium stems with a rough surface than with a smooth one was also reported recently by Hinrichs et al. [15]. In contrast to these findings, we found no difference between the two surfaces with regard to survivorship or subsidence, nor the incidence of osteolysis, in the prospective comparative study including 127 MS-30 stems with a matt and 128 MS-30 stems with a polished surface over a 6.5-year observation period (24) (◘ Tables 8.16, 8.17 and 8.18).

Even in the prospective study (Nr. 1) no revision for aseptic loosening of a MS-30 stem with matt surface had

Table 8.16. Incidence and cause of revisions of the MS-30 stem

Follow-up study No.	1	2	3	4
Surface characteristics	matt	matt/polished	polished	matt
No. of hip joints/patients	126/123	127/116, 128/117	197/193	333/318
No. of surgeons	13	15	1	36
Revisions (total) N/%	0	2, 1	1.5%	12 (3.6%)
for aseptic loosening (%)	0	1, 0	1.5%	3 (0.9%)
Infection N/%	0	0, 0	0	6 (1.8%)
Periprosthetic fracture	0	0, 0	0	1 (0.3%)
Recurrent dislocation N/(%)	0	1 (0.8%) 1 (0.8%)	0	2 (0.6%)
Overall surv./obs.time (%)	10y/100%	5.5y/98.4% 5.5y/99.2%	10 y/98.5%	6.5y/96.1
Survival: asept. loosening	100%	99.2% 100%	98.5%	98.8%

Table 8.17. Clinical results (Harris Hip Score, HHS)

Follow-up study No.	1	2	3	4
Surface characteristics	matt	matt/polished	polished	matt
No. of clin. + radiol. FU	90	109/108	95	195
Preoperative	73 (49–83)	67 (44–84)	48(24/77)	–
postoperative (median)	98	93	90	80
from – to (points)	72–100	67–100	68–100	26–100

Table 8.18. Radiological evaluation

Follow-up study No.	1	2	3	4
Surface characteristics	matt	matt/polished	polished	matt
No. of clin. + radiol. FU	90	109/108	95	195
Thin cement mantle	–	–	2	2/3
Osteolysis N	6 (Zones 5–7)	3 (Z.1/6/7)/3 (Z. 6/7)	3 (Z.6–7)	–
Radiolucencies N/%	20 (18%)	16 (17%), 15 (16%)	28 (26%)	44 (23%)
Axis (varus/valgus >3°)	var. 7 (5.5%) valg.1 (0.8%)	7 (6.4%), 6 (5.5%) 0, 0	10 (5.1%) 3 (1.5%)	– –
Subsidence: mm (%)	4–5: 5 (5.5%) ≤4: 17 (22.5%)	≥3 mm: ≥3 mm 7 (6.5%),7 (6.5%)	≥3 mm 4 (4.2%)	≥3 mm 21 (11%)

to be performed over a 10-year period. Neither the rate of revision (total and for aseptic loosening) nor the rate of osteolysis and/or radiolucencies had increased in the meantime. However, an increased number of stems with debonding and slight subsidence of less than 4 mm could be observed in relation to the comparative study of MS-30 stems with a matt and a polished surface with a follow-up time of 6.5 years. In the prospective consecutive series of 197 hips with the polished MS-30 stem with an average follow-up of 9.2 years (study Nr. 3), a revision rate for aseptic loosening of only 1% (2 out of 197) is reported.

Subsidence of a tapered, collarless stem within the cement mantle takes place, as a rule, mainly within the first two years after surgery [4, 21], then becomes slower or even completely stops after this time. Continued subsidence after the 2nd year of more than 5 mm (which is combined with a fracture of the cement mantle as a rule) must be considered definitive loosening [2, 13, 35, 36]. No such case was detected in the studies 1, 2 or 3.

When designing the MS-30 stem, the main goal was to improve the quality of the cement mantle without abandoning the proven concept of a tapered design, i.e.

the press-fit principle, realised for example in the Müller straight stem or in the Exeter stem. The rationale to allow a tapered stem to subside is the recognition of the fact that subsidence within the cement mantle has not only no correlation with regard to pain [10, 35, 37] but also allows the stem to re-stabilize. This has also been shown by the tapered Müller straight stem – a self-locking phenomenon, that we call »second line of defense« (◻ Fig. 8.22). Subsidence also results in a reduction in cement tensile and shear strain, and increases cement strain in compression. Cement is much stronger in compression than in either tension or shear. On the other hand, according to studies of stem surface roughness and creep-induced subsidence by Norman et al. [33], it appears that the stem subsidence is not important for the maintenance of a »taper-lock«, and creep-induced subsidence does not result in an increase of normal stress patterns at the stem/cement interface [22].

With a straight stem, the risk of a thin cement mantle in the zones 6 and 7 [35, 37] and 8 [5] is increased. In order to avoid the risk of metal/bone contact in zone 8, Wroblewski et al. [39] consider a low-neck osteotomy and aggressive removal of the posterior calcar femorale a necessity. Breusch et al. [5] have emphasised the importance of posterior canal entry (▶ chapter 5.2) and preparation to minimise the risk of thin cement mantles in Gruen zones 8/9 when using a straight stem. But with a low resection of the femoral neck, rotational stability is seriously compromised [11, 34]. Since loosening of a femoral stem rotates the stem into retroversion, and since a high neck resection secures the prosthesis stem effectively against migration into retroversion, we preferred the »high«, i.e. 30° instead of 45° resection. This is part of the »fixation rationale« of the MS-30 stem.

Conclusion

The reported follow-up studies show that excellent results with a 10 year survivorship of the MS-30 stem of 100% can be achieved. The results also show that for the MS-30 stem – at least when fixed with Palacos does not give rise to an increased rate of osteolysis and aseptic loosening – even not after 10 years. There is no more doubt that the quality of the bone cement also contributes much to the excellent outcome of the MS-30 stem. Several studies, especially the Implant Registers of Sweden and Norway and our own experience and experimental data showed that use of Palacos (with and without Gentamicin) correlates with the best results [5, 14, 25, 29, 32, 38].

Take Home Messages

- The reported follow-up studies show that excellent results with a 10-year survivorship of the MS-30 stem of 100% can be achieved.
- The outcome of a THR not only depends on the design of the implant but also on the conditions of its surface, the material and last but not least the operative, and especially the cementing technique.
- The surgeon still is the greatest variable!
- Since an optimal cement mantle completely surrounds the femoral stem and does not allow bone-metal contact and especially the Gruen zones 6/7 and 8/9 are at risk for a thin cement mantle or even bone-metal contact in the radiological assessment of THRs with a straight stem the evaluation must be performed both on an a.-p. and lateral X-ray of the proximal femur (▶ chapter 16).
- The results of the multi-surgeon study also show that even the Fe alloy MS-30 stem with a matt surface – at least when fixed with Palacos bone cement – does not give rise to an increased rate of aseptic loosening, even not after 10 years, though there is slight but not significant tendency to a higher incidence of osteolysis and radiolucencies.

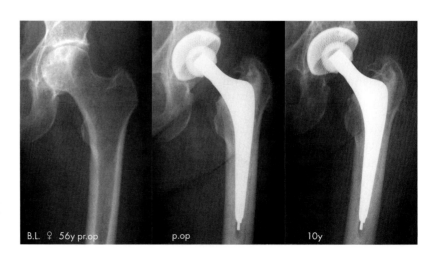

◻ **Fig. 8.22.** Ten year result of a matt MS-30 stem with the Morscher press-fit cup in a 56 year old woman (at operation) with avascular necrosis. The patient has no pain and an excellent range of movement

B.L. ♀ 56y pr.op   p.op   10y

References

1. Acklin YP, Berli BJ, Frick W, Elke R, Morscher EW. Nine-year results of Müller cemented titanium straight stems in total hip replacement. Arch Orthop Trauma Surg 2001;121:391–398

2. Alfaro-Adrián J, Gill HS, Murray DW. Cement migration after THR. A comparison of Charnley elite and Exeter femoral stems using RSA. J Bone Joint Surg [Br] 1999;81-B:130–134

3. Alfaro-Adrián J, Gill HS, Murray DW. Should total hip arthroplasty femoral components be designed to subside? A radiostereometric analysis study of the Charnley elite and Exeter stems. J Arthroplasty 2001;16:598–606

4. Berli B, Elke R, Morscher EW. The cemented MS-30 stem in total hip replacement, matte versus polished surface: minimum of five years of clinical and radiographic results of a prospective study. In: Winters GL, Nutt MJ (eds) Stainless steels for medical and surgical applications. ASTM STP 1438, 2003:249–261

5. Breusch SJ, Lukoschek M, Kreutzer J, Brocai D, Gruen TA. Dependency of cement mantle thickness on femoral stem design and centralizer. J. Arthroplasty 2001: 16–5: 648–57

6. Brooker AF, Bowerman JW, Robinson RA, Riley LH Jr. Ectopic ossification following total hip replacement. Incidence and a method of classification. J Bone Joint Surg [Am] 1973;55-A:1629–1632

7. Draenert K, Draenert Y. Die Adaptation des Knochens an die Deformation durch Implantate – Strain-Adaptive Bone Remodelling. Art & Science München, 1992

8. Ebramzadeh E, Sarmiento A, McKellop HA, Llinas A, Gogan W. The cement mantle in total hip arthroplasty. J Bone Joint Surg [Am] 1994;76-A:77–87

9. Estok DM, Orr TE, Harris WH. Factors affecting cement strains near the tip of a cemented femoral component. J Arthroplasty 1997;12:40–4

10. Fowler JL, Gie GA, Lee AJ, Ling RS: Experience with the Exeter total hip replacement since 1970. Orthop Clin North Am 1988: 19–3: 477–89

11. Freeman MAR. Why resect the neck? J Bone Joint Surg [Br] 1986;68-B:346–349

12. Gruen TA, McNeice GM, Amstutz HC. Modes of failure of cemented stem-type femoral components. A radiographic analysis of loosening. Clin Orthop 1979;141:17–2

13. Harris WH, McCarthy JC, O'Neill DA. Femoral component loosening using contemporary techniques of femoral cement fixation. J Bone Joint Surg [Am] 1986;68-A:1064–1066

14. Havelin, Engesaeter LB, Espehaug B, Furnes O, Lie SA, Vollset SE. The Norwegian Arthroplasty Register: 11 years and 73'000 arthroplasties. Acta Orthop. Scand. 2000, 71: 337–353

15. Hinrichs F, Kuhl M, Boudriot U, Griss P. A comparative clinical outcome evaluation of smooth (10–13 year results) versus rough surface finish (5–8 year results) in an otherwise identically designed cemented titanium alloy stem. Arch Orthop Trauma Surg 2003;123:268–272

16. Howie DW, Middleton RG, Costi K. Loosening of matte and polished cemented femoral stems. J Bone Joint Surg [Br] 1998;80-B:573–576

17. Iwase T, Wingstrand I, Persson BM, Kesteris U, Hasegawa Y, Wingstrand H. The ScanHip total hip arthroplasty: radiographic assessment of 72 hips after 10 years. Acta Orthop Scand 2002;73:54–59

18. Johnston RC, Fitzgerald RH, Harris WH, Poss R, Müller M.E, Sledge CB. Clinical and radiographic evaluation of total hip replacement. J Bone Joint Surg [Am] 1990;72-A:161–168

19. Joshi RP, Eftekhar NS, McMahon DJ, Nercession OA. Osteolysis after Charnley primary low-friction arthroplasty. J Bone Joint Surg [Br] 1998;80-B:585–590

20. Kelly AJ, Lee MB, Wong NS, Smith EJ, Learmonth ID. Poor reproducibility in radiographic grading of femoral cementing technique in total hip arthroplasty. J Arthroplasty 1996;11:525–528

21. Kiss J, Murray DW, Turner-Smith AR, Bithell J, Bullstrode CJ. Migration of cemented femoral components after THR: Roentgen stereophotogrammetry analysis. J Bone Joint Surg [Br] 1996;78-B:796–801

22. Lee AJC, Perkins RD, Ling RSM. Time dependent properties of polymethylmethacrylate bone cement. In: John O (ed) In implant bone interface. Springer New York, 1990:85–90

23. Ling RS. The use of a collar and precoating in cemented femoral stems is unnecessary and detrimental. Clin Orthop 1992;285:73–83

24. Malchau H, Herberts P. Prognosis of total hip replacement. Revision and re-revision rate in THR: A revision risk study of 148, 359 primary operations. Scientific exhibition, 65th Annual Meeting AAOS, February 19–23, 1998, New Orleans/USA

25. Malchau, Sodermann P, Herberts P. Swedish Hip Registry: Results with 20 Year Follow-up with Validation Clinically and Radiographically. 2000 Orlando, Presented at the 67th Annual Meeting of the American Academy of Orthopaedic Surgeons

26. Maloney WJ: Natiional Joint Replacement Registries: has the time come? J Bone Joint Surg Br 1997, 79–2: 254–7

27. Markolf KL, Amstutz HC. A comparative experimental study of stresses in femoral total hip replacement components: the effects of prosthesis orientation and acrylic fixation. J Biomech, 1976;9:73–79

28. Miller J, Johnson A. Advances in cementing techniques in total hip arthroplasty. In: Stilwell WT (ed) The art of total hip arthroplasty, Grunde & Stratton, 1987:277–292

29. Morscher EW, Wirz D. Current state of cement fixation in THR. Acta Orthop Belg 2002;68:1–12

30. Morscher EW, Spotorno L, Mumenthaler A, Frick W. The cemented MS-30 stem. In: Morscher EW (ed) Endoprosthetics. Springer Berlin, New York, 1995:211–219

31. Mulroy RD, Harris WH: The effect of improved cementing techniques on component loosening in total hip replacement. A 11 year radiographic review. J Bone Surg Br 1990, 72–5: 757–60

32. National Institute of Health. Conventions in total hip arthroplasty. Ministry of Health, London, GB 1998

33. Normann TL, Thyagarajan G, Saligrama VC, Gruen TA, Blaha JD. Stem surface roughness alters creep induced subsidence and »taper-lock« in a cemented femoral hip prosthesis. J Biomech 2001;34:1325–1333

34. Nunn D, Freeman MAR, Tanner KE, Bonfield W. Torsinal stability of the femoral component of hip arthroplasty. Response to an anteriorly applied load. J Bone Joint Surg [Br] 1989;71-B:452–455

35. Räber DA, Czaja S, Morscher EW. Fifteen-year results of the Müller CoCrNiMo straight stem. Arch Orthop Trauma Surg 2001;121:38–42

36. Søballe K, Toksvig-Larson S, Gelinek J. Migration of hydroxyapatite coated femoral prostheses: a roentgen stereophotogrammetric study. J Bone Joint Surg [Br] 1993; 75-B:681–687

37. Wilson-MacDonald J, Morscher E. Comparison between straight- and curved-stem Müller femoral prostheses; 5- to 10-year results of 545 total hip replacements. Arch Orthop Trauma Surg 1989;109:14–20

38. Wirz D, Zurfluh B, Goepfert B et al. Results of in vitro studies about the mechanism of wear in the stem-cement interface of THR. In: Winters GL, Nutt MJ (ed) Stainless steels for medical and surgical applications. ASTM STP 1438, 2003:222–234

39. Wroblewski BM, Siney PD, Fleming PA, Bobak P. The calcar femorale in cemented stem fixation in total hip arthroplasty. J Bone Joint Surg [Br] 1979;82-B:842–845

Femoral Components: Outcome with a Tapered, Polished, Anatomic Stem

Lee J. Taylor, Gyanendra Singh, Michael Schneider

Introduction

Failure of a cemented total hip arthroplasty (THA) is a rare event even in the long term. With improved cementing techniques, excellent and consistent long-term outcome has been achieved with a number of different femoral stem designs [1, 11, 21, 25, 32, 36, 37, 42]. However, some implants seem to perform better than others [32] and some very different design and anchorage philosophies [24, 40] can be identified (▶ chapter 7.1). A modern stem design should be easy and reproducible to implant for any surgeon including the trainee, but should also forgive minor mistakes and provide long-term survival of at least 95% after 10 years [33]. For long-term survival a complete cement mantle of adequate thickness [19, 28, 29] is of significant importance. There is no doubt that a thin or deficient cement mantle can lead to cracks, which create a pathway for wear particles to induce osteolysis and loosening [24, 26, 31]. Hence, it is considered important to create not only a sound cement interlock, but also an optimal cement mantle around the femoral stem at operation. It is the surgeon who »manufactures« the cement mantle, which also depends on a variety of factors (▶ chapter 5.2) including femoral anatomy, bone preparation, stem design and size and centralizer usage [10].

Most stem designs are straight and an obvious dilemma exists, if one considers the femoral anatomy in the lateral plane, which is curved [15]. Accordingly, a typical sagittal »mal-alignment« pattern of straight stems has been identified both clinically and experimentally [10, 15, 35] on lateral radiographs. This inevitably leads to areas at risk for producing thin cement mantles [10].

To address this anatomical fact and to minimise the risk of a deficient cement mantle, the Olympia hip stem, an anatomical, tapered and highly-polished design, has

been developed and used clinically since 1996. This chapter describes the 9-year survival and radiographic outcome of the Olympia stem in the first 120 consecutive cases implanted between 1996 and 1998.

Design Rationale

The Olympia stem (Biomet UK Ltd.) is tapered, of anatomic shape (left and right), with a highly-polished surface finish with a mean surface roughness (Ra) of 10 nm. (◉ Fig. 8.23). The modular design is manufactured from forged high Nitrogen Stainless Steel (to ISO 5832 part 9) and has a 12/14 neck taper.

- *Anatomic shape:* The stem is anatomically shaped (◉ Fig. 8.23) and available in 7 sizes (0 to 6), separated for the right and left side. The standard CCD is 134–137° depending on the stem size with a standard true offsets ranging from 40 to 46,55 mm. Lateralised offset stems are also now available (CCD 129–133°) with an incremental offset from 43 to 50,4 mm. The reduced neck diameter ensures an improved range of motion and minimises the dislocation risk to due to impingement
- *Polished*: The highly-polished surface (Ra 10 nm) reduces tensile stresses and cement abrasion at the stem-cement interface. Current evidence suggests that all stems, regardless of their design features, debond eventually and move within the cement mantle. With minimal distal migration of the stem, the tapered shape provides wedge fixation and loading of the surrounding cement in compression.
- *Tapered design:* The stem is 3-dimensionally tapered: the oval metaphyseal part provides rotational locking. A double reduced taper limits subsidence and increases intrinsic rotational stability.

- *In-built anteversion:* The 3-dimenstional geometry follows the natural femoral torque and provides a natural anteversion within the implant. As a consequence the proximal oval diameter even provides an even cement mantle
- *Centralizer:* Although a natural centralisation of the stem in the femoral canal is afforded by virtue of the shape of the stem, additionally a set of 4 distal PMMA centralizers, to prevent stem tip bone contact, is provided with each stem sizes to allow a selection depending on the canal diameter.
- *Cement mantle friendly:* The anatomic shape in both planes (reduced shoulder and proximal curve in lateral view) reduces the risk of thin cement mantles in all Gruen zones. The stem has no corners, which could act as a stress riser for the cement mantle. Templates with

2 and 3 mm outlines ensure stem size selection to produce a minimal cement mantle thickness of 2–3 mm distally and 4–7 mm proximally (medial calcar).
- *Abductor and approach friendly:* The stem shape and the simple instruments protect the abductors, especially in an antero-lateral approach, and allow MIS techniques.

Patients

Between November 1996 and October 1998 the first author implanted 120 Olympia stems in 111 consecutive patients at King Edward VII Hospital Midhurst (◘ Fig. 8.24). There were 40 males and 71 females (mean age 74,2 years; range 51–91). Preoperative diagnoses consisted of 116 primary osteoarthritis (OA), 3 femoral neck fractures and

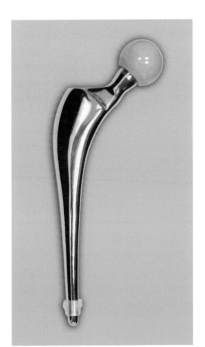
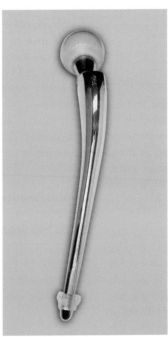

◘ **Fig. 8.23.** Photograph of Olympia stem indicating the anatomical shape in both planes

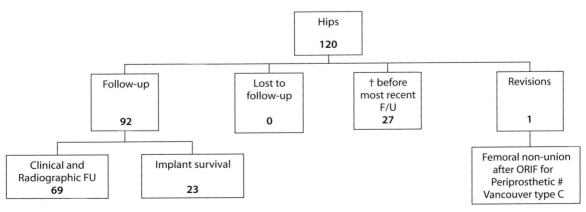

◘ **Fig. 8.24.** Patient follow-up data

1 posttraumatic OA. No patient had undergone previous hip surgery.

All operations were performed in a laminar flow theatre with a three dose prophylactic antibiotic regime, the same first assistant and anaesthetist being present at all operations. Using a lateral transgluteal Hardinge approach in lateral decubitus position, all Olympia stems were implanted with Palacos–Gentamicin cement using a modern cementing technique with distal femoral cement restrictor, pulsatile jet lavage and proximal pressurisation. In this initial series, no distal centralizers were used (not available). A stem size was chosen to allow a minimum cement mantle of 4–5 mm proximally-medially and 2–3 mm distally (templates). Size 3 (34%) and size 4 (30%) stems were used in the majority of cases. Modular metal head diameters were used: 28 mm (80%), 32 mm (16%) and 22 mm (4%). Both cemented and cementless acetabular cups had been implanted: cemented Ogee (11%), cemented Elite (56%) (DePuy International Ltd) and cementless Spotorno's expansion cup (33%) (Zimmer Inc., Warsaw).

Methods

This is a consecutive, prospective series of the first 120 Olympia stems ever implanted and includes therefore the learning curve with this design. All patients were traced for follow-up (FU), but some were unwilling to attend for radiographic review due to travelling time and 'inconvenience'. None had pain and all were still satisfied with their hip. There was no patient lost to follow-up regarding implant survival (◘ Fig. 8.24).

Clinical evaluation was done using the Harris hip score [23] and patient functional assessment using Oxford hip questionnaire [16]. Radiographs taken before, after operation and at final review and were examined by an independent experienced reviewer [M.S.]. The radiograph of the latest follow-up was also examined for any radiolucent lines at the cement/bone interface, measurable stem subsidence and significant cup migration. The integrity of the cement mantles was graded according to the Barrack classification [7]. Cement mantle was examined for cement fractures and cement mantle thickness was measured ap and lateral in all 14 Gruen zones [22, 27]. The stem was checked for varus/valgus and sagittal malalignment of the stem, which was defined as a deviation from the longitudinal axis of 3 or more degrees [29]. Osteolysis was defined as a newly developed, cystic lesion with endosteal scalloping [12].

Statistical Analysis

Survival analysis was performed using life-table analysis as detailed by Armitage and Berry [4]. The endpoint was defined as revision surgery with implant removal for any reason. All statistical calculations were performed with SPSS Version 12.0 (SPSS Inc., Chicago, Illinois).

Implant Survival

119 of the original 120 implants were not revised at latest follow-up. 25 patients (27 implants) had died, but their implants were in situ at the time of death. Mean implant survival was 6,7 years (range 0,2–9 years; median 7 years).

There were no dislocations or infections, but 3 reoperations were performed for periprosthetic fractures after a fall with adequate trauma. All 3 fractures were subprosthetic and classified class C according to the Vancouver-Classification [9] with the implants all well fixed. All fractures were treated with plate fixation. One fracture went on to non-union and removal of the well fixed stem was necessary for revision to a distally locked, long uncemented stem.

Overall-survival for aseptic loosening was 100% after 7–9 years and 99.2% for implant survival for all reasons (◘ Fig. 8.25; standard deviation for cumulative surviving 0,0092%).

At the time of review no stem was considered at risk for loosening. There have been no revisions for acetabular cup loosening or wear to date.

Clinical Results

Harris Hip Score

The score for the reviewed patients was a mean of 87.4 (range 67–91± 5.31). 52% of patients had a score above 90 with 92% scoring 80 or greater.

Oxford Hip Score

Functional outcome was measured by the patient administered Oxford hip questionnaire. The mean score at 5 years follow up was 13.2 (SD=1.67) with a range of 12–21. 51% of patients scored 12 (excellent) with only 2% scoring >24. Therefore, 98% of patients were classified at good or excellent at 5+ years.

Radiographic Assessment

All patients had AP and lateral radiographs at follow up. At latest follow up, during the study period 2004/05, only 69/92 hips were available for assessment. No measurable stem subsidence or the development of radiolucent lines

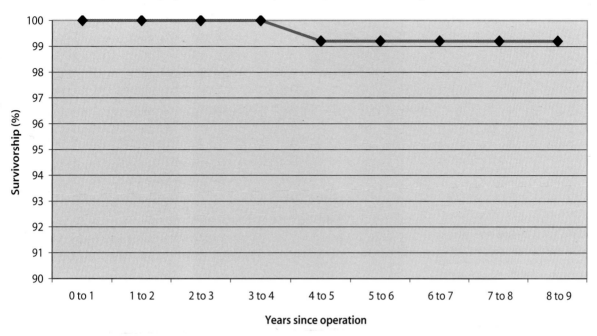

Fig. 8.25. Overall-survival for aseptic loosening was 100% after 7–9 years and 99.2% for implant survival for all reasons (standard deviation for cumulative surviving 0.0092%).

around the stem or cement bone interface was found. There was no femoral or acetabular osteolysis. There were radiolucent lines <2 mm in zone I DeLee and Charnley [17] in 21% of the cemented cups, but no migration of any cemented or uncemented cup. Visual examination and measurements of radiographs did not show any detectable polyethylene wear.

Stem

AP-alignment revealed neutral position ±3° in 76.4% of the reviewed cases, varus in 5.9% and valgus in 17.7%. No stem showed more than 5° deviation from neutral. Alignment on lateral views showed neutral position ±3° in 75.7%, anterior position in 2.7% and posterior tip orientation in 21.6% of the cases.

Table 8.19 shows cement mantle thickness according to Gruen zones 1–14. In more than 4/5 of cases excellent stem alignment with complete cement mantle were documented (Fig. 8.26). In 17.1% there was a thin, but complete cement mantle <2 mm in Gruen zones 8/9 and in 8.6% in zone 12 posterior at the stem tip.

In 67.6% of radiographs examined the cement mantle was classified as Barrack A with the appearance of a complete »white out« and in the remainder as Barrack B (32.4%). There were no poor gradings C or D in this review.

Table 8.19. Postoperative cement mantle thickness (%) in Gruen zones 1–14 [22, 27]

Zone	≥2 mm	<2 mm	≤1 mm
1	100	0	0
2	100	0	0
3	98,5	1,5	0
4	100	0	0
5	91,2	4,4	4,4 (valgus)
6	98,5	1,5	0
7	100	0	0
8	82,9	17,1	0
9	94,3	5,7	0
10	100	0	0
11	100	0	0
12	91,4	8,6	0
13	100	0	0
14	94,3	5,7	0

Discussion

This prospective, consecutive single-surgeon series of the first 120 Olympia stems revealed excellent implant survival, radiographic and clinical outcome. No stem had failed up to 9 years and there was no revision for aseptic loosening. Although no 10-year results are yet available, the likelihood of significantly worse results then, is ex-

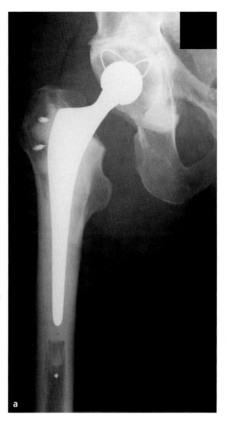
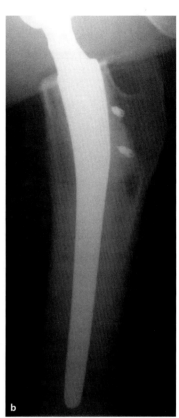

Fig. 8.26. a Postoperative radiograph at FU after 8,5 years with no evidence for subsidence, loosening or osteolysis of the stem. The cup remains well fixed despite a non-progressive radiolucent line in zone I [17]. The lateral radiographic view (**b**) shows optimal alignment and a complete cement mantle even in the anterior Gruen zones 8/9 at the level of the proximal femoral bow. *N.B. The suture anchors were used for reattachment of the vasto-gluteal flap*

tremely low, in particular as relevant stem subsidence was not detected. It therefore seems justified to expect a survival rate of at least 95% after 10 years (aseptic loosening) as recommended by the NIH [33].

It is certainly not possible to predict whether this anatomic design will show superior survival in its 2nd decade in comparison to straight stem designs. However, this study has provided further radiographic evidence, that an anatomic stem carries a lower risk of thin cement mantles in the sagittal plane (even with antero-lateral approach) in comparison to the published radiographic cement mantle analysis for some straight stem designs [13, 20, 35]. A recent multi-surgeon midterm study with a straight stem design revealed a high incidence (64.2%) of thin/deficient cement mantles in zone 8 on lateral radiographs. At midterm, the thin cement mantles had, however, not led to osteolysis or failure, but the authors had classified this group as »stems at risk« [13].

Surprisingly, a comprehensive cement mantle analysis, which includes the second plane, does not exist for the majority of femoral implants. Conventional stem designs make it difficult to achieve an optimal cement mantle due to the proximal femoral anatomy in the sagittal plane [10, 35, 39]. Even if a distal centralizer is used to centralise the stem tip, which is now done routinely, this has no preventive effect on the proximal/anterior Gruen zones 8/9 [10]. Valdivia et al. [39] also confirmed this

relationship in a cadaveric study with 6 different stem designs and identified this as an area »prone to deficient cement mantles«.

Thin or deficient cement mantles can reduce implant survival and are less able to absorb energy and may crack and fail [19, 24, 26, 31]. Only a deficient cement mantle can allow wear particles access to the cement-bone interface. In the presence of wear localised granuloma formation at the cement-bone interface and osteolysis can result as a consequence [3, 26, 31]. In this context, joint-fluid pressure has been found to play an important role for particle migration and osteolysis [5, 6]. Osteolysis is associated with a high risk of periprosthetic fracture, which represents one important mechanism for late failure [8, 14] of THA.

This study has some limitations which have to be considered. Implantation was performed by a single experienced surgeon, who achieved good to excellent cement gradings in all patients. Furthermore, the power of the radiographic analysis is reduced, as radiographs were not available for all patients.

Although we did not find any evidence for stem subsidence, it must be criticised that no Röntgen Stereometric Analysis (RSA) study, which would provide the most accurate measurement method [30], has yet been performed. On the other hand, it has been documented for the polished Exeter stem, that a mean migration of up to 2 mm [2, 38] did not adversely affect survivorship at 8–12 years [41]. Hence, the view that early migration is an indicator of long-term loosening [34] does not seem to be applicable to all femoral stem designs and geometries. It may well be that posterior migration, i.e. retroversion, detected by RSA, will prove to be the more significant predictor [30]. The significance of stem subsidence remains a controversial issue, but it is clear that subsidence may still cause cement mantle damage, which has been confirmed in human retrieval analysis [18]. It seems logical to assume that an undamaged cement mantle increases the chance of long-term performance.

Take Home Messages

- The anatomic Olympia stem revealed excellent radiographic results at 7–9 years and survival of 100% for aseptic loosening and 99.2% for all reasons.
- Radiographic analysis showed a low rate of thin cement mantles, in particular in the high risk Gruen zones 8/9 (on lateral radiographs).
- No measurable subsidence, radiolucent lines or osteolysis were found.
- Based on current results the continued clinical use of this polished, tapered, anatomic design seems justified.

References

1. Aamodt A, Nordsletten L, Havelin LI, Indrekvam K, Utvag SE, Hviding K: Documentation of hip prostheses used in Norway: a critical review of the literature from 1996–2000. Acta Orthop Scand 2004; 75(6): 663–76
2, Alfaro-Adrian J, Gill HS, Murray DW: Cement migration after THR. A comparison of Charnley Elite and Exeter femoral stems using R.S.A. J Bone Joint Surg 1999; 81-B: 130–34
3. Anthony PP, Gie GA, Howie CR, Ling RSM: Localised endosteal bone lysis in loosening of total hip replacement. J Bone Joint Surg 1990; 72-B: 971–79
4. Armitage P, Berry G: Statistical methods in medical research. 3rd ed. Blackwell Scientific Publications, Oxford 1994
5. Aspenberg P, Van der Vis H: Fluid pressure may cause periprosthetic osteolysis. Particles are not the only thing. Acta Orthop Scand 1998; 69 (1): 1–4
6. Aspenberg P, Van der Vis H: Migration, particles, and fluid pressure. A discussion of causes of prosthetic loosening. Clin Orthop 1998; 352: 75–80
7. Barrack RL, Mulroy RD, Harris WH: Improved cementing technique and femoral component loosening in young patients with hip arthroplasty. A 12 year radiographic follow up. J Bone Joint Surg 1992; 74-B: 385–89
8. Berry DJ: Priprosthetic fractures associated with osteolysis. J Arthroplasty 2003; 18(3) Suppl. 1: 107–11
9. Brady OH, Garbuz DS, Masri BA, Duncan CP: Classification of the hip. Orthop Clin N Am 1999; 30: 215–20
10. Breusch SJ, Lukoschek M, Kreutzer J, Brocai D, Gruen TA: Dependency of cement mantle thickness on femoral stem design and centralizer. J Arthroplasty 2001; 16(5): 648–57

11. Britton AR, Murray DW, Bulstrode CJ, McPherson K, Denham RA: Long-term comparison of Charnley and Stanmore design total hip replacements. J Bone Joint Surg 1996; 78-B: 802–8
12. Brooker AF, Bowerman JW, Robinson RA, Riley LH Jr: Ectopic ossification following total hip replacement. Incidence and a method of classification. J Bone Joint Surg 1973; 55-A: 1629–32
13. Clauss M, Reitzel T, Pritsch M, Schlegel U, Ewerbeck V, Mau H, Breusch SJ: Mid-term results after implantation of a cemented MS-30 stem. A multisurgeon series of 333 consecutive cases at 6–10 years. Der Orthopäde; submitted for publication
14. Clohisy JC, Calvert G, Tull F, McDonald D, Maloney WJ: Reasons for revision hip surgery – a retrospective review. Clin Orthop 2004; 429: 188–92
15. Crawford RW, Psychoyios V, Gie G, Ling R, Murray D: Incomplete cement mantles in the sagittal femoral plane: an anatomical explanation. Acta Orthop Scand 1999; 70(6): 596–98
16. Dawson J, Fitzpatrick R, Carr A, Murray D: Questionnaire on the perceptions of patients about total hip replacement. J Bone Joint Surg 1996; 78-B: 185–90
17. DeLee JG, Charnley J: Radiological demarcation of cemented sokets in total hip replacement. Clin Orthop 1976; 121: 20–32
18. Draenert KD, Draenert YI, Krauspe R, Bettin D: Strain adaptive bone remodelling in total joint replacement. Clin Orthop 2005; 430: 12–27
19. Ebramzadeh E, Sarmiento A, McKellop HA, Llinas A, Gogan W: The cement mantle in total hip arthroplasty. J Bone Joint Surg 1994; 76-A: 77–87
20. Garellick G, Malchau H, Regner H, Herberts P: The Charnley versus the Spectron hip prosthesis: radiographic evaluation of a randomized, prospective study of 2 different hip implants. J Arthroplasty 1999; 14(4): 14–25
21. Gerritsma-Bleeker CL, Deutman R, Mulder TJ, Steinberg JD: The Stanmore total hip replacement. A 22-year follow-up. J Bone Joint Surg 2000;82-B(1): 97–102
22. Gruen TA, McNeice GM, Amstutz HC. Modes of failure of cemented stem-type femoral components. A radiographic analysis of loosening. Clin Orthop 1979;141:17–27
23. Harris WH: Traumatic arthritis of the hip after dislocation and acetabular fractures: treatment by mold arthroplasty. An end-result study using a new method of result evaluation. J Bone Joint Surg 1969; 51-A: 737–55
24. Huiskes R: Some fundamental aspects of human joint replacement. Analyses of stresses and heat conduction in bone-prosthesis structures. Acta Orthop Scand 1980; Suppl. 185: 109–200
25. Issack PS, Botero HG, Hiebert RN, Bong MR, Stuchin SA, Zuckerman JD, Di Cesare PE: Sixteen-year follow-up of the cemented spectron femoral stem for hip arthroplasty. J Arthroplasty 2003;18(7): 925–30
26. Jasty MJ, Floyd WE, Schiller AL, Goldring SR, Harris WH: Localized osteolysis in stable, non-septic total hip arthroplasty. J Bone Joint Surg 1986; 68-A: 912–19
27. Johnston RC, Fitzgerald RH, Harris WH, Poss R, Müller M.E, Sledge CB. Clinical and radiographic evaluation of total hip replacement. J Bone Joint Surg 1990; 72-A: 161–68
28. Joshi AB, Porter ML, Trail IA: Long-term results of Charnley low friction arthroplasty in young patients. J Bone Joint Surg 1993;75-B: 616–23
29. Joshi RP, Eftekhar NS, McMahon DJ, Nercession OA: Osteolysis after Charnley primary low-friction arthroplasty. A comparison of two matched paired groups. J Bone Joint Surg 1998; 80-B: 585–90
30. Kärrholm J, Nivbrant B, Thanner J, Anderberg C, Börlin N, Herberts P, Malchau H: Radiostereometric Evaluation of Hip Implant Design and Surface Finish. Presented at the AAOS Orlando, USA 2000. March 15–19,2000

31. Kwak BM, Lim OK, Kim YY, Rim K: An investigation of the effect of cement thickness on an implant by finite element analysis. Inter Orthop (SICOT) 1979; 2: 315–19

32. Malchau H, Herberts P, Eisler T, Garellick G, Soderman P: The Swedish Total Hip Replacement Register. J Bone Joint Surg 2002; 84-A Suppl 2: 2–20

33. National Institute of Health. Conventions in total hip arthroplasty. Ministry of Health, London, UK 1998

34. Nilsson NG, Kärrholm J. RSA in the assessment of aseptic loosening. J Bone Joint Surg. 1996; 78-B: 1–3

35. Östgaard HC, Helger L, Regner H, Garellick G: Femoral alignment of the Charnley stem: a randomized trial comparing the original with the new instrumentation in 123 hips. Acta Orthop Scand 2001; Jun 72(3): 228–32

36. Raber DA, Czaja S, Morscher EW. Fifteen-year results of the Muller CoCrNiMo straight stem. Arch Orthop Trauma Surg 2001; 121(1–2): 38–42

37. Savilahti S, Myllyneva I, Pajamaki KJ, Lindholm TS: Survival of Lubinus straight (IP) and curved (SP) total hip prostheses in 543 patients after 4–13 years. Arch Orthop Trauma Surg 1997; 116(1–2): 10–13

38. Stefansdottir A, Franzen H, Johnsson R, Ornstein E, Sundberg M: Movement patterns of the Exeter femoral stem, a radiosteriometric analysis of 22 primary hip arthroplasties followed for 5 years. Acta Orth. Scan 2004; 75 (4): 408–14

39. Valdivia GG, Dunbar MJ, Parker DA, Woolfrey MR, MacDonald SJ, McCalden RW, Rorabeck CH, Bourne RB: The John Charnley Award: Three-dimensional analysis of the cement mantle in total hip arthroplasty. Clin Orthop 2001; 393: 38–51

40. Verdonschot N, Huiskes R: The effect of cement-stem debonding in THA on the long term probability of cement. J Biomech 1997; 30 (8): 795–802

41. Williams HD, Browne G, Gie GA, Ling RS, Timperley AJ, Wendover NA: The Exeter universal cemented femoral component at 8 to 12 years. A study of the first 325 hips. J Bone Joint Surg 2002; 84-B: 324–33

42. Wroblewski BM, Fleming PA, Siney PD: Charnley low-frictional torque arthroplasty of the hip. 20-to-30 year results. J Bone Joint Surg 1999; 81-B: 427–30

Femoral Components: The French Paradox

Gareth Scott, Michael Freeman, Marcel Kerboull

Summary

In this chapter, clinical and experimental evidence is reviewed with respect to implant survival in relation to cement mantle thickness. The so-called French paradox of excellent survival with thin cement mantles is discussed. Cement mantles perceived as »thin« may in fact by thicker than expected.

Introduction

It has become generally accepted that the cement surrounding a proximal femoral implant should be not less than 2 mm thick and that it should be complete i.e. without any 'windows' in the mantle. The widely used Barrack grading for cementing included no comment on the thickness of the cement mantle on its introduction in 1992 [1]. The following year the 'A' grade was qualified by the addition of the minimal thickness of 2 mm to its requirements [7]. Certain considerations arise:

- If a rectangular section tapered implant is used, distally the cement is unlikely to be uniform in thickness. At the corners of the prosthesis in all probability the cement will be thin at a site exposed to the increased torsional forces. Is this desirable? Amongst the contributing authors there is no consensus. On one hand it is felt that a rectangular cross section to the stem dissipates the torsional moment within cement mantle at the bone cement interface. On the other hand a stem rounded in the diaphyseal region would transfer torsional load in the metaphyseal region and risk cement cracking. This latter concern has been specifically addressed in one stem reported here by intentionally retaining of the femoral neck [2].

- If the medullary canal is narrow in the presence of thick cortices either extensive reaming of cortical bone or the use of a very thin stem would be necessary. Are either desirable? Two recent publications have questioned whether the 2 mm minimum thickness is the only way to successfully stabilize a proximal femoral component.

The Evidence

The credit for questioning this approach to cement handling lies with the observations of Marcel Kerboull. In 1971, with only a 2 year experience using the original Charnley stem, he noted a high rate (24%) of debonding associated with a longitudinal superomedial crack in the cement mantle which appeared to be associated with subsequent stem subsidence. Surprisingly, this problem was not observed in the dysplastic femur where the tightly fitted straight stem left room for only a thin cement layer. From this experience, changes were made to produce the Charnley Kerboull prosthesis which was polished, tapered and with the neck angle increased to 130 degrees. A sufficient range of sizes was available so that after removal of the cancellous bone the implant selected most accurately restored the hip architecture. It was not considered essential to take always the largest stem but rather to use the size that best suited the patient's requirement. If a large stem were required, little room would remain for the cement which may indeed contain windows [6].

It was considered that in this way the desired component alignment could be reproducibly obtained and the cement maintained in compression. Even when the stem produced a thin cement mantle on the anteroposterior radiograph, it might be thicker on the lateral view and sometimes the cement would be uniformly greater than 2 mm in thickness. Outcome studies summarised in a recent paper [5] have shown that this philosophy has produced excellent long-term results (except when fashion determined changes in the surface roughness where made). The MK, mark I had an aseptic loosening rate of 1 to 2% at 20 years and the MK III a zero percent aseptic loosening rate at 10 years [4]. It is not without interest that this technique did not succeed when the stem was considerably roughened in the CMK III with 21% aseptic loosening at 10 years [5]. This is analogous to the behaviour of the Exeter stem when it is roughened [3]. It would seem that the success of the Kerboull approach lies partly on the considerable compression of the cement generated by hammering a tightly fitting implant into the dough like material producing an interlock with the femur and partly (but more importantly in MK's opinion) on the polished surface finish which even in the event that debonding occurs will not produce particulate debris, and a tapered geometry that will continue to exert compressive forces on the cement bone interface under load.

A visiting French surgeon introduced the concept of 'thin' cement to Michael Freeman and it has been taught as the method for securing his neck retaining prosthesis when cement is used. This prosthesis is tapered in its proximal section where it engages the retained metaphyseal bone and polished distally in its conical section. As the femur is prepared by milling tools, a precise cavity is prepared of the same dimensions as the intended implant. However, it should be noted that unlike the Kerboull method, there is no emphasis on removing all the proximal cancellous bone. When the implant is introduced into the cement filled femur it creates pressurisation as there is nowhere for the cement to escape and the implant is forced to line up correctly in the prepared bone. A further difference is that the conical distal portion of the stem is not intended to produce a distal jammed press-fit with minimal cement augmentation as resistance to torsional forces is afforded by the retained neck, hence the distal section is not required to have a rectangular section. A clinical and experimental report [8] compared the results of cementing this implant after deliberately 'over-reaming' by 2 mm to provide space to accommodate a minimum thickness of 2 mm cement mantle and an alternative method of using the implant after reaming to size and cementing directly without any space reserved for cement. The clinical study showed no significant difference in the clinical outcome or in the survival rate (approximately 98% at 10 years) of the two methods. Thigh pain was not observed. Estimates for thickness could not be made reliably from radiographs due to the variability within particular zones and in places the lack of distinction between the margin of the cement and the surrounding cortical bone (whiteout). What was found was a higher incident of radiolucent lines and lytic lesions in the »over-reamed« group. A cadaveric study involved examining transversely sectioned femora which had been either 2 mm over-reamed or reamed to size prior to cementing a Freeman stem.

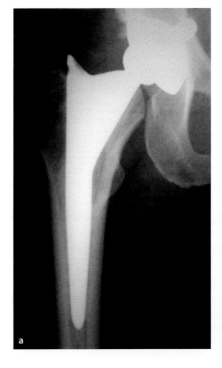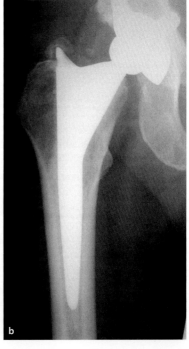

◘ Fig. 8.27. a Freeman stem immediately postoperatively with »thin« cement. **b** The same implant as **a** 10-years postoperatively

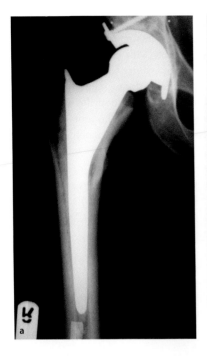

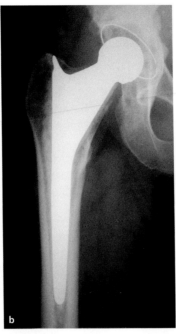

Fig. 8.28. a Freeman stem with »thick« cement immediately postoperatively. **b** The same implant as **a** 12 years post-operatively following an isolated acetabular revision

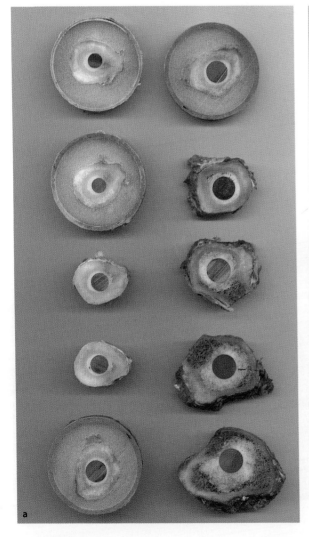

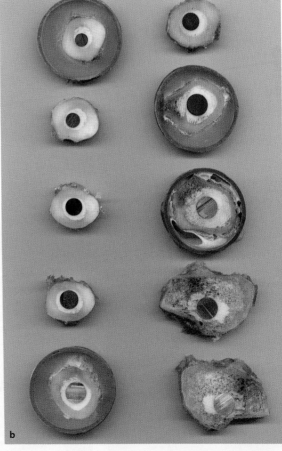

Fig. 8.29. a Transverse cuts of a cadaveric femur with »thin« cement showing the presence of windows at various locations. **b** As in **a** but with thick cement. (Note in both specimens on some slices the epoxy resin used to surround the femur to enable cutting is still in place)

These sections showed that around the proximal half of the implant the cement thickness was not significantly different between the two methods of femoral preparation with an average cement mantle of 3 to 4 mm in thickness. The lack of difference could only have arisen due to greater ingress of the cement in the less reamed femur. In turn this greater penetration must have occurred because greater pressurization was achieved. It was only in the distal conical section that the »over-reamed« femora had a significantly thicker cement mantle. Further, in both groups but more commonly with thin cement, windows were found in the cement which would not have been detected on an anteroposterior radiograph.

Thus, these observations give room for controversy. By attempting to emulate the method of Kerboull it transpires the Freeman 'thin' techniques conforms to the

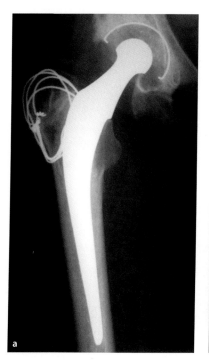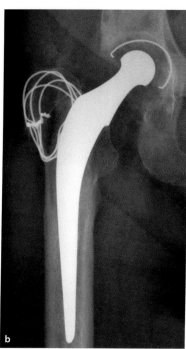

Fig. 8.30. a MK, mark I stem at 1 year post op with 'thick' cement. **b** Same prosthesis as **a** at 22 years post operatively

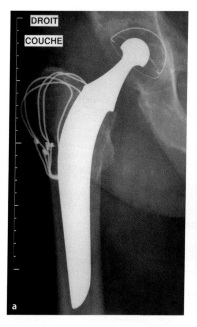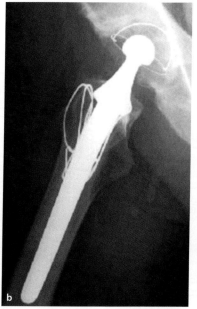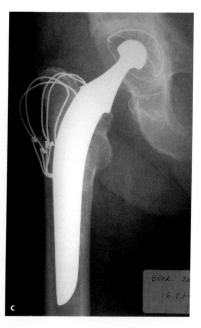

Fig. 8.31. a,b AP and lateral views of a large MK III stem at 6 years post op. **c** The same prosthesis as **a,b** at 16 years post operatively

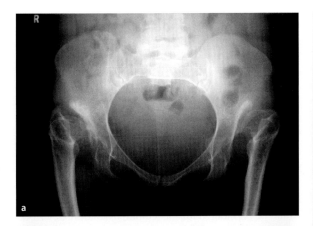

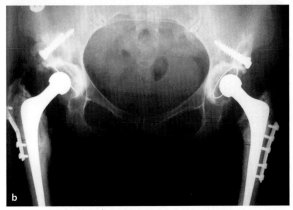

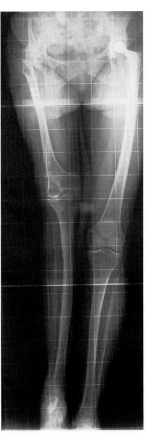

Fig. 8.32a,b. High dislocation brought down with osteotomy 8 years post surgery (acetabular grafts probably unnecessary)

Fig. 8.33. Surgically lengthened femur where accurate leg lengths may be difficult to achieve

Leg Length

It can be extremely difficult to ascertain true leg length both preoperatively and post surgery. Clinically, the pelvis may have been used in childhood as roof graft and significant positional deformity may be present both of which will result in extreme difficulty with accurate measurement. Furthermore, it should be noted that any surgery on the limb in childhood may result in relative overgrowth of the limb leading to an unexpected over lengthening after reconstruction to a normal hip. Occasionally the other limb may have undergone surgery to restrict growth to prevent significant discrepancy in childhood (**Fig. 8.33).

The surgeon, as part of preoperative assessment, should ensure that he has assessed the true leg lengths and that the lumbar spine deformity is correctable (by checking the seated position). As a general rule full correction is neither possible nor desirable in cases of high dislocation (greater than 4 cm), as the patient will feel extremely long if fully corrected. It is probably wise to correct offset and as a result reduce joint reaction force (and wear) rather than length. Patients do not feel comfortable overcorrected. We counsel all our patients that the length will be significantly better but not perfect.

Nerve Palsies

There is considerable debate as to the causes and incidence of nerve palsy (femoral or sciatic) following THA for DDH, with the range from 3–15% not all of which recover [6]. Most authors associate this devastating complication with leg lengthening of greater than 4 cm however just as important is the presence of pre-existing scarring from previous surgery. In a series of 27 sciatic palsies post THA from Finland [15] only 8 were associated with lengthening however 9 were in patients undergoing surgery for DDH. 8 patients recovered fully, 7 had a fair result and 12 had a poor long-term result. A further paper [5] concludes that nerve damage is caused by direct damage not stretching. While intra-operative monitoring has been suggested we review nerve tension and mobilise the nerve from around osteotomy sites (usually pelvic) at the time of surgery. Full exposure may not be necessary (and may interfere with the nerves blood supply) however the nerve should at least be palpated and protected. In our series of 132 Primary THA's for DDH no case had a persisting nerve palsy, several had transient palsies mostly femoral, and in every case the patient had undergone multiple pelvic and femoral surgeries previously and no significant lengthening had been carried out. We routinely use a posterior approach and identify but do not dissect the nerve.

Uncemented Series

There are a number of reports of uncemented stem replacement in the presence of DDH (11) including some where custom designed implants have been used (7). Recent reports of soft tissue lengthening followed by uncemented primary surgery have reported on 56 cases with 9 revisions (5 for polyethylene wear) [9]. This interesting paper showed that considerable lengthening could be carried out using an external fixator as the first stage procedure.

Paavilainen et al. [13] described osteotomy and fixation with a specially designed straight uncemented stem in 67 cases (including a number of cases where a longitudinal osteotomy was carried out to increase the femoral diameter). Many of these cases included severely deformed post surgical femora. With a three to five year follow up 4 stems were loose and 2 had been revised. Recently using a technique similar to Paavilainen et al [13], Carlsson et al. [2] reported an extended osteotomy by removing the trochanter and shortening the femur followed by insertion of a conical titanium stem all with good mid-term results. Della Valle et al. [4] using an extended trochanteric osteotomy in 6 patients with maximum 4-year follow-up and an uncemented stem had one non-union but all implants were stable. Masonis et al. [10] described 10 cemented and 11 uncemented hip replacements with a follow-up of 5–8 years and 91% of the osteotomies had united. They reported 3 dislocations and that one-cemented stem had

been revised for loosening. Decking et al. [13] reported 12 cases with femoral osteotomy using an uncemented stem, 2 stems had been revised, one for leg lengthening and one for cup loosening. Huo et al. [8] described an oblique osteotomy using a cementless stem in 26 cases, but only three were primary cases with a follow up of 3 to 5 years. The technique involved distal fix and distal osteotomies. There was a 24% failure rate, though it is not clear what the results were for the three primaries. Cameron [1] reported 71 cases using a distal fit and adjustable proximal segment, which can customised at the table to fit the proximal fragment. However only 17 were Crowe grade 4 and would be considered for the femoral osteotomy described here. Of these 17 there was a 50% complication rate with 2 sciatic palsies, one femoral fracture and one osteotomy collapse. Only two of these cases had a shortening osteotomy the anteversion being corrected by the customisable proximal segment. A report of osteotomy in severe deformity [17] in 28 cases using uncemented stems was presented: two developed non unions and they recommended grafting the osteotomy site. This was an interesting series where the stem size used was 10–13 mm, larger than many of the medullary canals met in our practice though they reported no fractures (◻ Table 8.20).

Own Results Using a Cemented Stem

We will report on a modified version of the technique (◻ Fig. 8.34) described by Reikeraas et al. [16] and outlined earlier in this book (▶ chapter 2.3). In his original series Reikeraas et al. reviewed 25 cases using a press fit uncemented prosthesis and found one sciatic palsy, one

◻ **Table 8.20.** Comparison of published series

Authors	Femoral Implant	Special Technique	N=	FU	Loosening	Non-union	Revisions
Paavalainen [13]	uncemented	Various osteotomies	67	3–5 y	4	0	2
Carlsson [2]	uncemented	Ext. trocht. Osteot.	22	8–94 mos	0	0	5
Lai [9]	uncemented	Ext. fixator	56	Avge 147 mos	0	0	9
Della Valle [4]	uncemented	Extended troch osteotomy	6	Avge 50 mos4	0	1	1
Huo [8]	uncemented	Custom made stem Oblique osteotomy	26	3–5	5	1	6
Matsui [11]	uncemented	Custom stem	51	5–9	18	N/A	2
Masonis [10]	uncemented cemented	Sub trochanteric osteotomy Sub-trochanteric osteotomy	11 10	5–9 5–9	1	2	2 1
Decking [13]	uncemented	Straight stem, sub-trochanteric	12	Mean 5.1 yrs	1	0	2
Sener [17]	uncemented	Step cut osteotomy	28	7–92 mos	4	2	3
Howie	cemented	Subtrochanteric; straight stem	40	6–120 mos	0	0	3

non-union and one malunion. Yasgur et al. [19] also reported the technique augmented by cables and strut grafts with uncemented stems with similar results.

We have undertaken 40 femoral osteotomies in primary cemented total hip replacements for DDH (from a series of 132 cases) to correct length, rotational or align-ment problems. 5 had retained metalwork (Fig. 8.35) at the time of osteotomy and the osteotomy was used to remove some of the metalwork. The femoral loosening rate in those cases without metalwork removal is zero, the deep infection rate zero, we had no osteotomy non-unions and no cases of aseptic loosening. However using

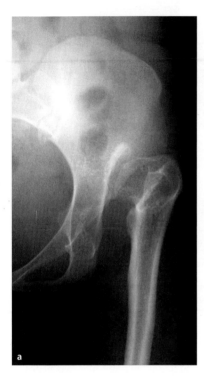
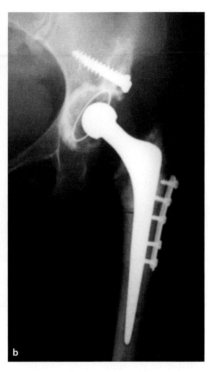

 Fig. 8.34a,b. High dislocation treated with femoral osteotomy and acetabular grafting

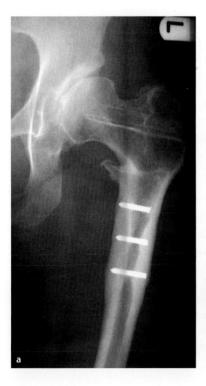
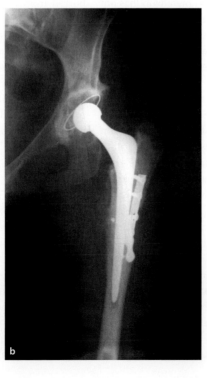

 Fig. 8.35. Femoral osteotomy removing screws from inside and retaining plate to support cortex

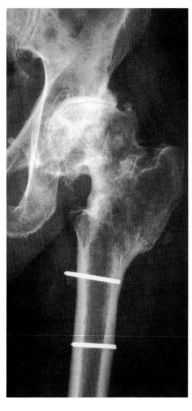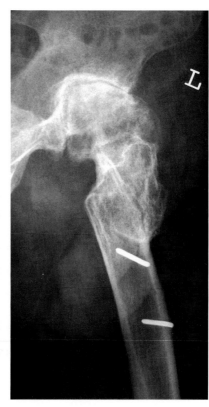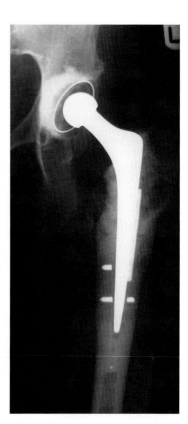

☐ Fig. 8.36. Ugly femur post osteotomy for SUFE (not included in this series) showing deformity, corrective osteotomy and cutting of screws from within (via osteotomy). On the post operative film note retained screw parts in both cortices

the double taper stem we have subsidence of the stem within the cement mantle. This gives 100% stem survival at 6 months to 10 year follow up when metalwork has not been removed and femoral osteotomy has been carried out (accepting two late periprosthetic fractures treated successfully by plating and retention of the hip implant). The grafted osteotomy site, however, has taken up to 2 years to show evidence of union.

In cases where ingrown metalwork was present at the time of hip replacement there were some difficult complications, in one case reactivation of a previous infection at the osteotomy site occurred, resulting in two stage revision and successful proximal femoral replacement. In another the distal femur fractured on insertion of the implant through holes created by the removal of screws and subsequently became infected, again resolving after a two stage revision. In both cases the plate and screws lay entirely within bone at the time of surgery, but staged removal would have resulted in fracture of the femur. Intraoperative fracture or perforation of the femur can occur because of the thin and abnormal anatomy. Often the risks are increased by the presence of metalwork or holes created by the previous removal of metalwork. Some have suggested prophylactic wiring and strut grafting of the femur, particularly when using uncemented implants

[14]. Our current practice is that any ingrown plates or irremovable screws are left where possible and the screws burred from the inside if necessary leaving the cortical segments to reduce stress risers and maintain femoral tube integrity. Of the five cases with retained metalwork two became infected and were revised (20%) the other three all healed without event.

Two patients in our series, both with united osteotomies, have fallen and sustained late (greater than 9 months post THR) periprosthetic fractures which have both been successfully treated with plating.

Conclusion

Full correction of leg length is less desirable than increasing offset, soft tissue tightness is more marked in the adductors and soft tissue structures leaving the pelvis than the abductors. Abductor release is rarely if ever required. Complications of all varieties are more common and the soft tissue continuity between abductors and Vastus lateralis should be maintained. It is our belief that the hip should be made to look normal (by osteotomy) then the surgeon should implant his normal device to obtain good long term results.

Take Home Messages

- Shortening osteotomy in CDH is required to correct deformity.
- Restoration of offset is important – leg length is secondary.
- Non-union and fracture can occur after osteotomy.
- Small implant sizes must be available.
- Both uncemented and cemented femoral stems are successful.

References

1. Cameron HU, Botsford DJ, Park YS: Influence of the Crowe rating on the outcome of total hip arthroplasty in congenital hip dysplasia. J. Arthroplasty 1996; 11:582–587

2. Carlsson A, Bjorkman A, Ringsberg K, von Schewelov T. Untreated congenital and posttraumatic high dislocation of the hip treated by replacement in adult age: 22 hips in 16 patients followed for 1–8 years. Acta Orthop Scand 2003;74(4):389–96

3. Decking J, Decking R, Schoellner C, Fuerderer S, Rompe JD, EckardtA. Cementless total hip replacement with subtrochanteric femoral shortening for severe developmental dysplasia of the hip. Arch Orthop Trauma Surg 2003; 123(7):357–62

4. Della Valle CJ, Berger RA, Rosenberg AG, Jacobs JJ, Sheinkop MB, Paprosky WG. Extended trochanteric osteotomy in complex primary total hip arthroplasty. A brief note.J Bone Joint Surg 2003;85A(12):2385–90

5. Eggli S, Hankemayer S, Muller ME. Nerve palsy after leg lengthening in total replacement arthroplasty for developmental dysplasia of the hip. J Bone Joint Surg 1999;81B(5):843–5.

6. Haddad FS, Masri BA, Garbuz DS, Duncan CP. Primary total replacement of the dysplastic hip. Instr Course Lect. 2000;49:23–39

7. Huo MH, Salvati EA, Lieberman JR, Burstein AH, Wilson PDJr: Custom-designed femoral prostheses in total hip arthroplasty done with cement for severe dysplasia of the hip. J. Bone and Joint Surg 1993; 75-A:1497–1504

8. Huo MH, Zatorski LE, Keggi KJ: Oblique femoral osteotomy in cementless total hip arthroplasty. Prospective consecutive series with a 3-year minimum follow-up period. J. Arthroplasty 1995;10:319–327

9. Lai KA, Shen WJ, Huang LW, Chen MY. Cementless total hip arthroplasty and limb-length equalization in patients with unilateral Crowe type-IV hip dislocation. J Bone Joint Surg 2005;87A(2):339–45

10. Masonis JL, Patel JV, Miu A, Bourne RB, McCalden R, Macdonald SJ, Rorabeck CH. Subtrochanteric shortening and derotational osteotomy in primary total hip arthroplasty for patients with severe hip dysplasia: 5-year follow-up. J Arthroplasty 2003;18(3 Suppl 1):68–73

11. Matsui M, Nakata K, Masuhara K, Ohzono K, Sugano N, Ochi T: The metal-cancellous cementless Lübeck total hip arthroplasty. Five-to-nine-year results. J. Bone and Joint Surg 1998; 80B(3):404–410

12. Noble PC, Kamaric E, Sugano N, Matsubara M, Harada Y, Ohzono K, Paravic V Three-dimensional shape of the dysplastic femur: implications for THR. Clin Orthop 2003;(417):27–40

13. Paavilainen T, Hoikka V, Paavolainen P: Cementless total hip arthroplasty for congenitally dislocated or dysplastic hips. Technique for replacement with a straight femoral component. Clin. Orthop 1993; 297:71–81

14. Papagelopoulos PJ, Trousdale RT, Lewallen DG: Total hip arthroplasty with femoral osteotomy for proximal femoral deformity. Clin Orthop 1996; 332:151–162

15. Pekkarinen J, Alho A, Puusa A, Paavilainen T. Recovery of sciatic nerve injuries in association with total hip arthroplasty in 27 patients J Arthroplasty. 1999;14(3):305–11

16. Reikeraas O, Lereim P, Gabor I, Gunderson R, Bjerkreim I: Femoral shortening in total arthroplasty for completely dislocated hips: 3–7 year results in 25 cases. Acta Orthop Scand 1996; 67:33–3

17. Sener N, Tozun IR, Asik M. Femoral shortening and cementless arthroplasty in high congenital dislocation of the hip. J Arthroplasty 2002;17(1):41–8

18. Sugano N, Noble PC, Kamaric E, Salama JK, Ochi T, Tullos HS. The morphology of the femur in developmental dysplasia of the hip. J Bone Joint Surg 1998;80B(4):711–9

19. Yasgur DJ, Stuchin SA, Adler EM, DiCesare PE: Subtrochanteric femoral shortening osteotomy in total hip arthroplasty for high-riding developmental dislocation of the hip. J. Arthroplasty 1997; 2:880–888

Acetabular Components: Is It Justified to Cement All Sockets?

A. John Timperley, Graham A. Gie, Robin S.M. Ling

Summary

Cemented sockets have provided good long-term outcome with lower overall re-operation rates than cementless designs. Results of cementless sockets implanted with polyethylene liners have been disappointing with increased wear rates and a higher incidence of pelvic and femoral osteolysis. Re-operation rates for problems on the socket side have been higher in almost all reports of cementless socket results. There are no long-term results of using highly cross-linked polyethylene liners; likewise, the fate of hard on hard bearings with contemporary socket design is not known. Results using cemented sockets are further improved when contemporary surgical techniques are used, with published evidence of a low risk for revision at more than fifteen years. With cemented sockets, the likelihood of long term success can be estimated on the first postoperative radiograph and there is strong evidence that the longevity of any socket with regard to mechanical loosening is determined by the surgeon and his/her team on the day of surgery.

Introduction

The operation of total hip replacement was popularised in the 1960's using self-curing polymethylmethacrylate as the material to fix a polyethylene socket to the pelvis. That this method of fixation has evolved and is still widely used today. It is testament to the clinical success of the concept. With the implantation of hundreds of thousand of hips it is inevitable that some will loosen and, with advances in materials and technology in all fields of medical science, it is natural that surgeons will explore alternative socket designs to try to improve further on what has already

proven to be a hugely successful procedure. Some of the alternative designs look promising in the short term, others have already been shown to give significantly poorer results than the »golden standard« cemented polyethylene socket. This chapter explores the results that have emerged from using cement to fix the socket and describes the fundamental importance of using good surgical technique for the best clinical outcome. The use of sockets implanted without cement fixation has generally led to a higher need for re-operation.

Establishing and Comparing Results of Implants in the Acetabulum

There are many problems in assessing whether changes in socket design and alternative methods of fixation are successful. A prosthetic socket rarely needs revising in the first decade for any indication and it therefore takes more than ten years to compare results adequately. The modes of failure and the indications for re-operation have changed with alternative methods of fixation and bearing surfaces and therefore different end-points for comparison may be applicable. For example, it is acknowledged that revision for aseptic loosening at ten years is lower with many designs of cementless sockets with polyethylene liners when compared with cemented sockets. However, the re-operation rate for other indications such as polyethylene wear, pelvic lysis and failure of the locking mechanism of the cup often means the overall re-operation rate for the patients is significantly increased.

To add to the difficulties in comparing results, sockets that have failed radiologically are very often asymptomatic and therefore the headline re-operation rate does not reflect the real failure rate of the device. Patients may have

Chapter 9.1 · Acetabular Components: Is It Justified to Cement All Sockets?

261

9

lost a lot of bone stock around a failing implant before presenting for, or indeed accepting, revision surgery.

Comparative Studies: Cemented Versus Cementless

The best quality outcome data available is from randomised, prospective clinical studies and such studies do exist comparing cemented and cementless sockets. Most published studies have been conducted for relatively short periods and no difference in clinical success has been noted in the near-term [25]. However, metal-backed cemented sockets show more evidence of compromised fixation [10] whereas uncemented devices show a greater frequency and severity of pelvic osteolysis [25]. At a mean 5 years, a comparison using RSA showed no difference in migration or wear rate between a cemented socket and a press-fit design [22]. With longer follow-up, another randomised prospective study demonstrated a statistically significantly greater wear rate of an uncemented cup design and other publications record the increasing problem of accelerated wear and osteolysis around some designs of uncemented cup implanted with UHMW polyethylene liner [8]. In a randomised prospective study comparing a cementless acetabular component with a cemented all-polyethylene cup when the same femoral implant was used, the mean wear rate observed with cementless cups was 0.15 mm per year compared with 0.07 mm per year with the cemented design. The difference in wear was significant (p<0.0001) [20].

Havelin et al. compared the performance of two hydroxyapatite-coated acetabular cups with Charnley cups in the Norwegian Hip Register and found the revision rates of the uncemented design were increased compared with the cemented cup. The results using a stainless steel head were worse than with an alumina head on polyethylene in an uncemented shell [13]. Revision because of wear and osteolysis was more common with both designs of uncemented HA cup. In a report of 73,000 arthroplasties it has been noted that uncemented cups with more than 6 years of follow-up have an increased overall revision rate, compared to cemented cups due to wear and osteolysis and this is especially the case in young patients [12].

Results Using Cementless Sockets

Cementless sockets have evolved in an effort to improve the results in the young and active patients, but although fixation has not been an issue for many designs of implant, an increased wear rate (▶ chapter 10) and an unacceptable incidence of pelvic osteolysis has been reported in almost all designs of cementless socket used in combination with

a UHMWP liner and they have not yet been shown to confer any benefit in the longer term [27].

Aseptic Loosening Versus Wear, Osteolysis and Liner Exchange

A cohort of 120 patients in whom a cementless Harris-Galante cup was inserted have been reported with 15 years follow-up [8]. These sockets showed better durability in terms of fixation than a series of cemented sockets with which they were compared, but if failure of the device was defined as acetabular revision *for any reason* the survival rate was only 81%. In addition, average linear wear rate was high (0.15 mm) and the osteolysis rate was 7.1% leading the authors to express concern that revision related to these appearances may increase dramatically in the second decade after implantation. Results of the Harris Galante I socket were also reported for a cohort of 204 hips at more than 15 years follow-up [5]. The survival rate, defined as revision of the acetabular metal shell because of aseptic loosening or radiographic evidence of definite loosening, was 99% at 15 years. However, this figure gives a misleading idea of the success of the implant. 10 hips (5%) of the 204 hips had required a new polyethylene liner, 5 (2.5%) other shells had been revised as well as one loose acetabular shell (0.5%). By the time of the 15–18 year follow-up, 36 (18%) of hips had had a liner exchange at the time of a femoral revision. At eighteen years, survivorship analysis revealed that 25% of the metal shells were associated with radiographic evidence of osteolysis. The authors reported an increased number of re-operations because of liner wear and osteolysis with increasing follow-up.

The Mayo clinic reported the results of 5371 primary hip replacements when uncemented sockets from a variety of manufacturers were inserted between 1984 and 1998 [18]. The 10-year survivorship of the shell was 85.1% but survivorship of the liner was 77.3% [18]. This figure for re-operation is much higher than for most reported series of cemented sockets at ten years.

Increased Wear Rates in Cementless Sockets – New Bearings

Attempts have been made to discover why the polyethylene wear is increased with cementless devices and various designs features have been blamed including the presence of holes in the shell, backside polyethylene wear within the shell and poor locking mechanisms for the liners. However, one study of 6 different single-surgeon series of porous ingrowth acetabular components showed that the incidence of lysis was actually lower in the group assumed to be at increased risk (cup with screw holes, modular design). The authors agreed that the incidence of lysis (about 9%) was associated with larger head size and longer follow-up [27].

As the problem of increased wear and osteolysis associated with uncemented cups has been recognised, other bearing surfaces have been developed in an attempt at solving the problem. Cross-linked polyethylene cups have shown lower wear rates in vitro but the cross-linking process affects other material properties of the polyethylenes and any adverse effects of these changes are unclear. As with any change in the socket, it will take many years to define whether the change is an improvement or will lead to poorer results. Already, there are reasons to be concerned; in a retrieval study of 24 explanted liners made of highly cross-linked UHMWP, evidence of early surface deformation and surface change was found in every case [2]. The changes included surface cracking, abrasion, pitting or scratching. Although the devices had not failed clinically because of wear, this surface damage had not been predicted by in vitro hip simulator studies and the significance of the findings was unclear.

Ceramic-on-ceramic bearings are being actively promoted in an effort to obviate the problems ascribed to polyethylene wear, but a recent publication from a proponent of this material highlights the need for caution. Although wear rates at the articulation are dramatically reduced compared with polyethylene, migration of the rigid cementless socket within the pelvis may be higher and the problem of lysis may be exchanged for one of implant loosening. At 20 years Hamadouche et al. [11] reported a survival rate of cementless alumina cups of 86% for re-operation but only 51% if radiographic loosening was chosen as the endpoint. The authors noted the need for improved socket fixation. Whether the results will be improved in the long term by the use of metallic shells or bioactive coatings is not known. If the problem is the stiffness mismatch between implant and pelvis and the process of loosening is a mechanical phenomenon, then an improvement in results cannot be assumed [11].

Results Using Cemented Sockets

The clinical results of using cemented sockets in hip arthroplasty have been extensively reported in the literature as the science and the art of hip-replacement surgery have evolved. Since Sir John Charnley described the low friction arthroplasty, there have been changes to the method of preparation of the bony acetabulum, the handling and application of acrylic bone cement, the geometry and design of the implant and there have been improvements to the instruments employed to effect each stage of the operation. Results have therefore depended on the era in which the index operation was performed and the surgical »culture« of the time. Other factors affecting the outcome relate to the demographic distribution of the cohort of patients being reported since results are known to be influenced by the age, sex, diagnosis and activity level of the individual and the presence of any co-morbidities.

Data Interpretation

The best quality data for analysing results comes from randomised prospective studies, but the value of these may be limited as surgical techniques change during the period the trials are running and the implants and instruments compared are often obsolete by the time the study is reported. Good quality data is available from National Joint Registries, particularly those from the Nordic countries that have been in existence over the longest period. However, these too give incomplete information and have methodological limitations. The definition of failure in most registers is the exchange or removal of a hip prosthesis, but it is estimated that the number of patients with pain or unsatisfactory function – who are not revised – is roughly equal to the number who are revised [14]. Also, when a hip is revised it is not always made clear which side of the articulation has failed and led to the revision procedure. This makes it very difficult to report the results of the acetabulum separately from those of the stem.

A very significant contribution of the Swedish Registry has been the demonstration of how changes in surgical technique have affected the clinical outcome with regard to aseptic loosening. However, this data on technique changes has to be interpreted with care since each clinic in Sweden is only asked once a year to define the surgical method practiced at that institution. It has been assumed that all surgeons operate on all patients using the same technique. Details of the surgical technique used in the socket are not provided in detail.

To report the outcome of arthroplasties accurately and relevantly, both clinical and radiological results will need to be considered wherever they are reported. The radiological results are important because Hodgkinson et al. [16] showed a correlation between radiological demarcation of a cemented implant and loosening. The more extensive the demarcation, the more likely a socket is to be loose. He demonstrated that radiographic demarcation of the cemented socket is a prognostic sign for eventual failure.

Long-Term Survival of Cemented Sockets

The 20–30 year results of the low-friction arthroplasty have been reported from Wrightington [30]. 320 LFAs with a mean follow-up of 22 years 10 months were reviewed. 4.1% of cemented sockets were revised for loosening. Radiologically, 18.5% of sockets were designated as loose. The clinical scores did not predict the state of fixation of the arthroplasty.

263   9

Chapter 9.1 · Acetabular Components: Is It Justified to Cement All Sockets?

Wroblewski et al. [32] identified that with the LFA a high wear rate of the socket was associated with socket loosening. High wear (>0.2 mm/yr) and increased socket loosening were seen in active men with unilateral hip disease whose primary diagnosis was osteoarthritis. Low wear was defined as less than 0.02 mm per year. The position of the cup in relation to the acetabular rim or the floor of the acetabulum had an effect on load and wear. Medialisation of the cup, as advocated by Charnley [3], reduces the medial lever arm thus reducing both load and wear whereas lateralisation of the centre of rotation had the opposite effect.

Technique Dependent Outcome

Results from single surgeon series have generally been reported as giving better results than multi-surgeon series. A cohort of patients having a cemented Charnley socket inserted by a single surgeon between 1970 and 1972 using first generation techniques has been reported with a minimum follow-up of 25 years [8]. The survivorship at 25 years with end-point revision for aseptic acetabular loosening was over 90% although if the end point was changed to include radiological loosening this fell to 55% over the same period of follow-up. The wear rate was 0.09 mm year.

The results from Exeter have been reported for the 433 patients who had their hips inserted by multiple surgeons between 1970 and 1975. The sockets were machined out of RCH1000 bar stock and were asymmetrical in geometry – a poor design now known to produce an increased turning moment at the interfaces. After 33 years, 37 cups had been revised giving an overall revision rate of 8.54%. Of interest is the fact that 23 out of these 37 sockets had significant early post-operative radiolucencies suggesting poor mechanical fixation at the time of surgery (vide infra). Primitive surgical techniques were used in this era. In this series there was no correlation between loosening of either component and socket wear which was low at less then 0.1 mm per year for the whole series. The survivorship at 33 years with the end-point of revision for mechanical socket loosening was 72% (◻ Fig 9.1) although the confidence interval at this length of follow-up was wide.

Outcome of Cemented Sockets in Young Patients

Younger, more active patients have had poorer long-term results [19] and these patients are the most severe test for the fixation of the implant. The results of the Charnley low friction arthroplasty in patients aged less than 51 has been reported in a series of 1434 hips [30]. This series of young patients who had their surgery before 1990 includes patients from Sir John's »first 500« who had operations between 1962 and 1965. The stems fared rather better than the sockets. 10.6% of sockets had been revised at an average 15 year follow-up. Unfortunately, survivorship of the stem and socket were not reported separately. Sur-

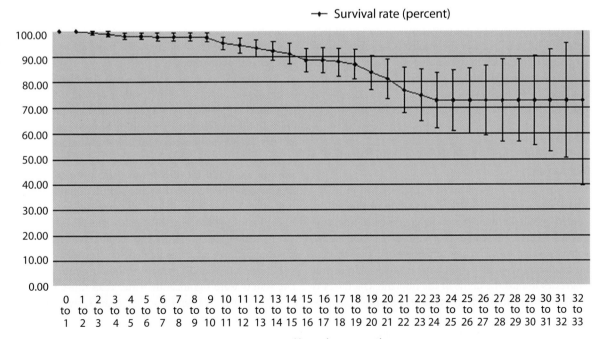

◻ **Fig. 9.1.** Original Exeter cups 1970; survivorship with end-point revision for aseptic cup loosening

vivorship of the hip overall was 93.7% at ten years, 84.7% at 15 years, 74.3% at 20 years, and 55.3% at 27 years with wide confidence limits at the last follow-up. The authors warn that the clinical results may not reflect the mechanical state of the arthroplasty and highlight the need for a radiological review of all implants. They reported a correlation between the depth of penetration of the 22 mm femoral head into the polyethylene of the socket, the incidence of migration of the cup and the outcome of a revision procedure for aseptic loosening of the cup.

Factors Important in Determining Loosening of Cemented sockets

Importance of Surgical Technique

There is more detailed data in the literature on the long-term radiological outcome of cemented sockets when original, unsophisticated surgical techniques were employed. Garcia-Cimbrello [9] studied 680 cemented sockets inserted between 1971 and 1979. Traditional Charnley reamers stabilised in a central pilot hole were used to deepen and expand the acetabulum. Only two further 12.5 mm fixation holes were drilled, one each into the ilium and ischium. No attempt was made to graft bony defects and cement was packed into the cavity digitally before an unflanged Charnley socket was implanted. Using this technique it is unsurprising that radiolucent lines at the cement bone interface were common, 47% of cases having a radiolucent line in Zone 1 at 6 months' follow-up. The incidence of radiolucent lines more than 2 mm increased gradually to reach 27% at 16 years. Overall, radiological loosening of the implant was apparent in 19% of cases at 18 years; 48% of these sockets loosened within ten years. Clinical failure was noted in 76% of the cases that were seen to fail early on X-ray. The authors noted that this »early loosening« was usually associated with deficient structure of the bone of the acetabulum.

Radiolucent Lines – Evidence for Poor Surgical Technique

It has been suggested that late aseptic loosening of cemented acetabular components is governed by the progressive, three-dimensional resorption of the bone immediately adjacent to the cement mantle [26]. This process begins circumferentially at the intraarticular margin and progresses toward the dome of the implant. The thesis is supported by the frequent appearance of a radiolucent line at the edge of DeLee zone 1 that tends to extend with time further around the interface from the periphery. Whilst it is possible to achieve good penetration of trabecular bone and sound mechanical fixation in the central portion of

the acetabulum, it is extremely difficult to achieve good mechanical interlock at the periphery since the bone here can be very sclerotic and thin.

Radiolucent lines seen on the first post-operative radiograph reflect both the pre-operative architecture of the bony acetabulum and also technical faults at the time of surgery. In a group of 185 cemented Charnley hips reported by Ritter [24], 6.5% were loose and 4.8% revised at a mean of 11.7 years follow-up. The authors found that where the initial radiograph showed a radiolucency in DeLee and Charnley zone 1 the incidence of acetabular loosening was 21.2% compared to 0.7% where no such radiolucency was evident. There is, therefore, a 38.8 fold increased risk for revision if the surgeon has employed a surgical technique that results in a radiolucent line being evident at the lateral cement-bone interface on the post-operative film.

Interpretation of Published Outcome – How Well Were They Really Cemented?

Some papers purported to be showing the effect of changes in cementing technique in the socket are misleading. Harris and colleagues [28] reported results of »second generation« cementing techniques at 18 years. The rate of revision for the cemented all-polyethylene components increased from 7% at 10 years to 14% at 18 years. If these revised cases were combined with those designated to be radiologically loose, then overall 27% of sockets were deemed to have failed. However, evolution in surgical technique on the acetabular side was not defined and it is clear from the illustrative X-rays that the methods of cementing in the socket were primitive. These results should therefore be considered to be those achieved using first generation methods.

Bourne [1] reported results when the Harris HD-2 eccentric socket was inserted with a revised cementing technique in 195 hips with a mean follow-up time of 12 years. In these cases, the subchondral bone was preserved and 10–15 five millimetre deep holes were made with a cebatome at the periphery of the socket. A lavage system was used and the socket was dried prior to cement application. The 42 mm diameter circular handle of the acetabular holder was used to pressurise the cement but it is unclear how effective this single diameter instrument was in sealing the mouth of the acetabulum or for how long the pressure was maintained. The revision rate was low at 3% and the radiographic loosening rate was 9%. The results were significantly better than those reported by Mulroy et al. [21] and this discrepancy highlights the fact that the different »generations« of cement technique have never been defined. Radiolucent lines were observed in zone I around 38% acetabular components, in zone II around 23%, and in zone III around 41%.

265   9

Chapter 9.1 · Acetabular Components: Is It Justified to Cement All Sockets?

Better Technique – Lower Risk of Revision

It is now widely recognised that it is technically demanding to implant a cemented socket and yet the longevity of a cemented socket depends fundamentally on the quality of surgical techniques employed at the time of implantation of the device [4, 14].

The importance of surgical technique in determining the outcome of hip arthroplasty with regard to mechanical loosening is highlighted in publications from the Swedish Hip Registry [14]. The incidence of revision for loosening has decreased three times in the decade-and-a-half up to the millennium as improved surgical techniques have been adopted by Swedish surgeons. Failure for loosening has fallen from 9% for the 1979 cohort of patients to 2.8% for the 1990 cohort after 10 years [19].

In the Norwegian Register most revisions for mechanical failure at ten years were for loosening of the stem rather than the socket [6]. The type of cement used for fixation was found to be important; with the best cements socket survivorship was 98% at ten years in the last cohort of patients where newer cementing techniques would have been employed.

Experience and Volume

The early outcome of hip-replacement surgery varies with the number of replacements undertaken by the consultant firm. In the UK, the risk of failure in patients operated on by a consultant whose firm carried out 60 or more THRs in 1990 was 25% of that of patients under the care of a consultant whose firm undertook less than 30 [7].

Influence of Cemented Cup Design

Hodgkinson and his colleagues [15] reviewed the X-rays of 302 primary Charnley arthroplasties to determine the effect of the flanged socket on the appearance of the bone–cement interface. The most significant finding on the post-operative X-rays was the reduction in radiolucency when the flanged cup had been inserted. The interface was line-free in 82% of flanged cups and 60% of unflanged sockets. Lucencies in zone I were also reduced with an incidence of 14.7% and 36.8%, respectively. At ten years it was statistically significant that more of the flanged group were free of radiolucencies compared with the unflanged group. However, approximately 50% of *both* groups demonstrated progression of demarcation lines over the review period. They concluded that the improved long-term radiological result was due to the superior cement-bone interface created at the time of implantation.

Kobayashi et al. [17] also studied the effect of a flange but in this series of patients the method of bone preparation was also modified. As with other reported series from this era, there would have been neither pulsatile lavage of the bone surface nor any formal attempt at pressurisation of cement prior to socket insertion. Kobayashi compared a group of patients in whom the socket had been decorticated and one or two 12.5 mm drill holes made, with a second cohort in which the subchondral bone was left intact and multiple 6 mm holes were made. In the second group a flanged socket was inserted. On the 5-year radiographs the authors showed a statistical correlation between socket demarcation and socket fixation technique with *no* demarcation being evident in 33% of the later group with a flanged socket compared with 80% of the earlier, unflanged group. In making a change to both the surgical technique and the geometry of the implant, it is not certain what was the main contributory factor to the differences observed.

Outcome with Modern Cementing Techniques

Results when more modern techniques are employed in the acetabulum have been described from Exeter. In a cohort of 325 patients who underwent surgery between 1998 and 1991, the survivorship of the socket at 12 years was 96.8% with no case lost to follow-up (Fig. 9.2). Most of the sockets implanted had a metal-backing – a design now obsolete since the results in the literature have generally been inferior to those when an all polyethylene ultra-high molecular weight polyethylene socket has been inserted. Even in the young patients the results have been better when more advanced techniques of bone preparation and pressurisation have been employed. In a multi-surgeon cohort of 88 hips in patients aged 50 or under using the same design of metal-backed implant, 9 (10.3%) had been revised or were awaiting revision at 15 years. The survivorship with end-point aseptic loosening of the socket was 87% at fifteen years (Fig. 9.3).

An »interface bioactive bone cement technique« has been advocated for use in both the knee and the hip in an attempt to improve the results when cement is used for fixation and Oonishi et al. have reported excellent results using this technique for socket fixation with 10.3 years average follow-up [23]. This type of material warrants further investigation since its use may lead to improved results for the future.

Conclusion

Modern fixation techniques with cement have led to better results compared to uncemented designs [14]. Uncemented devices from the 1990s have shown improved stability, equal to cemented fixation [29]. However, the incidence of wear and lysis with most of these designs has been daunting. The long-term results of modern uncemented implants with alternative bearing surfaces are unknown, and it is quite possible that their use will exchange one set of problems with regard to longevity for a different set of complications as yet to emerge. The results of new designs cannot be reliably predicted outside the human body. What has been demonstrated, however, is the improved result of using modern cementing techniques and it is our belief in Exeter that there are further major advances in socket preparation and cementing to come in the future. The surgeon should be aware that ultimately the success of the surgery is defined by the surgeons and their team on the day of the implantation.

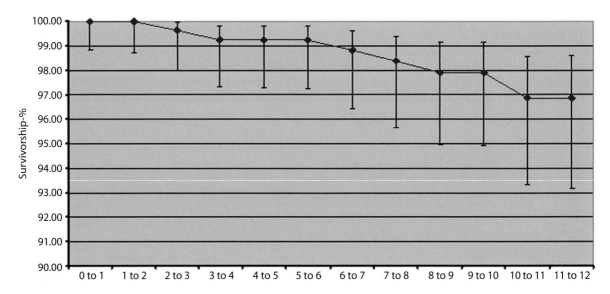

Fig. 9.2. Exeter Universal Series: Survivorship with endpoint re-operation for aseptic cup loosening; (95% confidence limits obtained using the Rothman equation).

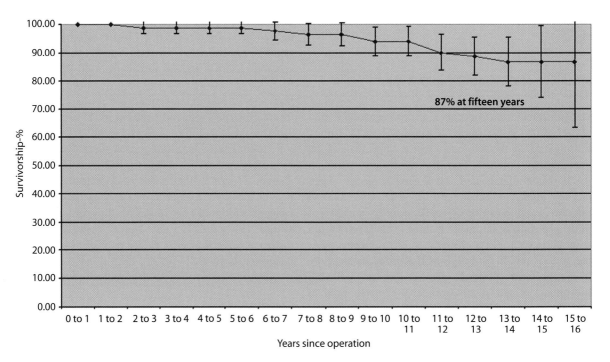

Fig. 9.3. Survivorship with end point as: Aseptic cup loosening in young patients (< 50 years)

Chapter 9.1 · Acetabular Components: Is It Justified to Cement All Sockets?

267   9

Take Home Messages

- Cemented sockets provide good long-term outcome with lower overall re-operation rates than cementless designs.
- The risk of wear and osteolysis (and the risk) for re-operation is higher with cementless fixation.
- Results using cemented sockets are significantly improved when contemporary surgical techniques are used.
- Cemented sockets implanted by the experienced surgeon with meticulous bone preparation technique, pulsatile lavage and sustained pressurisation carry a very low risk for revision at more than fifteen years (also in young patients).
- With cemented sockets, the likelihood of long term success (i.e. absence of re-operation) can be estimated on the first postoperative radiograph.
- The longevity of any socket with regard to mechanical loosening is determined by the surgeon and his/her team on the day of surgery.

References

1. Bourne RB, Rorabeck CH, Skutek M, Mikkelsen S, Winemaker M, Robertson D. The Harris Design-2 total hip replacement fixed with so-called second-generation cementing techniques. A ten to fifteen-year follow-up. J. Bone Joint Surg 1998; 80-A(12):1775–80
2. Bradford L, Baker DA, Graham J, Chawan A, Ries MD, Pruitt LA. Wear and surface cracking in early retrieved highly cross-linked polyethylene acetabular liners. J. Bone Joint Surg 2004;86-A(6):1271–82
3. Charnley J. Low friction arthroplasty of the hip – theory and practice. Springer, Berlin, Heidelberg New York, 1979. p 66
4. Crites BM, Berend ME, Ritter MA. Technical considerations of cemented acetabular components: a 30-year evaluation. Clin Orthop 2000;381:114–9
5. Della Valle CJ, Berger RA, Shott S, Rosenberg AG, Jacobs JJ, Quigley L et al. Primary total hip arthroplasty with a porous-coated acetabular component. A concise follow-up of a previous report. J. Bone Joint Surg 2004;86-A(6):1217–22
6. Espehaug B, Fumes O, Havelin LI, Engesaeter LB, Vollset SE. The type of cement and failure of total hip replacements. J. Bone Joint Surg 2002;84-B(6):832–8
7. Fender D, van der Meulen JH, Gregg PJ. Relationship between outcome and annual surgical experience for the charnley total hip replacement. Results from a regional hip register. J. Bone Joint Surg 2003;85-B(2):187–90
8. Gaffey JL, Callaghan JJ, Pedersen DR, Goetz DD, Sullivan PM, Johnston RC. Cementless acetabular fixation at fifteen years. A comparison with the same surgeon's results following acetabular fixation with cement. J. Bone Joint Surg 2004;86-A(2):257–61
9. Garcia-Cimbrelo E, Munuera LL. Early and late loosening of the acetabular cup after low friction arthroplasty. J Bone Joint Surg 1992;74-A:1119–29
10. Garellick G, Malchau H, Regner H, Herberts P. The Charnley versus the Spectron hip prosthesis: radiographic evaluation of a randomized, prospective study of 2 different hip implants. J. Arthroplasty 1999;14(4):414–25
11. Hamadouche M, Boutin P, Daussange J, Bolander ME, Sedel L. Alumina-on-alumina total hip arthroplasty: a minimum 18.5-year follow-up study. J Bone Joint Surg 2002;84-A(1):69–77
12. Havelin, L. I., Engesoeter, L. B., Espehaug, B., Furnes, O., Lie, S. A., and Vollset, S. E. The Norwegian Arthroplasty Register: 11 years and 73,000 arthroplasties. Acta Orthop Scand 2000;71(4):337–53
13. Havelin LI, Espehaug B, Engesaeter LB. The performance of two hydroxyapatite-coated acetabular cups compared with Charnley cups. From the Norwegian Arthroplasty Register. J. Bone Joint Surg 2002;84-B(6):839–45
14. Herberts P, Malchau H. Long-term registration has improved the quality of hip replacement. A review of the Swedish THR Register comparing 160,000 cases. Acta Orthop Scand 2000;71(2):111–21
15. Hodgkinson JP, Maskell AP, Paul A, Wroblewski BM. Flanged acetabular components in Charnley hip arthroplasty. Ten year follow-up of 350 patients. J Bone Joint Surg 1993;75-B:464–7
16. Hodgkinson JP, Shelley P, Wroblewski BM. The correlation between the roentgenographic appearance and operative findings at the bone-cement junction of the socket in Charnley low friction arthroplasties. Clin Orthop1988;228:105–9
17. Kobayashi S, Terayama K. Factors influencing survival of the socket after primary low-friction arthroplasty of the hip. Arch.OrthopTrauma Surg. 1993;112(2):56–60
18. Lewallen D.G., Berry D.J., Cabanela M.E., Hanssen A.D., Pagnano M.W., Trousdale R.T. Survivorship of Uncemented Acetabular Components Following Total Hip Arthroplasty. 69th Annual Meeting of the American Academy of Orthopaedic Surgeons, Feb 13–17, Dallas, TX.; 2002
19. Malchau, H., Herberts, P., Garellick, G., Soderman, P., and Eisler, T. Prognosis of total hip replacement. update of results and risk-ratio analysis. Scientific exhibit at the 69th Annual Meeting of the American Academy of Orthopaedic Surgeons, Dallas, USA, 2002. 2002
20. McCombe P, Williams SA. A comparison of polyethylene wear rates between cemented and cementless cups. A prospective, randomised trial. J. Bone Joint Surg 2004; 86-B(3):344–9
21. Mulroy WF, Estok DM, Harris WH. Total hip arthroplasty with use of so-called second-generation cementing techniques. A fifteen-year-average follow-up study. J Bone Joint Surg 1995;77-A(12):1845–52
22. Onsten I, Carlsson AS, Besjakov J. Wear in uncemented porous and cemented polyethylene sockets: a randomised, radiostereometric study. J. Bone Joint Surg 1998;80-B(2):345–50
23. Oonishi H, Kadoya Y, Iwaki H, Kin N. Total hip arthroplasty with a modified cementing technique using hydroxyapatite granules. J Arthroplasty 2001;16(6):784–9
24. Ritter MA, Zhou H, Keating CM, Keatinge EM, Faris PM, Meding JB et al. Radiological factors influencing femoral and acetabular failure in cemented Charnley total hip arthroplasties. J Bone Joint Surg 1999;81-B(6):982–6
25. Rorabeck CH, Bourne RB, Mulliken BD, Nayak N, Laupacis A, Tugwell P, Feeney D. The Nicolas Andry award: comparative results of cemented and cementless total hip arthroplasty. Clin Orthop 1996;325:330–44
26. Schmalzried T.P., Kwong L.M., Jasty M., Sedlacek R.C., Haire T.C., O'Connor D.O. et al. The mechanism of loosening of acetabular components in total hip arthroplasty. Analysis of specimens obtained at autopsy. Clin Orthop 1992;274:60–78
27. Schmalzried TP, Brown IC, Amstutz HC, Engh CA, Harris WH. The role of acetabular screw holes and/or screws in the development of pelvic osteolysis. J Engin Med 1999;213:147–53
28. Smith SW, Estok DM, Harris WH. Total hip arthroplasty with use of second-generation cementing techniques. An eighteen-year-average follow-up study. J. Bone Joint Surg1998;80-A(11):1632–40
29. Thanner J. The acetabular component in total hip arthroplasty. Evaluation of different fixation principles. Acta Orthop Scand.Suppl 1999;286:1–41
30. Wroblewski BM, Fleming PA, Siney PD. Charnley low-frictional torque arthroplasty of the hip. 20-to-30 year results. J. Bone Joint Surg 1999;81-B(3):427–30
31. Wroblewski BM, Siney PD, Fleming PA. Charnley low-frictional torque arthroplasty in patients under the age of 51 years. Follow-up to 33 years. J Bone Joint Surg 2002;84-B(4):540–3
32. Wroblewski BM, Siney PD, Fleming PA. Wear of the cup in the Charnley LFA in the young patient. J.Bone Joint Surg 2004; 86(4):498–503

Acetabular Components: Long-Term Success of a Well-Cemented Flanged Ogee Cup

John Older

Summary

This chapter is entirely devoted to the flanged Ogee cup. Initially, it presents evaluation of a cohort of 268 Ogee cups inserted by a single surgeon in a continuous series of primary Charnley low-friction arthroplasties. Clinically at 20 years, the revision rate for aseptic loosening of the Ogee cup was 2% a probability of 96.8% survival. Radiological evaluation at 13 years showed 89% of cups to have perfect bonding at the bone cement interface. The X-rays at 20 years are still being evaluated, but data suggests the excellent radiological bonding is being preserved.

Explanation of the design emphasises that the flange of the Ogee cup has two main functions. It assists pressurisation of the cement and stabilises the cup against the bony rim of the acetabulum. From the clinical and radiological evidence available, the use of the flanged Ogee cup is assisting sound bonding between cup and host bone in the acetabulum.

Introduction

The Ogee cup is a flanged cup developed by Charnley between 1979–1982. It was named Ogee because the double curvature of the plan of the face of the flange passing from concave to convex, resembles in cross section the type of curve best illustrated in the Ogee Arch of Gothic architecture (Oxford English Dictionary: »Ogee: Sinuous line of two opposite curves as in letter S«).

Material and Methods

At King Edward VII Hospital, Midhurst, West Sussex, Charnley personally used the first developmental Ogee cup on the 29 November 1979. There followed a period of experimentation before the Ogee cup went into production. The surgeon author used an Ogee cup for the first time on 29 June 1982. This is a review of a continuous series of primary Charnley low friction arthroplasties (LFA) using the Ogee cup, inserted by one surgeon, between June 1982 and December 1984.

There were 232 patients, 36 had bilateral LFAs, 28 simultaneous and 8 interval, giving 268 Ogee cups for review. The vast majority of patients (97.6%) had the LFA for primary osteoarthrosis. The age at operation ranged from 30 to 88, with a mean of 67 years (SD± 9.4). Females dominated with a ratio 3:1.

Operative Technique

Each operation took place in a Charnley Howarth Ultra-clean air enclosure with a body exhaust system. The procedure was a classical Charnley low friction arthroplasty, lateral approach with trochanteric osteotomy. The acetabulum was deepened transversely using a medial pilot hole which was covered with wire mesh as a cement restrictor. Ebonated bone was left intact in the roof of the acetabulum. Three anchor holes 12.5 mm in diameter were made in pubic, ilial and ischial directions. In addition, a multiplicity of 6-mm holes were distributed randomly over the acetabulum especially in the areas of dense, ebonated bone in the superior roof. The operative technique also involved assiduous irrigation with a syringe and sucker. A power-driven rotary nylon brush was used to help remove fibrous tissue and clean out soft marrow tissue from cancellous spaces, to leave the cancellous bone with a coarse texture to accept the cement (► chapter 2.2).

CMW 1 polymethylmethacrylate cement rendered radio-opaque with 10% barium sulphate with no antibiotics was used in 97% of cups. The remaining cups were fixed with Palacos R cement.

The cups used in this series were machined from compression moulded sheets of Chirulen ultra high molecular weight polyethylene manufactured by Hoechst in Germany. The flanges were moulded from silane crosslinked medium density polyethylene. The finished cups were sterilised by gamma irradiation in an air environment using a dose range of 25–40 kGy.

Review

Two reviews have taken place. The initial review was at 12–14 years; data at 20–22 years is at present being analysed. At 20 years, 151 patients had died all from causes unrelated to the implant, 5 (2%) of patients were lost to follow-up. There were therefore 76 patients alive, available for study.

Clinical Results

Excluding 9 revision patients, there were 130 patients alive with their Ogee cups at 12 years. One hundred and fifteen patients (89%) judged the procedure to be near perfect. Eleven patients (8%) were less pleased, but still considered the arthroplasty satisfactory. Only four patients (3%) thought the result less satisfactory than they had hoped. These figures had not changed at 20 years.

Prior to surgery, regarding subgroups 3 on the d'Aubigne-Postel scale [2,] patients were graded A – 90%, B – 8% and C – 2% the majority of hips were grade 3. This indicated severe pain when attempting to walk and very limited activity. At the first evaluation the majority of patients had improved to grade 6, a universal relief of pain over an average of 13 years, which did not vary between subgroups A, B and C. Assessment of the whole group showed their grading moved from an average pre-operative level of 333 to 665 and were maintained at this level. The only change at the 20 year evaluation was that 20% of the patients had become frail and subgroup C with a functional grade of 3 or 4. However, these hips remained pain free with a good range of movement. The Ogee cup was good and functional in 96% of patients until death or review.

Radiological Evaluation

At review, all patients had antero-posterior X-rays at two penetrations and oblique lateral views of the acetabulum. At the first review, there were radiographs of 137 Ogee cups available for assessment. The X-rays were reviewed independent of the surgeon. Using the modified DeLee-Charnley method [3], grade I is considered perfect ac-

ceptance of cement with no demarcation of radio opaque cement from the bone of the acetabulum. This occurred in 89%. Slight or moderate demarcation affecting the upper quadrant only (grade II) occurred in 6%. Severe demarcation (grade III) involving the whole circumference of the cup was seen in 5 (4%). There was only one cup with radiological evidence of migration.

At 20 years there are 55 radiographs available of patients with their original Ogee cup. At going to press, analysis of their radiographs is still in progress. The initial data suggests grade I, no demarcation is present in 78%. Radiological evaluation continues and the results await further publication.

True Failure Requiring Revision Surgery

There have been 15 revisions. One patient had a fall and fractured the shaft of the femur around the stem of the femoral component. This was revised and replaced. The Ogee cup functioned well both clinically and radiologically for 18 years. A second patient had a periprosthetic femoral fracture at 17 years. Both components were replaced, the cup for wear with no sign of aseptic loosening.

Two cups have been revised for infection. One patient with psoriasis had a bilateral simultaneous LFA. Within months one hip became infected. It was revised as a one stage procedure. Both the original and revised Ogee cups continued to give good service for 17 years.

The other patient, 14 years after the original LFA, developed septicaemia from an abdominal abscess secondary to Crohn's disease. This led to an abscess in the thigh around the LFA. A Girdlesone excision arthroplasty was performed and later revised to a LFA using impacted morsellised allograft bone to reconstruct the acetabulum and proximal femur.

True aseptic loosening requiring revision surgery has occurred in 11 patients. Six of these patients had femoral component problems; four had both components replaced, but only the Ogee cup for wear, with no sign of aseptic loosening. The other two had the femoral stem only replaced, both Ogee cups are good.

Five patients had revision of the Ogee cup for aseptic loosening. Two patients had only the cup replaced, the other 3 had both implants changed. Of these 5 patients, 3 were revised at 12 years and the remaining 2 at 20 years. This represents 1% revision of the Ogee cup at 16 years and 2% at 22 years for aseptic loosening.

Survivorship Analysis and Summary

This is a study to assess the outcome of the Ogee cup in the primary Charnley LFA. It gives a unique insight into the outcome, both clinical and radiological at 20–22 years of 76 patients alive, 95% have their original ogee Cup. The subjective patient satisfaction is high with 91% having excellent or good hips. This includes those patients too frail to travel to hospital for X-ray. The follow-up has been 98% and the Ogee Cup was good and functional in 96% of patients until death or review.

The Kaplan-Meier survivorship estimates, taking failure as revision of any component for any cause, shows a 93% probability of survival at 13 years. The 15 hips that required revision surgery for any cause, represent 5.6% of 268 LFA's at 20–22 years. A probability of survivorship of 88% at 20 years. However, the revision rate for aseptic loosening was 5/268, representing 2% at 22 years, i.e. a 96.8% probability at 20 years. We cannot extrapolate beyond 20 years, as there are not enough cases to balance the revisions.

Review of the Literature

Garellick and colleagues [5, 6] evaluated clinically and radiologically a randomised, prospective study comparing the Charnley prosthesis using the all polyethylene flanged Ogee cup with a Spectron metal back cup. The aim of this study was to evaluate the influence of prosthetic design on early and long term clinical and radiographic outcomes. After 7–11 years the Ogee cup performed remarkably well with no revision, a 100% survivorship at 11 years. Four Spectron Cups were revised, survivorship of 97.4%. In contrast, no Spectron femoral stem required revision, but five Charnley femoral prostheses were revised. Radiological evaluation revealed 23 Spectron cups to be loose, but only 4 Ogee cups were radiographically loose; these patients were satisfied and without pain. This is the only paper so far published giving long-term data on the Ogee cup. The disparity both clinically and radiographically illustrates that the design differences in these two implants had a significant influence on revision rates. As well as the flanged cup another contributing factor to the difference in cup revisions might be that the larger circumference femoral heads (Spectron 32 mm) have been shown to create greater frictional torque [4] and hence higher stresses on the bone-cement interface [5, 6].

Other reports on the flanged cup have been scanty. Wroblewski [12] claimed revision for socket loosening has been reduced to 3% by the introduction of the Ogee flanged socket. Hodgkinson [7] reported a radiological review at 9–11 years comparing unflanged with flanged cups in Charnley cemented arthroplasties. The incidence of radiological demarcation at the cement-bone interface was significantly reduced in early radiographs after the use of a flanged socket and the advantage maintained in the long term results.

The same year, 1993, that Wroblewski and Hodgkinson published, Kobayashi [8], in a 5–18 year review of 267 primary Charnley low friction arthroplasties, presented evidence that preservation of the subchondral bone plate or eburnated bone in the acetabular roof, multiple 6 mm anchor holes and two steps of evolution in socket design, the flanged and later Ogee socket, benefited radiological socket survival. Valle [11] has presented the most up to date review, 123 consecutive primary hip arthroplasties by a single surgeon using cemented all polyethylene flanged cups. These were the first generation flanged cups before the Ogee cup. At a minimum of 20 years, 40 hips in 33 patients were alive and available for study. Two cups (5%) had been revised for aseptic loosening at 13.5 and 21.3 years post operation. Four additional cups had definite evidence of radiographic loosening. They concluded that the use of a cemented all polyethylene flanged acetabular component was associated with a low rate of repeat surgery.

All the surgical procedures in the cohorts reviewed by Kobayashi and Valle [8, 11] were performed by a single surgeon, Terayama and Lazansky, trained by the originator of the LFA and Ogee cup, Charnley. This also applies to the author of this chapter. The surgical technique may have played a factor in the results observed.

Theory

The design of the cup has evolved in a series of stages since high density polyethylene was first used for cups in November 1962. Initially it was rimless. The conventional design of cup, which is basically a simple hemisphere, has three disadvantages. It pressurises and injects cement only when pressed into the acetabulum in a direction perpendicular to its face, at 45° to the long axis of the body. If pressed into the cement transversely, to keep the centre of the cup at a normal low level, a crescent of cement must appear between it and the superior lip of the acetabulum. It will continue to 'wobble' while the cement is soft. This instability in the soft cement imposes a great strain on the surgeon attempting to hold it stationery while the cement is setting.

The pressure injection flanged cup was introduced in 1976 to overcome these disadvantages. This was the first design of cup to have a semi-flexible flange, which could be trimmed with scissors to fit the mouth of the reamed acetabulum. It restricts the escape of cement and enhances compression of the soft cement, especially around the rim of the acetabulum during the last few millimetres of pressing into position. It gives the cup a positive location in the acetabulum, produces mechanical stability so that the cement can polymerise without the cup 'wobbling'.

A criticism of this first pattern of trimmable pressure injection flange was its failure to use a narrow strip of bone surface available in the most lateral part of the posterior wall of the acetabulum. Consider the anatomy of the socket seen as a transverse section of the acetabulum viewed vertically in a standing patient. The anterior wall of the normal acetabulum is shorter than the posterior wall. This shortness is frequently very marked. Neutral anteversion leaves a gap anteriorly and unused bone surface of the acetabulum posteriorly.

The Ogee socket makes use of the maximum area of bone surface on the posterior wall of the acetabulum, at the same time avoiding anteversion of the central part of the face. While the anterior part of the Ogee cup flange remains medially directed as in the previous patterns, the posterior part of the flange is directed somewhat laterally. Trimming the rim of the flange is critical and must take account of the design of the flanged cup and the anatomy of the acetabulum. If the flange is not trimmed enough, it will 'rim out' – the rim may come against bone and prevent further pressurisation. If trimmed too much, the cup may 'bottom out' and prevent further pressurisation.

Shelley [10] evaluated the Ogee flange socket experimentally to determine its efficacy in pressurisation of the acetabular cement and compare it with unflanged cup. The Ogee socket gave a consistently high injection pressure which could be maintained throughout the process of polymerisation. The importance of maintaining a continuous pressure on the cement throughout polymerisation was emphasised.

Parsch and colleagues [9] have evaluated the effects of an acetabular flange on cement pressurisation and cement penetration in 12 cadavers. The flanged cups produced greater intra acetabular peak pressures than the unflanged cups, but did not increase the average intra acetabular pressure. The cement penetration did not differ significantly between the two groups. They interpreted their findings as not supporting the use of flanged cups as the sole means of cement pressurisation in the acetabulum. The use of the word 'sole' is very significant. The definition of 'sole' is 'one and only, exclusive, unique'. The use of the flanged Ogee Cup is not solely to increase pressurisation. A major concept of the flange is meticulous trimming of the rim to obtain accurate contact with the irregular rim of the acetabulum. This stabilises the cup and prevents bottoming out. Maintaining pressure on the cup until the cement has polymerised is essential to cause intrusion of viscoelastic cement into small cancellous bone.

Conclusions

The long term radiological study of the behaviour of bone in contact with cement, is a more important criteria of long-term success, than patient satisfaction. The behaviour of cement and bone in the femur has been gratifying. However, in prospective studies of the cement – bone interface, Charnley in 1979 [1] observed radiological demarcation of cement in the acetabulum in roughly 60% of hips after an average period of 14 years. In 25% there was, with passage of time, progressive, severe demarcation and migration of cups. These were disturbing facts. The corollary that 40% of hips showed no demarcation, even after an average of 14 years was important, because if demarcation was caused by a basic problem such as too great a discrepancy between the elastic moduli of cement and bone, then 100% of cups ought to demarcate. That 40% of cups appeared to have a perfect bone-cement interface could be explained by some factor of better technique in these perfect cases.

Nevertheless, Charnley [1] suggested we could not consider ourselves in control of the situation until a technique of using cement in the acetabulum significantly reduced the incidence of demarcation, to make it as rare as in the femur. Have the changes in the cup and technique over 20 years ago improved the long term results?

In this series, the radiological appearances of the cement – bone interface in the acetabulum demonstrated that 89% of cups at 13 years were perfectly accepted. At going to press, the definitive radiological analysis at 22 years is still in progress and will await further publication. It appears, however, that sound radiological bonding at the cement bone interface in the acetabulum is being maintained. This is surely cause for optimism and supports the idea that there is no fundamental defect in the principal of using cement in the acetabulum. Radiological loosening in other series may therefore be a reflection of unsophisticated cement technique, poor acetabular components and adjacent bone, rather than the fault of cement.

The clinical and especially radiological long term results of the Ogee cup are excellent. It must answer Charnley's original request in 1979 to control the situation in the acetabulum by significantly reducing the incidence of demarcation at the interface. Why are the results so good? I suggest that the clinical use of the flanged Ogee cup endorses the experimental results of Shelly and Charnley's original conception of the flanged cup. The flange firstly provides injection pressure on cement during insertion, giving better bone-cement bonding. Secondly, positive location in the acetabulum giving stability whilst cement is setting. There is a third hypothesis, which may be impossible to prove. The rim, if correctly trimmed to sit precisely on the bone of the acetabulum, acts as a seal – the cement is confined and particles of cement cannot escape.

There is a fourth factor for success. It is now universally recognised that surgical technique is a fundamental factor in the longevity of all hip prostheses. The preparation of the bony bed of the acetabulum, correct trimming of the flange, together with accurate insertion of the cement and cup, are all essential to long term success.

> **Take Home Messages**
>
> - Clinical review of Ogee cup at 20 years revealed a revision rate for aseptic loosening of 2% and a probability of survivorship of 96.8%.
> - Radiological review of Ogee Cup at 13 years showed that 89% of cups had perfect radiological bonding at bone cement interface.
> - X-rays at 20 years are being evaluated. Data suggests excellent radiological bonding is being preserved.
> - The flange of the Ogee cup restricts escape of cement, enhances pressurisation of cement, gives the cup a positive location in the acetabulum and maintains mechanical stability against the bone of the acetabulum.

References

1. Charnley J. Low friction arthroplasty of the hip. Springer, Berlin, 1979
2. D'Aubigne MR, Postel M. Functional results of hip arthroplasty with acrylic cement. J Bone Joint Surg 1954: 36A:451
3. De Lee JG, Charnley J. Radiological demarcation of cemented sockets in total hip replacement. Clin Orthop 1976; 121:20
4. Frankel A, Balderston RA, Booth RE, Rothman RH. Radiographic demarcation of the acetabular bone cement interface. J Arthroplasty 5 (Suppl) 1990; 1
5. Garellick G, Malchau H, Herberts P. The Charnley versus the Spectron hip prosthesis. Clinical evaluation. J Arthroplasty 1999; 4:407–413
6. GarellickG, Malchau H, Regner H, Herberts P. The Charnley versus the Spectron hip prosthesis. Radiographic evaluation. J Arthroplasty 1999; 4: 414–425
7. Hodgkinson JP, Maskell AP, Paul A, Wroblewski BM. Flanged acetabular components in cemented Charnley hip arthroplasty. J Bone Joint Surg 1993; 75B: 464–467
8. Kobayashi S, Terayama K. Factors influencing survival of the socket after primary low friction arthroplasty of the hip. Arch Orthop Trauma Surg 1993: 112; 56–60
9. Parsch D, Diehm C, Schneider S, New A, Breusch SJ. Acetabular cementing technique in THA – flanged versus unflanged cups, cadaver experiments. Acta Orthop Scand 2004; 75(3): 269–275
10. Shelley P, Wroblewski BM. Socket Design and Current Pressurisation in the Charnley Low Friction Arthroplasty. J Bone Joint Surg 1988; 79B: 358–363
11. Valle CJD, Kaplan K, Jazrawi A, Ahmed S, Jaffe WL. Primary Total Hip Arthroplasty with a Flanged Cemented All-Polyethylene Acetabular Component. J Arthroplasty 2004: 19: 23–26
12. Wroblewski B M, Siney PD. Charnley low-friction arthroplasty of the hip. Long term results. Clin Orthop 1993: 292; 191–201

Acetabular Components: Long-Term Survival of Cemented Sockets with Roof Graft

Colin Howie

Summary

In this chapter, we will review the results of cemented acetabulae, where the acetabulum has required grafting to obtain good cover. The dysplastic acetabulum where no augmented support is necessary should have the same results as acetabular components in general. However, as will be presented, the results when graft augmentation is required are less successful. In addition, the dysplastic acetabulum is often small and special implants and bearings may be required if non cemented options are chosen.

Anatomical and Technical Considerations

John Charnley [3] noted that the acetabular bone stock is best in the true acetabulum, though this may not always be true following pelvic surgery. Local experience suggests that Chiari osteotomy may appear to antevert and medialise the true acetabulum making the anterior column seem small. While peri-acetabular osteotomy has been reported to improve head cover, this does not cause problems at time of hip replacement [26]. However, in some cases the posterior wall may be made functionally reduced by repositioning what bone is available after previous surgery.

In the high false acetabulum, while superior cover appears to be good, the anterior and posterior aspects of the acetabulum are often formed by osteophytes. The depth of the false acetabulum is limited by the thickness of the wing of ilium. Charnley [3] noted in the true acetabulum of the high dislocation in the Caucasian population that there is often sufficient AP width to insert an implant of 40 mm outside diameter with no need for a superior rim graft. This was subsequently confirmed by others [31]. Crowe et al. [5] pointed out that when the acetabulum is over-reamed to prepare an elongated false acetabulum then the anterior and/or posterior wall is reamed away leading to instability and early failure of the acetabulum. Therefore, it must be anticipated in most cases of DDH that small implants will be required, sized to the AP diameter of the true acetabulum.

Where an uncemented acetabular component is used, the reduced AP dimension restricts outer cup diameter and thus the inner liner dimensions. Inevitably, this reduces the bearing surface thickness available to the surgeon. Because the dislocation rate for total hip replacement in the presence of DDH is known to be higher, the surgeon may be tempted to use larger head size to reduce the likelihood of dislocation. This will further reduce bearing thickness. Where large head sizes have been used in uncemented cups using polyethylene bearings, this has left the polyethylene-bearing surface extremely thin. Therefore, it is our belief that when uncemented components are used in the presence of DDH, a hard-on-hard bearing should be considered. However, in our practice we use cemented all-polyethylene cups with a 22 mm diameter head to maintain as much polyethylene thickness as possible.

Roof Cover and Hip Centre

The survival of an acetabular component in the presence of DDH depends on the amount of host–bone contact that has been achieved at the primary surgery. Perhaps the most sensible comment on acetabular fixation was made by Wolfgang [33] who suggested that adequate host–bone cover predicts failure and suggested that 80% cover was adequate, supporting Linde's earlier observation [20]. There have been a number of publications which have considered the amount of cup cover necessary for long-term survival. Mulroy and Harris [22] believe that 70% host bone is required. Schuller et al. [30] showed that lack of superior cover results in abnormal stresses and a poor mechanical construct.

More recent long-term follow-up data would suggest that these earlier statements are true [4].

Russotti and Harris recommended using a high hip centre to place the implant in living host bone [29]. This paper pointed out that the centre of rotation should not be lateralised as this led to early failure – perhaps through increased joint reaction force and lack of AP support with 16% cup failure at 11 years. Keeping the implant proud of the femur could compensate leg length.

Yoder et al. [34] noted that high cup placement caused a significant increase in stem loosening. In a mathematical model Johnston et al. [18] showed that forces through the acetabulum were greatest when the cup was placed superior, posterior or lateral; all of which would theoretically increase loosening and wear. This work was confirmed in a laboratory model by Doehring et al. [6]. More recently, Pagnano et al. [25] noted that both the cup and the stem became loose if the cup centre was placed higher than 15 mms from the true centre. Crowe [5] noted that high cup placement meant increased and more persistent Trendelenburg gait and recommended anatomical placement. ◘ Figure 9.4 shows, that high cup placement in the totally dislocated hip will often destroy the true roof of the acetabulum. While this may make the initial THR possible, any subsequent revision will then be extremely difficult as the bone loss will be compounded.

Cotyloplasty

Hartofilakidis et al. [12] advocated medial cotyloplasty of the acetabulum using a technique originally described by Dunn and Hess [7]. In this technique, the medial wall of the pelvis is fractured in a controlled way (◘ Fig. 9.5).

Graft augmentation of the medial defect is carried out and protected weight bearing is encouraged for 3–4 months. In the original series of 86 hips with a mean follow-up of 7 years using an offset bore Charnley cup, they described no failures of the acetabular component, though 14% had radiolucent lines and 81% showed evidence of graft incorporation. Subsequently, Hartofilakidis et al. [13] described excellent, though deteriorating results with 15% revision rates in the dysplastic hips, 21% in the low dislocation and 14% in the high dislocation with a minimum 7 year follow up. This technique medialises the centre of rotation and concerns about long-term survival of the offset bore cup have been raised elsewhere [17]. While medialisation reduces joint reaction force and gives good anterior and posterior cover, the main weight-bearing force vector is placed medial to the roof of the acetabulum and a surgically produced protrusio has been accepted. In rheumatoid protrusio, however, medialisation is known to result in an increased risk of acetabular loosening [28]. In the author's opinion, this technique is not favourable.

High hip centre

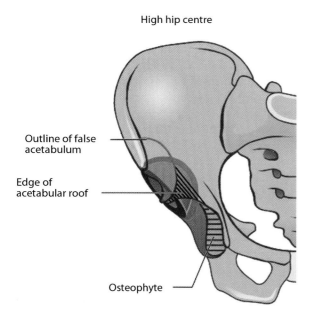

Outline of false acetabulum

Edge of acetabular roof

Osteophyte

◘ **Fig. 9.4.** This diagram shows that reaming high hip centre destroys the acetabular true roof

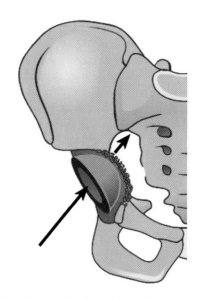

◘ **Fig. 9.5.** Cotyloplasty showing medialised force vector

Reconstruction with Cement

Reconstructing the centre of rotation in its anatomical position by augmenting the rim of the acetabulum has been described in a variety of ways. Cement augmentation can produce good short-term results; however, poor intermediate and long-term results have been reported with 14% revision and 32% radiographically loose at 16 years [21] conversely for Hartofilakidis grade 1. Okamoto et al. [24] showed that cementing alone provided good results.

Allograft and Reinforcement Rings

Acetabular augmentation in the true acetabulum using bone grafts has been described in a variety of ways. Initial reports involved bulk allograft bolted onto the pelvis as described by Mulroy and Harris with 46% failure at 12 years [22] with late fatigue failure of the allograft the likely mode of failure. Compaction grafting has been described with acetabular rim mesh being applied to the outside of the pelvis and the natural head morcellised and impacted in place before cementing [2] in an acetabulum. Using this technique in 27 patients at an average follow up of 7 years (maximum 12 years), 2 had been revised. Acetabular ring augmentation has recently been reported using the Ganz cage with some success [10] though 4 of 33 failed relatively early.

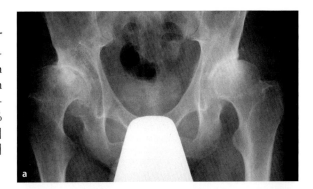

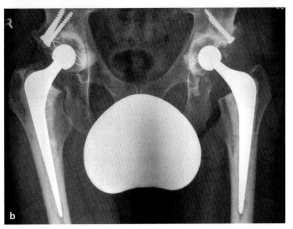

Fig. 9.6a,b. Grade 2 acetabulae treated with roof graft radiographs at 5 years

Uncemented Sockets

There are a few large long-term studies of uncemented cups below graft. Although a number of papers report good results in DDH, only few include large numbers with significant acetabular grafts: 39 uncemented hips below acetabular grafts were reported with an average follow up of 7.6 years showing graft incorporation in all and two cases of loosening [14]. A more recent paper reported excellent results in 44 hips followed for a mean 7.5 years with 4 acetabular revisions, 2 for polyethylene wear, one for loosening and one for fracture of a shell [32]. In a further series of 39 acetabular reconstructions, two sockets had been revised and two other cases showed graft resorption at an average of 7 years [15]. Paavilainen et al. [27] noted a high failure rate with threaded cups and suggested press-fit, and whilst a number of the illustrations showed graft, the article does not divide out the cases with graft.

Roof Graft and Cemented Cups

It is difficult to be sure about the long-term survival of cemented acetabular components as many series do not give adequate breakdown of long-term results based on acetabular cover. Garvin et al. followed up 6 hips from Crowe's original series with acetabular grafts and found no loosening at 14 years [9]. Mackenzie et al. [21] reported 32% radiographic acetabular loosening at 15 years. Sochart et al. [31] described 63% of acetabulae that survived 20 years. Chougle et al. [4] have recently reported again from Wrightington on 292 DDH hips with an overall cup survival of 78% at 2–31 years follow up with aseptic loosening as the principle cause of failure. This paper noted the incidence of failure was related to the grading of the acetabular dysplasia/dislocation and not to the presence of graft. Numair et al. [23] described a series of 190 patients with cemented acetabulae and an acetabular revision rate of 12% at a mean duration of 9.9 years.

The author's preferred technique is to augment any acetabular defect with bone from the patient's own femoral head by placing the autograft femoral head graft back into the defect from which it came, screwing the graft into position (► chapter 2.3). This technique was originally described by Wolfgang in 1990 [34] and has been further outlined by Iida et al. [16], who presented a 95% 12-year survival and a series of elegant longitudinal observations showing that the graft undergoes union, partial resorption and subsequent remodelling over time. A more up to date follow up [19] described 38 hips in 37 patients with graft; all had graft union but it was noted, that slight proximal placement was helpful if less than 50% host cover was possible in the true acetabulum and accepted up to 1 cm proximal placement of the acetabulum in these circumstances.

Author's Results

The author's series includes 132 hips (average age 46.2 years) undergoing cemented THA for significant DDH. Only 53 of the 132 had no associated acetabular graft or femoral osteotomy at the time of index-hip replacement. All of these cases (without osteotomy or graft) required small DDH components. 31 of the 132 had undergone previous acetabular osteotomy and 57 previous femoral osteotomy. Follow up is short (6 months to 10 years) but complete. Overall the dislocation rate was 6.2% and there have been two infections (both associated with removal of metalwork and femoral osteotomy, ▶ chapter 8.7, one grew the same organism isolated at time of femoral osteotomy years before). There have been three other revisions, one for cup loosening and two for recurrent dislocation. 81 patients have undergone acetabular grafting using the technique described earlier (▶ chapter 2.3), the only acetabular reconstruction technique used in this series. In all patients with acetabular grafts both union and integration have occurred. There has been one loose cup revised at 6 years and a further 6 acetabulae have a lucent line in one or more zones. Both revisions for recurrent dislocation occurred in cases where no graft was used and cup positioning may have been compromised.

Dislocation remains an issue with rates varying from 5–11% [11]. In the author's series of primary THA for DDH some of the dislocations have been associated with anterior impingement of the trochanter on a displaced anterior-inferior iliac spine particularly when the patient had previously undergone a pelvic osteotomy prior to hip replacement (▣ Fig. 9.7).

We attempt to avoid impingement on the displaced anterior inferior spine by using as great an offset as possible and removing the inferior spine at the time of surgery. Occasionally, anterior dislocation has occurred when the acetabular cup position was accepted slightly open in an attempt to avoid acetabular rim graft – this is always a mistake. We do not perform trochanteric osteotomy as part of the approach – which is associated with a non union rate of 10–29% [11] – but trochanteric drift and loss of soft-tissue integrity must increase the dislocation rate. Rarely, when necessary, we prefer the extended trochanteric osteotomy preserving the vasto-gluteal sling.

In our practice when the defect is less than 10%, we ignore the defect; when the defect is up to 20%, we use

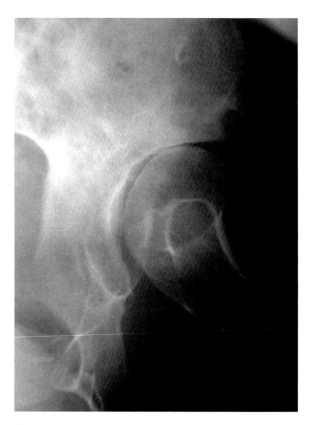

▣ **Fig. 9.7.** Preoperative oblique radiographic view of pelvis post Chiari osteotomy showing displaced anterior inferior spine and thin diameter of pelvic bone

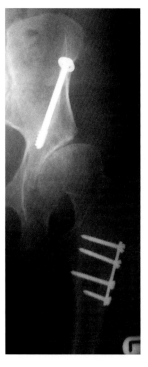
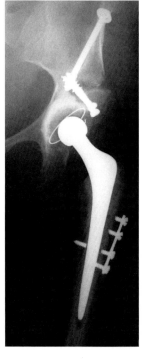

▣ **Fig. 9.8.** Ugly acetabulum and femur pre-operatively and two years post reconstruction with autogenous roof graft

a flanged cup to maintain the centre of rotation with superior cement support. Greater than 20% uncovering, we use an antero-superior autograft block graft. This restores bone stock for future revision surgery, restores the hip centre and restores limb length in an anatomical way. Occasionally, we will accept up to 10 mm of proximal placement either to avoid graft altogether or reduce the amount of graft cover necessary to below 50%.

We would suggest that cemented acetabular components using an all polyethylene component with a 22 mm head augmented by antero-superior roof graft and fixed with 2 screws as described in the earlier chapter using a technique originally described by Wolfgang [34] with long-term follow-ups by Iida [16], Kobiashi [19] and ourselves and also similar techniques using block autograft described by Wroblewski [1], support the continued use of reconstruction of the true centre of rotation of the hip with block autograft. Many of these patients will be young at the time of surgery and are therefore likely to heavily use the hip and are known to have a high risk of long-term loosening [8].

This concept is also supported by experience from revisional surgery. In our series of 39 revision THA's in patients, who had previously undergone THA for OA secondary to DDH, those cases, where the hip centre had been left high, presented with much more severe bone loss and required multiple procedures to recreate the acetabulum adequately. The 15 cases, where the acetabulum had been placed anatomically, were »routine« revisions and though dislocation occurred none have required further revision.

Take Home Messages

- An anatomic hip centre should be achieved at the time of THA for DDH to improve function, to reduce the risk of early failure and to prepare for an easier revision.
- If you think or are in doubt about roof graft, do it!
- In DDH, small sockets sizes are common (PE thickness!).
- Cemented sockets with roof grafts provide excellent long-term outcome.

References

1. Bobak P, Wroblewski BM, Siney PD, Fleming PA, Hall R Charnley low-friction arthroplasty with an autograft of the femoral head for developmental dysplasia of the hip. The 10- to 15-year results. JBJS 2000; 82(4):508–11
2. Bolder SB, Melenhorst J, Gardeniers JW, Sloof TJ, VethRP, Schreurs BW. Cemented total hip arthroplasty with impacted morcellized bone-grafts to restore acetabular bone defects in congenital hip dysplasia. J Arthroplasty 2001;16(8 Suppl 1):164–9
3. Charnley J, Low friction arthroplasty in congenital subluxation of the hip Clinic Orthopaedics 1973; 91:98–113
4. Chougle A, Hemmady MV Hodgkinson JP. Severity of hip dysplasia and loosening of the socket in cemented total hip replacement. A long term follow up, JBJS 2005; 87-B:16–20
5. Crowe JF, Mani VJ, Ranawat CS: Total hip replacement in congenital dislocation and dysplasia of the hip. JBJS 1979; 61-A:15–23
6. Doehring TC, Rubash HE, Shelley FJ, Schwendeman LJ, Donaldson TK, Navalgund YA: Effect of superior and superolateral relocations of the hip center on hip joint forces. An experimental and analytical analysis. J Arthroplasty 1996; 11:693–703
7. Dunn HK, Hess WE: Total hip reconstruction in chronically dislocated hips. JBJS 1976; 58-A:838–845
8. Furnes O, Lie SA, Espehaug B, Vollset SE, Engesaeter LB, Havelin LI. Hip disease and the prognosis of total hip replacements. A review of 53,698 primary total hip replacements reported to the Norwegian Arthroplasty Register 1987–99. JBJS 2001; 83(4):579–86
9. Garvin KL, Bowen MK, Salvati EA, Ranawat CS: Long-term results of total hip arthroplasty in congenital dislocation and dysplasia of the hip. A follow-up note. JBJS 1991; 73-A:1348–1354
10. Gill TJ, Siebenrock K, Oberholzer R, Ganz R: Acetabular reconstruction in developmental dysplasia of the hip: results of the acetabular reinforcement ring with hook. J Arthroplasty 1999; 14:131–137
11. Haddad FS, Masri BA, Garbuz DS, Duncan CP. Primary total replacement of the dysplastic hip. Instr Course Lect. 2000; 49:23–39
12. Hartofilakidis G, Stamos K, Karachalios T, Ioannidis TT, Zacharakis N: Congenital hip disease in adults. Classification of acetabular deficiencies and operative treatment with acetabuloplasty combined with total hip arthroplasty. JBJS 1996; 78-A:683–692
13. Hartofilakidis G, Karachalios T. Total hip arthroplasty for congenital hip disease. JBJS 2004;86-A(2):242–50
14. Hartwig CH, Beele B, Kusswetter W. Femoral head bone grafting for reconstruction of the acetabular wall in dysplastic hip replacement. Arch Orthop Trauma Surg 1995;114(5):269–73
15. Hintermann B, Morscher EW: Total hip replacement with solid autologous femoral head graft for hip dysplasia. Arch Orthop Trauma Surg 1995; 114:137–44
16. Iida H, Matsusue Y, Kawanabe K, Okumura H, Yamamuro T, Nakamura T. Cemented total hip arthroplasty with acetabular bone graft for developmental dysplasia. Long-term results and survivorship analysis. JBJS 2000;82(2):176–84
17. Izquierdo-Avino, Siney PD, Wroblewski BM. Polyethylene wear in the Charnley offset bore acetabular cup. A radiological analysis. JBJS 1996;78-B(1):82–4
18. Johnston RC, Brand RA, Crowninshield RD: Reconstruction of the hip. A mathematical approach to determine optimum geometric relationships. JBJS 1979; 61-A:639–652
19. Kobayashi S, Saito N, Nawata M, Horiuchi H, Iorio R, Takaoka K. Total hip arthroplasty with bulk femoral head autograft for acetabular reconstruction in DDH. Surgical technique. JBJS 2004;86-A Suppl 1:11–7
20. Linde F. Jensen J. Socket loosening in arthoplasty for congenital dislocation of the hip. Acta Orthop Scand 1988; 59(3) 254–257
21. MacKenzie JR, Kelley SS, Johnston RC: Total hip replacement for coxarthrosis secondary to congenital dysplasia and dislocation of the hip. Long-term results. JBJS 1996; 78-A:55–61
22. Mulroy, RD Jr, Harris WH.: Failure of acetabular autogenous grafts in total hip arthroplasty. Increasing incidence: a follow-up note. JBJS 1990; 72-A:1536–40
23. Numair J, Joshi AB, Murphy JC, Porter ML, Hardinge K Total hip arthroplasty for congenital dysplasia or dislocation of the hip. Survivorship analysis and long-term results. JBJS 1997; 79-A:1352–1360
24. Okamoto T, Inao S, Gotoh E, Ando M: Primary Charnley total hip arthroplasty for congenital dysplasia. Effect of improved techniques of cementing. JBJS 1997; 79-B(1):83–86

25. Pagnano MW, Hanssen AD, Lewallen DG, Shaughnessy WJ: The effect of superior placement of the acetabular component on the rate of loosening after total hip arthroplasty. Long-term results in patients who have Crowe type-II congenital dysplasia of the hip. JBJS 1996; 78-A:1004–10

26. Parvizi J, Burmeister H, Ganz R. Previous Bernese periacetabular osteotomy does not compromise the results of total hip arthroplasty. Clin Orthop. 2004;(423):118–22

27. Paavilainen T, Hoikka V, Paavolainen P. Cementless total hip arthroplasty for congenitally dislocated or dysplastic hips. Technique for replacement with a straight femoral component. Clin. Orthop 1993; 297:71–81

28. Poss R, Maloney JP, Ewald FC, Thomas WH, Batte NJ, Hartness C, Sledge CB Six- to 11-year results of total hip arthroplasty in rheumatoid arthritis. Clin Orthop 1984;182:109–16

29. Russotti GM, Harris WH: Proximal placement of the acetabular component in total hip arthroplasty. A long-term follow-up study. JBJS 1991; 73-A:587–592

30. Schüller HM, Dalstra M, Huiskes R, Marti RK: Total hip reconstruction in acetabular dysplasia. A finite element study. JBJS 1993; 75-B:468–474

31. Sochart DH, Porter ML: The long-term results of Charnley low-friction arthroplasty in young patients who have congenital dislocation, degenerative osteoarthrosis, or rheumatoid arthritis. JBJS 1997; 79-A:1599–1617

32. Spangehl MJ, Berry DJ, Trousdale RT, Cabanela ME. Uncemented acetabular components with bulk femoral head autograft for acetabular reconstruction in developmental dysplasia of the hip: results at five to twelve years. JBJS 2001; 83-A; 1484–9

33. Wolfgang GL.: Femoral head autografting with total hip arthroplasty for lateral acetabular dysplasia. A 12-year experience. Clin. Orthop. 1990; 255:173–185

34. Yoder SA, Brand RA, Pedersen DR, O'Gorman TW: Total hip acetabular component position affects component loosening rates. Clin. Orthop. 1988; 228:79–87

9

What Bearing Should We Choose?

Christian Heisel, Mauricio Silva, Thomas P. Schmalzried

Summary

New bearings for total hip arthroplasty (THA) have been introduced with the aim of reducing the number of biologically active wear particles. Crosslinked polyethylene, metal-on-metal, and ceramic-on-ceramic bearings have all demonstrated lower *in vivo* wear rates than conventional metal-on-plastic couples. The degree of wear reduction is promising, but it may not directly translate into greater longevity of a THA for all patients. Each new material needs to be evaluated clinically. The surgeon has to decide for each individual patient which bearing surface option is the most favourable.

Introduction

Osteolysis associated with polyethylene wear has become the limiting factor for implant fixation [45, 54]. Except in cases where the bearing may actually wear-through, wear is practically important only if it induces progressive osteolysis. Hips are generally not revised for wear; they are revised for osteolysis associated with wear (and the generation of wear particles). Patient-related factors contribute to implant wear regardless of the bearing material [108]. Higher patient activity results in higher wear rates [108].

New bearings for THA have been introduced with the aim of reducing the number of biologically active wear particles. There are two approaches: one is to improve the wear resistance of polyethylene through crosslinking [82] and the other is to utilise alternative bearings. This has fueled the development and reintroduction of new ceramic-on-ceramic and metal-on-metal bearings. It is the generic goal of all bearing combinations to reduce wear below a clinically significant level. For practical purposes,

this is a level that does not induce osteolysis or another outcome that necessitates revision surgery. Although helpful as a prognostic tool, caution should be taken in the use of surrogate variables such as age, gender or wear rate to predict the outcome of a total joint arthroplasty [10, 16, 38, 53, 142].

Crosslinked Polyethylene Acetabular Bearings

Ultrahigh molecular weight polyethylene (UHMWPE or PE) has been the preferred acetabular bearing material for more than 30 years. The aggregate clinical experience indicates a low probability for gross material failure in this application and, despite evidence of systemic distribution; there are no clinically apparent systemic consequences. The fundamental limitation is wear resistance.

Polyethylene Basics

Ethylene is a gaseous hydrocarbon, composed of two carbon atoms and four hydrogen atoms, C_2H_4. Polyethylene is a long chain polymer of ethylene molecules, in which all of the carbon atoms are linked, each of them holding its two hydrogen atoms [1]. The mechanical properties of UHMWPE are strongly related to its chemical structure, molecular weight, crystalline organisation and thermal history [71].

UHMWPE microstructure is a two-phase viscoplastic solid, consisting of crystalline domains embedded within an amorphous matrix [8, 71]. Connecting the crystalline domains are bridging tie molecules, that provide improved stress transfer and physical strength [8]. UHMWPE is defined as polyethylene with an average molecular weight of greater than 3 million g/mol [71]. The UHMWPE currently used in orthopaedic applications has a molecular weight of 3–6 million g/mol, a melting point of 125–145 ºC and a density of 0.930–0.945 g/cm^3 [71, 72]. Calcium stearate is an additive in the manufacturing process of many polyethylene resins, which acts as a corrosion inhibitor [71, 135], whitening agent [72], and lubricant to facilitate the extrusion process [71, 122, 135].

Sterilisation

Clinical and laboratory research has revealed that sterilisation methods can dramatically affect the in vivo performance of a polyethylene component [83]. Polyethylene components can be sterilised using gamma irradiation, gas plasma or ethylene oxide (EtO) (◘ Table 10.1). Gamma irradiation in an air environment was the industry standard since the early 1970's, using doses between 2.5 and 4 Mrad, most commonly between 3.0 and 3.5 Mrad. Gamma radiation breaks covalent bonds, including those in the polyethylene molecules. This produces unpaired electrons from the broken covalent bonds, called free radicals. These highly reactive moieties can combine with oxygen (if present) during the irradiation process, during shelf-storage, and in vivo.

Oxidation of the polyethylene molecule is a chemical reaction that results in chain scission (fragmentation and shortening of the large polymer chains) and introduction of oxygen into the polymer [72]. The net result lowers the molecular weight of the polymer, reduces its yield strength, reduces ultimate tensile strength, reduces elongation to break (more brittle), reduces toughness, and increases density (lowers volume) [29, 85, 98, 120].

In general, oxidation and crosslinking (see below) are competing reactions. As crosslinking increases, oxidation decreases and vice versa [86, 114]. For components that have been gamma irradiated in air, the relative amount of oxidation and crosslinking varies with depth from the surface of the component [114]. This results in a corresponding variation in the wear resistance of the material as a function of depth from the surface [86]. Once implanted, the component is exposed to dissolved oxygen in body fluids. Free radicals in the polyethylene will react with the available oxygen over time. There is relatively little known about the rate of oxidation of polyethylene in vivo. It appears that the rate of oxidation in vivo is lower than that in vitro, but there is debate as to how much lower and there is likely an interplay of several factors.

Crosslinking

Crosslinking has been utilised to improve the wear resistance of polyethylene and can be accomplished us-

ing peroxide chemistry, variable-dose ionising radiation, or electron beam irradiation [117]. Crosslinking occurs when free radicals, located on the amorphous regions of polyethylene molecules, react to form a covalent bond between adjacent polyethylene molecules. It is believed that crosslinking of the polyethylene molecules resists inter-molecular mobility, making it more resistant to deformation and wear in the plane perpendicular to the primary molecular axis. This has been demonstrated to dramatically reduce wear from crossing-path motion, as occurs in acetabular components [9, 81]. Crosslinking has a detrimental effect on yield strength, ultimate tensile strength and elongation to break [82]. The decrease in these properties is proportional to the degree of crosslinking. This fact has generated debates on the optimal degree of crosslinking. Wear simulator studies indicate that with crosslinking the type of wear that occurs in acetabular components can be reduced by more than 95% [69, 82, 131].

Heat Treatment

Methods have been developed to produce components that have increased wear resistance due to crosslinking and that do not oxidise on the shelf or in the body. Free radicals created in polyethylene by ionising radiation can be driven to a crosslinking reaction by heating the polymer to above the melting temperature (125–135 °C) [82]. Components made from such re-melted material have no residual free radicals and thus there is no potential for oxidation when the component is subsequently sterilised by EtO or gas plasma. Heat annealing does not reach melting temperature and free radicals remain in the material [28, 90]. Re-melting induces changes in the crystalline structure of the material that are associated with a decrease in some material properties, which do not occur with annealing. This fact has resulted in controversy as to the relative detriment of re-melting compared to the retention of residual free radicals.

Clinical Results

The manufacturing processes of the currently available products differ in dose and type of irradiation (gamma radiation or electron beam), thermal stabilization (re-melting or annealing), machining, and final sterilization [84] (see ◘ Table 10.1). For this reason, each material should be considered separately and the specific wear characteristics of each established through clinical studies.

Re-operation for any reason is the primary definition of failure of a THA. Unfortunately, this often requires a long follow-up period in order to demonstrate statisti-

⬛ Table 10.1. Commercially available polyethylene inserts

Manufacturer	Resin	Manufacturing Method	Irradiation	Method	Sterilization	Heat Stabilization
Highly crosslinked						
Stryker Howmedica (Crossfire)	GUR 4050	Ram extrusion	7.5 Mrad (cumulative 10.5 Mrad)	Gamma irradiation	Gamma in N_2 2.5–3.5 Mrad	Annealed (= below melting temp.)
Zimmer (Longevity)	GUR 1050	Compression molded sheets	10 Mrad	e-beam, cold (CIAM)	Gas plasma	Remelted (= above melt. temp.)
Smith & Nephew (ReflectionXLPE)	GUR 1050	Extruded bar	10 Mrad	Gamma irradiation	EtO	Remelted
Centerpulse/Zimmer (Durasul)	GUR 1050	Compression molded sheets	9.5 Mrad	e-beam, warm (WIAM)	Ethylenoxid (EtO)	Remelted
Moderately crosslinked						
DePuy (Marathon)	GUR 1050	Ram extrusion	5 Mrad	Gamma irradiation	Gas plasma	Remelted
Partially crosslinked						
Biomet (Arcom)	1900H	Compression molded	–	–	Gamma/Argon 2.5–4 Mrad	–
DePuy (Pinnacle GVF)	GUR 1020	Ram extrusion	–	–	Gamma/vacuum up to 4 Mrad	–
DePuy (Enduron)[1]	GUR 1050	Ram extrusion	–	–	Gamma in N_2 up to 4 Mrad	–
Zimmer (standard)	GUR 1050	Compression molded sheets	–	–	Gamma in N_2 2.5–3.5 Mrad	–
Centerpulse/Zimmer (Sulene)	GUR 1020	Compression molded sheets	–	–	Gamma in N_2 2.5–3.5 Mrad	–
Aesculap (standard)	GUR 1020	Molded sheets	–	–	Gamma in N_2 2.5–3.5 Mrad	–
Stryker Howmedica (Duration)	GUR 4050	Ram extrusion	–	–	Gamma in N_2 2.5–3.5 Mrad	55 deg. for 5 days
Stryker Howmedica (N2Vac)	GUR 4050	Ram extrusion	–	–	Gamma in N_2 2.5–3.5 Mrad	–
Link Orthopaedics (standard)	GUR 1020	Compression molded sheets	–	–	Gamma in N_2 2.5–2.9 Mrad	–
Not crosslinked						
DePuy (Enduron)[1]	GUR 1050	Ram extrusion	–	–	Gas plasma	–
Wright Medical Tech. (Duramer)	GUR 1050	Compression molded	–	–	EtO	–
Smith & Nephew (standard)	GUR 1050	Extruded bar	–	–	EtO	–

[1] Manufacturing method dependent on shell design

cal and practical differences between implant systems. Shorter-term in vivo wear studies may help to predict long-term outcomes. Increased volumetric wear has been associated with component loosening and osteolysis [22, 89, 92, 103, 106].

Penetration of the femoral head into the acetabular polyethylene is due to a combination of creep and wear. Because of creep, short-term linear penetration rates tend to be higher than those seen over the longer term. Because creep decreases exponentially with time, it is generally accepted that the majority of the linear penetration that occurs after the first one or two years is due to wear [35, 139].

There are data available from clinical trials with small patient groups that show a reduction in wear rate associated with crosslinking [51, 58, 61, 78, 94, 99, 139].

A study which measured short-term in vivo wear in correlation to patient activity found a 72% wear reduction of crosslinked PE in combination with cementless acetabular components in comparison to gamma-in-air sterilised PE [58]. These results were comparable to hip-simulator wear rates with the same materials.

Other studies showed a reduction between 53 and 93% [36, 61, 77, 78] with different cup designs and PE liners included in their investigations. One has to be careful if different studies are compared because all available crosslinked PE liners differ in the manufacturing process and they are compared to different conventional polyethylenes (see ◘ Table 10.1). All the data represent short-term studies and the influence of creep on the results has to be considered for each study.

Cemented Versus Cementless Cup Fixation

Most studies investigate wear rates with only one mode of fixation. Two randomised trials tried to compare the cemented with the cementless fixation [79, 93]. Onsten et al. [93] could not find a difference in wear rates and in cup migration with RSA after five years. The second study by McCombe et al. [79] found a lower wear rate after six years with cemented cups compared to cementless acetabular components. The drawback even in these randomised studies is the comparison of two different cup designs in each study and the lack of identifying the influence of patient related factors in both groups (e.g. patient activity). There may be a slightly lower wear rate in cemented cups compared to modular cementless implants. This may not be related to the type of fixation but to the modular design. Young et al. [143] found a higher wear rate in modular cups compared to monoblock designs. Backside wear probably contributes significantly to the total amount of particle load. Further studies are necessary to answer the remaining questions regarding fixation method and modularity.

Ceramic Femoral Heads

Another approach to reduce polyethylene wear is to improve the wear characteristics of the femoral head. McKellop et al. [81] demonstrated in a hip-simulator study that lower surface roughness reduces polyethylene wear. The ceramic material is much harder than CoCr and can be polished to a lower surface roughness (made smoother). Alumina (Al_2O_3) heads have both a higher hardness and strength, which makes them more difficult to scratch, and this can reduce abrasive wear [30, 42, 118]. Another important issue is the better wettability of the material. Ceramics are more hydrophilic and have improved lubrication and lower friction.

Hip-simulator and clinical studies indicate that the wear of a ceramic-on-polyethylene bearing is at least equivalent to [13, 35, 70, 121] or better [27, 95, 139, 145] than that of a metal-on-polyethylene bearing. Wear reduction of up to 50% has been reported [27, 42, 95, 118, 145].

Ceramics are brittle materials creating the possibility of fracture of a ceramic head. A review of more than 500,000 current generation alumina femoral heads indicates a fracture rate of 0.004% (4:100,000) [136]. Even if the number of unreported cases is assumed to be three times higher [136], the fracture rate of ceramic heads is still much lower than that of femoral stems, which is around 0.27% (270:100,000) [57]. Following a specific change in their manufacturing process in 1998, there was an increased rate of fracture of zirconia heads from one manufacturer (Prozyr, SGCA Desmarquest, Vincennes Cedex, France, www.prozyr.com). It is important to recognise that the fracture risk of alumina or zirconia heads from other manufacturers was not affected by this occurrence.

Wear Particles

Differences in wear particles from crosslinked and non-crosslinked PE have been found in vitro. Crosslinked PE releases a relatively high number of submicron and nanometer size polyethylene particles and relatively fewer particles several microns in dimension [44, 63, 65, 97]. These submicron particles induce a greater inflammatory response in vitro than do larger particles [44, 63–65]. Additionally, the cellular response is dependent on the shape of the particles; elongated particles generated a more severe inflammatory reaction than globular particles [141] (◘ Fig. 10.1).

Illgen et al. [63] tried to correlate the volumetric wear to the biologic activity in vitro. They compared the wear of a crosslinked PE to a conventional PE measured in a hip simulator and tested afterwards the biologic activity of the isolated particles in cell cultures. They found a reduced relative biologic activity for the crosslinked poly-

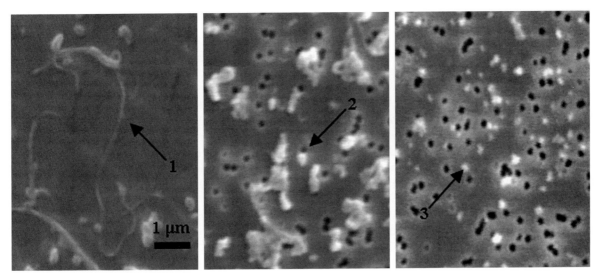

Fig. 10.1. Non-crosslinked PE produces high amount of large particles shaped in elongated fibrils (*arrow 1*). Most significant reduction in particle size is recognised between non-crosslinked and partially crosslinked (3.5 Mrad) PE (*arrow 2*). Partially crosslinked PE shows evidence of mostly round particles of sub-micrometre size and fibrils up to few micrometre in size. Highly crosslinked PE shows predominantly round particles in sub-micrometre size range (*arrow 3*)

ethylene. The association between volumetric wear and periprosthetic bone resorption appears to be related to the number and size of polyethylene wear particles generated and released into the effective joint space [104]. On this basis, a lower wear rate may not necessarily be clinically preferred if a higher number of biologically active wear particles are generated. As number, size and shape of particles released by crosslinked PE liners depend on the material used [64], the mode of crosslinking [97] and patient related wear factors [108]. Only clinical studies for each specific crosslinked polyethylene can answer the question as to whether crosslinked polyethylene offers a favourable benefit to risk ratio.

Metal-on-Metal Bearings

Re-Invention of Metal-on-Metal

Early loosening of prostheses with a metal-on-metal (MOM) bearing, which in the 70´s was assumed to be due to the MOM bearing, has now been recognised as due to sub-optimal implant design, inconsistent manufacturing, and surgical technique [4, 5, 84, 107, 109]. A review of 15 to 20 year results shows survivorship of MOM hip prostheses comparable to the Charnley and other metal-on-polyethylene (MOP) prostheses [68]. The failures have not been due to the wear properties of the bearing [2, 7, 20, 59, 67, 107, 109, 125, 144]. Retrieval studies indicate that the MOM McKee-Farrar prostheses produced significantly less wear than the conventional MOP bearings [84, 87, 110]. Hip-simulator studies with MOM bearings have

shown a significant reduction in volumetric wear rates compared to conventional polyethylene articulations (up to 200 fold) [6, 19, 26, 46, 50, 80, 96, 111]. Consequently, there is renewed interest in MOM bearings for total hip arthroplasty and there has been a revival of MOM bearing research and development, initially in Europe [91, 130, 132] and now in the United States [60, 102].

In 1988, Müller and Weber reintroduced the MOM bearing, and the development of this CoCr alloy bearing was sold under the brand name Metasul (Centerpulse/ Zimmer). With more than a decade of experience with second-generation MOM bearings, over 200,000 Metasul bearings have been implanted and this bearing technology has also been extended to large diameter surface replacement components [5, 129].

Lubrication and Wear

The interplay of material(s), macrogeometry (diameter and radial clearance), microgeometry (surface topography), and lubrication influence the wear of MOM bearings to a far greater degree than with MOP bearings [116]. Mixed-film lubrication appears to be the operative mechanism in most MOM hip joints. Fluid-film lubrication is encouraged by making the femoral head as large as practically possible (doing so increases the sliding velocity and pulls more fluid into the articulation), the clearance as small as practically possible, and the surface as smooth as practically possible. For MOM bearings, in distinction from polyethylene bearings, larger diameter bearings actually produce lower wear rates than smaller diameter bearings with similar manufacturing parameters [43, 119, 119].

Clinical Results

The clinical outcome of contemporary total hip systems with MOM bearings has generally been good [60, 130, 132]. There are no reports of re-operations for a problem directly attributable to the MOM articulation. There has been no evidence of run-away wear, and few metal particles are seen in histologic sections [129, 130, 132]. There have, however, been re-operations for infection, heterotopic ossification, instability, impingement, and aseptic loosening. Impingement wear can be a source of metallosis, especially if a titanium alloy neck impinges on the CoCr acetabular articulation [62]. Larger diameter bearings have a greater arc of motion, which decreases the risk of impingement.

Sieber et al. [115] reported on 118 Metasul components (65 heads and 53 cups) retrieved for dislocation (24%), loosening of the stem (17%), loosening of the cup (28%), and other reasons such as heterotopic ossification or infection (31%). None were revised for osteolysis. The mean time to revision was 22 months (range: 2 to 98 months). An update of this experience includes 297 retrieved head or cup components [140]. The time between implantation and revision in this group ranged from 1 to 117 months with a similar distribution of indications (21% dislocation, 39% loosening of any component, 40% other reasons). The mean annual linear wear rate was found to decrease with the time from insertion, being 25 and 35 µm for the running-in phase and reducing to a steady state of about 5µm after the third year in both studies. The volumetric wear after the run-in period was estimated to be 0.3 mm³/year, leading to the conclusion that these MOM bearings have a volumetric wear rate more than 100 times lower than that of conventional polyethylene bearings.

In clinical reports of hips with second generation MOM bearings, with short term follow-up of 2.2 to 5 years, osteolysis is rare [60, 129, 130, 132]. Beaulé at al. [11], however, have reported a case of a well-fixed, cementless THA with a Metasul bearing with progressive diaphyseal osteolysis occurring within two years. Histologically, there was minimal bearing surface wear and only a small number of inflammatory cells seen in the tissues. Absent evidence of a foreign-body reaction, it was hypothesised that this was a case of osteolysis secondary to transmission of joint fluid pressure, rather than particulate-induced osteolysis [100].

In the initial U.S. experience, 74 Metasul bearings in the Weber cemented cup were implanted with a variety of femoral components. With up to four years follow-up (average 2.2), the clinical results were good to excellent and no hips had loosened. Twenty-seven of these patients had a contralateral MOP bearing hip of similar design and none of these patients could detect a difference between the two hips [60]. Complete clinical and radiographic data on 56 of these patients (56 hips), with follow-up between 4 and 6.8 years (average 5.2 years) has also been reported [41]. Good to excellent clinical results were found in 99%. One patient required acetabular revision for loosening secondary to sub-optimal cementing technique. There were no loose or revised femoral components. There was no radiographically apparent osteolysis [41].

Wear Particles

Wear particles from metal-on-metal bearings are nanometres in linear dimension and substantially smaller than polyethylene wear particles [38, 39]. The size of metal particles reported by scanning electron microscopy (SEM) studies ranges from 0.1 to 5 µm. SEM studies have suggested that large metallic particles observed with light microscopy were agglomerates of smaller particles [39, 52].

There is little known about the rates of metallic particle production in vivo, lymphatic transport of metallic particles from the joint, or systemic dissemination [40, 88]. Utilising information on volumetric wear rate and average particle size, it has been estimated that 6.7×10^{12} to 2.5×10^{14} metal particles are produced per year, which is 13–500 times the number of polyethylene particles produced per year by a typical MOP joint [39]. The aggregate surface area of these metal wear particles is substantial and may have both local and systemic effects. Surface area has been identified as a variable affecting the macrophage response to particles [113]. However, the local tissue reaction around a MOM prosthesis, indicated by the number of histiocytes, is about one grade lower than that around a MOP prosthesis [39, 40]. Most of the histology is from (loose) cemented hips, which makes it difficult to assess the isolated effect of CoCr particles in vivo. There may be a difference in the relative proportion of metal wear particles that are retained locally vs. systemically distributed compared to polyethylene wear particles. Dissolution of metal particles results in elevation of the cobalt and chromium ion concentrations in erythrocytes, serum, and urine [75].

It appears that the ion levels are higher in the short term and decrease over time. This is consistent with a conditioning phase or running-in of the bearing [47]. Since wear of a metal-on-metal bearing cannot generally be measured on a radiograph, erythrocyte, serum, and urine metal ion concentrations may be useful indicators of patient activity and the tribological performance of these bearings. Unfortunately, the toxicological importance of these trace metal elevations has not been established yet.

Delayed-Type Hypersensitivity

Delayed-type hypersensitivity (DTH), an immune response from exposure to metal ions such as nickel, chromium, and cobalt, may develop in a small number of susceptible patients. Recently, some groups have described specific histological changes in the tissues around revised MOM prostheses [3, 34, 133, 134]. These immunological reactions are described with the term »aseptic lymphocytic vasculitis-associated lesions« (ALVAL) [34]. The clinical relevance of these findings is not clear yet, because only a small number of patients with MOM bearings have had to be revised so far and only a fraction of the revised cases show these histological changes.

Cancer Risk

There remains a theoretical increase in the risk of cancer [21, 24, 37, 66, 73, 124, 126–128]. The aggregate clinical data do not indicate an increase in the risk of cancer associated with MOM bearings. However, the majority of patients in these reports have less than 10 years of follow-up. The latency of known carcinogens, such as tobacco, asbestos and ionising radiation, is several decades. Longer follow-up of large patient groups is needed to better assess the risk of cancer with any implant system [123]. Since the goal of more wear resistant bearings is to reduce the need for re-operation, theoretical risks should be weighed against the known risks of revision total hip replacement. In the American Medicare population, the 90-day mortality following revision THA is 2.6%, which is significantly and substantially higher than that of primary total hip and directly related to the revision procedure [76].

Ceramic-on-Ceramic Bearings

Material Properties

Ceramic bearings have demonstrated the lowest in vivo wear rates to date of any bearing combination [18, 26]. The same principles of friction and lubrication reported for MOM bearings apply to ceramic-on-ceramic (COC) bearings. However, ceramics have two important properties that make them an outstanding material regarding friction and wear. Ceramics are hydrophilic, permitting a better wettability of the surface. This ensures that the synovial fluid-film is uniformly distributed over the whole bearing surface area. Secondly, ceramic has a greater hardness than metal and can be polished to a much lower surface roughness. Although the better wettability results in a slightly thinner fluid-film than with MOM bearings it is compensated by the reduced size of the asperities on the surface. Overall, this results in a favourable higher λ ratio

and in a reduced coefficient of friction [43]. This bearing combination is the most likely to achieve true fluid-film lubrication [43]. However, because of the hardness of ceramics, the wear characteristics are sensitive to design, manufacturing, and implantation variables. Rapid wear has also been observed, generally associated with sub-optimal positioning of the implants [25, 137].

Clinical Results

Ceramic-on-ceramic bearings currently in clinical use are made of alumina. Developments in the production process (sintering) have improved the quality of the material [12]. Modern alumina ceramics have a low porosity, low grain size, high density, and high purity. Thus, hardness, fracture toughness, and burst strength increased [12, 15, 112].

The current generation of COC bearings is frequently being utilised with implant systems that have demonstrated long-term successful fixation and excellent clinical results with a MOP bearing. A long-term follow-up study from Europe showed excellent results with a survivorship after 9 years of 94% [14].

Two prospective, randomised multicentre trials are being performed in the United States with more than 300 patients enrolled in each study. Garino [48] reported the short term experience with the Transcend system (Wright Medical Technology) which was implanted with a modular cementless acetabular component in 333 cases, with either a cemented or cementless stem. With follow-up of 18 to 36 months (mean 22 mo.) 98.8% of the implants are still in situ. The second trial utilises the ABC-System (Stryker-Howmedica-Osteonics), which was implanted in 349 cases [31, 33]. D`Antonio et al. [31] reported the most recent results of the six participating surgeons with the highest number of enrolled patients. This sub-group consists of 207 patients with 222 hips with a mean follow-up of 48 months. Five patients have been revised, with 97.7% of the implants in place. As an additional non-randomised study arm, the Trident system (Stryker Howmedica-Osteonics) was included in this multicentre study with 209 patients enrolled. One hundred seventy-five patients in the Trident group have a minimum of 2 years follow-up with a revision rate of 1.4% (3 revisions) [32].

One potential complication with these implants, which a surgeon should recognise, is liner chipping during insertion. This happened in 3 (1%) cases in the Transcend group and in 9 (2.6%) cases [32] in the ABC study group. The Trident bearing has a metal-backed ceramic insert with an elevated titanium liner rim and no intraoperative liner chipping has been reported in this group [31].

Including the original study groups and additional implantations, at this time 1,361 ceramic inserts have been implanted in these studies and there have been no failures due to the bearing [31, 48]. No fractures of the implanted liners or ceramic heads have been reported. Fracture of a current generation ceramic head happens with an incidence of 4 in 100,000 [136]. It is too early to make a comparable statement about the acetabular inserts as more data with a higher number of implants are needed. Results from the multicentre studies are encouraging with no liner fractures reported to date.

Wear Particles

Ceramic materials may have better bio-compatibility than metal alloys [23], but the relative size, shape, number, re-activity, and local vs. systemic distribution of the respective wear particles has not been fully determined. Hatton et al. [56] reported a bimodal size-range of particles isolated from tissue around failed COC total hip arthroplasties. They found a large amount of small particles between 5–90 nm (mean: 24 nm) but also bigger particles between 0.05–3.2 μm. Ceramic debris may not be bio-inert as initially assumed because osteolysis has been described in some patients with a COC bearing [138, 142]. Recently, some studies describe inflammatory and cytotoxic reactions on the cellular level, but the relationship to material, size, and particle number remains uncertain [49, 55, 56, 74]. It seems that there is less inflammatory reaction compared to MOM or MOP bearings in well-functioning prostheses [17]. Ion toxicity is not an issue with ceramics because of their high corrosion resistance [17].

Take Home Messages

- Crosslinked polyethylene, metal-on-metal, and ceramic-on-ceramic bearings have all demonstrated lower in vivo wear rates than conventional metal-on-plastic couples.
- The degree of wear reduction is promising, but it may not directly translate into greater longevity of a total hip arthroplasty for all patients.
- The possibility to use bigger femoral heads with new materials offers a solution where joint stability is an issue. Bigger femoral heads improve joint stability and range of motion. Additionally, bigger femoral heads in MOM or COC couples offer better wear characteristics and improve fluid-film lubrication.
- Bearing wear, osteolysis and aseptic loosening can limit the durability of total hip replacements, irrespective of the material combination used [101, 105], given that the biomechanical reconstruction and fixation are satisfactory.
- It has to be recognised that the products from different manufacturers have different material properties and characteristics due to different manufacturing processes and design features. Each new material needs to be evaluated clinically. The surgeon has to decide for each individual patient which bearing surface option is the most favourable (◻ Table. 10.2).
- For the typical patient undergoing a fully cemented THA the bearing combination metal/ceramic head on polyethylene remains the standard.

◻ **Table 10.2.** Benefits and risks of bearing combinations used in total hip arthroplasty

Bearing Material:	Benefits	Risks

Polyethylene (combined with metal or ceramic femoral head)	relatively low cost
	no toxicity
	different liner options(elevated rim, face angle)
	1. conventional PE:
	  – long in vivo experience
	  – no gross material failure
	2. crosslinked PE
	  – high wear resistance
	  – long in vitro experience
	  – larger head diameter possible
	  – no free radicals = no oxidation
		particles induce osteolysis
		1. conventional PE
		  – oxidation in vivo and in vitro increases wear
		  – aging (longer shelf life) increases wear
		2. crosslinked PE
		  – unknown in vivo wear resistance
		  – larger number of small particles
		  – change in other material properties (>brittleness)

Metal-On-Metal	very high wear resistance larger head diameter possible (bigger head = lower wear) long in vivo experience	systemic ion release toxicity DLH (delayed hypersensitivity) potentially carcinogenic manufacturer binding for head and cup (no mix and match) high cost
Ceramic-On-Ceramic	best wear resistance no toxicity low inflammatory response to particles best wettability = improved fluid-film lubrication often larger head diameter possible (bigger head = lower wear)	position sensitivity fracture risk/liner chipping head size dependent on shell diameter/liner thickness manufacturer binding for head and cup (no mix and match) highest costs

References

1. Plastics and Polyolefins.Petrothene Polyolefins: A processing guide,3 ed., pp. 6–12. New York, NY, National Distillers and Chemical Corporation, 1965.

2. Ahnfelt, L., Herberts, P., Malchau, H., and Andersson, G.B.: Prognosis of total hip replacement. A Swedish multicenter study of 4,664 revisions. Acta Orthop. Scand. Suppl. 238:1–26, 1990

3. Al-Saffar, N.: Early clinical failure of total joint replacement in association with follicular proliferation of B-lymphocytes: a report of two cases. J. Bone Joint Surg. Am. 84-A:2270–2273, 2002

4. Amstutz, H.C.: History of metal-on-metal articulations including surface arthroplasty of the hip. In Rieker, C., Oberholzer, S., and Wyss, U. (eds),World Tribology Forum in Arthroplasy, pp. 113–123. Bern, Hans Huber, 2001

5. Amstutz, H.C. and Grigoris, P.: Metal on metal bearings in hip arthroplasty. Clin. Orthop. 329 Suppl:S11-S34, 1996

6. Anissian, H.L., Stark, A., Gustafson, A., Good, V., and Clarke, I.C.: Metal-on-metal bearing in hip prosthesis generates 100-fold less wear debris than metal-on-polyethylene. Acta Orthop. Scand. 70:578–582, 1999

7. August, A.C., Aldam, C.H., and Pynsent, P.B.: The McKee-Farrar hip arthroplasty. A long-term study. J. Bone Joint Surg. Br. 68-B:520–527, 1986

8. Ayers, D.C.: Polyethylene wear and osteolysis following total knee replacement. Instr. Course Lect. 46:205–213, 1997

9. Baker, D.A., Hastings, R.S., and Pruitt, L.: Study of fatigue resistance of chemical and radiation crosslinked medical grade ultrahigh molecular weight polyethylene. J. Biomed. Mater. Res. 46:573–581, 1999

10. Bauer, T.W.: Particles and periimplant bone resorption. Clin. Orthop. 405:138–143, 2002

11. Beaule, P.E., Campbell, P., Mirra, J., Hooper, J.C., and Schmalzried, T.P.: Osteolysis in a cementless, second generation metal-on-metal hip replacement. Clin. Orthop. 386:159–165, 2001

12. Bierbaum, B.E., Nairus, J., Kuesis, D., Morrison, J.C., and Ward, D.: Ceramic-on-ceramic bearings in total hip arthroplasty. Clin. Orthop. 405:158–163, 2002

13. Bigsby, R.J., Hardaker, C.S., and Fisher, J.: Wear of ultra-high molecular weight polyethylene acetabular cups in a physiological hip joint simulator in the anatomical position using bovine serum as a lubricant. Proc. Inst. Mech. Eng. [H.]. 211:265–269, 1997

14. Bizot, P., Hannouche, D., Nizard, R., Witvoet, J., and Sedel, L.: Hybrid alumina total hip arthroplasty using a press-fit metal-backed socket in patients younger than 55 years. A six- to 11-year evaluation. J. Bone Joint Surg. Br. 86:190–194, 2004

15. Bizot, P., Nizard, R., Lerouge, S., Prudhommeaux, F., and Sedel, L.: Ceramic/ceramic total hip arthroplasty. J. Orthop. Sci. 5:622–627, 2000

16. Bohler, M., Kanz, F., Schwarz, B., Steffan, I., Walter, A., Plenk, H., Jr., and Knahr, K.: Adverse tissue reactions to wear particles from Co-alloy articulations, increased by alumina-blasting particle contamination from cementless Ti-based total hip implants. A report of seven revisions with early failure. J. Bone Joint Surg. Br. 84-B:128–136, 2002

17. Bos, I. and Willmann, G.: Morphologic characteristics of periprosthetic tissues from hip prostheses with ceramic-ceramic couples: a comparative histologic investigation of 18 revision and 30 autopsy cases. Acta Orthop. Scand. 72:335–342, 2001

18. Boutin, P., Christel, P., Dorlot, J. M., Meunier, A., de Roquancourt, A., Blanquaert, D., Herman, S., Sedel, L., and Witvoet, J.: The use of dense alumina-alumina ceramic combination in total hip replacement. J. Biomed. Mater. Res. 22:1203–32, 1988

19. Brill, W.: Comparison of different bearing surfaces in new and retrieved total hip prostheses. In Rieker, C., Oberholzer, S., and Wyss, U. (eds),World Tribology Forum in Arthroplasty, pp. 105–109. Bern, Hans Huber, 2001

20. Brown, S.R., Davies, W.A., DeHeer, D.H., and Swanson, A.B.: Long-term survival of McKee-Farrar total hip prostheses. Clin. Orthop. 402:157–163, 2002

21. Case, C.P., Langkamer, V.G., James, C., Palmer, M.R., Kemp, A.J., Heap, P.F., and Solomon, L.: Widespread dissemination of metal debris from implants. J. Bone Joint Surg. Br. 76-B:701–712, 1994

22. Cates, H.E., Faris, P.M., Keating, E.M., and Ritter, M.A.: Polyethylene wear in cemented metal-backed acetabular cups. J. Bone Joint Surg. Br. 75-B:249–253, 1993

23. Christel, P.S.: Biocompatibility of surgical-grade dense polycrystalline alumina. Clin. Orthop. 282:10–18, 1992

24. Clark, C.R.: A potential concern in total joint arthroplasty: systemic dissemination of wear debris. J. Bone Joint Surg. Am. 82-A:455–456, 2000

25. Clarke, I.C.: Role of ceramic implants. Design and clinical success with total hip prosthetic ceramic-to-ceramic bearings. Clin. Orthop. 282:19–30, 1992

26. Clarke, I.C., Good, V., Williams, P., Schroeder, D., Anissian, L., Stark, A., Oonishi, H., Schuldies, J., and Gustafson, G.: Ultra-low wear rates for rigid-on-rigid bearings in total hip replacements. Proc. Inst. Mech. Eng. 214:331–347, 2000

27. Clarke, I.C. and Gustafson, A.: Clinical and hip simulator comparisons of ceramic-on-polyethylene and metal-on-polyethylene wear. Clin. Orthop. 379:34–40, 2000

28. Collier, J.P., Currier, B.H., Kennedy, F.E., Currier, J.H., Timmins, G.S., Jackson, S.K., and Brewer, R.L.: Comparison of cross-linked polyethylene materials for orthopaedic applications. Clin. Orthop.289–304, 2003

29. Collier, J.P., Sperling, D.K., Currier, J.H., Sutula, L.C., Saum, K.A., and Mayor, M.B.: Impact of gamma sterilization on clinical performance of polyethylene in the knee. J. Arthroplasty. 11:377–89, 1996

30. Cuckler, J.M., Bearcroft, J., and Asgian, C.M.: Femoral head technologies to reduce polyethylene wear in total hip arthroplasty. Clin. Orthop. 317:57–63, 1995

31. D'Antonio, J. and Capello, W.: Alumina ceramic bearings for total hip arthroplasty. Semin. Arthroplasty. in press: 2002

32. D'Antonio, J., Capello, W., Manley, M., and Bierbaum, B. Alumina/alumina ceramic bearings in THA. Hip Society Meeting. 2002

33. D'Antonio, J., Capello, W., Manley, M., and Bierbaum, B.: New experience with alumina-on-alumina ceramic bearings for total hip arthroplasty. J. Arthroplasty. 17:390–397, 2002

34. Davies, A., Willert, H., Campbell, P., and Case, P. Metal-on-metal bearing surfaces may lead to higher inflammation. 70th Annual Meeting of the American Academy of Orthopaedic Surgeons. 2003

35. Devane, P. A. and Horne, J. G.: Assessment of polyethylene wear in total hip replacement. Clin. Orthop. 369:59–72, 1999

36. Digas, G., Thanner, J., Nivbrant, B., Rohrl, S., Strom, H., and Karrholm, J.: Increase in early polyethylene wear after sterilization with ethylene oxide: radiostereometric analyses of 201 total hips. Acta Orthop. Scand. 74:531–541, 2003

37. Dobbs, H.S. and Minski, M.J.: Metal ion release after total hip replacement. Biomaterials. 1:193–198, 1980

38. Doorn, P.F., Campbell, P.A., and Amstutz, H.C.: Metal versus polyethylene wear particles in total hip replacements. A review. Clin. Orthop. 329 Suppl:S206-S216, 1996

39. Doorn, P.F., Campbell, P.A., Worrall, J., Benya, P.D., McKellop, H.A., and Amstutz, H.C.: Metal wear particle characterization from metal on metal total hip replacements: transmission electron microscopy study of periprosthetic tissues and isolated particles. J. Biomed. Mater. Res. 42:103–111, 1998

40. Doorn, P.F., Mirra, J.M., Campbell, P.A., and Amstutz, H.C.: Tissue reaction to metal on metal total hip prostheses. Clin. Orthop. 329 Suppl:S187-S205, 1996

41. Dorr, L.D., Wan, Z., Longjohn, D.B., Dubois, B., and Murken, R.: Total hip arthroplasty with use of the Metasul metal-on-metal articulation. Four to seven-year results. J. Bone Joint Surg. Am. 82-A:789–798, 2000

42. Dowson, D.: A comparative study of the performance of metallic and ceramic femoral head components in total replacement hip joints. Wear. 190:171–183, 1995

43. Dowson, D. New joints for the millennium: wear control in total replacement hip joints. Proc.Inst.Mech.Eng.[H.] 215, 335–358. 2001

44. Endo, M., Tipper, J.L., Barton, D.C., Stone, M. H., Ingham, E., and Fisher, J.: Comparison of wear, wear debris and functional biological activity of moderately crosslinked and non-crosslinked polyethylenes in hip prostheses. Proc. Inst. Mech. Eng. [H.]. 216:111–122, 2002

45. Engh, C.A.J., Claus, A.M., Hopper, R.H..J., and Engh, C.A.: Long-term results using the anatomic medullary locking hip prosthesis. Clin. Orthop. 393:137–146, 2001

46. Firkins, P.J., Tipper, J.L., Ingham, E., Stone, M.H., Farrar, R., and Fisher, J.: A novel low wearing differential hardness, ceramic-on-metal hip joint prosthesis. J. Biomech. 34:1291–1298, 2001

47. Firkins, P.J., Tipper, J.L., Saadatzadeh, M.R., Ingham, E., Stone, M.H., Farrar, R., and Fisher, J.: Quantitative analysis of wear and wear debris from metal-on-metal hip prostheses tested in a physiological hip joint simulator. Biomed. Mater. Eng. 11:143–157, 2001

48. Garino, J.P.: Modern ceramic-on-ceramic total hip systems in the United States: early results. Clin. Orthop. 379:41–47, 2000

49. Germain, M.A., Hatton, A., Williams, S., Matthews, J.B., Stone, M.H., Fisher, J., and Ingham, E.: Comparison of the cytotoxicity of clinically relevant cobalt-chromium and alumina ceramic wear particles in vitro. Biomaterials. 24:469–479, 2003

50. Greenwald, A.S. and Garino, J.P.: Alternative bearing surfaces: the good, the bad, and the ugly. J. Bone Joint Surg. Am. 83-A:68–72, 2001

51. Grobbelaar, C.J., Weber, F.A., Spirakis, A., and et al.: Clinicial experience with gamma irradiation-crosslinked polyethylene. A 14 to 20 year follow-up report. S. Afr. Bone Joint Surg. IX:140–147, 1999

52. Hanlon, J., Ozuna, R., Shortkroff, S., Sledge, C.B., Thornhill, T.S., and Spector, M. Analysis of metallic wear debris retrieved at revision arthroplsty. [Implant Retrieval Symposium of the Society for Biomaterials]. 1992. St. Charles, Illinois

53. Harris, W.H.: The problem is osteolysis. Clin. Orthop. 311:46–53, 1995

54. Hartley, W.T., McAuley, J.P., Culpepper, W.J., Engh, C.A.J., and Engh, C.A., Sr.: Osteonecrosis of the femoral head treated with cementless total hip arthroplasty. J. Bone Joint Surg. Am. 82-A:1408–1413, 2000

55. Hatton, A., Nevelos, J.E., Matthews, J.B., Fisher, J., and Ingham, E.: Effects of clinically relevant alumina ceramic wear particles on TNF-alpha production by human peripheral blood mononuclear phagocytes. Biomaterials. 24:1193–1204, 2003

56. Hatton, A., Nevelos, J. E., Nevelos, A.A., Banks, R.E., Fisher, J., and Ingham, E.: Alumina-alumina artificial hip joints. Part I: a histological analysis and characterisation of wear debris by laser capture microdissection of tissues retrieved at revision. Biomaterials. 23:3429–3440, 2002

57. Heck, D., Partridge, C.M., Reuben, J.D., Lanzer, W.L., Lewis, C.G., and Keating: Prosthetic component failures in hip arthroplasty surgery. J. Arthroplasty. 10:575–80, 1995

58. Heisel, C., Silva, M., dela Rosa, M.A., and Schmalzried, T P.: Short-term in vivo wear of cross-linked polyethylene. J. Bone Joint Surg. Am. 86-A:748–751, 2004

59. Higuchi, F., Inoue, A., and Semlitsch, M.: Metal-on-metal CoCrMo McKee-Farrar total hip arthroplasty: characteristics from a long-term follow-up study. Arch. Orthop. Trauma Surg. 116:121–124, 1997

60. Hilton, K.R., Dorr, L.D., Wan, Z., and McPherson, E. J.: Contemporary total hip replacement with metal on metal articulation. Clin. Orthop. 329 Suppl:S99–105, 1996

61. Hopper, R.H., Jr., Young, A.M., Orishimo, K F., and McAuley, J.P.: Correlation between early and late wear rates in total hip arthroplasty with application to the performance of marathon cross-linked polyethylene liners. J. Arthroplasty. 18:60–67, 2003

62. Iida, H., Kaneda, E., Takada, H., Uchida, K., Kawanabe, K., and Nakamura, T.: Metallosis due to impingement between the socket and the femoral neck in a metal-on-metal bearing total hip prosthesis. A case report. J. Bone Joint Surg. Am. 81-A:400–403, 1999

63. Illgen, R.L., Laurent, M.P., Watanuki, M., Hagenauer, M.E., Bhambri, S.K., Pike, J.W., Blanchard, C.R., and Forsythe, T.M.: Highly crosslinked vs. conventional polyethylene particles--an in vitro comparison of biologic activities. Trans. Orthop. Res. Soc. 28: 2003

64. Ingram, J., Matthews, J.B., Tipper, J., Stone, M., Fisher, J., and Ingham, E.: Comparison of the biological activity of grade GUR 1120 and GUR 415HP UHMWPE wear debris. Biomed. Mater. Eng. 12:177–188, 2002

65. Ingram, J.H., Fisher, J., Stone, M., and Ingham, E.: Effect of crosslinking on biological activity of UHMWPE wear debris. Trans. Orthop. Res. Soc. 28: 2003

66. Jacobs, J.J., Hallab, N.J., Urban, R., and Skipor, A.: Systemic implications of total joint replacement. In Rieker, C., Oberholzer, S., and Wyss, U. (eds),World Tribology Forum in Arthroplasty, pp. 77–82. Bern, Hans Huber, 2001

67. Jacobsson, S.A., Djerf, K., and Wahlstrom, O.: A comparative study between McKee-Farrar and Charnley arthroplasty with long-term follow-up periods. J. Arthroplasty. 5:9–14, 1990

68. Jacobsson, S.A., Djerf, K., and Wahlstrom, O.: Twenty-year results of McKee-Farrar versus Charnley prosthesis. Clin. Orthop.S60-S68, 1996

69. Jasty, M., Bragdon, C.R., O'Connor, D.O., Muratoglu, O.K., Permnath, V., and Merrill, E.: Marker improvement in the wear resistance of a new form of UHMWPE in a physiologic hip simulator. Trans. Soc. Biomat. 20:157, 1997

70. Kim, Y.H., Kim, J.S., and Cho, S.H.: A comparison of polyethylene wear in hips with cobalt-chrome or zirconia heads. A prospective, randomised study. J. Bone Joint Surg. Br. 83-B:742–750, 2001

71. Kurtz, S.M., Muratoglu, O. K., Evans, M., and Edidin, A. A.: Advances in the processing, sterilization, and crosslinking of ultra-high molecular weight polyethylene for total joint arthroplasty. Biomaterials. 20:1659–1688, 1999

72. Li, S. and Burstein, A.H.: Ultra-high molecular weight polyethylene. The material and its use in total joint implants. J. Bone Joint Surg. Am. 76-A:1080–90, 1994

73. Lidor, C., McDonald, J.W., Roggli, V.L., and Vail, T P.: Wear particles in bilateral internal iliac lymph nodes after loosening of a painless unilateral cemented total hip arthroplasty. J. Urol. 156:1775–1776, 1996

74. Lohmann, C.H., Dean, D.D., Koster, G., Casasola, D., Buchhorn, G.H., Fink, U., Schwartz, Z., and Boyan, B.D.: Ceramic and PMMA particles differentially affect osteoblast phenotype. Biomaterials. 23:1855–1863, 2002

75. MacDonald, S.J., McCalden, R.W., Chess, D.G., Bourne, R.B., Rorabeck, C.H., Cleland, D., and Leung, F.: Metal-on-metal versus polyethylene in hip arthroplasty: a randomized clinical trial. Clin. Orthop. 406:282–296, 2003

76. Mahomed, N.N., Barrett, J.A., Katz, J.N. et al.: Rates and outcomes of primary and revision total hip replacement in the United States medicare population. J. Bone Joint Surg. Am. 85-A:27–32, 2003

77. Manning, D., Chiang, P., Martell, J., and Harris, W.H.: In vivo comparison of traditional vs. highly crosslinked polyethylene wear. J. Arthroplasty. 19:262, 2004

78. Martell, J.M., Verner, J.J., and Incavo, S.J.: Clinical performance of a highly cross-linked polyethylene at two years in total hip arthro-

plasty: a randomized prospective trial. J. Arthroplasty. 18:55–59, 2003

79. McCombe, P. and Williams, S.A.: A comparison of polyethylene wear rates between cemented and cementless cups. A prospective, randomised trial. J. Bone Joint Surg. Br. 86:344–349, 2004

80. McKellop, H., Park, S.H., Chiesa, R., Doorn, P., Lu, B., Normand, P., Grigoris, P., and Amstutz, H.: In vivo wear of three types of metal on metal hip prostheses during two decades of use. Clin. Orthop. 329S:128–40, 1996

81. McKellop, H., Shen, F.W., DiMaio, W., and Lancaster, J.G.: Wear of gamma-crosslinked polyethylene acetabular cups against roughened femoral balls. Clin. Orthop. 369:73–82, 1999

82. McKellop, H., Shen, F.W., Lu, B., Campbell, P., and Salovey, R.: Development of an extremely wear-resistant ultra high molecular weight polyethylene for total hip replacements. J. Orthop. Res. 17:157–167, 1999

83. McKellop, H., Shen, F.W., Lu, B., Campbell, P., and Salovey, R.: Effect of sterilization method and other modifications on the wear resistance of acetabular cups made of ultra-high molecular weight polyethylene. A hip-simulator study. J. Bone Joint Surg. Am. 82-A:1708–1725, 2000

84. McKellop, H.A.: Bearing surfaces in total hip replacements: state of the art and future developments. Instr. Course Lect. 50:165–179, 2001

85. McKellop, H.A., Shen, F.W., Campbell, P., and Ota, T.: Effect of molecular weight, calcium stearate, and sterilization methods on the wear of ultra high molecular weight polyethylene acetabular cups in a hip joint simulator. J. Orthop. Res. 17:329–339, 1999

86. McKellop, H.A., Shen, F.W., Yu, Y.J., Lu, B., Salovey, R., and Campbell, P.A.: Effect of sterilization method and other modifications on the wear resistance of UHMWPE acetabular cups.Polyethylene Wear in Orthopaedic Implants Workshop, pp. 20–31. Society for Biomaterials, 1997

87. Medley, J.B., Bobyn, J.D., Krygier, J.J., Chan, F.W., Tanzer, M., and Roter, G.E.: Elastohydrodynamic lubrication and wear of metal-on-metal hip implants. In Rieker, C., Oberholzer, S., and Wyss, U. (eds),World Tribology Forum in Arthroplasty, pp. 125–136. Bern, Hans Huber, 2001

88. Merritt, K. and Brown, S. A.: Distribution of cobalt chromium wear and corrosion products and biologic reactions. Clin. Orthop. 329 Suppl:S233-S243, 1996

89. Morrey, B.F. and Ilstrup, D.: Size of the femoral head and acetabular revision in total hip-replacement arthroplasty. J. Bone Joint Surg. Am. 71-A:50–55, 1989

90. Muratoglu, O.K., Merrill, E.W., Bragdon, C.R., O'Connor, D., Hoeffel, D., Burroughs, B., Jasty, M., and Harris, W.H.: Effect of radiation, heat, and aging on in vitro wear resistance of polyethylene. Clin. Orthop.253–262, 2003

91. Müller, M.E.: The benefits of metal-on-metal total hip replacements. Clin. Orthop. 311:54–59, 1995

92. Nashed, R.S., Becker, D.A., and Gustilo, R.B.: Are cementless acetabular components the cause of excess wear and osteolysis in total hip arthroplasty? Clin. Orthop. 317:19–28, 1995

93. Onsten, I., Carlsson, A.S., and Besjakov, J.: Wear in uncemented porous and cemented polyethylene sockets: a randomised, radiostereometric study. J. Bone Joint Surg. Br. 80:345–350, 1998

94. Oonishi, H., Kadoya, Y., and Masuda, S.: Gamma-irradiated cross-linked polyethylene in total hip replacements--analysis of retrieved sockets after long-term implantation. J. Biomed. Mater. Res. 58:167–171, 2001

95. Oonishi, H., Wakitani, S., Murata, N., Saito, M., Imoto, K., Kim, S., and Matsuura, M.: Clinical experience with ceramics in total hip replacement. Clin. Orthop. 379:77–84, 2000

96. Rieker, C., Shen, M., and Kottig, P.: In-vivo tribological performance of 177 metal-on-metal hip articulations. In Rieker, C., Oberholzer, S., and Wyss, U. (eds) World Tribology Forum in Arthroplasty, pp. 137–142. Bern, Hans Huber, 2001

97. Ries, M.D., Scott, M.L., and Jani, S.: Relationship between gravimetric wear and particle generation in hip simulators: conventional compared with cross-linked polyethylene. J. Bone Joint Surg. Am. 83-A Suppl 2:116–122, 2001

98. Rose, R.M., Crugnola, A., Ries, M., Cimino, W.R., Paul, I., and Radin, E. L.: On the origins of high in vivo wear rates in polyethylene components of total joint prostheses. Clin. Orthop. 145:277–286, 1979

99. Sakoda, H., Voice, A.M., McEwen, H.M., Isaac, G.H., Hardaker, C., Wroblewski, B.M., and Fisher, J.: A comparison of the wear and physical properties of silane cross-linked polyethylene and ultra-high molecular weight polyethylene. J. Arthroplasty. 16:1018–1023, 2001

100. Schmalzried, T.P., Akizuki, K.H., Fedenko, A.N., and Mirra, J.: The role of access of joint fluid to bone in periarticular osteolysis. A report of four cases. J. Bone Joint Surg. Am. 79-A:447–452, 1997

101. Schmalzried, T.P. and Callaghan, J.J.: Wear in total hip and knee replacements. J. Bone Joint Surg. Am. 81-A:115–136, 1999

102. Schmalzried, T.P., Fowble, V.A., Ure, K.J., and Amstutz, H.C.: Metal on metal surface replacement of the hip. Technique, fixation, and early results. Clin. Orthop. 329 Suppl:S106-S114, 1996

103. Schmalzried, T.P., Guttmann, D., Grecula, M., and Amstutz, H.C.: The relationship between the design, position, and articular wear of acetabular components inserted without cement and the development of pelvic osteolysis. J. Bone Joint Surg. Am. 76-A:677–688, 1994

104. Schmalzried, T.P., Jasty, M., and Harris, W.H.: Periprosthetic bone loss in total hip arthroplasty. Polyethylene wear debris and the concept of the effective joint space. J. Bone Joint Surg. Am. 74-A:849–863, 1992

105. Schmalzried, T.P., Jasty, M., Rosenberg, A., and Harris, W.H.: Polyethylene wear debris and tissue reactions in knee as compared to hip replacement prostheses. J. Appl. Biomater. 5:185–190, 1994

106. Schmalzried, T.P., Kwong, L.M., Jasty, M., Sedlacek, R.C., Haire, T.C., O'Connor, D.O., Bragdon, C.R., Kabo, J.M., Malcolm, A.J., and Harris, W.H.: The mechanism of loosening of cemented acetabular components in total hip arthroplasty. Analysis of specimens retrieved at autopsy. Clin. Orthop. 274:60–78, 1992

107. Schmalzried, T.P., Peters, P.C., Maurer, B.T., Bragdon, C.R., and Harris, W.H.: Long-duration metal-on-metal total hip arthroplasties with low wear of the articulating surfaces. J. Arthroplasty. 11:322–331, 1996

108. Schmalzried, T.P., Shepherd, E F., Dorey, F.J. et al.: Wear is a function of use, not time. Clin. Orthop. 381:36–46, 2000

109. Schmalzried, T.P., Szuszczewicz, E.S., Akizuki, K.H., Petersen, T.D., and Amstutz, H.C.: Factors correlating with long term survival of McKee-Farrar total hip prostheses. Clin. Orthop. 329 Suppl:S48-S59, 1996

110. Schmidt, M., Weber, H., and Schon, R.: Cobalt chromium molybdenum metal combination for modular hip prostheses. Clin. Orthop. 329 Suppl:S35-S47, 1996

111. Scholes, S.C., Green, S.M., and Unsworth, A.: The wear of metal-on-metal total hip prostheses measured in a hip simulator. Proc. Inst. Mech. Eng. [H.]. 215:523–530, 2001

112. Sedel, L.: Evolution of alumina-on-alumina implants: a review. Clin. Orthop. 379:48–54, 2000

113. Shanbhag, A.S., Jacobs, J.J., Black, J., Galante, J. O., and Glant, T.T.: Macrophage/particle interactions: effect of size, composition and surface area. J. Biomed. Mater. Res. 28:81–90, 1994

114. Shen, F.W. and McKellop, H.A.: Interaction of oxidation and cross-linking in gamma-irradiated ultrahigh molecular-weight polyethylene. J. Biomed. Mater. Res. 61:430–439, 2002

115. Sieber, H.P., Rieker, C.B., and Kottig, P.: Analysis of 118 second-generation metal-on-metal retrieved hip implants. J. Bone Joint Surg. Br. 81-B:46–50, 1999

116. Silva, M. and Schmalzried, T.P.: Alternate Bearing Materials: Metal-on-Metal. In Shanbhag, A., Rubash, H.E., and Jacobs, J.J. (eds) Joint Replacements and Bone Resorption: Pathology, Biomaterials and Clinical Practice, pp. in press. Marcel Dekker, 2002

117. Silva, M. and Schmalzried, T.P.: Polyethylene in Total Knee Arthroplasty. In Callaghan, J.J., Rosenberg, A.G., Rubash, H.E., Simonian, P.T., and Wickiewicz, T.A. (eds), Lipincott Williams & Wilkins, 2002

118. Skinner, H.B.: Ceramic bearing surfaces. Clin. Orthop. 369:83–91, 1999

119. Smith, S.L., Dowson, D., and Goldsmith, A.A.J.: The effect of diametral clearances, motion and loading cycles upon lubrication of metal-on-metal hip replacements. Proc. Inst. Mech. Eng. [C]. 215:1–5, 2001

120. Sutula, L.C., Collier, J.P., Saum, et al.: Impact of gamma sterilization on clinical performance of polyethylene in the hip. Clin. Orthop. 319:28–40, 1995

121. Sychterz, C.J., Engh, C.A.J., Young, A.M., Hopper, R.H.J., and Engh, C.A.: Comparison of in vivo wear between polyethylene liners articulating with ceramic and cobalt-chrome femoral heads. J. Bone Joint Surg. Br. 82-B:948–951, 2000

122. Tanner, M.G., Whiteside, L.A., and White, S.E.: Effect of polyethylene quality on wear in total knee arthroplasty. Clin. Orthop. 317:83–88, 1995

123. Tharani, R., Dorey, F.J., and Schmalzried, T.P.: The risk of cancer following total hip or knee arthroplasty. J. Bone Joint Surg. Am. 83-A:774–780, 2001

124. Urban, R.M., Jacobs, J.J., Tomlinson, M.J., Gavrilovic, J., Black, J., and Peoc'h, M.: Dissemination of wear particles to the liver, spleen, and abdominal lymph nodes of patients with hip or knee replacement. J. Bone Joint Surg. Am. 82-A:457–476, 2000

125. Visuri, T.: Long-term results and survivorship of the McKee-Farrar total hip prosthesis. Arch. Orthop. Trauma Surg. 106:368–374, 1987

126. Visuri, T. and Koskenvuo, M.: Cancer risk after Mckee-Farrar total hip replacement. Orthopedics. 14:137–142, 1991

127. Visuri, T. and Pukkala, E.: Does metal-on-metal total hip prosthesis have influence on cancer? In Rieker, C., Oberholzer, S., and Wyss, U. (eds),World Tribology Forum in Arthroplasty, pp. 181–187. Bern, Hans Huber, 2001

128. Visuri, T., Pukkala, E., Paavolainen, P., Pulkkinen, P., and Riska, E. B.: Cancer risk after metal on metal and polyethylene on metal total hip arthroplasty. Clin. Orthop. 329 Suppl:S280-S289, 1996

129. Wagner, M. and Wagner, H.: Preliminary results of uncemented metal on metal stemmed and resurfacing hip replacement arthroplasty. Clin. Orthop. 329 Suppl:S78-S88, 1996

130. Wagner, M. and Wagner, H.: Medium-term results of a modern metal-on-metal system in total hip replacement. Clin. Orthop. 379:123–133, 2000

131. Wang, A., Essner, A., Polineni, V. K., Sun, D.C., Stark, C., and Dumbleton, J.H.: Wear mechanisms and wear testing of ultra-high molecular weight polyethylene in total joint replacements.Polyethylene Wear in Orthopaedic Implants Workshop, pp. 4–18. Society for Biomaterials, 1997

132. Weber, B.G.: Experience with the Metasul total hip bearing system. Clin. Orthop. 329 (Suppl): S69-S77, 1996

133. Willert, H., Buchorn, G., Fayaayazi, A., and Lohmann, C.: Histopathological changes around metal/metal joints indicate delayed type hypersensitivity. Primary results of 14 cases. Osteologie. 9:2–16, 2000

134. Willert, H.G., Buchhorn, G.H., Fayyazi, A., and Lohmann, C.H.: Histopathological changes in tissues surrounding metal/metal joints – Signs of delayed type hypersensitivity (DTH)? In Rieker, C., Oberholzer, S., and Wyss, U. (eds),World Tribology Forum in Arthroplasty, pp. 147–166. Bern, Hans Huber, 2001

135. Willie, B.M., Gingell, D.T., Bloebaum, R.D., and Hofmann, A.A.: Possible explanation for the white band artifact seen in clinically retrieved polyethylene tibial components. J. Biomed. Mater. Res. 52:558–566, 2000

136. Willmann, G.: Ceramic femoral head retrieval data. Clin. Orthop. 379:22–28, 2000

137. Winter, M., Griss, P., Scheller, G., and Moser, T.: Ten- to 14-year results of a ceramic hip prosthesis. Clin. Orthop. 282:73–80, 1992

138. Wirganowicz, P.Z. and Thomas, B.J.: Massive osteolysis after ceramic on ceramic total hip arthroplasty. A case report. Clin. Orthop. 338:100–104, 1997

139. Wroblewski, B.M., Siney, P.D., Dowson, D., and Collins, S.N.: Prospective clinical and joint simulator studies of a new total hip arthroplasty using alumina ceramic heads and cross-linked polyethylene cups. J. Bone Joint Surg. Br. 78-B:280–285, 1996

140. Wyss, U. and Rieker, C. Metal-on-metal hip articulation. 32nd Annual Course, Advances in Hip and Knee Arthroplasty. 2002

141. Yang, S.Y., Ren, W., Park, Y., Sieving, A., Hsu, S., Nasser, S., and Wooley, P.H.: Diverse cellular and apoptotic responses to variant shapes of UHMWPE particles in a murine model of inflammation. Biomaterials. 23:3535–3543, 2002

142. Yoon, T.R., Rowe, S.M., Jung, S.T., Seon, K.J., and Maloney, W.J.: Osteolysis in association with a total hip arthroplasty with ceramic bearing surfaces. J. Bone Joint Surg. Am. 80-A:1459–1468, 1998

143. Young, A.M., Sychterz, C.J., Hopper, R.H.J., and Engh, C.A.: Effect of acetabular modularity on polyethylene wear and osteolysis in total hip arthroplasty. J. Bone Joint Surg. Am. 84-A:58–63, 2002

144. Zahiri, C.A., Schmalzried, T.P., Ebramzadeh, E., Szuszczewicz, E.S., Salib, D., Kim, C., and Amstutz, H.C.: Lessons learned from loosening of the McKee-Farrar metal-on-metal total hip replacement. J. Arthroplasty. 14:326–332, 1999

145. Zichner, L.P. and Willert, H.G.: Comparison of alumina-polyethylene and metal-polyethylene in clinical trials. Clin. Orthop. 282:86–94, 1992

10

The Evidence from the Swedish Hip Register

Henrik Malchau, Göran Garellick, Peter Herberts

Summary

The Swedish Total Hip Arthroplasty (THA) Register was initiated in 1979. The primary reason was to document failures and the need for revision surgery to improve and redefine the primary indication, surgical technique and implant choice. The hypothesis is that feedback of data stimulates participating clinics to reflect and improve their health care accordingly. In addition to revision, which has been used as end-point definition to date, patient based outcome measures and radiographic results will be included in the future to improve sensitivity. The national average 7-year survival (revision as end-point), has improved from 93.5% (±0.15) to 95.8 (±0.15) between the two periods 1979–1991 and 1992–2003. The Swedish results are based on more than 90%, all cemented THA. National implant registers define the epidemiology of primary and revision surgery. In conjunction with individual, subjective, patient data and radiography they contribute to the development of evidence-based THA surgery.

Introduction

The rapid growth of new surgical techniques in conjunction with an accelerating development of new hip implant technology warrants a continuous and objective monitoring of the results paralleled with precise educational efforts. For many years, the purpose of the Swedish National Hip Arthroplasty register was to monitor surgical techniques and prophylactic measures to minimise complications by persisting continuous feed-back to all THA-performing units and to provide a warning system for rapid implant failures. A substantial part of the feed-back system (reporting), all publications, annual reports and scientific exhibitions, are communicated via www. jru.orthop.gu.se. All 81 orthopaedic units in Sweden, both public and private, participate voluntarily in the register. The vast majority of the clinics are reporting data directly via the Internet. Ninety percent of THAs and 75% of re-operations are reported immediately online. There is a short delay in reporting for the remaining units. Copies of complete medical records from all re-operations/revisions are collected for further scientific studies.

The current end point of revision or re-revision is easy to define but leaves many questions regarding the true outcome. The low sensitivity of this end-point has prompted implementation of more sensitive alternatives such as individual health outcome (captured by the EQ-5D questionnaire) and a basic radiographic analysis. These measures are now being implemented in a project that is continuously expanding to involve most parts of Sweden and eventually the entire country. This effort parallels the national health care providers' (The Swedish Board of Health and Welfare) demand that individual patient outcome should be reported from all national quality registries.

This chapter present an extract of the latest report from the Swedish National Register and preliminary experiences with implementation of patient based outcome measures.

Materials and Methods

Primary THA

The register contains information on primary hip arthroplasties performed in Sweden since 1979. From 1979 until 1991 the number of primary operations and the type of implant used were recorded from each unit. The distribution of age, gender and index diagnoses was estimated through a corrective formula based on diagnosis-specific incidence and prevalence figures given by Statistics Sweden (www.scb.se). From 1992 onwards, data has been collected on an individual basis regarding information on the primary procedure and any subsequently open procedure by the use of the patient's social security number (Swedish PNR number). The diagnosis is registered with the ICD-9 and ICD-10 codes. All implant parts are registered separately for e.g. cup/liner and stem/head as well as the method of fixation and type of cement. The register's web application was introduced in January 1999. It uses article bar codes supplied by the manufacturer's catalogues to ensure correct implant identification and cement brand. The type of incision is also registered per surgical procedure. 77 of the 81 hospitals (96%) report via the Internet and the remainder within a week after surgery. We know now that the estimations made from 1979 until 1992 were valid [12], and at present 229,031 primary hip arthroplasties have been registered.

End-Points

The current failure end-point in the analyses is revision of either of the components. The revision burden, defined as the fraction of revisions in relation to all primary and revision procedures is used as a crude figure for national and international comparisons. Starting with 2003 annual

report (www.jru.orthop.gu.se), all results are presented according to the Kaplan-Meier survival method using the date of death (provided by the Swedish Cause-of-Death Register). Separate survival analyses for cup and stem are presented (example see ◘ Fig. 11.1). In the survival analysis for the cup the definition of failure is the exchange of the cup or total revision. The analysis for the stem is performed in a similar way. When a total revision is performed, the register does not display information on which of the components failed. Based on a consensus meeting within the profession in 1996, implant survival for the individual units is public data.

Multivariate Cox´s regression and Poisson regression are used for more complex risk models. However, whatever complex multivariate analyses we undertake, it is important to note that the register's advantage *and* drawback is that its results depict the performance of »the average surgeon«.

Other open surgical procedures, apart from revisions, constitute only 10% of re-operations. Since 2000 we ceased registration of closed reduction of implant dislocation due to a suspected, systematically under-reporting of this procedure.

To increase the sensitivity of the register, patient-related outcome parameters and a radiographic analysis are now included. A standardised follow-up protocol was introduced as a pilot project in 2001 in the Western region in Sweden. All patients completed a questionnaire containing 10 items including Charnley's functional categories (A, B and C) [1], a pain visual analogue scale (VAS) (0–100, none to unbearable) and the EQ-5D [13]

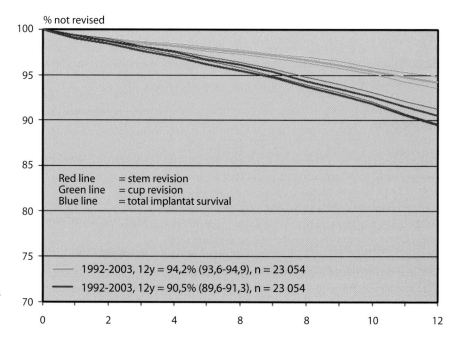

◘ **Fig. 11.1.** Survival for all diagnoses and all reasons for revision. The survival rate and 95% confidence limit are indicated for the Charnley stem (*red line*) and the Ogee all poly, cemented cup (*green line*). The *blue line* indicates the survival rate for both components preoperatively and at 1 year, with the intention to repeat the measurement at 6 and 10 years. The functional class will allow for correction of comorbidity. The EQ-5D is a global health index, with a weighted total value for health, with the lowest value –0.594 and a maximum of 1.0. When the index is used for cost-utility analyses, all negative values are set to 0.0. As a complement to the follow-up instrument a satisfaction VAS (0–100, satisfied to dissatisfied) has been added. Data are preoperatively entered via an internet application either by a secretary or by the patient via a touch screen.

At the clinical follow-up (1, 6 and 10 years) the questionnaire is mailed to the patient. Each unit can log in with a password and obtain the EQ-5D index, Charnley category and pain and satisfaction VAS results in real time and compare their results with the remaining users. The Internet site also includes a feature allowing the individual unit to download its own data at any time.

No results from the EQ-5D data will be presented in this chapter.

Results

Primary THA – Patient Demographics

The annual THA incidence in Sweden is approximately 12,500 procedures (7.7–10.2 per 10,000 inhabitants).

More women than men are operated on and the women are at a slightly higher age. Generally, indications for THA have been remarkably stable over the past 20 years although with a different distribution in patients under 50 years of age (◘ Table 11.1).

Primary THA – Implants Used

There has been a marked concentration to fewer well-functioning prosthetic systems for all three fixation principles over the past 10 years. Among cemented systems, the Lubinus SP II dominates and has increased continuously during the last five years, followed by the Exeter and the Spectron prostheses. More than 90% of the total hip replacements performed in Sweden have been all cemented reflecting a rather conservative and evidence based attitude among Swedish orthopaedic surgeons. Four uncemented prosthetic systems, comprising 580 THAs in 2003 and all with well a documented survival in the medium-term, account for some 80%. Hybrid implants accounted for 512 hips in 2003. The Trilogy cup in combination with Spectron and Lubinus stems are currently dominant. The number of uncemented and hybrid arthroplasties have been increasing during the last two years (◘ Figs. 11.2 to 11.5). The specific age, fixation- and diagnosis-related distribution (1992–2003) are presented in ◘ Tables 11.1 and 11.2.

◘ **Table 11.1.** Diagnoses at the index operation 1992–2003. Diagnoses are indicated for age groups: <50 years, 50–59 years, 60–75 years and older than 75 years

Diagnoses	<50 Years		50–59 Years		60–75 Years		>75 Years		Total	
	[n]	[%]	[n]	[%]	[n]	[%]	[n]	[%]	[n]	[%]
Primary osteoarthritis	3,129	52.0	13,067	78.2	51,775	80,5	27,584	66.9	95,555	74,5
Fracture	207	3.4	686	4.1	5,106	7,9	8,658	21.0	14,657	11,4
Inflammatory disease	1,058	17.6	1,140	6.8	2,770	4,3	927	2.2	5,895	4,6
Avascular necrosis	374	6.2	456	2.7	1,298	2,0	1,569	3.8	3,697	2,9
Childhood disease	762	12.7	636	3.8	489	0,8	116	0.3	2,003	1,6
Secondary osteoarthritis	95	1.6	110	0.7	469	0,7	619	1.5	1,293	1,0
Tumour	71	1.2	127	0.8	234	0,4	125	0.3	557	0,4
Traumatic osteoarthritis	51	0.8	48	0.3	121	0,2	115	0.3	335	0,3
(Missing)	274	4.6	437	2.6	2,094	3,3	1,542	3.7	4,347	3,4
Total	6,021	100	16,707	100	64,356	100	41,255	100	128,339	100

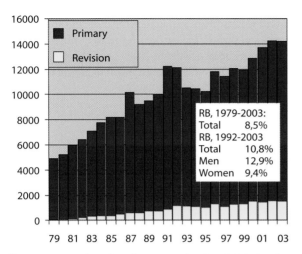

Fig. 11.2. Annual number of primary and revision THR in Sweden 1979–2003. The revision burden (*RB*) is indicated for all observations and for 1992–2003 with separate RB for women and men

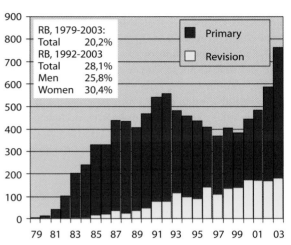

Fig. 11.4. Annual number of uncemented primary THR and the revisions generated from uncemented replacements in Sweden 1979–2003. The revision burden (*RB*) is indicated for all observations and for 1992–2003 with separate RB for women and men

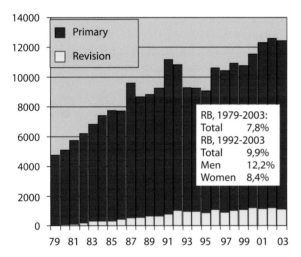

Fig. 11.3. Annual number of cemented primary THR and the revisions generated from cemented replacements in Sweden 1979–2003. The revision burden (*RB*) is indicated for all observations and for 1992–2003 with separate RB for women and men

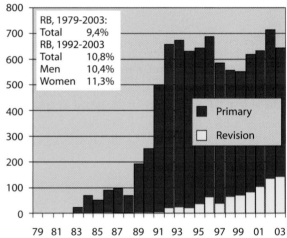

Fig. 11.5. Annual number of hybrid primary THR and the revisions generated from hybrid replacements in Sweden 1979–2003. The revision burden (*RB*) is indicated for all observations and for 1992–2003 with separate RB for women and men

Table 11.2. Type of fixation at the index operation 1992–2003. Fixation in four categories: cemented, hybrid (uncemented cup/cemented stem), uncemented and reverse hybrid is indicated for age groups: <50 years, 50–59 years, 60–75 years and older than 75 years

Type of Fixation	<50 Years		50–59 Years		60–75 Years		>75 Years		Total	
	[n]	[%]	[n]	[%]	[n]	[%]	[n]	[%]	[n]	[%]
Cemented	2,807	46.6	11,403	68.3	60,971	94.7	40,679	98.6	115,860	90.3
Hybrid	1,354	22.5	2,812	16.8	2,247	3.5	287	0.7	6,700	5.2
Uncemented	1,532	25.4	1,894	11.3	665	1.0	15	0.0	4,106	3.2
Inverse hybrid	273	4.5	513	3.1	271	0.4	33	0.1	1,090	0.8
(Missing)	55	0.9	85	0.5	202	0.3	241	0.6	583	0.5
Total	6,021	100	16,707	100	64,356	100	41,255	100	128,339	100

Primary THA – Regions and Units

The number of primary procedures is increasing in rural hospitals, which might reflect the political ambition to concentrate prosthetic surgery to fewer elective units. Since 2001, these units have performed more THAs than the county hospitals. There is a reciprocal decrease in the regional and university hospitals.

Figures 11.6 and 11.7 illustrate the changes over time in crude prosthetic survival for each participating unit. The average national 10-year survival has improved from 89.4% (±0.15) to 92.5% (±0.15) between the observation periods 1979–1991 and 1992–2003. During the period 1979–1991, 27% of the units did not differ significantly from the national average; 19% performed worse, and 44% performed better. For the period 1992–2003, 53% did not statistically differ from the national average, only 13% performed worse and 34% were above average.

Revision Burden

The revision burden for the period 1992–2003 was 9.9% for cemented implants, 28.1% for uncemented implants and 10.8% for hybrid implants (see Figs. 11.2 to 11.5). For 1979–2003 the total revision burden for cemented implants was 7.8%. During the last ten-year period, the revision burden has been higher for men than that for women with the exception of uncemented and hybrid fixations. The revision burden for the uncemented and hybrid implants had a decelerating increase.

Re-Operations and Revision

Revision was the dominant subsequent procedure, accounting for 86% of all re-operations. Among the revisions aseptic loosening (73.9%), deep infection (7.9%), dislocation (7.5%) and periprosthetic fractures (5.7%) are the primary causes (Table 11.3). A small, but continuous reduction of the total number of revisions has been observed over the past 5 years, which might indicate a trend of improved national quality, since the number of patients at risk is constantly increasing. Patients with index diagnoses of rheumatoid joint disease and sequel to childhood hip disease are overrepresented in the group of multiple revisions as are those revised due to deep infection, periprosthetic fractures and dislocation (Tables 11.3 and 11.4).

The reasons for revision have been relatively stationary during recent years, except for revisions due to dislocation and/or technical reasons which have increased. For patients with 5 years' follow-up the cumulative revision rate is 5–6 times higher for the group operated on in 1998 compared to those operated on in 1984 (Fig. 11.8). During the entire period the quality has improved in terms of fewer revisions because of aseptic loosening (Fig. 11.9)

For cemented implants the results for the stem are generally better than the cup, with the flanged Charnley cup (see Fig. 11.1) as the sole exception. In uncemented and hybrid implants, the stem results are generally good, whereas the cups show poorer result.

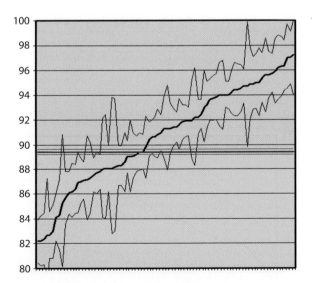

Fig. 11.6. Survival rate with 95% confidence limits 1979–1991 for the individual units/hospitals in Sweden. All diagnoses and all reasons for revision are included. Each tick mark on the x axis indicates one hospital unit. The national average 89.4% is shown with *horizontal red line* (95% confidence limits indicated). 44% of the units had a result significant above the average and 19% below

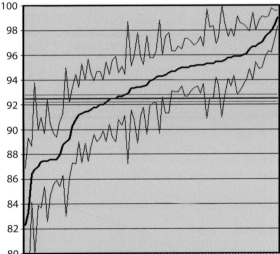

Fig. 11.7. Survival rate with 95% confidence limits 1992–2003 for the individual units/hospitals in Sweden. All diagnoses and all reasons for revision are included. Each tick mark on the x axis indicates one hospital unit. The national average 92.5% is shown with *horizontal red line* (95% confidence limits indicated). 34% of the units had a result significant above the average and 13% below

Table 11.3. Diagnoses at index operation 1979–2003 in Sweden. The diagnoses at the index operation are indicated for first revisions and for 1, 2 and >2 repeated revisions

Diagnose at Index Operation	0		1		2		>2		Total	
	[n]	[%]	[n]	[%]	[n]	[%]	[n]	[%]	[n]	[%]
Primary osteoarthritis	13,252	74.1	2,034	71.6	361	69.4	82	65.1	15,729	73.6
Fracture	1,684	9.4	233	8.2	36	6.9	6	4.8	1,959	9.2
Inflammatory disease	1,451	8.1	272	9.6	61	11.7	15	11.9	1,799	8.4
Childhood disease	843	4.7	182	6.4	38	7.3	15	11.9	1,078	5.0
Avascular necrosis	280	1.6	46	1.6	9	1.7	2	1.6	337	1.6
Traumatic osteoarthritis	150	0.8	45	1.6	9	1.7	6	4.8	210	1.0
Secondary osteoarthritis	49	0.3	6	0.2	1	0.2	0	0.0	56	0.3
Tumour	23	0.1	5	0.2	2	0.4	0	0.0	30	0.1
(Missing)	149	0.8	17	0.6	3	0.6	0	0.0	169	0.8
Total	17,881	100	2,840	100	520	100	126	100	21,367	100

Table 11.4. Reason for revision 1979 – 2003 in Sweden. The reason for revisions is indicated for first revisions and for 1, 2 and >2 repeated revisions.

Reason for Revision	0		1		2		>2		Total	
	[n]	[%]	[n]	[%]	[n]	[%]	[n]	[%]	[n]	[%]
Aseptic loosening	13,581	76.0	1,829	64.4	319	61.3	59	46.8	15,788	73.9
Infection	1,292	7.2	316	11.1	64	12.3	26	20.6	1,698	7.9
Dislocation	1,176	6.6	325	11.4	69	13.3	27	21.4	1,597	7.5
Periprosthetic fracture	966	5.4	221	7.8	38	7.3	2	1.6	1,227	5.7
Technical reason	447	2.5	71	2.5	17	3.3	2	1.6	537	2.5
Implant fracture	276	1.5	45	1.6	7	1.3	3	2.4	331	1.5
Miscellaneous	86	0.5	24	0.8	5	1.0	6	4.8	121	0.6
Pain only	57	0.3	9	0.3	1	0.2	1	0.8	68	0.3
Total	17,881	100	2,840	100	520	100	126	100	21,367	100

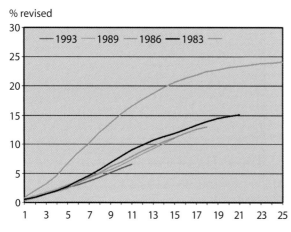

Fig. 11.8. Cumulative revision rate for all diagnoses and all reasons for revision for 1979, 1983, 1986, 1989 and 1993

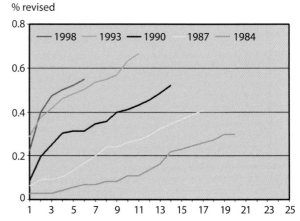

Fig. 11.9. Cumulative revision rate for recurrent dislocation for 1979, 1983, 1986, 1989 and 1993

Regions

The unadjusted procedure frequency per 100,000 inhabitants for patients aged 50 years and older and with the diagnosis of primary osteoarthritis is shown for the period 1992–2003. The national average is given for comparisons between the different regions (◘ Fig. 11.10). The variation in procedure frequency (77–102/100 000 inhabitants) can be explained by a real difference in incidence of osteoarthritis requiring treatment but more likely also reflects limited resources, as for example in the Western region.

Discussion

The overall aim for the national register is to improve the quality of THA. The register can generate hypotheses suitable for either a specific study based on register data [5] or a carefully planned prospective clinical study. This is in accordance with the experience from the Norwegian Register [3]. The failure end-point definition used in registries has traditionally been revision. Revision is a well-defined event, but can potentially bias the result as use of both patient satisfaction and radiographic changes probably would give an inferior outcome [4]. In the 2003 report from the Swedish Total Hip Arthroplasty Register (www.jru.orthop.gu.se) the results are based on data for each primary procedure, as this has been captured since 1992, and adjustment for death is made on-line, which is a major improvement compared with to previous reports where part of the statistics were based on assumptions and estimates [11]. The improved failure definitions and accuracy in the epidemiological data will also facilitate comparisons and benchmarking among different national registries. Many countries have used registries for several years (Finland, Norway, Denmark, New Zealand, Hungary, Australia, Canada, and Romania) and others have started recently or are in the planning phase (Czech Republic, Turkey, Slovakia, Moldova, Austria, England and Wales, France, Germany and the USA). Revision burden is one of the possible key figures that will enable crude comparison between different countries. It is important to clearly define and internationally agree on which key features that should be presented from national registers in order to make comparisons unbiased. An international Register Society could facilitate this process and there are ongoing efforts to initiate this.

A new and important development in the Swedish National THA Register during the past 3–4 years is the integration of individual patient related outcome data as well as the effort to register basic radiographic data. The Swedish health authorities encourage the registers current in function to give high priority for registration and inclusion of patient reported outcome [8].

General Swedish Trends in THA

The number of surgical procedures performed is probably too low to meet the future demands in an ageing population [9]. The regional variation in surgical procedures performed can be explained by local differences in patient demographics, incidence of disease, indications and economical restrictions.

For patients operated on in 1993, only about 5% are revised after 10 years. The proportion revised for the most common complication (aseptic loosening) has decreased to one third. In contrast, we see an increase in revision due to dislocation. This worrisome development may be related to an increase in primary THA for displaced cervical femoral fractures in the elderly, which is in contrast to a long tradition of using percutaneous techniques with screws or pins as the primary intervention [10]. Another explanation is the equally long tradition in Sweden with use of small head sizes (22 or 28 mm). Besides these possible reasons surgical education, choice of surgical technique and implant design are factors that need a more detailed analysis in future studies. It is of particular importance to establish whether there has been deterioration in the teaching of surgical techniques. At present, only some of these factors can be evaluated from the register data, but this is an example of a hypothesis generated from register data where a more detailed analysis could provide answers.

The openness in the register provides a basis for further discussions locally, as each orthopaedic unit receives (in the confidential report) revision data, no matter where in Sweden the patients have been revised. Since the register started, it has been anticipated that a continuous improvement will follow. Although we do not exactly know the true impact of the register, the rate of implant survival has improved from 89.4% to 92.5% between the two periods 1979–1991 and 1992–2003. It is very satisfying that the proportion of orthopaedic units lying

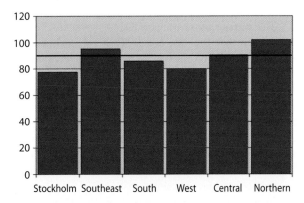

◘ **Fig. 11.10.** The unadjusted procedure frequency per 100,000 inhabitants. Six regions and patients aged 50 years and older with the diagnosis primary osteoarthritis are shown for the period 1992–2003. The national average 92 THR/100,000 is indicated with a *horizontal line*

significantly below the national average has decreased. However, the individual units' patient profiles influence their results and in the analyses case-mix differences are not taken into account. Still, these crude revision rates only give a rough idea.

There is a potential conflict of interest between hip implant manufacturers and results reported from the register. Several manufactures have expressed concern that the register inhibits evolution, market introduction and clinical use for better functioning implants and surgical techniques. Therefore the register, for more than 10 years, has invited all Swedish hip-implant manufacturers to their annual meetings. At these meetings, the current findings in the register are presented and discussed as well as any future projects. The companies can obtain on-line information about the results for their products. We have found this cooperation very rewarding.

The incidence of THA varies considerably between different regions as well as between different hospital types. There are systematic variations in choice of fixation mode because university and regional hospitals tend to use more unproven devices and mainly in prospective evaluations. Research implies closer clinical and radiographic follow-up. Such monitoring might result in earlier re-operations due to polyethylene wear and osteolysis without any apparent symptoms or gross loosening.

The revision burden (RB) in the different regions varies between 8.9% and 11.5%. The lowest RB is noted in the Northern regions. One explanation might be that mostly well-documented implants have been used, but cultural differences, patients' expectations and so-called patient's delay might play important roles as well. An important bias lays in the fact that even if general practitioners find patients with failed implants, the patients may still hesitate to be referred for additional surgery. Furthermore, there is a consistently higher RB for men compared to women. This difference is accentuated inter-regionally, with a variation for men between 14.3% and 10.2%. This finding may be related to greater body weight and higher activity level followed by increased implant wear.

The average age at primary THA is generally higher for women than for men except when the indication is sequel to childhood disease. Whether this reflects different access to surgery for women or that women systematically tend to seek orthopaedic consultancy later is not clear, but it is important to analyse this phenomenon further. However, sequel to childhood disease and rheumatoid joint disease, mostly in younger patients, are both over-represented in the multiple revision groups, indicating that such patients should prompt extra care both in the primary and revision situation.

In a public health economy subjected to financial restrictions computation of cost-utility is important in order to allocate resources as optimally as possible. THA has advantageous cost-effectiveness when compared with other medical treatments. League tables of different health care interventions, calculated by cost utility analyses, have been reported in the literature [6, 7, 14]. If a cost-utility table is going to be used as an instrument for allocating health-care resources, the studies should preferably be done at the same time, with use of identical outcome and cost evaluation methods. The current reported 10 years QALY cost of USD 3,000 (SEK 22,000) is very low compared to the Swedish threshold value USD 71,000 [2].

Summary and Conclusion

During recent years our ambition has been to improve the value of the register by analysing the patient's own opinion of the results of THA. The preoperative routine has shown and confirmed that the unoperated patient with osteoarthritis is suffering from severe pain and has low general health related quality of life. The prospective 1-year results show extremely good pain relief and very high patient satisfaction, and a self-rated quality of life (EQ5D) that is equal to that of an age-matched normal population. At present we can show a very good cost–utility result and assert THA in comparisons with other medical interventions when priorities and resource allocation are discussed. Increased sensitivity of the register analysis and creation of routines that can reduce the number of follow-up visits after hip-replacement surgery and late revision cases with severe bone stock deficiencies is desirable. Further validation of our follow-up instruments combined with development of new instruments for adequate economic evaluations of THA surgery may provide powerful tools to further optimise the results of THA.

In the Swedish population, cemented THA has given an excellent result with decreasing revision frequency despite an increasing number of patients at risk. This is probably a combined result of both adequate and contemporary surgical and cementing techniques as well as use of well-documented implants. The cemented THA is still a primary choice for the majority of Swedish patients in need of a THA.

> **Take Home Messages**
>
> - The purpose of the Swedish National Hip Arthroplasty Register is to monitor surgical techniques and prophylactic measures to minimise complications by persisting continuous feed-back to all THA-performing units and to provide a warning system for rapid implant failures.
> - All 81 orthopaedic units in Sweden, both public and private, participate voluntarily in the register. The vast majority of the clinics are reporting data directly via the Internet.

- All participating units have agreed to display their results open and public. However, the individual units' patient profiles influence their results and in the analyses case-mix differences are not taken into account.
- Although we do not exactly know the true impact of the register, the rate of overall implant survival (including poor designs) has improved from 89.4% to 92.5% between the two periods 1979–1991 and 1992–2003.
- The revision burden for cemented implants is considerable lower than for uncemented implant and even recent hybrid combinations. This is probably related to inferior liner fixation and polyethylene quality of the contemporary uncemented implants used in Sweden.
- Cemented THA constitutes more than 90% of the implant surgeries in Sweden and remains a primary choice for the majority of Swedish patients.
- The surgical technique is of outmost importance and must be implemented through extensive educational efforts.

References

1. Charnley J. The low friction arthroplasty of the hip. Springer, New York, 1979
2. Eichler H, Kong SX, Gerth WC, Mavros P, Jönsson B: Use of cost-effectiveness analysis in health-care resource allocation decision-making: how are cost-effectiveness thresholds expected to emerge? Value in Health 2004, 7(5):518–28
3. Furnes OH, Havelin LI, Espehaugh B, Engesæter LB, Lie SA, Vollset SE: Det norske leddproteseregistret – 15 nyttige år for pasienterne og helsevesenet. Tidskr Nor Lægeforen, 2003, 123:1367–69
4. Garellick G, Malchau H, HerbertsP: Survival of hip replacements. A comparison of a randomized trial and a registry. Clin Orthop 2000(375):157–67
5. Havelin LI, Espehaug B, Engesæter LB: The performance of two hydroxyapatitecoated acetabular cups compared with Charnley cups. From the Norwegian Arthroplasty Register. J Bone Joint Surg Br 2002, 84B:839–45.
6. Laupacis A, Bourne R, Rorabeck C, Feeny D, Wong C, Tugwell P, Leslie K, Bullas R: Costs of elective total hip arthroplasty during the first year. J Arthroplasty, 1994. 9: p. 481–92.
7. Maynard A: Developing the health care market. Econ J 1991, 101:1277
8. National Health Care. Quality Registries in Sweden 1999. 2000, Stockholm: Information Department, The Federation of Swedish County Councils
9. Ostendorf M, Johnell O, Malchau H, Dhert WJ, Schrijvers AJ, Verbout AJ. The epidemiology of total hip replacement in The Netherlands and Sweden: present status and future needs. Acta Orthop Scand, 2002, 73(3):282–6
10. Rogmark C, Carlsson A, Johnell O, Sernbo I: A prospective randomized trial of internal fixation versus arthroplasty for displaced fractures of the neck of the femur. Functional outcome for 450 patients at two years. j Bone Joint Surg Br, 2002, 84-B(2):183–88
11. Soderman P: On the validity of the results from the Swedish National Total Hip Arthroplasty register, in Dept. of Orthopaedic Surgery. Institute of Surgical Sciences. 2000, University of Gothenburg: Gothenburg
12. Soderman P, Malchau H, Herberts P, Johnell O. Are the findings in the Swedish National Total Hip Arthroplasty Register valid? A comparison between the Swedish National Total Hip Arthroplasty Register, the National Discharge Register, and the National Death Register. J Arthroplasty, 2000, 15(7):884–9
13. »The_EuroQol_Group«, EuroQol – a new facility for the measurement of health-related quality of life. Health Policy, 1990, 16(3):199–208
14. Williams A: Economics of coronary artery bypass grafting. Br Med J, 1985, 291:326–34

Part V   **Perioperative Management,
Complications and Prevention**

Chapter 12   **We Need a Good Anaesthetist
for Cemented THA   – 302**
A. Dow

Chapter 13   **Perioperative Management – Rapid Recovery
Protocol   – 307**
A.V. Lombardi, K.R. Berend, T.H. Mallory

Chapter 14   **Prevention of Infection   – 313**
L. Frommelt

Chapter 15   **Pulmonary Embolism in Cemented
Total Hip Arthroplasty   – 320**
M. Clarius, C. Heisel, S.J. Breusch

Chapter 16   **How Have I Done It? Evaluation Criteria   – 332**
E. Morscher

Chapter 17   **Mistakes and Pitfalls with Cemented Hips   – 340**
G. von Foerster

Chapter 18   **Revision is Not Difficult!   – 348**
T. Gehrke

We Need a Good Anaesthetist for Cemented THA

Alasdair Dow

Summary

In this chapter, the perioperative management of cemented total hip arthroplasty is presented from the anaesthetic point of view. Guidelines for selection, risk factors, type of anaesthetic and postoperative care are given.

The provision of anaesthesia for cemented hip arthroplasty can be considered under a number of sections:

- Preoperative selection and preparation
- Anaesthetic practice, including monitoring
- Postoperative care, including analgesia and blood loss strategies

Preoperative Selection and Preparation

The aim of the preoperative assessment process should be to provide an efficient throughput of patients, to minimise the number of operation-day cancellations. Patients should receive sufficient information to allow them to decide on the risks and benefits that their proposed surgery offers. The ideal arrangement would be to have a preoperative assessment clinic, which is staffed by an experienced anaesthetist in the adjacent area. Ideally, the anaesthetist would either be likely to provide anaesthesia for that patient, or else be in regular communication with the anaesthetists that do. It would be ideal for every patient to be seen by an anaesthetist at the time of booking for surgery. However, this approach would require the provision of considerable anaesthetic input. A more practical approach is to ask the surgeon or referring family physician to »flag-up« any particular problems that may influence outcome from surgery. It is hard to be proscriptive about such situations, and it is preferable to allow the surgeon to refer those patients that cause concern for whatever reason. A useful aide-memoire, that is not exclusive, would include:

- previous cardiac or thoracic surgery,
- unstable angina, angina at rest,
- exercise limited prior to hip disease to less than 100 metres flat walking,
- those unable to sleep with less than 3 pillows,
- recurrent transient ischaemic attacks (TIAs),
- known severe peripheral vascular disease,
- previous documented anaesthetic problems,
- prolonged previous admission to intensive care.

The preoperative assessment clinic should include a discussion on:

- the type of anaesthetic proposed,
- likely need for augmented postoperative care e.g. ICU, HDU,
- the associated risks of morbidity and mortality.

The provision of a figure for predicted mortality is a difficult and subjective issue. The quoted mortality for primary total hip arthroplasty (THA) is as low as 0.1% in some series [13]. A more commonly quoted figure of around 0.3–0.4% is supported by other studies [16]. However, these figures are an overall guide, and do not take into account the effect on an individual of coexisting disease. One strategy for quantifying risk for the patient is to discover the 30-day mortality rate for primary arthroplasty for the local unit, or a regional figure where there is no local figure. Fit patients can then be quoted this figure, while multiples of this figure are used for those with co-existing disease. It is important to point out to patients that the figure is an average, and that no certainty exists for the safe provision of anaesthesia or surgery.

Operative Practice

The choice of anaesthetic technique is usually based on the following factors:
- preference of anaesthetist and surgeon,
- duration and associated problems of surgery,
- patient preference,
- associated medication and medical conditions.

It is unrealistic to suggest that an ideal anaesthetic exists for hip arthroplasty. However, the following points may influence practitioners, with regard the unique features of hip arthroplasty.

General Anaesthesia/Sedation/Awake

The choice of the degree of sedation depends on a number of factors. General anaesthesia will be required if regional block is not employed, or if the block used is inadequate for surgical anaesthesia. Lumbo-sacral plexus block falls into the latter category: It provides an acceptable method of postoperative analgesia, but may not be adequately »dense« to avoid the need for balanced general anaesthesia.

The practice of having an awake patient may be safer for patients with certain types of medical problems. Thus, patients with known airway problems such as sleep apnoea or difficult anatomical airways will be unlikely to develop airway problems if sedation is avoided. Further, patients with severe respiratory disease may deteriorate if consciousness is lost. In practice, however, these problems are rarely so severe that sedation cannot be cautiously used. Further, an awake patient does not guarantee the absence of such problems. Many patients prefer to be sedated or unconscious, and fear the noises associated with arthroplasty. Additionally, many surgeons find it distracting to have patients talking throughout the case, and such interaction may make the surgical task harder. A specific criticism of the awake technique is that conscious patients will often cough at the point of cement insertion, which can cause operative site movement. This is undesirable during insertion of either femoral or acetabular components.

Thus, many practitioners include sedation or general anaesthesia as part of the anaesthetic technique for arthroplasty. General anaesthesia has the advantage that it can be continued for any duration of time, whereas sedation often becomes ineffective after 2–3 hours. This is because many patients find the lateral position (where used) too uncomfortable, and so the technique may have to be converted into general anaesthesia during the procedure. This may be technically difficult, and it is preferable to select general anaesthesia from the outset for operations of uncertain duration.

Choice of Regional Block

The methods of local anaesthesia block for hip arthroplasty include:
- spinal (subarachnoid) anaesthesia,
- epidural anaesthesia,
- lumbo-sacral plexus block,
- femoral/sciatic/lateral cutaneous nerve of thigh.

There are advantages to each of the techniques, and also rare but potentially serious side effect from each type of block. The central neural axis blocks, epidural and spinal, have the benefit of inducing hypotension, and also increasing pelvic venous blood flow. This results in lower operative blood loss [3]. Further, the incidence of DVT and PE is reduced, although this benefit may not be as great as previously described [7]. Many of the studies looking at these blocks and the association with thrombo-embolism, are studies that pre-date the introduction of foot pumps, low molecular weight heparin, thrombo-embolism stockings and early mobilisation. It is unclear what their place is in today's practice, but they still confer some benefit in reducing the risk of DVT/PE. The major (but rare) complication of central neural block is neural axis damage, either of the spinal cord/cauda equina or a spinal nerve root. The practice of inserting the block awake has not been shown to reduce the prevalence of such injury [12]. However, the occurrence of pain in an awake patient during needle or catheter insertion, would alert the operator to a potential nerve root or cord injury. There are some clinical conditions where block insertion may be easier in the asleep patient, and the practice should be influenced by local/national best practice guidance.

The lumbo-sacral plexus block has the benefit of no risk of central axis injury. However, injury to the plexus has been reported and it should not be assumed that it is a technique without risk [2]. This block does not provide the same degree of intraoperative hypotension as a central axis block, and there is little data to suggest it confers the same benefit on the incidence of thrombo-embolism. Despite this, the medico-legal climate in some countries may make it an attractive option, given the high costs of claims for central neural axis damage [4].

The femoral/sciatic/lateral cutaneous nerve of thigh block has similar advantages and disadvantages to the lumbo-sacral plexus block. It generally takes longer to perform than a central axis block, and will usually require the addition of general anaesthesia.

The authors own practice is to administer spinal anaesthesia plus light general anaesthesia, for the majority of patients undergoing primary hip arthroplasty. The addition of drugs like clonidine or morphine/diamorphine to the CSF provides more prolonged analgesia than local anaesthetic alone [1]. However, there is a higher incidence of nausea and vomiting with the addition of opiates [9]. This complication needs to be considered against more modern techniques of balanced postoperative analgesia (see below).

Prevention of Complications During Cement Insertion

The problem of »cement reaction« was first described more than 30 years ago [6], as a sudden drop in blood pressure following the insertion of cement, particularly into the femoral canal. The current theory on the likely mechanism suggests that pressurisation of cement increases pressure in the femoral canal or acetabulum (► chapter 15). This leads to fat or air being forced into the circulation, which then reaches the pulmonary circulation via the right side of the heart. This creates a fat or air pulmonary embolism, which results in right heart strain and failure, as well as drop in pulmonary blood flow. The systemic arterial oxygen level drops because of low pulmonary blood flow, and systemic blood pressure drops because of low cardiac output. Patients with limited cardiac reserve, especially the elderly, and those who are hypovolaemic, are unable to compensate for the drop in pressure by systemic vasoconstriction. The resultant fall in blood pressure, especially diastolic, may lead to myocardial ischaemia or cardiac arrest.

The prevention of this problem is based on an understanding of the aetiology. This relies on:
- reduction of pressure within the air chamber distal to the cement,
- better fluid loading to increase the response to low cardiac output,
- use of vasoconstrictors/inotropes when hypotension occurs,
- recognition of at-risk patients.

The pressure in the air pocket in the femoral canal may be reduced by inserting a suction catheter into the distal femur, and aspirating on it as cement is introduced into the femur. This catheter is then removed as the cement is inserted, and this should produce a reduced pressure at the cement/marrow vessel interface [10].

Aggressive fluid-loading usually means the use of colloid or crystalloid infusion prior to cement insertion. The volume of fluid used is less critical in the fit patient, but the patient with poor cardiac reserve may require closer control. This can be done by the use of a CVP or PA catheter, although both take time to insert and have associated risks. A newer technique is the use of pulse or arterial waveform analysis to assess cardiac filling. The oesophageal Doppler probe allows an estimate to made of cardiac filling from the corrected flow time (FTC) of the aortic signal close to the oesophagus. This probe is cheap, and quick and easy to insert. It does suffer from operator and inter-patient variability, but the trend in FTC is a useful guide to cardiac filling [14].

The other major risk factor for the development of severe arterial hypotension following cement impaction appears to be poor cardiac reserve, and increasing age. These two risk factors often co-exist. The presence of cardiac failure, or known LV dysfunction in patients over the age of 80 years, is indicative of high risk for the development of a marked drop in cardiac output following cement impaction.

Closer control of filling volume, when combined with generous use of vasoconstrictors and inotropes, may prevent marked falls in blood pressure and cardiac output following cement impaction. Thus, the anaesthetist should monitor the cardiac filling state by use of a device such as the oesophageal Doppler. IV fluids should be given to a normal filling pressure in advance of cement impaction to try to reduce the reduction in cardiac output. The anaesthetist needs to anticipate the timing of cement impaction, and ensure that inotropes and vasoconstrictors are immediately available. The use of an arterial line will allow prompt and early detection of hypotension, but many anaesthetists feel that this form of invasive monitoring represents an unnecessary risk for the majority of hip arthroplasty patients. However, high-risk patients, as described above, may benefit from such monitoring to give early warning of potential cardio-vascular collapse.

Postoperative Care

The majority of primary hip arthroplasty patients will be mobilised later on the operative day, or on the first postoperative day. The anaesthetic technique should ensure that this goal is possible, and there are a number of considerations to allow this to occur.

Nausea and Vomiting

There is no anaesthetic technique that avoids nausea or vomiting in all patients. There is good evidence that a subset of patients is likely to vomit regardless of the anaesthetic technique employed, or the surgery performed. Such patients may be identified preoperatively from their history, and may benefit from an anaesthetic technique that is aimed at maximum reduction in nausea and vomiting. This would include anti-emetic premedication, avoidance of nitrous oxide and opiates where possible. In addition, regular anti-emetics can be used, including the use of some newer $5HT_3$ antagonists such as ondansetron. Two older agents, dexamethasone and cyclizine have been shown to be highly cost-effective, and may be useful as adjuncts or alternatives to other modern therapies [11].

Postoperative Analgesia

The current trend in analgesia for hip arthroplasty favours the following sequence [15]:

- use of non-opiate analgesics preoperatively,
- use of spinal/epidural/regional local anaesthetic,
- infiltration of a mixture of local anaesthetic/non-steroidal/morphine into the wound at the end of surgery,
- prescription of regular non-opiate analgesics in the post-operative period rather than an as-required basis,
- use of i.v. or oral opiates on a rescue basis for patients with severe pain unrelieved by the above methods.

The choice of mixture to infiltrate into the wound at the end of surgery is a matter for personal preference. However, the author favours the use of 60–80 ml of bupivacaine 0.125% with adrenaline 1 in 400,000, with the addition of an injectable COX-2 analgesic, and 10 mg of morphine. This mixture can provide analgesia for 18–24 hours, although additional analgesics may be required. It avoids the problems associated with prolonged epidural analgesia, and the limitation of leg movement that this induces.

Blood Conservation/Transfusion

There is a variety of ways to limit the use of banked blood in the patient undergoing primary hip arthroplasty. These include:

- reduction of perioperative blood loss,
- return of shed blood in the perioperative period (autologous transfusion),
- protocols to control the administration of banked blood.

The perioperative blood loss may be influenced by both the surgical and anaesthetic technique. The use of intraoperative hypotension reduces loss from the arterial tree, and contributes to a reduced total blood loss. It is impossible to be proscriptive about an acceptable level of perioperative blood pressure that is safe: the majority of the morbidity from excessive hypotension is renal or neurological and is very rare. The author's own practice is to allow the systolic BP to fall as low as the level of the preoperative diastolic pressure, for the shortest time possible. The rationale behind this is that hypertensive patients have impaired cerebral and renal vascular autoregulation, and do not tolerate falls in blood pressure as well as their normotensive comparators. In addition, it is important to note that operative site blood loss is not just influenced by the systemic arterial pressure. The downstream venous pressure that drains the operative site may be just as important, and is influenced by the operative position, and the venous tone. The posterior approach in association with a lateral position reduces blood loss in comparison to other operative techniques. Further, the use of spinal or epidural blockade leads to improved pelvic venous blood flow, and is associated with reduced operative loss [8].

Return of shed blood can be achieved by the use of cell-washing devices in the perioperative phase, and re-infusion drains that are inserted for postoperative care. The cost of these techniques may limit their value, although cost is not the only reason to favour re-infusion of the patient's own blood over banked blood transfusion. Further, some surgeons prefer to avoid the use of a drain as part of their technique, and so this method may not apply. The use of a red cell salvage/wash technique in the operative period may require a certain minimum volume to allow the first wash cycle. For many units this minimum volume is not routinely shed, and the cost of disposables and labour to retrieve this unused shed blood is not justified. Thus, the technique may be useful in selected patients who are anticipated to have higher blood loss, or routinely where banked blood is scarce or contraindicated. Patients with a preoperative haemoglobin level of less than 12 g/dl have a high chance of requiring postoperative transfusion. Thus, it is advisable to employ a cell salvage system for these patients, as the cost and blood saving is more likely to justify the expense of the cell salvage technique.

The guidance on the haemoglobin threshold for transfusion depends on a number of factors:

- availability of banked blood,
- patient preference,
- associated cardio-respiratory disease,
- preoperative haemoglobin.

Generally, most practitioners accept national guidance that an absolute trigger of Hb <7 g/dl, and a relative trigger of <8 g/dl are reasonable thresholds [5]. However, the final decision depends on the individual patient, and their response/tolerance of postoperative anaemia. In the author's experience, it is often the size of the drop in haemoglobin rather than the final figure that influences the need for postoperative banked blood transfusion.

> **Take Home Messages**
>
> - Preoperative identification of at-risk patients allows better use of resources, including operative time.
> - The addition of a central axis local anaesthetic blockade reduces the incidence of thrombo-embolism, and the magnitude of operative blood loss.
> - A combination approach to analgesia in the postoperative period, including reduction of opioid use, can reduce postoperative nausea and assist in earlier discharge.
> - The threshold for blood transfusion varies between patients, and is influenced by associated disease, and preoperative haemoglobin.

References

1. Abuzaid H, Prys-Roberts C et al. The influence of diamorphine on spinal anaesthesia induced with isobaric 0.5% bupivacaine. Anaesthesia 1993;48(6):492–5

2. Aveline C, Bonnet F. Delayed retroperitoneal haematoma after failed lumbar plexus block. Br J Anaesth 2004; 93(4):589–91

3. Bannister GC, Young SK et al. Control of bleeding in cemented arthroplasty. J Bone Joint Surg Br 1990: 72(3):444–6

4. Buckenmaier CC 3rd, Xenos JS et al. Lumbar plexus block with perineural catheter and sciatic nerve block for total hip arthroplasty. J Arthroplasty 2002; 17(4):499–502

5. Hardy JF. Should we reconsider triggers for red blood cell transfusion? Acta Anaesthesiol Belg 2003; 54(4):287–95

6. Kepes ER, Underwood PS et al. Intraoperative death associated with acrylic bone cement. Report of two cases. JAMA 1972; 222(5):576–7

7. McKenzie PJ, Wishart HY et al. Effects of anaesthetic technique on deep vein thrombosis. A comparison of subarachnoid and general anaesthesia. Br J Anaesth. 1985; 57(9):853–7

8. Modig J. Regional anaesthesia and blood loss. Acta Anaesthesiol Scand Suppl. 1988; 89:44–8

9. Parlow JL, Costache I et al. Single-dose haloperidol for the prophylaxis of postoperative nausea and vomiting after intrathecal morphine. Anesth Analg. 2004; 98(4):1072–6

10. Parvizi J, Holiday AD et al. The Frank Stichfield Award. Sudden death during primary hip arthroplasty. Clin Orthop. 1999; 369:39–48.

11. Rollins G. Guidelines outline strategies to reduce post-operative nausea and vomiting. Rep Med Guidel Outcome Res. 2002; 13(8):9–10.

12. Rosen M. Regional anaesthesia – awake or asleep? Anaesthesia. 1999; 54(5):510

13. Sharrock NE, Cazan MG et al. Changes in mortality after total hip and knee arthroplasty over a ten-year period. Anaesth Analg 1995; 80(2):242–8

14. Sinclair S, James S et al. Intraoperative intravascular volume optimisation and length of hospital stay after repair of proximal femoral fracture: randomised controlled trial. BMJ. 1997; 315(7113):909–12.

15. Skinner HB, Shintani EY. Results of a multimodal analgesic trial involving patients with total hip or total knee arthroplasty. Am J Orthop. 2004; 33(2):85–92.

16. Warwick D. Thromboprophylaxis and death after total hip replacement. J Bone Joint Surg Br 1998; 80(2):370–1

Perioperative Management – Rapid Recovery Protocol

Adolph V. Lombardi, Keith R. Berend, Thomas H. Mallory

Summary

The perioperative care of the total hip-arthroplasty (THA) patient has undergone a significant evolution similar to advancements in the technical performance of the operative procedure itself. The concept of a rapid recovery protocol is the establishment of aggressive perioperative programmes with the distinct intention to speed recovery, reduce morbidity and complications, and create a programme of efficiency while maintaining the highest level of patient care. The establishment of a focused care plan will align short-term goals of THA with long-term goals which are to relieve pain, increase function, provide stability, and maintain durability.

Introduction

Total hip arthroplasty (THA) has evolved into one of the most successful operative interventions in the field of orthopaedics. The past three decades have witnessed significant technical improvements in the actual surgical procedure. THA consistently provides pain relief and improvement in the quality of life which is sustained into the second and third decades of follow-up [2]. However, THA represents a significant event in a patient's life. It is incumbent upon health-care providers to develop and provide a comprehensive perioperative care plan for the patient and his family. During the past three decades, the authors have developed and refined a rapid recovery protocol for patients undergoing THA. The outline of this protocol is presented in ◘ Table 13.1.

◘ **Table 13.1.** Fundamentals of the joint implant surgeons rapid road to recovery

1	Comprehensive review of patient's past medical history
2	Preoperative orthopaedic evaluation
3	Preoperative education with educational materials
4	Surgery scheduling
5	Comprehensive medical evaluation
6	Informational videos and surgical consent
7	Preoperative review of entire perioperative protocol with patient and family
8	Preoperative physical therapy evaluation and commencement of rehabilitation
9	Perioperative nutrition and smoking cessation
10	Discharge planning and home requirements
11	Preoperative radiographic planning conference
12	Pre-emptive analgesia
13	Multimodal perioperative analgesia
14	Efficient and accurate surgery
15	Wound-healing adjuncts
16	Clinical pathways focused on early mobilisation
17	Full weight-bearing with crutches or walker for 3 to 4 weeks, then cane as needed
18	Hospital discharge planning for postoperative day 1 or 2
19	Post-discharge nursing contact
20	6 week follow-up clinical evaluation

Preoperative Assessment, Education and Pre-Arthroplasty Rehabilitation

The initial assessment of the patient commences with a comprehensive review of the patients past medical history. Detailed »review-of-systems« forms have been created which can be completed by the patient prior to or at the time of initial consultation. The accuracy and completeness of this information must be documented by the health-care provider at the time of initial assessment. With the appropriate transfer of information, this assessment can be utilised not only at the time of orthopaedic consultation but also at the time of preoperative medical evaluation as well as admission to the hospital in an effort to avoid the often all too frequent repetition of questioning [20]. The patient should be requested to complete standardised outcome measures. A thorough and complete orthopaedic evaluation must be performed and documented, and a preoperative assessment score calculated.

Once the patient's need for THA has been established, preoperative education should commence. Patient education materials have become readily available and include a multimedia approach. Printed perioperative brochures outline details of the entire operative intervention. These brochures deal with a number of topics ranging from »frequently asked questions« to »intimacy following THA.« Educational videos and interactive computer-based programmes can assist patients in comprehension of both preoperative and postoperative expectations. Videos of the actual surgical procedure can be created for more inquisitive patients who wish to have an in-depth understanding. Frequently, patients will request to see and handle an actual prosthesis, and demonstration models are available in the clinic. Personalised guide books for THA which outline pre- and postoperative exercises, perioperative nutrition, and review what to expect and how to prepare, are extremely beneficial in assisting patients and their families. Additionally, the World Wide Web serves as a source of information for many patients and families. Physicians should direct patients and their families to appropriate online sources. Scheduling for the surgical procedure begins after the pros and cons of the surgical intervention and potential complications have been reviewed with the patient.

A comprehensive medical evaluation should be performed preoperatively. This should include an assessment of co-morbidities and appropriate interventions to optimise the patient's preoperative medical status [11]. While this can be performed by the patient's family or internal medicine practitioner, we have obtained better results by establishing a relationship with a group of internal medicine hospitalists who specialise in the preoperative and perioperative medical management of joint-replacement patients. Upon optimisation of the patient's preoperative medical status, a review of the entire perioperative protocol should be performed with the patient and family. This discussion should include discharge planning and home requirements. A comprehensive physical therapy evaluation should be performed in an effort to establish a baseline and to determine ultimate goals. Patients are instructed before surgery in a preoperative physical therapy conditioning programme and the requisite postoperative exercise regimes.

The benefit of preoperative multi-media education of patients and family and pre-arthroplasty rehabilitation is not only an enhanced comprehension of the entire operative intervention which will concomitantly allay anxiety and facilitate a smoother transition through the entire perioperative period. Liebergall et al. [17] evaluated the effects of preadmission social-work interventions in the form of education, discharge planning and hospital length of stay. Patients who received intense preadmission screening with psychosocial evaluation, discharge planning, coordination of nursing and physical therapy interventions and monitoring of medical testing before elective THA had reduced hospital stays compared with those who did not receive preadmission screening. They concluded that an emphasis on preoperative education and assessments is one method to decrease hospital stay. Crowe and Henderson [5] evaluated the effectiveness of an individually tailored preoperative rehabilitation programme in patients undergoing THA. This preoperative multi-disciplinary rehabilitation and education included information about the hospital stay, early discharge planning, and home preparation. The authors demonstrated that patients who received this focused preoperative rehabilitation rapidly achieved discharge criteria and had shorter hospital stays. In addition to reducing hospital length of stay, Daltroy et al. [6] noted that preoperative education including psychoeducational preparation also reduced pain medication utilisation. It is apparent from the literature that preoperative education focused on informing patients on all aspects of perioperative period combined with perioperative rehabilitation exercises can enhance the patient's ability to progress uneventfully through the perioperative period. Of further note is that reduced hospital stays are obtainable without altering results or complications.

Nutritional Status and Tobacco Utilisation

A number of studies have documented that the patient's nutritional status correlates with perioperative complications following THA. Perioperative malnutrition has been noted to be predictive of delayed or complicated wound healing and has been associated with increased morbidity and increased length of hospitalisation. Del Savio et al. [7] found that patients with low preoperative serum albumin had significant longer hospitalisation than those with normal serum levels. Gherini et al. [10] evaluated nutritional status of patients undergoing THA using serum albumin and serum transferrin levels. Low preoperative transferrin levels were shown to be predictive of delayed wound healing. When combined with bilateral surgery, which causes a higher metabolic demand on the perioperative period, and advancing age, also associated with poor nutrition, serum transferrin levels resulted in predicting delayed wound healing in 79% of the cases. Similarly, Lavernia et al. [15] found that lower preoperative nutritional parameters such as serum transferrin also were predictive of increased hospital charges, longer surgical and anaesthetic times, and an increased length of stay. These authors along with the current authors suggest that preoperative education regarding nutrition and efforts at supplements or hyperalimentation may help prevent perioperative complications and perhaps improve outcomes.

Multiple studies have noted the adverse effects of cigarette utilisation on the perioperative period. Smoking has been shown to compromise blood supply and decrease both collagen synthesis and osteosynthesis. As a result, multiple studies have documented that smokers are prone to increased cardiopulmonary events, increased intensive care utilisation, higher rate of wound complications, increased surgical times, and longer hospital stays [14, 21, 22]. Smoking cessation protocols have been shown to reduce this increased preoperative morbidity. In a randomised clinical trial, Moller et al. [21] investigated the affects of a smoking-cessation intervention programme on the outcomes of THA and TKA. Sixty patients were randomised into a smoking-intervention group with education, nicotine-replacement therapy and smoking cessation, and compared with 60 patients who were not enrolled in a smoking-intervention programme. The overall complication rate was reduced from 52% in the control group to 18% in the intervention group. Wound related complications dramatically reduced from 31% in the control group to 5% in the intervention group. Furthermore, this six- to eight-week programme reduced the number of secondary surgeries from 15% in the control group to 4% in the intervention group.

Multimodal Perioperative Pain Management

Effective management of perioperative pain is a critical part of the rapid recovery protocol for THA. Pain is a complex conundrum of interactions between the central nervous system, the different pathways and the local site of injury. Peripheral pain like that associated with THA has two sources: neurogenic and inflammatory. Neurogenic pain is a result of the stimulus produced by the surgical trauma and inflammatory pain is a result of the cascade of events involving cytokines, prostaglandins and various chemical mediators [27]. The most significant shortcoming of conventional treatment of surgical pain is that it commences postoperatively. Traditionally, nothing was done to reduce or block the inciting events which cause neurogenic and inflammatory aspects of post surgical pain. These conventional methods have been abandoned and multimodal pain management strategies have been adopted. Multimodal management pain involves pre-emptive analgesia, or pre-treatment of pain prior to the initiat-

ing event that results in central nervous-system excitability and local wound and extremity inflammation [19, 27].

We have been involved and have reported our ongoing efforts at addressing pain management following THA in a multimodal systemic and pre-emptive fashion [18, 19]. The cumulative results of the aforementioned studies suggest that a combined programme of postoperative anti-inflammatory medications, namely non-steroidal anti-inflammatory drugs, regional anaesthetics to include spinal, epidural and blocks [9], anti-emetic medications and local wound soft-tissue infiltration with a cocktail of local anaesthetics, anti-inflammatory agents and narcotics provides safe and effective postoperative pain control [18]. These measures are supplemented with long-acting and short-acting oral narcotics. Several studies have documented that patients undergoing THA can achieve near immediate mobilisation with the establishment of such pain-control management programmes. ◘ Table 13.2 outlines the authors' current recommended perioperative pain-control pathway. The incorporation of this pain-control programme has facilitated early mobilisation and early discharge. Patients undergoing THA are mobilised within 24 hours of the operative intervention, with the majority mobilised within six hours. This early mobilisation facilitates early discharge to home within 48 hours of the operative intervention in the majority of patients undergoing THA.

Clinical Pathways for THA Patients

The establishment of specific protocols for the care and treatment of patients undergoing THA can provide efficient and effective service. Commonly referred to as clinical pathways or care maps, these outlines of care provide a framework by which the patient's postoperative care is managed. It is believed that by defining a sequence of events and goals with a map of care, the patient may be able to meet these goals more efficiently and thus experience reduced and uncomplicated hospital stays. THA is a relatively routine procedure when performed on a healthy individual; therefore, clinical pathways can be standardised easily.

Numerous publications have examined the role and effectiveness of these clinical pathways. Kim et al. [13] performed a meta-analysis and identified 11 articles which met the criteria for review. They specifically addressed the reported effectiveness of clinical pathways on perioperative complications, functional rehabilitation, hospital cost and length of stay. As a result of this review, they concluded that implementation of a clinical pathway for elective THA can result in a reduction of the incidence of complications. Furthermore, clinical pathways tended to reduce hospital cost and decrease length of stay without compromise of the clinical result. In a randomised

Table 13.2. Perioperative pain management pathway

Time Period	Component
Preoperative	Cyclooxygenase-2 inhibiting non-steroidal anti-inflammatory, day before and day of surgery
Intraoperative	Spinal anaesthesia using: ■ Bupivacaine 0.75% (7.5 mg to 12 mg based on patient height and weight) ■ Duramorph (200 mcg to 300 mcg based on patient height and weight) Intra-articular soft-tissue injection following closure of fascial muscular periarticular layer using: ■ Ropivacaine 0.5% (60 cc) (slightly above recommended dosage due to Epinephrine effect with local anaesthesia) ■ Epinephrine 1:1,000 (0.5cc) ■ Toradol 30 mg
Post-anaesthesia care unit	Dilaudid IV PRN breakthrough pain (dosage based on patient's pain level, height and weight)
Postoperative inpatient unit	
Day of surgery	■ Oxycontin (Oxycodone SR) 20 mg PO q 12 hours x 4 doses (initiate within 2 hours of arrival to unit) OR ■ If >70 years, Oxycontin (Oxycodone SR) 10 mg PO q 12 hours x 4 doses (within 2 hours of arrival to unit) ■ Oxycodone (Roxicodone) 5 mg PO q 4 hours PRN breakthrough pain > 5 on pain scale; may repeat × 1 (notify physician if pain is not relieved after 3rd PRN within 6 hours) ■ If unable to tolerate PO medication within first 24 hours postoperatively, morphine 2 mg IVP q 2 minutes up to a maximum of 10 mg in 1 hour for pain. Notify physician if pain not relieved
Postoperative day 1	Cyclooxygenase-2 inhibiting non-steroidal anti-inflammatory (Celebrex 200 mg PO bid) × 10 days
After 48 hours on unit	After Oxycontin and Oxycodone are discontinued as above, begin: Hydrocodone/APAP (Vicodin) 5/500 mg 2 tabs PO q 4 hours PRN for pain 6–10 on pain scale Hydrocodone/APAP (Vicodin) 5/500 mg 1 tab PO q 4 hours PRN for pain 1–5 on pain scale Give no more than 4000 mg of acetaminophen in 24 hours

prospective study of 163 patients who either entered a clinical pathway or represented a control group, Dowsey et al. [8] demonstrated that clinical pathways resulted in a significant reduction in hospital length of stay, early ambulation, reduction of readmission rate, and more accurate matching of the patient discharge destination as determined by preoperative planning. Clinical pathways should, therefore, be an integral part of the rapid recovery protocol to facilitate the perioperative care of the patient undergoing THA.

Wound-Healing Adjuncts

There is increasing evidence that the use of growth factors in the form of the autologous platelet gel may facilitate wound healing [3, 24]. Autologous platelet gel is a type of tissue adhesive that is derived from the patient's own platelet-rich plasma. This material was originally introduced in the early 1990's and is known to have excellent haemostatic and tissue sealant properties when combined with thrombin and calcium. This byproduct of blood collection techniques has proven to be an excellent source of beneficial cytokines, such as platelet derived growth factor (PDG) and transforming growth factor-data (TGF-D). By activating the platelets and causing degranulation, the calcium thrombin combination creates a glue-like

substance which promotes osteogenesis, speeds wound healing, promotes haemostatsis and may also decrease postoperative pain.

Several manufacturers within the orthopaedic industry have noted these beneficial effects and are currently marketing products to assist in the harvesting of the patient's own platelets from a sample of whole blood (GPS, Biomet Inc., Warsaw, Indiana USA; Symphony, DePuy Inc., Warsaw, Indiana USA). The efficacy of these wound-healing adjuncts is surfacing in arthroplasty. Mooar et al. [23] performed a retrospective evaluation examining the outcome of autologous platelet gel usage. Patients were selected to receive autologous platelet gel applied to the synovium, bony ends and wound prior to closure following TKA. These patients were compared with patients who did not receive the gel. Several distinct differences were noted. The study group experienced significantly less blood loss, had improved range of motion and required significantly less intravenous and oral narcotics than the control group. This study is preliminary and certainly further studies are required to validate the effect of autologous platelet gel. However, no adverse effects currently appear to exist from autologous platelet gel and there is potential benefit in terms of enhanced wound healing, pain relief, diminished blood loss and early hospital discharge. Therefore, the use of wound healing adjuncts should be considered as part of a rapid recovery protocol.

Postoperative Physiotherapy and Rehabilitation

Concomitant with the aggressive and effective multi-modal pain management is aggressive physiotherapy and rehabilitation. Despite concerns regarding weight-bearing status following THA, especially with cementless designs, the data would suggest that immediate weight bearing as tolerated with an assistive device has no negative impact on prosthetic stability or osteointegration [25]. Certainly this is not a concern with cemented THA. The benefits of early mobilisation are well-recognized especially with respect to enhancement of pulmonary function [12], facilitation of gastrointestinal motility and prophylaxis against deep venous thrombosis [1]. Several authors have described a multi-modal approach to prophylaxis again deep venous thrombosis in patient undergoing THA which includes early mobilization [19, 26]. This multimodal approach has been shown to be efficacious and avoids the concomitant perioperative wound complications which are present with chemical prophylaxis.

Results of the Utilization of the Rapid Recovery Protocol in Patients Undergoing THA

Over the past decade, our concept of the road to recovery following THA has evolved into what is now referred to as rapid recovery. Patients are therefore achieving postoperative milestones at significantly earlier times. The average length of stay of 10 days in the early 1990's is now diminished to a little over two days. A retrospective review was performed to examine the perioperative effects of the rapid recovery programme. The control group consists of all primary unilateral THA performed by joint implant surgeons during a six-month period from February 1997 through June 1997. The study group included all primary unilateral THA performed by joint implant surgeons for a consecutive six-month period after implantation of the rapid recovery program (January 2003 to June 2003). Patient demographics, length of hospital stay, discharge disposition and readmission rates were compared between the control and study groups. The control group consisted of 168 THA and the study group was 128 THA. No statistically significant differences were noted between groups for height, weight or age (p <0.05). The length of stay was significantly reduced from 4.0 days in 1997 (range 2–9 days; standard deviation 1.1) to 2.7 days in 2003 (range 1–7 days; standard deviation 0.86; p >0.001). Furthermore, the rate of readmission to the hospital within three months of surgery was significantly lower in the study group (3.9% versus 8.3%; p=0.05).

Conclusion

Total hip arthroplasty (THA) continues to be an evolving science. Numerous debates exist with respect to technique and implants utilised. There is continued controversy regarding issues of cementless versus cemented fixation, appropriate surface finish for cemented implants, and the ideal bearing surface. There is an increasing focus on surgical approaches for THA with is a keen interest in minimally invasive or less invasive surgical procedures. The World Wide Web and lay press are inundated with descriptions of new surgical approaches which facilitate rapid return of function. This chapter has outlined a multifactorial rapid recovery protocol which will enhance the patient's ability to successfully undergo THA. It is our distinct impression that rapid return of function is not limited to the size of the incision but rather to the development of a comprehensive program to guide patients through the perioperative period.

Take Home Messages

- Preoperative assessment, patient education and pre-arthroplasty rehabilitation are essential tools for the implementation of a multifactorial rapid recovery protocol.
- Perioperative malnutrition and smoking are predictive of delayed or complicated wound healing and have been associated with increased morbidity and increased length of hospitalisation.
- Effective management of perioperative pain is a critical part of the rapid recovery protocol for THA. The incorporation of a special pain control programme has facilitated early mobilisation and early discharge.
- Standardised clinical pathways play an important role in the effectiveness of rapid recovery in THA.
- Implementing a multifactorial rapid recovery protocol, the length of stay and the rate of readmission to the hospital within three months of surgery could be significantly reduced.

References

1. Berend KR, Lombardi AV Jr et al. (2004) Ileus following total hip or knee arthroplasty is associated with increased risk of deep venous thrombosis and pulmonary embolism. J Arthroplasty 19(7 Suppl 2):82–86

2. Berry DJ, Harmsen WS (2002) Twenty-five year survivorship of two-thousand consecutive primary Charnley total hip replacements. J Bone Joint Surg 84-A(2):171–177

3. Breuing K, Andree C (1997) Growth factors in the repair of partial thickness porcine skin wounds. Plast Reconstr Surg 100(3):657–664

4. Buvanendran A, Kroin JS (2003) The effect of peri-operative administration of a selective cyclooxygenase-2 inhibitor on pain

management and recovery of function after knee replacement: a randomized controlled trial. JAMA 290(19):2411–2418

5. Crowe J, Henderson J (2003) Pre-arthroplasty rehabilitation is effective in reducing hospital stay. Can J Occup Ther 70(2):88–92

6. Daltroy LH, Morlino CI (1998) Preoperative education for total hip and knee replacement patients. Arthritis Care Res 1(6):469–478

7. Del Savio GC, Zelicof SB (1996) Pre-operative nutritional status and outcome of elective total hip replacement. Clin Orthop 326:153–161

8. Dowsey MM, Kilgour ML (1999) Clinical pathways in hip and knee arthroplasty: a prospective randomized controlled study. Med J Aust 170(2):59–62

9. Fournier R, Van Gessel E (1998) Post-operative analgesia with »3-in-1« femoral nerve block after prosthetic hip surgery. Can J Anaesth 45(1):34–38

10. Gherini S, Vaughn BK et al. (1993) Delayed wound healing and nutritional deficiencies after total hip arthroplasty. Clin Orthop 293:188–195

11. Huddleston HM, Long KH et al. (2004) Medical and surgical comanagement after elective hip and knee arthroplasty: a randomized, controlled trial. Ann Intern Med 141(6):28–28

12. Kamel HK, Iqbal MA et al. (2003) Time to ambulation after hip fracture surgery: relation to hospitalization outcomes. J Gerontol A Biol Sci Med Sci 58(11):1042–5.

13. Kim S, Losina E (2003) Effectiveness of clinical pathways for total knee and total hip arthroplasty. Literature review. J Arthroplasty 18(1):69–74

14. Lavernia CJ, Serra RJ (1999) Smoking and joint replacement. Resource consumption and short term outcome. Clin Orthop 367:172–180

15. Lavernia CJ, Sierra RJ (1999) Nutritional parameters and short term outcome in arthroplasty. J Am Coll Nutr 18(3):274–278

16. Leali A, Fetto J et al. (2002) Prevention of thromboembolic disease after non-cemented hip arthroplasty. A multimodal approach. Acta Orthop Belg 68(2):128–134

17. Liebergall M, Soskolone V (1999) Preadmission screening of patients scheduled for hip and knee replacement: impact on length of stay. Clin Perform Qual Health Care 7(1):17–22

18. Lombardi AV Jr, Berend KR et al. (2004) Soft-tissue and intra-articular bupivacaine, epinephrine and narcotic injection in knee arthroplasty. Clin Orthop (paper accepted, in preparation)

19. Mallory TH, Lombardi AV Jr et al. (2002) Pain management for joint arthroplasty: preemptive analgesia. J Arthroplasty 17(4 Suppl 1):129–133

20. Mansfield JA, Dodds KL et al. (2001) Linking the orthopaedic office-hospital continuum: Results before and after implementation of an automated patient health history project. Orthopaedic Nursing 20(2):51–60

21. Moller AM, Villebro N (2002) Effect of pre-operative smoking intervention on post-operative complications: a randomised clinical trial. Lancet 359(9301):114–117

22. Moller AM, Pedersen T (2003) Effect of smoking on early complications after elective orthopaedic surgery. J Bone Joint Surg 85-B(2):178–181

23. Mooar PK, Gardner MJ (2000) The efficacy of autologous platelet gel in total knee arthroplasty. AAOS 67th Annual Meeting March 15–19, Orlando, USA

24. Oz MC, Jeevanandam V (1992) Autologous fibrin glue from intra-operatively collected platelet-rich plasma. Ann Thorac Surg 53:530–531

25. Rao RR, Sharkey PF et al. (1998) Immediate weightbearing after uncemented total hip arthroplasty. Clin Orthop 349:156–162

26. Sarmiento A, Goswami AD (1999) Thromboembolic prophylaxis with the use of aspirin, exercise, and graded elastic stockings or intermittent compression devices in patients managed with total hip arthroplasty. J Bone Joint Surg Am 81(3):339–346

27. Woolf CJ, Chong MS (1993) Pre-emptive analgesia-treating post-operative pain by preventing the establishment of central sensitization. Anesth Analg 77:362–379

Prevention of Infection

L. Frommelt

Summary

This chapter deals with precautions to prevent surgical-site infection in patients undergoing total hip arthroplasty. The precautions are divided into three groups: general, preoperative and precautions in the operating theatre. Measures taken in the theatre are categorised as precautions that avoid contamination of the wound and those which prevent bacterial contamination from inducing postoperative infection. Procedures to improve the host's own defence and perioperative prophylaxis with antimicrobial agents are discussed, and recommendations for proper use of antibiotics with respect to choice, timing and frequency of administration are given. The different measures are categorised by level of evidence as proposed by the US Agency for Health Care Policy and Research.

Introduction

Periprosthetic infection of total hip arthroplasty (THA) is a rare complication after this frequently performed surgical procedure. It may lead to disaster for the patient. Patients undergo total hip arthroplasty in order to get rid of pain and regain their mobility. What they get, if infection occurs, is immobility, pain and a condition that may even be life-threatening.

Every operation harbours the risk of surgical infection because it is impossible to completely avoid bacterial contamination in the operating theatre. The source of these infections is human bacterial flora. Whether contamination leads to infection depends on the number of bacteria introduced during surgery, the virulence of the bacteria and the condition of the host's defence. If the host's defence is unable to balance the bacterial attack, surgical infection will result. Unfortunately, the presence of foreign material suppresses the host's defence locally. Thus, the total joint prosthesis is at risk of being infected even by low grade pathogens such as coagulase-negative staphylococci and propioni bacteria.

Avoiding microbial contamination and defeating periprosthetic infection before it becomes established is the most effective way of protecting orthopaedic devices from infection.

One of the outstanding advantages of THA is that in most cases it is an elective procedure that can be planned. This gives the orthopaedic surgeon the opportunity for meticulous preoperative management.

Unfortunately, most precautions against periprosthetic infection are not based on medical evidence. They are mostly empiric, sometimes of low value and expensive.

These precautions will be discussed with respect to the pathogenesis of periprosthetic infection and commonly accepted standards.

Pathogenesis of Periprosthetic Infection

Periprosthetic infection is a foreign-body associated infection. The problems result from the interaction between the foreign body and host defence and also between bacteria and the foreign body. The site of infection is primarily the interface between the bone and the foreign material.

In most cases, micro-organisms from human bacterial flora gain access to the surface of the prosthesis during the THA procedure. Blood-borne infections and infections which reach the site of infection from other sources are less frequent. Lidwell and co-workers stated that more than

90% of infections during the first year after implantation are due to bacterial contamination during surgery [22].

Bacteria, Host Defence and Foreign-Material Surfaces

To understand how periprosthetic infection starts it is necessary to understand that bacterial interaction with the foreign-material surface is a crucial factor. Specialised bacteria are able to colonise surfaces by forming a biofilm (◘ Fig. 14.1). This biofilm protects them from the host's defence mechanisms and these sessile bacteria are also highly resistant to antimicrobial agents [9, 18, 39]. Inside the biofilm, bacteria may spread along the surface of the implant. Periprosthetic infection begins when some of them switch back to planktonic forms and induce infection in the adjacent tissue – periprosthetic osteomyelitis [16]. The period between colonisation and clinically detectable infection may last for months, even up to about three years.

In the presence of foreign bodies, a contamination as low as 100 colony-forming units (CFU) is sufficient to induce an infection in contrast to 10,000 CFU without foreign material [12]. This effect is due to the diminished clearing capacity of phagocytosis by leucocytes in the presence of foreign material [39].

Precautions to Prevent Periprosthetic Infection

Prophylaxis against periprosthetic infection consists of several elements: choosing a period for prosthesis implantation when the host's own defence is in optimal condition, avoiding contact between the patient and germs adapted to the hospital environment, and avoiding bacterial contamination in the operating theatre. The second approach is to reduce bacterial contamination in number and if possible to prevent bacteria from colonising the prosthetic device.

Quite a large number of precautionary measures are taken. Some of them have the quality of rituals and there is little or no evidence that these procedures are of any value. Some of them are useless for preventing surgical-site infection, but they are of some value in the sense that they enhance the awareness of operating theatre staff for this problem and thus induce appropriate behaviour.

The procedures are categorised and ranked in order of evidence levels. The definitions of the types of evidence are those used by the US Agency for Health Care Policy and Research [1].

Levels of evidence:

Ia Evidence obtained from meta-analysis of randomised controlled trials.

Ib Evidence obtained from at least one randomised controlled trial.

IIa Evidence obtained from at least one well-designed controlled study without randomisation.

IIb Evidence obtained from at least one other type of well-designed quasi-experimental study.

III Evidence obtained from well-designed non-experimental descriptive studies, such as comparative studies, correlation studies and case studies.

IV Evidence obtained from expert committee reports or opinions and/or clinical experiences of respected authorities.

General Precautions

Most pathogens in periprosthetic infections originate from human bacterial skin flora. Therefore, the length of time patients are exposed to germs in the hospital environment should be as short as possible in order to avoid colonisation by these bacteria.

Patients undergoing THA should be separated from patients treated in general surgery. If epidemiology shows a high prevalence of multi-resistant pathogens, like methicillin-resistant Staphylococcus aureus (MRSA), patients should be screened for these organisms and decontaminated preoperatively. Biant and co-workers [3] stated that these precautions lead to a significant reduction in the number of infections by MRSA in a British hospital (Cat. Ib).

The blood glucose of patients suffering from diabetes mellitus must be monitored meticulously, pre- and postoperatively. Blood–glucose levels exceeding 300 mg/dL postoperatively increase the odds for surgical-site infection (SSI) from 2.54 to 3.32 compared with patients with glucose levels lower than 250 mg/dL (Cat.Ib) [3].

In patients treated with immunosuppressive drugs, the dose should be reduced to a tolerable amount. If possible, immunosuppressive therapy should be discontinued

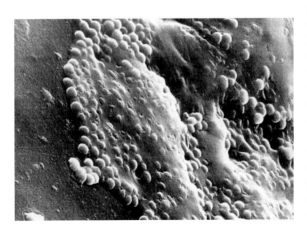

◘ **Fig. 14.1.** Electronmicroscopy of *staphylococcus* with biofilm formation. (Reprinted with permission from Peters G (1998) 'Plastikinfektionen' durch Staphylokokken. Dt.Ärztebl 85:C-204–C-208)

perioperatively. Bacterial infections such as urinary-tract infection, infected teeth, pyoderma or other bacterial lesions should be treated before THA is performed.

Precautions Before Operation

Shaving the Site of Operation

There is a long tradition of removing hair at the operation site in order to reduce the risk of wound infection. Cruise and Foord [10] showed that shaving may itself be a risk factor because of micro-lesions in the skin. Several studies have found no strong evidence against preoperative hair removal. However, there was strong evidence to recommend that when hair removal is considered necessary, it should not be removed by shaving but by a depilatory cream or electric clipping, preferably immediately before surgery (Cat. Ia).

Preoperative Showering

The patient's skin is a major source of bacterial contamination in clean operations. Traditionally, patients are asked to bathe or shower with or without disinfectant soap. Cruise and Foord [10] found no significant reduction of the postoperative infection rate. Ayliffe [2] showed that preoperative washing with an antiseptic did not reduce the infection rate even though there was evidence that the bacterial burden of the skin was temporarily reduced. Many other studies have also come to the conclusion that antiseptic showers do not reduce the incidence of surgical-site infection (Cat. Ib).

Precautions in the Operating Theatre

Reducing Bacterial Contamination of the Wound

Preoperative Hand Hygiene of the 'Scrub' Team. Hand decontamination is an important contribution to reducing infections. Unfortunately, there is no evidence as to which method is more effective in reducing postoperative infection rates. Alcoholic disinfectants are appropriate for reducing skin bacteria. Rehork and Rüden [32] suggested initial hand-washing for 5 minutes followed by disinfection using an alcoholic disinfectant for 3 minutes. If further decontamination is necessary within the next 60 minutes, no hand-washing is necessary but alcoholic hand-rubbing for 1 minute is required. If the time exceeds 60 minutes, the whole procedure has to be repeated. In the British Medical Journal editorial is was recommended that alcohol hand rubs should replace washing as the recommended method of hand hygiene [35]. However, hand decontamination before operation is recommended on the evidence level of Category IV, because it is impossible to design studies without the knowledge of strong theoretical rationale.

Preparation of the Patient's Skin. For disinfection of the skin at the site of operation, aqueous iodophore preparations have an excellent bactericidal effect comparable with alcohol preparations. Some preparations combine the alcohol with iodophore or chlorhexidine.

The ideal antiseptic should be effective on a broad spectrum of pathogens; in particular it should have a rapid and persistent effect on gram-negative and gram-positive bacteria, on fungi and also viruses. It should be resistant to inactivation on organic material like blood or discharge. It should be non-toxic and initiate no allergic reaction.

Skin antiseptics must be supplied in ready-for-use dilution in small, single-use containers. Multiple-use containers can be contaminated by resistant micro-organisms which can be dispersed to the next patient. If multi-use bottles are used, they must be marked with the date of first use and the local infection control committee should give recommendations for a 'use by date' which is different from the manufacturer's expiry date. These containers must not be refilled. Alcohol-based preparations must be allowed enough time to dry completely; otherwise the patient is at the risk of burns when electro-surgery is used (Cat. Ib).

Protecting the Wound. Adhesive incisional films were first used in the early 1960s. The idea was to prevent bacteria from the patient's own skin flora from contaminating the surgical wound. These films adhere to the complete operative field and are surrounded by linen or disposable drapes. However, there is no evidence that these incise drapes are able to reduce the incidence of post-operative wound infection. A similar approach is the use of incise films with antiseptic impregnation. These reduce re-colonisation of the skin, but they do not appear to reduce the incidence of surgical-site infection as well [6]. In conclusion, there is no benefit or evidence that incisional drapes reduce the incidence of SSI (Cat. IIb).

Textiles in the Theatre. Textiles are used for garments and drapes in the theatre. Linen is used for different purposes in operating departments:

- surgical suits which staff change into when entering the department
- garments worn by patients
- sterile gowns worn by the 'scrub' team
- sterile drapes used around the operation incision.

Surgical suits and patient's linen have to be clean but not sterile. Sterile coats worn by the 'scrub' team and drapes are used as a barrier to prevent micro-organisms from passing from operating theatre staff through garments to the surgical wound, or, if the clothing becomes wet, by capillary action called bacterial strike-through. Standard cotton fabrics with a pore size of 80–100 μm are not suitable because bacteria are dispersed into the air by small epithelial cell fragments measuring about 20 μm. To prevent bacterial strike-through, the textile material must be waterproof [27]. Fabrics used for surgical purposes have to prevent fluid penetration and need a pore size smaller than 20 μm whether they are woven or not. Nowadays, non-woven disposable clothing is more frequently used.

The barrier also protects staff from infections which can be acquired from patients such as hepatitis or HIV infection.

In conclusion, theatre gowns and drapes must be sterile and should be made of waterproof material with a pore size of less than 20 μm. Disposable material is preferable. Other surgical linen needs to be clean, but not sterile (Cat. Ib).

Facemasks. There is no reliable evidence that facemasks reduce postoperative infections. However, they should be used in joint replacement, where even low numbers of pathogens are able to induce foreign-body infection.

On the other hand, facemasks protect operating theatre staff from splash infections, which can be caused by blood and discharge. Masks should be worn exclusively in the operating room and must be changed if they become damp or contaminated, and for the next operation in any case.

Facemasks should be worn in the theatre for the protection of the wearer. Unfortunately, there is only insufficient evidence that they also contribute to protection of the wound, but theoretical rationale makes it reasonable to wear facemasks during total joint replacement procedures (Cat. IIb).

Gloves. In joint replacement surgery double gloves should be worn by the 'scrub' team. Gloves act as a barrier between the wearer and the wound. They protect the wound from becoming contaminated by bacteria from the surgeon's hands and they prevent the surgical team from viral infections. Double gloves are necessary because surgical gloves are not as fluid-proof as one might expect. Randomised studies have shown that the leakage for water can be reduced by three to nine times if two pairs of gloves are used [11]. In conclusion: Wearing double gloves is reasonable for the 'scrub' team and enhances the barrier function of gloves (Cat. Ia).

Theatre Ventilation. Periprosthetic infection can be induced by a small number of pathogens and also by low-grade pathogens, which play only a small role in the pathogenesis of infections not associated with foreign bodies. Even though most of these infections originate directly from the patients' own skin flora, studies suggest that some of these infections are airborne and can be prevented by ultra-clean air ventilation systems like vertical laminar air flow [15, 23, 30]. Laminar air-flow units in combination with body exhausts are very effective in re-

ducing airborne pathogens in number, but the number of infections caused by airborne pathogens is probably low anyway. Evidence for the reduction of the postoperative infection rate exists only for artificial joint-replacement procedures. In 1970, Charnley, who introduced ultra-clean air supply into artificial joint replacement surgery, suggested that the concept of laminar air flow should be revised. He pointed out that it is crucial to avoid contamination of air in the theatre by means of clothing that is impermeable and does not allow the passage of skin particles (contaminated with bacteria). Furthermore, the operation field should be separated from other parts of the theatre [7]. In conclusion, ultra-clean air units are beneficial in artificial joint replacement, but some surgeons and bacteriologists are of the opinion that it might be possible to obtain the same effect with less technical effort. If laminar air flow is used, it must be stable against influences from the surrounding areas and the deposit for sterile surgical instruments has to be in the clean area as well. Ultra-clean units may serve Category Ib, but a retrospective study by the Norwegian Register [13] suggests that there is no difference between ordinary ventilation of the operating theatre and theatres with laminar flow ventilation (Cat. III).

Improving the Host's Own Defence

The following precautions cannot avoid bacterial contamination of the wound but they are able to reduce subsequent surgical-site infection to a certain extent and are therefore of supplementary value.

Normothermia during Operation. Patients in operating theatres are chilled by mechanical ventilation systems because they are only lightly dressed. If body temperature drops by a mean of 1.5 °C, the rate of postoperative infections including surgical-site infection is higher. Patients can preferably be warmed up by warmed air in the theatre [19, 24]. The mechanism is that normothermia avoids stress, which can lead to hormonal suppression of the host's defence. Melling and co-workers [26] reported a reduction in the incidence of infection of about 50% in clean surgery. Although this has not been investigated for total joint-replacement surgery, the principle is convincing and well studied (Cat. IIb for THA).

Oxygen During Operation. Some studies suggest that providing 80% oxygen instead of 30% during the operation reduces the incidence of postoperative wound infection by 50% [17, 31]. These studies were performed in colorectal surgery. The mechanism behind this theory is that macrophages are activated by oxygen-dependent stimulation. O'Connor [29] mentioned liberal postoperative use of oxygen as a co-factor for successful and uncomplicated wound healing. If this is true, this principle should work in joint replacement as well (Cat. IIa).

Defeating Bacteria Before Infection Becomes Established

Perioperative Antibiotic Prophylaxis

It is well known that antimicrobial agents are useful in preventing postoperative wound infection. Nevertheless, antibiotics are used not only as a therapy against already existing infections but also to prevent an infection that has a good chance of becoming established on a prosthetic device. In view of increasing bacterial resistance to antibiotics, prophylactic use should be prudent and based on reasonable arguments. The problems involved in prophylactic use are which antimicrobial agents should be given, when and for how long.

Timing the Administration of Antimicrobial Agents for Prophylactic Use. The knowledge that correct timing determines the efficacy of perioperative antibiotic prophylaxis goes back to the early sixties. Burke [5] studied the timing in animal experiments. The study was designed as follows: He set a standardised skin lesion and inoculated this lesion with living staphylococci or with dead bacteria of the same strain. In addition, he applied antibiotics according to a time schedule. The animals were exposed to only one dose of antimicrobial agents. The animals were examined at intervals of one hour before incision to six hours afterwards. He found out that the result in the animals inoculated with living bacteria was as good as in animals inoculated with dead bacteria, provided antibiotics were given one hour before incision. Antibiotics administered six hours after incision had no effect at all. The results in this group were equal to those of the animals inoculated with living bacteria but not given antibiotics. Several studies were carried out in humans and showed the same results, even in placebo-controlled studies [34]. Classen and co-workers [8] showed that administration of antibiotics three hours before incision was as worthless as administration six hours after incision. Good timing is therefore an important principle in all types of surgery. This applies to THA as well (Cat. Ia).

Duration of Antimicrobial Application for Prophylactic Use. In the past, the duration of antimicrobial prophylaxis was the subject of controversial discussion. Antibiotics were used for three days to three weeks. Nelson [28] showed that in orthopaedic surgery 7 days of antibiotics is no better than one day. Williams [36] showed that 3 days is as no better than one day. A lot of studies in other surgical specialities support these findings. In compliance with the recommendations of the American Academy of Orthopedic Surgeons (AAOS), perioperative prophylactic use of antibiotics should be discontinued within 24 hours (Cat. Ia).

How Many Doses of Antibiotics? Theory suggests that supplementary doses according to the half-life of the antimicrobial agent used are beneficial. Unfortunately, there are no studies supporting this theory on a good evidence level. Well-designed studies are required to support the expertise of opinion leaders and advisory committees. Until then, this practice corresponds to evidence level IV.

The concentration of prophylactic antibiotics is reduced by blood loss or transfusion of replacement serum, especially if this occurs during the first hour of surgery when the drug levels are high [33, 37]. An additional dose of prophylactic agent is therefore necessary if the blood loss exceeds 1,500 mL during surgery or haemodilution is above 15 mL/kg (Cat. II a/b).

Choice of Antimicrobial Agents in Artificial Joint Replacement. To prevent postoperative infection after surgery, first- and second-generation cephalosporins, especially cefazoline, are recommended as the first-line agent by most guidelines. If a patient is allergic to beta-lactam agents, vancomycin is recommended as a second-line antibiotic. Vancomycin may also be chosen when the epidemiologic situation suggests a prevalence of pathogens resistant to cephalosporins (Cat. Ia).

The increasing prevalence of *Staphylococcus aureus* (MRSA) raises the issue of glycopeptide prophylaxis against MRSA and methicillin resistant *Staphylococcus epidermidis* (MRSE) infections in artificial joint replacement. However, clinical trials have failed to show that glycopeptides are superior to beta-lactam drugs in combating MRSE [37]. It is conceivable that beta-lactam drugs are still effective against infections by MRSE or MRSA. Widespread use of glycopetide agents harbours the additional risk of increasing the prevalence of vancomycin resistant enterococci (VRE) and the induction of vancomycin resistant MRSA or MRSE.

Additional Doses After the End of the Operation. Administration of additional doses of antimicrobial agents for prophylactic use has been discussed as controversially as the duration of prophylaxis. A large study of 2,651 hip replacements in the Netherlands found no difference between cefuroxime prophylaxis used once or three times. Joint infection occurred less often in the three dose group (0.45% versus 0.83%) but the difference was not statistically significant [38] (Cat. Ib). Another more recent retrospective study carried out by the Norwegian Register suggests that three and even four doses within 24 hours are more effective than one dose alone (► chapter 3.7). It is astonishing that this refers to all complications leading to removal of the prosthesis, whereas the differences for periprosthetic infection were only slight [13] (Cat. III). As long as there are no prospective randomised studies available there is no high-level evidence regarding postoperative administration of supplementary doses of prophylactic antibiotics, and it is difficult to give proper recommendation. The problem stays unresolved at the moment and surgeons should be free to give supplementary doses within 24 hours after surgery.

Preventing Bacteria from Colonising the Surface

The idea of incorporating antibiotics in PMMA-bone-cement as a prophylactic measure against infection was introduced by Buchholz and led to gentamicin-impregnated bone cement [4]. In a study comparing gentamicin-loaded bone cement versus systemic antibiotic prophylaxis, the results were in favour of local application of gentamicin (Cat. IIa). Another retrospective study by the Norwegian Register suggests that the combination of local application of antibiotics and systemic antibiotics is more efficient for prophylaxis than local antibiotics in bone-cement or systemic administration of antimicrobial agents alone [14] (Cat. III). The Norwegian Register studies almost exclusively total joint replacement fixed with bone cement. It is therefore prudent to use gentamicin-loaded bone cement in combination with systemic antibiotics for perioperative prophylaxis. There is no equivalent for cementless implants and there are no studies suggesting that cemented joint replacement has more favourable results with regard to surgical-site infection.

Conclusion

Prevention of foreign-body associated infections means reducing the rate of contamination, which may lead to colonisation of prosthetic devices. Whether infection occurs or not depends on several circumstances: the extent of bacterial contamination, the reduction of the number of pathogens contaminating the wound, and the vigilance of the host's own defence. There are therefore three principle approaches to the prevention of periprosthetic infection:

- separation of the surgical wound from sources of potential contamination like theatre gowns, gloves, drapes and ventilation systems;
- measures to enhance the host's own defence, like maintenance of normothermia during surgical procedure, high-level oxygen supply to the patient during the procedure or meticulous perioperative control of serum glucose levels;
- the use of antimicrobial agents for perioperative prophylaxis according to current guidelines.

Not all precautionary measures are supported by good levels of evidence and there are some, which can be omitted because there is no evidence that they are of any value. Most of the practices contribute to the prevention of surgical-site infection. Success results from a cascade of small steps in the same direction. The contribution made by one of the single steps may be not spectacular, when all steps are added together they result in a better outcome.

Most THA procedures are elective. This gives orthopaedic surgeons the opportunity to ensure optimal preoperative management. At the time of operation, the patient should be in a good state of health. Distant sites of infection like urinary-tract infection or pyoderma should be treated before the patient is admitted for THA. Pre-existing metabolic disorders like diabetes mellitus should be controlled as far as possible.

The preoperative stay of the patient in hospital should be as short as possible. Diagnostic or preoperative procedures should be performed on an outpatient basis whenever possible.

Hazardous techniques like shaving the site of operation the evening before THA should be avoided.

Operating theatre staff should take all precautionary measures to separate the surgical wound from bacterial contamination. Staff must be aware that that their behaviour in the theatre contributes to the reduction of postoperative wound sepsis.

Perioperative antimicrobial prophylaxis is not a substitute for this behaviour, but prophylaxis with antimicrobial agents is of supplementary benefit for the patient if handled properly.

It is impossible to avoid all surgical-site infections, but quite a large number can be avoided if the right steps are taken at the right time.

Take Home Messages

- Periprosthetic infection in total hip arthroplasty is a rare complication after this frequently performed procedure, but when it occurs it can mean disaster for the patient. Therefore, all measures to avoid postoperative infection must be taken.
- Precautions start at the time of patient's first contact with the surgeon. The aim is to reduce risks that derive from the patient's concomitant diseases and choose a period for THA when the patient is in an optimal state of health.
- Most pathogens leading to infection originate from the human skin flora but some derive from the environment adjacent to the wound. Procedures that influence the intactness of the patient's own skin flora, like shaving the evening before operation, may be omitted. Reasonable precautions to separate the wound from bacterial contamination must be taken.
- Precautions that reduce bacterial contaminants in number and improve the host's own defence are beneficial. The most effective measure is perioperative prophylaxis using antimicrobial agents.
- Timing, the choice of antimicrobial agent and duration of administration are crucial for the success of perioperative antibiotic prophylaxis.

References

1. AHCPR. Acute Pain Management: Operative or Medical Procedures and Trauma Clinical Practice Guideline No. 1 (1992) AHCPR Publication No. 92–0032: February 1992. Rockville, MD: Agency for Health Care Policy and Research (AHCPR)

2. Ayliffe GA (1984) Surgical scrub and skin disinfection. Infect Control 5: 23–27

3. Biant LC, Teare EL, Williams WW, Tuite JD (2004) Eradication of methicillin resistant Staphylococcus aureus by »ring fencing« of elective orthopaedic beds. Br Med J 329:149–151

4. Buchholz HW, Engelbrecht H (1970) Über die Depotwirkung einiger Antibiotika bei Vermischung mit dem Kunstharz Palacos. Chirurg 41:511–515

5. Burke JF (1961) The effective period of preventive antibiotic action in experimental incisions and dermal lesions. Surgery 50:161–168

6. Byrne DJ, Napier A, Buscheri A (1990) Rationalizing whole body disinfection. J Hosp Infect 15: 183–187

7. Charnley J (1970) Operating-theatre ventilation. Lancet i:1053–10

8. Classen DC, Evans RS, Pestotnik SL, Horn SD, Menlove RL, Burke JP (1992) The timing of prophylactic administration of antibiotics and the risk of surgical-wound infection. N Engl J Med 326:281–286

9. Costerton JW, Stewart PS, Greenberg EP (1999) Bacterial biofilm: a common cause of persistent infections. Science 284:1918–1322

10. Cruse PJ, Foord R (1973) A five-year prospective study of 23,649 surgical wounds. Arch Surg 107: 206–210

11. Doyle PM, Alvi S, Johanson R (1992) The effectiveness of double gloving in obstetrics and gynaecology. Br J Obstet Gynaecol 99: 83–84

12. Elek SD, Conen PE (1957) The virulence of staphylococcus pyogenes for man: a study of the problems of wound infection. Br J Exp Pathol 38:573–586

13. Engesæter LB, Lie SA, Espehaug B, Furnes O, Vollset SE, Havelin LI (2003) Antibiotic prophylaxis in total hip arthroplasty: effects of antibiotic prophylaxis systemically and in bone cement on the revision rate of 22,170 primary hip replacements followed 0–14 years in the Norwegian Arthroplasty Register. Acta Orthop Scand. 74:644–651

14. Espehaug B, Engesæter LB, Vollset SE, Havelin LI, Langeland N (1997) Antibiotic prophylaxis in total hip arthroplasty. Review of 10,905 primary cemented total hip replacements reported to the Norwegian Arthroplasty Register, 1987–1995. J Bone Joint Surg (Br) 79B:590–595

15. Fitzgerald RH Jr, Brechtol CO, Eftekhar N, Nelson JP (1979) Reduction of deep sepsis after total hip arthroplasty. Arch Surg 114:803–804

16. Frommelt L (2000) Periprosthetic Infection – Bacteria and the interface between prosthesis and bone. In: Learmonth ID (ed) Interfaces in total hip arthroplasties. Springer, London. pp 153–161

17. Greif R, Akca O, Horn E, Kurz A, Sessler DI, for the Outcomes Research Group (2000) Supplemental perioperative oxygen to reduce the incidence of surgical-wound infection. N Engl J Med.3 42:161–169

18. Gristina AD (1987) Biomaterial-centred infection: microbial adhesion versus tissue integration. Science 237:1588–1595

19. Kurz A, Sessler DI, Lenhardt R (1996) Perioperative normothermia to reduce the incidence of surgical-wound infection and shorten hospitalization. N Engl J Med. 334:1209–1216

20. Latham R, Lancaster AD, Covington JF, Priolo LS, Thomas CS (2001) The association of diabetes and glucose control with surgical-site infection among cardiothoracic surgery patients. Control Hosp Epidemiol 22:607–612

21. Levy M, Egersegi P, Strong A et al. (1990) Pharmacokinetic analysis of cloxacillin loss in children undergoing major surgery with massive bleeding. Antimicrob Agents Chemother 34:1150–1153

22. Lidwell OM, Lowbury EJL, Whyte W, Blowers R, Stanley SJ, Lowe D (1982) Effect of ultraclean air in operating rooms on deep sepsis in the joint after total hip or knee replacement: a randomised study. Br Med J 285:10–14

23. Lidwell OM, Lowbury EJL, Whyte W, Blowers R, Stanley SJ, Lowe D (1983) Airborne contamination of wounds in joint replacement operations: the relationship to sepsis rates. J Hosp Inf 4:111–131

24. Mahoney C, Odom J (1999) Maintaining intraoperative normothermia: a meta-analysis of outcomes with costs. AANA Journal 67:155–164

25. Mangram AJ, Horan TC, Pearson ML, Silver LC, Jarvis WR (1999) The Hospital Infection Control Practices Advisory Committee. Guidelines for prevention of surgical site infection 1999. Infect Control Hosp Epidemiol 20:247–280

26. Melling AC, Ali B, Scott EM, Leaper DJ (2001) Effects of preoperative warming on the incidence of wound infection after clean surgery: a randomised controlled trial. Lancet 358:876–880

27. Mitchell NJ, Evens DC, Kerr A (1978) Reduction of skin bacteria in the theatre air with comfortable, non-woven disposable clothing for the operating-theatre staff. Br Med J 1:696–698

28. Nelson CL, Green TG, Porter RA, Warren RD (1983) One day versus seven days of preventive antibiotic therapy in orthopedic surgery. Clin Orthop. 176:258–263

29. O'Connor MI (2004) Wound healing problems in TKA: just when you thought it was over! Orthopedics 27:983–984

30. Peersman G, Laskin R, Davis J, Peterson M (2001) Infection in total knee replacement: a retrospective review of 6,489 total knee replacements. Clin Orthop 392:15–23

31. Pryor KO, Fahey TJ 3rd, Lien CA, Goldstein PA (2004) Surgical site infection and the routine use of perioperative hyperoxia in a general surgical population: a randomized controlled trial. 291:79–87

32. Rehork B, Rüden H (1991) Investigations into the efficacy of different procedures for surgical hand disinfection between consecutive operations. J Hosp Infect 19:115–127

33. Sanderson PJ (1998) Prophylaxis in orthopaedic implant surgery – should we use a glycopeptide? J Antimicrob Chemother 41: 322–325

34. Stone HH, Hooper CA, Colb LB, Geheber CE, Dorkins EJ (1976) Antibiotic prophylaxis in gastric, bilary and colonic surgery. Ann Surg 184: 443–452

35. Teare L, Cookson B, Stone S (2001) Hand hygiene. Br Med J 323: 411–412

36. Williams DN, Gustilo RB (1984) The use of preventive antibiotics in orthopaedic surgery. Clin Orthop 190:83–88

37. Wollinsky KH, Buchele M, Oethinger M, Kluger P, Mehrkens HH, Marre R, Puhl W (1996) Influence of hemodilution on cefuroxime levels and bacterial contamination of intra- and postoperative processed wound blood during hip replacement. Beitr Infusionsther Transfusionsmed 33:191–195

38. Wymenga A, van Horn J, Theeuwes A, Muytjens H, Slooff T (1992) Cefuroxime for prevention of postoperative coxitis. One versus three doses tested in a randomized multicenter study of 2,651 arthroplasties. Acta Orthop Scand 63:19–24

39. Zimmerli W, Lew PD, Waldvogel FA (1984) Pathogenesis of foreign body infection – evidence for a local granulocyte defect. J Clin Invest 73:1191–1200

Pulmonary Embolism in Cemented Total Hip Arthroplasty

Michael Clarius, Christian Heisel, Steffen J. Breusch

Summary

Embolism is a well-known complication of cemented to-tal hip arthroplasty (THA). As a result of manipulations of the medullary cavity, the intramedullary pressure rises and fat, bone marrow and air embolises into the venous system and to the lung. Clinically, this is seen as acute hypotension, which can go as far as cardiac failure. Although a fatal outcome is rare, fat embolism is a serious complication. The most effective prophylactic measure to reduce the risk is a thorough lavage of the femoral cavity. The use of pulsatile jet-lavage can be regarded as an obligatory preparatory procedure before cement application. Fat and bone marrow are removed as potential embolic sources and, further, the cement-bone interface is enhanced.

Introduction

Deep vein thrombosis (DVT) and pulmonary embolism (PE) are feared and well known complications of THA [54]. Fat embolism comprises an entity amongst the group of PE and usually occurs in the early perioperative phase and is unrelated to DVT. The incidence of postoperative DVT as assessed by phlebography is reported in literature to be as high as 77% [68], although, in clinical practice, it is frequently underestimated and consequently not diagnosed. An important and life-threatening complication of DVT is secondary PE with an incidence estimated to be between 6–33% [28, 43, 68] confirmed by lung perfusion- and ventilation scans. Although effective anti-embolic and DVT prophylactic measures have been able to reduce these figures significantly, DVT and PE are still the most common causes of death after THA [54, 93].

Consequences of Pulmonary Embolism

Pulmonary embolism leads to an increase in pulmonary vascular resistance. The blockage of the pulmonary vascular system results in an increased AV-shunt and in pulmonary hypoperfusion [49, 60, 95]. The acute pressure increase in the pulmonary arteries [16, 17] causes the functional and structural alteration of a cor pulmonale to occur resulting in left ventricular hypovolaemia and a reduced cardiac output [1, 91]. Clinically, this is seen as acute hypotension, which can go as far as cardiac failure.

Cardiopulmonary Complications and Death During Total Hip Arthroplasty

Soon after introduction of methylmethacrylate (MMA) as bone cement towards the end of the 1960s, reports of adverse intraoperative complications were published and associated with the use of bone cement. Sir John Charnley [18] himself, who inaugurated MMA in orthopaedic surgery observed a drop in blood pressure immediately after implantation of the endoprosthesis in many of his patients for up to 5 minutes which was more pronounced during implantation of the stem than the cup. Some authors reported instances of intraoperative cardiac arrest [18, 25, 27, 66, 67, 69, 78, 88, 98], which were fortunately manageable with resuscitation. Such instances of so-called »cardiac arrest syndrome« [88] as a reaction to implantations of cemented implants was not, however, always reversible and a number of intraoperative deaths were reported in literature (❑ Table 15.1), mostly in patients with hip fracture. At autopsy 15/49 cases showed extensive pulmonary fat embolisation. An exact microscopic examination of lung tissue revealed an additional bone marrow emboli-

Table 15.1. Intraoperative cardiac arrests and deaths during total hip replacement reported in literature

Author	Diagnosis	Cardiac Arrest Syndrome	Death	Autopsy	Cause of Death
Charnley 1970	no information	4	2	–	–
Powell et al. 1970	hip fracture	3	–	–	–
Hyland, Robins 1970	hip fracture	1	1	1	air and fat embolism
Burgess 1970	hip fracture	1	1	1	fat embolism
Gresham et al. 1971	hip fracture	2	2	2	fat embolism
Schulitz et al. 1971	OA	3	2	1	fat embolism
Thomas et al. 1971	hip fracture	1	1	–	–
Cohen, Smith 1971	Revision	1	1	1	fat and bone marrow embolism
Phillips et al. 1971	hip fracture	1	1	1	fat and bone marrow embolism
Dandy 1971	hip fracture	4	2	2	fat embolism
Michelinakis et al. 1971	hip fracture	2	–	–	–
Sevitt 1972	hip fracture	2	2	2	fat embolism
Kepes et al. 1972	hip fracture	2	2	1	bone marrow embolism
Peebles et al. 1972	hip fracture	1	1	–	–
Newens, Volz 1972	hip fracture	1	–	–	–
De Angelis et al. 1973	Revision, OA	2	–	–	–
Nice 1973	hip fracture	1	1	–	–
Milne 1973	OA	1	–	–	–
Tronzo et al. 1974	no information	1	1	–	
Jones 1975	no information	1	1	–	fat embolism
Hyderally, Miller 1976	path. hip fracture	1	1	–	–
Beckenbaugh, Ilstrup 1978	no information	1	1	–	–
Engsaeter 1984	no information	1	1	1	fat embolism
Zichner 1987	no information	10	3		
Hochmeister et al. 1987	hip fracture	1	1	1	fat and bone marrow embolism
Maxeiner 1988	hip fracture	3	3	1	fat embolism
Egbert et al. 1989	path. hip fracture	1	1	1	fat and bone marrow embolism
Patterson et al. 1991	hip fracture	7	4	1	no evidence of embolism
Bogner, Landauer 1991	hip fracture	10	10	1	no evidence of embolism
Pietak et al. 1997	hip fracture	2	2	2	fat and bone marrow embolism
Tsujitou et al. 1998	no information	2	2	2	fat embolism
Parvizi et al. 1999	17 HF., 4 OA, 1 RA, 1 NU	23	23	13	11/13 bone marrow, 3/13 bone cement
Ortega et al. 2000	no information	5	1	1	fat embolism
Fallon et al. 2001	path. hip fracture	1	1	1	fat embolism
Leidinger 2002	hip fracture	12	12	12	1x fat embolism, 11x right heart failure
total		115	87	49	–

HF hip fracture, *OA* osteoarthritis, *RA* rheumatoid arthritis, *NU* non union.

sation alongside fat embolisms in 18 patients whereby the particles were found to even contain cancellous bone fragments.

Intraoperative Mortality

Intraoperative mortality during hip replacement was evaluated by Parvizi [77] in a large retrospective study involving 38,488 patients and found to be at around 0.06%. One particularly risk-laden group was the patient with fracture of the femoral neck with an intraoperative mortality of 0.18%, those with pertrochanteric fracture and cemented hip replacement suffered a 1.6% risk. Leidinger [61], though, published data in 2002 from 150 patients with fracture of the femoral neck for whom the intraoperative mortality was found to be much higher at 8%. Elective THA carries a risk well below 0.1%.

Diagnosis and Visualisation of Intraoperative Embolism

The intraoperative complications forced anaesthetists to monitor patients very carefully when hip replacement was undertaken. During intraoesophagal cardiac auscultation so-called »mill-wheel-murmurs« could be detected during prosthesis implantation [70]. These phenomena were accompanied by hypotensive episodes and blood aspiration via a Swan-Ganz catheter allowed Jones to establish the first diagnosis of fat embolism in 1975.

Visualisation of intraoperative embolism was first achieved using echocardiography [20, 22, 44, 92, 109]. The development of transoesophageal echocardiography (TEE) allowed a continuous high-quality monitoring of the patient intraoperatively without complicating influences such as breathing movements, adipositas or emphysema, because it is benefited by the close proximity of the oesophagus to the target organ the heart (◘ Fig. 15.1).

Continuous echocardiographic monitoring during cemented hip replacement operations allowed an assessment of the relative frequency of intraoperative embolic events [22, 41]. Therefore TEE is regarded as the most sensitive method to detect intraoperative embolism [39], although the less invasive transcranial Doppler has been advocated.

Pathomechanism

Cement »Toxicity«

Many attempts were made to explain the implantation syndrome [90]. Initially, bone cement was seen as the prime culprit and cause of cardiovascular complications.

Frost [37] suspected the heat emission during polymerisation as the primary cause of the observed losses in pressure. Other authors postulated a connection between the acute onset of hypotension and the release of monomeric MMA, which was assumed to cause peripheral vasodilatation and bradycardia accompanied by a negative inotropic effect when released during the hardening process [34, 53, 58, 62, 66, 69, 72, 79, 97, 104]. Radioactive marking of the monomer proved the influx of methylmethacrylate into the blood circulation, which permitted in vivo MMA measurements [50, 65].

Hypotension could be reproduced in animal models after intravenous injection of the monomer with a dose dependent relationship. Intraoperative measurements in patients showed in vivo concentrations from 0.3–5.9 mg/100 ml [50, 58, 65, 103, 114], but Bright [14] found that a measurable hypotensive effect was only attained at concentrations around the tenfold of those achieved in humans. Death occurred in the animal model after injection of doses correlating with the hundredfold MMA concentrations (125 mg/100 ml) [50]. However, clinically a statistical correlation between measured MMA concentrations and pressure drop could not be demonstrated.

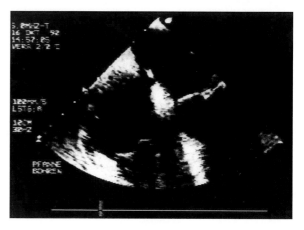

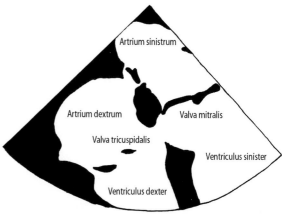

◘ **Fig. 15.1.** Normal cross-sectional view of the heart as seen during transoesophageal echocardiography

Not just the monomers, but also initiators of the dimethyl-p-toluidin type were accused of causing acute hypotensive crises. But Schlag [96] was able to demonstrate that initiators of this type were totally depleted during the polymerisation process.

It is therefore important to realise the cement itself is not the »toxic culprit«.

Intramedullary Pressure

Another line of argument in the explanation of the implantation syndrome was the pathogenetic intravasation of air, fat and bone marrow components and the autopsy findings mentioned above appeared to support this. Causal in this argument is the increase in intramedullary pressure during implantation of the prosthesis [19, 26, 40, 80, 94]. Experiments involving femora from deceased donors were able to show very high intramedullary pressure peaks of up to 1447 kPa as can be seen in ◘ Table 15.2. Values of up to 250 kPa were attained during intraoperative pressure measurement (◘ Table 15.2).

◘ **Table 15.2.** Intramedullary pressure during implantation of the femoral prosthesis

Author	Pressure (kPa)		Method
	Without Drill Hole	With Drill Hole	
Ohnsorge 1971	455	262	cadaver femur
Phillips et al. 1973	250		intraoperative
Hallin 1974	89		intraoperative
Breed 1974	114	13	animal model
Tronzo et al. 1974	75		intraoperative
Kallos et al. 1974	118	32	animal model
von Issendorff, Ritter 1977	504	96	cadaver femur
Indong et al. 1978	1282		cadaver femur
Drinker et al. 1981	1243		animal model
Engsaeter et al. 1984	76	4	intraoperative
Orsini et al. 1987	223		animal model
Wenda et al. 1988	131		intraoperative
Song et al. 1994	488		cadaver femur
Yee et al. 1999	1052		cadaver femur
McCaskie et al. 1997	157 667		intraoperative cadaver femur
Reading et al. 2000	131		cadaver femur
Dozier et al. 2000	486		cadaver femur
Churchill et al. 2001	1447		cadaver femur

The increase in intramedullary pressure during cement insertion and stem implantation causes an influx of air [2, 3, 5, 24], fat and bone marrow fragments via the linea aspera [31] into the venous system [45, 112]. A proportion of these particles embolise swiftly, the remainder adhere to vessel walls and initiate the development of a mixed thrombus [114]. It was Pelling and Butterworth [80], who finally proved the mechanism of fat displacement from the femur as the decisive mechanism. There was no difference in the extent of fat embolism between bone cement, bone wax and simple dough.

Irrespective of the operative approach chosen, the femoral vein is subject to a significant torsion as a result of flexion and rotation of the leg and this can lead to temporary total occlusion of the vessel [101]. Intraoperative phlebography has been able to confirm this phenomenon [87]. Such occlusion implies a complete cessation of blood flow, torsion of the femoral vein leads to damage of the endothelial wall, the trauma of the operation itself causes a higher propensity for blood to coagulate and thus the triad of factors postulated by Virchow in 1856 for the development of venous thrombus is fulfilled. This shows that the high incidence of postoperative deep venous thrombosis of the leg after hip replacement as well as the subsequent pulmonary embolic events can be explained to a high degree by the operative method itself. A further consequence of the operative method is that the act of relocation of the hip implies also the re-canalisation of the femoral vein from which the newly formed thrombi are released into the venous system [22]. The danger of cardiopulmonary complications rises and it becomes apparent why this moment can be regarded as particularly dangerous, even more so, as it closely follows the most critical moment, that of cement and stem implantation.

Multicentre Study

Our own investigations within the framework of a multicentre study included 96 cemented THA patients, which were continuously monitored using TEE. We were able to identify several intraoperative steps that were followed by embolic events. ◘ Figure 15.2 shows such a risk profile during a total hip replacement operation.

Our studies revealed that femoral stem implantation and relocation of the hip (i.e. unkinking of the femoral vein) were the most embolism-prone operative steps.

A so-called »snow flurry« (◘ Fig. 15.3), which is the echocardiographic correlate for an air embolism, was seen in virtually all patients immediately after cement and stem implantation. Diagnostic signs such as these are then frequently followed by a manifest embolus (◘ Fig. 15.4), which can then circulate in the right-side of the heart for up to 2 minutes before being swept out into the blood vessels of the lung (◘ Fig. 15.5 and 15.6).

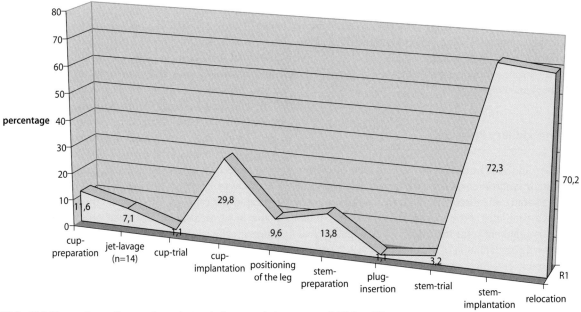

Fig. 15.2. Time and operative step dependent embolic events during cemented THA (n = 96)

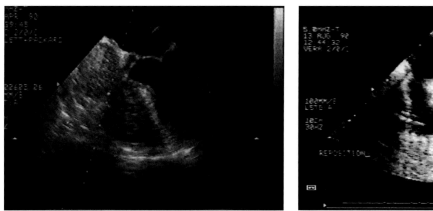

Fig. 15.3. »Snow flurry«, the echocardiographic correlate of air embolism

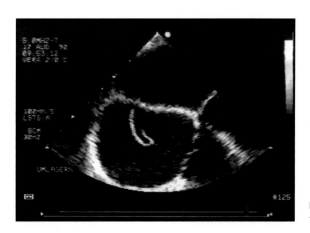

Fig. 15.4. Filamentous embolus in the right atrium

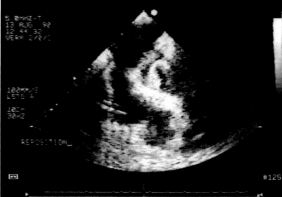

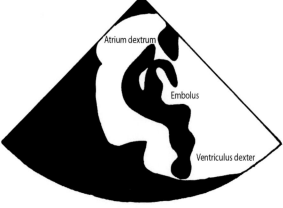

Fig. 15.5. Massive embolus circulating in the right heart for more than 40 seconds after trial reduction

»Snow flurries« were observed in 85% of stem implantations and emboli similarly, in 72%. Some very small emboli occurred during pulsatile lavage of the acetabulum in 1/14 patients [22]. At the moment of relocation of the implanted components, 93% of patients who were subject to echocardiographic monitoring displayed »snow flurries«, while embolic events could be found in 70%. It is, however, of note that no pulsatile lavage had been used in 82/96 patients in this multicentre study, hence representing a worse case scenario.

Cementing Techniques Influencing Intraoperative Embolism

There are several factors influencing intramedullary pressure and therefore intraoperative embolism. In a new animal model we were able to compare certain methods and operation/cementing techniques and it was possible to quantify the amount of fat and bone marrow intravasation.

Animal Model

A new sheep model was developed (◘ Fig. 15.6), which allowed for standardised bilateral, simultaneous cement pressurisation. The operative procedure involved bilateral placement of intravenous catheters into the external iliac veins via retroperitoneal approach (◘ Fig. 15.7). A specially designed cementing apparatus was used to allow for bilateral simultaneous cement pressurisation. Venous blood from both iliac catheters was then collected during cementing (◘ Fig. 15.8), anticoagulated and a quantitative and qualitative fat analysis was performed.

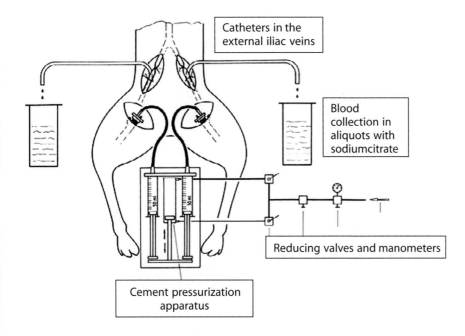

Catheters in the external iliac veins

Blood collection in aliquots with sodiumcitrate

Reducing valves and manometers

Cement pressurization apparatus

◘ **Fig. 15.6.** Schematic drawing of the sheep model which allows for bilateral simultaneous cement pressurization and collection of blood via the external iliac veins

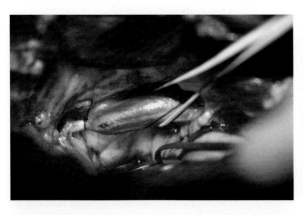
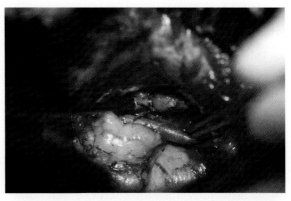

◘ **Fig. 15.7.** Intraoperative view of the retroperitoneal situs. On the left the ballooned iliac vein after proximal ligation is shown, on the right the catheter is placed and secured

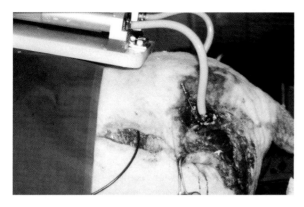

Fig. 15.8. Animal model setup during operation. On top cement apparatus with bilateral simultaneous pressurisation is shown. Via the retroperitoneal iliac vein catheter the draining blood could be collected during cementing to allow determination of the fatty contents

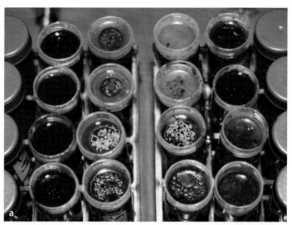

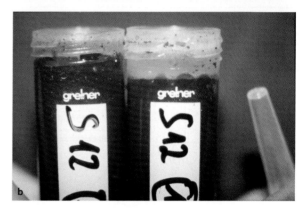

Fig. 15.9a,b. Macroscopic appearance of blood samples collected. **a** More supernatant fat on the blood surface in the syringe lavage group (*right*) than in pulsatile lavage group (*left*). **b** Higher magnification and comparison of pulsatile (*left*) versus manual lavage (*right*) groups

Influence of Pulsatile Lavage

Using the sheep model described above, we studied the effectiveness of both pulsatile and syringe lavage of equal volume with regard to their cleansing capabilities as measured by fat and bone-marrow intravasation. After randomisation, one side was lavaged with 250 ml irrigation using a bladder syringe, the contralateral femur with the identical volume but using a pulsatile lavage. Despite equal volume manual lavage produced significantly higher fat and bone marrow intravasation (p <0.001) than pulsatile lavage (Fig. 15.9) [12].

It is well known that lavage is necessary to clean the cancellous bone in order to obtain a strong bone-cement interface [11, 13]. Further, our model was able to demonstrate, that not only the volume but also the quality of bone lavage is an essential factor influencing the risk of fat embolism and adverse cardiorespiratory effects. Manual lavage carries a significantly increased risk of fat and bone-marrow intravasation [12].

Influence of Cement Viscosity

Pressurisation is necessary in order to force the cement into the bone. Bone cements displace blood and bone marrow when pushed into the medullary cavity. Little is known about the in vivo impact of cement viscosity on cement interdigitation and fat embolism.

Using this model, we also studied the influence of different cement viscosities on fat intravasation and cement penetration in vivo [8]. As high viscosity cement we used Palacos in comparison to low viscosity Osteopal cement.

In this model, low viscosity cement yielded significantly lower rates of microradiographically measured cement penetration under in vivo bleeding conditions despite adequate and sustained pressurisation. Cement application at a higher viscosity state carried a higher risk of fat embolism but resulted in improved cement interdigitation – a finding in contrast to many in-vitro cement studies! Cement applied at low viscosity state seems to take the path of least resistance into the venous system (Fig. 15.10) before deeper cement penetration into bone can occur [8]. Accordingly, three cases have been reported in literature of intraoperative death, where bone cement was found in the lung at autopsy [77].

Influence of Pressure and Pressurisation

Intramedullary, pressure is dependent upon a number of factors such as the magnitude of pressure, the duration of pressurisation, the cement viscosity as well as the stem design and the relationship between the prosthesis and the medullary cavity [21]. Tapered stem designs resulted in significantly higher pressures and higher intrusion rates. The larger the prosthesis in relation to the medullary cav-

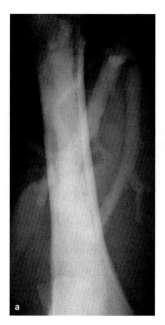

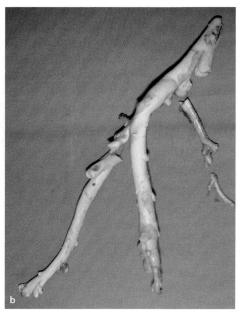

Fig. 15.10. a Postoperative radiograph taken after implantation and pressurisation of low viscosity bone cement showing cement intravasation into the venous system. **b** After dissection of the specimen the full extent of cement escape is revealed

ity, the higher is the measured pressure and the amount of embolised material. Large stem sizes should be inserted slowly and particular emphasis should lie on prior meticulous canal cleansing with pulsatile lavage.

Influence of a Cement Restrictor

Contemporary cementing techniques include the use of a cement restrictor to occlude the intramedullary canal to allow for cement containment, cement pressurisation and improvement of cement interdigitation [73]. These intramedullary plugs seal the distal medullary cavity and therefore lead to higher intramedullary pressures during pressurisation and implantation of the femoral prosthesis. A good cementation result requires the ability of the restrictor to withstand displacement forces during cementation [47]. In order to get a good fit in the femur, it is usually necessary to advance the plug distally with force, resulting in high intramedullary pressure peaks leading to pulmonary embolisation [22]. Obviously, there are differences between the designs of the cement restrictors. Our own investigations in cadaver femora, showed that expandable restrictors have favourable characteristics and the potential to reduce the risk of fat embolism [10]. In a further in-vivo animal study [46], utilising the same principle of venous blood collection and fat sampling, we found in eight of thirteen evaluated animals a peak in the fat intravasation caused by the application of the cement restrictor.

Our results emphasise the importance of a thorough preparation of the intramedullary canal, particularly when cemented fixation is performed. As a consequence of these studies we concluded that pulsatile lavage, which

should be considered a mandatory standard in cemented THA, should be implemented prior to the insertion of the cement restrictor (and even templating for it!) in order to further reduce the risk of fat embolism.

Influence of Femoral Cement Filling Technique

In the early years of hip replacement, cement was introduced in an antegrade fashion from the proximal end into the femoral cavity before insertion of the femoral component. Charnley's »thumbing« method induced intramedullary pressure peaks with cement alone [73, 74]. Use of a venting tube during cement introduction was able to reduce the pressure peaks [26, 74], it did, however, cause cement mantle defects [30].

Glen proposed as early as 1970, that holes could be drilled into the distal femur in order to relieve pressure build-ups [38]. This enabled a fourfold reduction in intramedullary pressure [7, 56, 74, 111] and furthermore provided a route via which material from within the marrow cavity could escape. Numerous animal models [7, 56] and clinical studies [44, 108] have established the efficacy of the distal venting hole.

The logical continuation of this concept was the vacuum technique according to Draenert [31]. The distal venting hole, as stipulated by many authors, is connected to a vacuum and thus sucks the cement into the cancellous bone and, additionally, should serve to reduce pressure during cement and stem implantation. A further cannula located proximally in the fossa piriformis was intended to improve the cement filling of cancellous honeycomb structures and at the same time reduce intramedullary pressure peaks. It could be proven using echocardiography that this method was superior to antegrade cement application (via syringe injection from the proximal end) in terms of reduction of embolism rates [59, 84–86]. The theoretical premise that vacuum-based techniques avert the possibility of intramedullary pressure increase and its accompanying cardiopulmonary complications could not be supported by our own findings [22], when comparing with the more common retrograde cement filling technique. Moreover, periprosthetic fractures had occurred at the same level as the distal vent hole [107]. The currently widely-used retrograde technique [9] with application from the distal end with a cement gun, the so-called »snorkel« method [32] represents an improvement over the antegrade technique in terms of embolism rate and is regarded as the safest method so far for the application of cement [102].

In a further animal experiment [110], in modification to the sheep model described above, we compared retrograde cement application, which is regarded as the golden-standard method, with the technically more challenging vacuum-application method (Draenert) with regard to in vivo cement-bone interface measured by cement penetration. Using pulsatile lavage in both groups, we could find no further reduction of fat-embolism risk between the groups and our results support the hypothesis, that prior cleansing is more important than the mode of cement application. However, antegrade cement technique without prior pulsatile lavage must be regarded as a high-risk procedure.

Influence of the Implantation of the Prosthesis

The moment in which the femoral stem is implanted implies an unavoidable further increase of intramedullary pressure. The cement is further driven into the medullary cavities by the volume of the femoral component und leads further bone-marrow extrusion (⬛ Fig. 15.11).

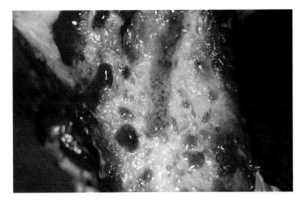

⬛ **Fig. 15.11.** Visible fat extrusion at the anterior aspect of the proximal femur during implantation of the femoral prosthesis

Prevention and Prophylaxis of Fat Embolism

The surgeon is faced with a dilemma, as the primary goal must be to achieve durability of the implant and an immediate capacity to withstand loading, which both demand an optimal penetration of cement into the bone. Many technical developments such as intramedullary plugs used to seal distally and proximal pressurising devices all necessarily raise (and aim to raise) intramedullary pressure. It seems a logical deduction from the outlined above, that minimising intramedullary pressure may be an important step to reduce the risk of fat embolism. This, however, is a wrong conclusion!

The only way in which to reduce the risk of fat embolism is thorough pulsatile lavage of the femoral cavity to reduce the volume of the embolic load. This washes out fat and bone marrow as potential embolic material and further enables an improved penetration of cement into bone. The use of pulsatile jet-lavage has been proven to be far superior to any other method and must be regarded as an obligatory preparatory procedure before cement application [11]. Pulsatile jet-lavage should be implemented before all manipulations of the intramedullary cavity, for example, prior to templating for and prior to the implantation of the distal cement restrictor [46]. Usually, 1 litre of irrigation should be used per femur.

The phenomenon of intraoperative embolisation during relocation of the hip is caused by the re-opening of the temporarily occluded femoral vein during operation. To avoid kinking and occlusion of the femoral vein, it is recommended to avoid extreme leg positioning (if access to the femur is possible) and to release the torsion of the leg as often as possible thus preventing prolonged venous stasis. Long operative durations should be avoided in this abnormal position.

In recognition of the high risk of intraoperative embolism, some authors prefer to implant cementless prostheses. From this point of view, our own investigations confirmed the hypothesis that cementless prosthetic replacement is associated with a lower risk of embolism than cemented THA [20]. In our animal model with intra-individual comparison, we could show that the amount of fat that passed into the venous draining system of the femur induced by cemented implantation was twice the amount than seen with cementless implantation [46]. However, the increased risk of fat embolism should not lead to change in fixation philosophy.

In conclusion, if the use of pulsatile is strictly implemented in cemented THA, the risk of perioperative fat embolism of clinical significance is very low, even if modern cementing techniques with high and sustained cement pressurisation are used.

References

1. Albrecht M, Frey L, Krüger P: Langdauernde pulmonal-vaskuläre Veränderungen bei alten Patienten nach Methyl-Acrylat-(Palacos)-Implantation. Anaesthesist 33:474, 1984
2. Andersen KH: Air aspirated from the venous system during total hip replacement. Anaesthesia 38:1175–8, 1983
3. Bachmann B, Biscoping J, Ratthey K, Krumholz W, Hempelmann G: Incidence of air embolism in implantation of hip prostheses. Z Orthop Ihre Grenzgeb 125:369–74, 1987
4. Beckenbaugh RD, Ilstrup DM: Total hip replacement. J Bone Joint Surg 60A:306–313, 1978
5. Bednarz F, Roewer N: Intraoperative detection of air embolism and corpuscular embolism using pulse oximetry and capnometry. Comparative studies with transesophageal echocardiography. Anasth Intensivther Notfallmed 24:20–6, 1989
6. Bogner C, Landauer B: Anaesthesiologische Aspekte bei Hüftprothesenoperationen. In: Vortrag beim 45. praktischen Seminar in der Orthopädie und Chirurgie des Bewegungsapparates. 31.5.1991 München, 1991
7. Breed AL: Experimental production of vascular hypotension, and bone marrow and fat embolism with methylmethacrylate cement. Traumatic hypertension of bone. Clin Orthop 0:227–44, 1974
8. Breusch S, Heisel C, Muller J, Borchers T, Mau H: Influence of cement viscosity on cement interdigitation and venous fat content under in vivo conditions: a bilateral study of 13 sheep. Acta Orthop Scand 73:409–15, 2002
9. Breusch SJ, Berghof R, Schneider U, Weiss G, Simank HG, Lukoschek M, Ewerbeck V: Status of cementation technique in total hip endoprostheses in Germany. Z Orthop Ihre Grenzgeb 137:101–7, 1999
10. Breusch SJ, Heisel C: Insertion of an expandable cement restrictor reduces intramedullary fat displacement. J Arthroplasty 19:739–44, 2004
11. Breusch SJ, Norman TL, Schneider U, Reitzel T, Blaha JD, Lukoschek M: Lavage technique in total hip arthroplasty: jet lavage produces better cement penetration than syringe lavage in the proximal femur. J Arthroplasty 15:921–7, 2000
12. Breusch SJ, Reitzel T, Schneider U, Volkmann M, Ewerbeck V, Lukoschek M: Cemented hip prosthesis implantation--decreasing the rate of fat embolism with pulsed pressure lavage. Orthopade 29:578–86, 2000
13. Breusch SJ, Schneider U, Kreutzer J, Ewerbeck V, Lukoschek M: Effects of the cementing technique on cementing results concerning the coxal end of the femur. Orthopade 29:260–70, 2000
14. Bright DS, Clark HG, McCollum DE: Serum analysis and toxic effects of methylmethacrylate. Surg Forum 23:455–7, 1972
15. Burgess DM: Cardiac arrest and bone cement. Br Med J 3:588, 1970
16. Byrick RJ, Kay JC, Mullen JB: Pulmonary marrow embolism: a dog model simulating dual component cemented arthroplasty. Can J Anaesth 34:336–42, 1987
17. Byrick RJ, Mullen JB, Mazer CD, Guest CB: Transpulmonary systemic fat embolism. Studies in mongrel dogs after cemented arthroplasty. Am J Respir Crit Care Med 150:1416–22, 1994
18. Charnley J: Acrylic Cement in Orthopaedic Surgery. Baltimore, Williams & Wilkins Company, 1970
19. Charnley J: Total hip replacement by low-friction arthroplasty. Clin Orthop 72:7–21, 1970
20. Christie J, Burnett R, Potts HR, Pell AC: Echocardiography of transatrial embolism during cemented and uncemented hemiarthroplasty of the hip. J Bone Joint Surg Br 76:409–12, 1994
21. Churchill DL, Incavo SJ, Uroskie JA, Beynnon BD: Femoral stem insertion generates high bone cement pressurization. Clin Orthop:335–44, 2001
22. Clarius M: Intraoperativer Embolienachweis mittels zweidimensionaler Echokardiographie beim künstlichen Hüftgelenkersatz. In: Institut für Chirurgische Forschung der Universität München, Zentrum für Orthopädische Wissenschaften München. München Germany, Dissertation. Ludwig-Maximilians-Universität, 1996
23. Cohen CA, Smith TC: The intraoperative hazard of acrylic bone cement: report of a case. Anesthesiology 35:547–9, 1971
24. Dambrosio M, Tullo L, Moretti B, Patella V, Simone C, Calo MN, Dalfino L, Cinnella G: [Hemodynamic and respiratory changes during hip and knee arthroplasty. An echocardiographic study]. Minerva Anestesiol 68:537–47, 2002
25. Dandy DJ: Fat embolism following prosthetic replacement of the femoral head. Injury 3:85–8, 1971
26. Dandy DJ: The safety of acrylic bone cement. Injury 5:169–74, 1973
27. De Angelis J, Kenneth J: Cardiac Arrest Following Acrylic-Cement Implants. Anaesth Analg 52:298–302, 1973
28. Dorr LD, Sakimura I, Mohler JG: Pulmonary emboli followed total hip arthroplasty: incidence study. J Bone Joint Surg Am 61:1083–7, 1979
29. Dozier JK, Harrigan T, Kurtz WH, Hawkins C, Hill R: Does increased cement pressure produce superior femoral component fixation? J Arthroplasty 15:488–95, 2000
30. Draenert K: Beobachtung zur Zementierung von Implantatkomponenten. Med Orthop Tech 106:200–205, 1986
31. Draenert K: Modern cementing techniques. An experimental study of vacuum insertion of bone cement. Acta Orthop Belg 55:273–93, 1989
32. Drinker H, Goel VK, Panjabi MM: Acute in vivo toxicity of methylmethacrylate pressurization. Trans Ortho Research 6:131, 1981
33. Egbert R, von Hundelshausen B, Gradinger R, Hipp E, Kolb E: Heart arrest in implantation of a cemented total hip joint endoprosthesis under spinal anesthesia – a case report. Anasth Intensivther Notfallmed 24:118–20, 1989
34. Ellis RH, Mulvein J: The cardiovascular effects of methylmethacrylate. J Bone Joint Surg Br 56:59–61, 1974
35. Engesaeter LB, Strand T, Raugstad TS, Husebo S, Langeland N: Effects of a distal venting hole in the femur during total hip replacement. Arch Orthop Trauma Surg 103:328–31, 1984

36. Fallon KM, Fuller JG, Murley -Forster P: Fat embolization and fatal cardiac arrest during total hip arthroplasty with methlmethacrylate. Can J Anaesth 48 (7):626–9, 2001

37. Frost PM: Cardiac arrest and bone cement. Br Med J 3:524, 1970

38. Glen ES: Cardiac Arrest and Bone Cement. Brit Med J 3:524, 1970

39. Glenski JA, Cucchiara RF, Michenfelder JD: Transesophageal echocardiography and transcutaneous O2 and CO2 monitoring for detection of venous air embolism. Anesthesiology 64:541–5, 1986

40. Gresham GA, Kuczynski A, Rosborough D: Fatal fat embolism following replacement arthroplasty for transcervical fractures of femur. Br Med J 2:617–9, 1971

41. Hagio K, Sugano N, Takashina M, Nishii T, Yoshikawa H, Ochi T: Embolic events during total hip arthroplasty: an echocardiographic study. J Arthroplasty 18:186–92, 2003

42. Hallin G, Modig J, Nordgren L, Olerud S: The intramedullary pressure during the bone marrow trauma of total hip replacement surgery. Ups J Med Sci 79:51–4, 1974

43. Harris WH, McKusick K, Athanasoulis CA, Waltman AC, Strauss HW: Detection of pulmonary emboli after total hip replacement using serial C15O2 pulmonary scans. J Bone Joint Surg Am 66:1388–93, 1984

44. Heinrich H, Kremer P, Winter H, Worsdorfer O, Ahnefeld FW: Transesophageal 2-dimensional echocardiography in hip endoprostheses. Anaesthesist 34:118–23, 1985

45. Heisel C, Clarius M, Schneider U, Breusch SJ: Thromboembolic complications related to the use of bone cement in hip arthroplasty--pathogenesis and prophylaxis. Z Orthop Ihre Grenzgeb 139:221–8, 2001

46. Heisel C, Mau H, Borchers T, Muller J, Breusch SJ: Fat embolism during total hip arthroplasty. Cementless versus cemented--a quantitative in vivo comparison in an animal model. Orthopäde 32:247–52, 2003

47. Heisel C, Norman TL, Rupp R, Mau H, Breusch SJ: Stability and occlusion of six different femoral cement restrictors. Orthopäde 32:541–7, 2003

48. Hochmeister M, Fellinger E, Denk W, Laufer G: Intraoperative fatal fat and bone marrow embolism of the lung in implantation of a hip endoprosthesis with polymethylmethacrylate bone cement. Z Orthop Ihre Grenzgeb 125:337–9, 1987

49. Hofmann S, Huemer G, Kratochwill C, Koller-Strametz J, Hopf R, Schlag G, Salzer M: Pathophysiology of fat embolisms in orthopedics and traumatology. Orthopäde 24:84–93, 1995

50. Homsy CA, Tullos HS, Anderson MS, Diferrante NM, King JW: Some physiological aspects of prosthesis stabilization with acrylic polymer. Clin Orthop 83:317–28, 1972

51. Hyderally H, Miller R: Hypotension and cardiac arrest during prosthetic hip surgery with acrylic bone cement. Ortho Rev 5:55–61, 1976

52. Indong OH, Carlson CE, Tomford WW, Harris WH: Improved fixation of the femoral component after total hip replacement using a methacrylate intramedullary plug. J Bone Joint Surg 60-A: 608–613, 1978

53. Johansen I, Benumof JL: Methylmethacrylate: A myocardial depressant and peripheral dilator. Anesthesiology 51:77, 1979

54. Johnson R, Green JR, Charnley J: Pulmonary embolism and its prophylaxis following the Charnley total hip replacement. Clin Orthop:123–32, 1977

55. Jones RH: Physiologic emboli changes observed during total hip replacement arthroplasty. A clinical prospective study. Clin Orthop:192–200, 1975

56. Kallos T, Enis JE, Gollan F, Davis JH: Intramedullary pressure and pulmonary embolism of femoral medullary contents in dogs during insertion of bone cement and a prosthesis. J Bone Joint Surg Am 56:1363–7, 1974

57. Kepes ER, Undersood PS, Becsey L: Intraoperative death associated with acrylic bone cement. Report of two cases. Jama 222:576–7, 1972

58. Kim KC, Ritter MA: Hypotension associated with methyl methacrylate in total hip arthroplasties. Clin Orthop 88:154–60, 1972

59. Koessler MJ, Pitto RP: Fat and bone marrow embolism in total hip arthroplasty. Acta Orthop Belg 67:97–109, 2001

60. Kratochwill C, Huemer G, Hofmann S, Koller-Strametz J, Hopf R, Schlag G, Salzer M: Monitoring of bone marrow spilling and cardiopulmonary changes in fat embolism syndrome. Orthopäde 24:123–9, 1995

61. Leidinger W, Hoffmann G, Meierhofer JN, Wolfel R: Reduction of severe cardiac complications during implantation of cemented total hip endoprostheses in femoral neck fractures. Unfallchirurg 105:675–9, 2002

62. Ling RS, James ML: Blood pressure and bone cement. Br Med J 2:404, 1971

63. Maxeiner H: Significance of pulmonary fat embolism in intra- and early postoperative fatal cases following femoral fractures of the hip region. Orthopäde 24:94–103, 1995

64. McCaskie AW, Barnes MR, Lin E, Harper WM, Gregg PJ: Cement pressurisation during hip replacement. J Bone Joint Surg B 1997; 79: 379–384

65. McLaughlin RE, DiFazio CA, Hakala M, Abbott B, MacPhail JA, Mack WP, Sweet DE: Blood clearance and acute pulmonary toxicity of methylmethacrylate in dogs after simulated arthroplasty and intravenous injection. J Bone Joint Surg Am 55:1621–8, 1973

66. Michelinakis E, Morgan RH, Curtis PJ: Circulatory arrest and bone cement. Br Med J 3:639, 1971

67. Milne IS: Hazards of acrylic bone cement. A report of two cases. Anaesthesia 28:538–43, 1973

68. Modig J, Borg T, Karlstrom G, Maripuu E, Sahlstedt B: Thromboembolism after total hip replacement: role of epidural and general anesthesia. Anesth Analg 62:174–80, 1983

69. Newens AF, Volz RG: Severe hypotension during prosthetic hip surgery with acrylic bone cement. Anesthesiology 36:298–300, 1972

70. Ngai SH, Stinchfield FE, Triner L: Air embolism during total hip arthroplasties. Anesthesiology 40:405–7, 1974

71. Nice EJ: Case report: cardiac arrest following use of acrylic bone cement. Anaesth Intensive Care 1:244–5, 1973

72. Nishioka K, Iwatsuki K: Effects of monomer of bone cement on the circulatory system and blood gases. Masui 24:787–92, 1975

73. Oh I, Carlson CE, Tomford WW, Harris WH: Improved fixation of the femoral component after total hip replacement using a methacrylate intramedullary plug. J Bone Joint Surg Am 60:608–13, 1978

74. Ohnsorge P: Experimentelle Untersuchungen zur Bestimmung des intramedullären Druckverlaufes im Femur beim Eindrücken von Knochenzement und beim Einbringen einer Femurschaftendoprothese. In: Dissertation Medizinischen Fakultät der Universität Köln. Köln, 1971

75. Orsini EC, Byrick RJ, Mullen JB, Kay JC, Waddell JP: Cardiopulmonary function and pulmonary microemboli during arthroplasty using cemented or non-cemented components. The role of intramedullary pressure. J Bone Joint Surg Am 69:822–32, 1987

76. Ortega S, Ortega JP, Pascual A, Fraca C, Garcia-Enguita MA, Arauzo P, Urieta-Solanas A: Heart arrest in cemented hip arthroplasty. Rev Esp Anestesiol Reanim 47:31–5, 2000

77. Parvizi J, Holiday AD, Ereth MH, Lewallen DG: The Frank Stinchfield Award. Sudden death during primary total hip arthroplasty. Clinical orthropaedics and Related Research 369:39–48, 1999

78. Patterson BM, Healey JH, Cornell CN, Sharrock NE: Cardiac arrest during hip arthroplasty with a cemented long-stem component. A report of seven cases. J Bone Joint Surg Am 73:271–7, 1991

79. Peebles DJ, Ellis RH, Stride SD, Simpson BR: Cardiovascular effects of methylmethacrylate cement. Br Med J 1:349–51, 1972

80. Pelling D, Butterworth KR: Cardiovascular effects of acrylic bone cement in rabbits and cats. Br Med J 2:638–41, 1973

15

81. Phillips H, Cole PV, Lettin AW: Cardiovascular effects of implanted acrylic bone cement. Br Med J 3:460–1, 1971

82. Phillips H, Lettin AWF, Cole PV: Cardiovascular effects of implanted acrylic cement. J Bone Joint Surg 55B:210, 1973

83. Pietak S, Holmes J, Matthews R, Petrasek A, Porter B: Cardiovascular collapse after femoral prosthesis surgery for acute hip fracture. Can J Anaesth 44:198–201, 1997

84. Pitto RP, Hamer H, Fabiani R, Radespiel-Troeger M, Koessler M: Prophylaxis against fat and bone-marrow embolism during total hip arthroplasty reduces the incidence of postoperative deep-vein thrombosis: a controlled, randomized clinical trial. J Bone Joint Surg Am 84-A:39–48, 2002

85. Pitto RP, Koessler M, Draenert K: The John Charnley Award. Prophylaxis of fat and bone marrow embolism in cemented total hip arthroplasty. Clin Orthop:23–34, 1998

86. Pitto RP, Schafer M, Schuster E: Performance of vacuum pumps used during implantation of hip endoprostheses with an innovative cementing technique--a comparative study. Biomed Tech (Berl) 44:176–81, 1999

87. Planes A, Vochelle N, Fagola M: Total hip replacement and deep vein thrombosis. A venographic and necropsy study. J Bone Joint Surg Br 72:9–13, 1990

88. Powell JN, McGrath PJ, Lahiri SK, Hill P: Cardiac arrest associated with bone cement. Br Med J 3:326, 1970

89. Reading AD, McCaskie AW, Barnes MR, Gregg PJ: A comparison of 2 modern femoral cementing techniques: analysis by cement-bone interface pressure measurements, computerized image analysis, and static mechanical testing. J Arthroplasty 15:479–87, 2000

90. Rinecker H: The bone cement inplantation syndrome. A special form of acute respiratory insufficiency. Fortschr Med 96:1553, 1978

91. Rinecker H: New clinico-pathophysiological studies on the bone cement implantation syndrome. Arch Orthop Trauma Surg 97:263–74, 1980

92. Roewer N, Beck H, Kochs E, Kremer P, Schroder E, Schontag H, Jungbluth KH, Schulte am Esch J: Detection of venous embolism during intraoperative monitoring by two-dimensional transesophageal echocardiography. Anasth Intensivther Notfallmed 20:200–5, 1985

93. Salzman EW, Harris WH: Prevention of venous thromboembolism in orthopaedic patients. J Bone Joint Surg Am 58:903–13, 1976

94. Sato I, Matsumoto N, Hanyu M, Sukie M, Hori T: Air embolism as the factor in cardiovascular changes in total hip arthroplasty. Masui 25:692–6, 1976

95. Schlag G: Mechanisms of cardiopulmonary disturbances during total hip replacement. Acta Orthop Belg 54:6–11, 1988

96. Schlag G, Schliep HJ, Dingeldein E, Grieben A, Ringsdorf W: Does methylmethacrylate induce cardiovascular complications during alloarthroplastic surgery of the hip joint? Anaesthesist 25:60–7, 1976

97. Schuh FT, Schuh SM, Viguera MG, Terry RN: Circulatory changes following implantation of methylmethacrylate bone cement. Anesthesiology 39:455–7, 1973

98. Schulitz KP, Koch H, Dustmann HO: Vital intrasurgical complications due to fat embolism after the installation of total endoprostheses with polymethylmethacrylate. Arch Orthop Unfallchir 71:307–15, 1971

99. Sevitt S: Fat embolism in patients with fractured hips. Br Med J 2:257–62, 1972

100. Song Y, Goodman SB, Jaffe RA: An in vitro study of femoral intramedullary pressures during hip replacement using modern cement technique. Clin Orthop:297–304, 1994

101. Stamatakis JD, Kakkar VV, Sagar S, Lawrence D, Nairn D, Bentley PG: Femoral vein thrombosis and total hip replacement. Br Med J 2:223–5, 1977

102. Svartling N: Detection of embolized material in the right atrium during cementation in hip arthroplasty. Acta Anaesthesiol Scand 32:203–8, 1988

103. Svartling N, Pfaffli P, Tarkkanen L: Methylmethacrylate blood levels in patients with femoral neck fracture. Arch Orthop Trauma Surg 104:242–6, 1985

104. Thomas TA, Sutherland IC, Waterhouse TD: Cold curing acrylic bone cement. A clinical study of the cardiovascular side effects during hip joint replacement. Anaesthesia 26:298–303, 1971

105. Tronzo RG, Kallos T, Wyche MQ: Elevation of intramedullary pressure when methylmethacrylate is inserted in total hip arthroplasty. J Bone Joint Surg 56:714–8, 1974

106. Tsujitou T, Ishiyama T, Dohi S: Pulmonary fat embolism during bipolar hip endoprosthesis. Masui 47:1338–43, 1998

107. Ulrich C: Klinische Risiken der femoralen Druckerhöhung und deren Prophylaxe – Vorstellung des Theodor Naegeli Award Papers. In: 42. Praktisches Seminar in der Orthopädie und Chirurgie des Bewegungsapparates. München Germany, 1991

108. Ulrich C: Value of venting drilling for reduction of bone marrow spilling in cemented hip endoprosthesis. Orthopade 24:138–43, 1995

109. Ulrich C, Burri C, Worsdorfer O, Heinrich H: Intraoperative transesophageal two-dimensional echocardiography in total hip replacement. Arch Orthop Trauma Surg 105:274–8, 1986

110. Ungethüm S. Vergleich von retrograder Zementapplikation und Vakuumzementierung hinsichtlich Zementpenetration und Fettembolie – eine tierexperimentelle Untersuchung. Inauguraldissertation 2004, Heidelberg.

111. von Issendorff WD, Ritter G: Untersuchungen zur Höhe und Bedeutung des intramedullären Druckes während des Einzementierens von Hüftendoprothesen. Unfallchirurgie 3:99–104, 1977

112. Wenda K, Ritter G, Ahlers J, von Issendorff WD: Detection and effects of bone marrow intravasations in operations in the area of the femoral marrow cavity. Unfallchirurg 93:56–61, 1990

113. Wenda K, Ritter G, Degreif J, Rudigier J: Pathogenesis of pulmonary complications following intramedullary nailing osteosyntheses. Unfallchirurg 91:432–5, 1988

114. Wenda K, Scheuermann H, Weitzel E, Rudigier J: Pharmacokinetics of methylmethacrylate monomer during total hip replacement in man. Arch Orthop Trauma Surg 107:316–21, 1988

115. Yee AJ, Binnington AG, Hearn T, Protzner K, Fornasier VL, Davey JR: Use of a polyglycolide lactide cement plug restrictor in total hip arthroplasty. Clin Orthop:254–66, 1999

116. Zichner L: Embolisms from the bone marrow canal following implantation of intramedullary femur head endoprostheses with polymethylmethacrylate. Aktuelle Probl Chir Orthop 31:201–5, 1987

How Have I Done It? Evaluation Criteria

Erwin Morscher

Summary

In this chapter, the relevant tools for outcome and quality assessment after cemented THA are presented. Success can be measured very differently and both patient and surgeon perception are important. The value of clinical scoring systems and the importance of serial radiographic assessment are discussed. The quality of the cement mantle has a greater significance on long-term outcome than the design of the prosthesis. The surgeon remains the greatest variable!

Introduction

The quality of a hip arthroplasty can be assessed very differently, depending whether it is judged by the patient, the surgeon, or the prosthesis manufacturer. The patient is mostly interested, whether his or her expectations for the operation have been met. The surgeon wonders how well he has performed the operation, and the prosthesis manufacturer is satisfied if early complications are not attributable to prosthesis design or manufacture.

The primary goals of an arthroplasty, i.e., absence of pain and improvement of mobility and ability to walk, are almost always achieved and have actually been achieved from the very beginning, after Charnley [6] introduced his »low friction arthroplasty« more than 40 years ago. The patients were, compared with those still treated with an intertrochanteric osteotomy or an arthrodesis at that time, very happy about the regained freedom of pain and the quickly restored mobility. As a result, even early catastrophes were accepted and were due to excessive abrasion of the Teflon cups or prostheses fractures in early designs, and could not stop the triumphal march of the total joint

prosthesis. Consequently, the advances made in endoprosthetics since then are not primarily advances from good to better endoprosthetics but have mainly consisted of a drastic reduction in complications – aseptic implant loosening included. »Good endoprosthetics« thus means first of all: no perioperative and postoperative complications!

Aside from the patient-related, individual factors, such as age, gender, etiology of the coxarthrosis, etc., four basic factors always play a role in the survival length of an artificial hip joint. These factors influence each other and are dependent on each other. They are:
- the mechanical design,
- the characteristics of the implant surface,
- the material properties of the implant, in the case of cemented endoprostheses the quality of the cement mantle, and
- the operative and cementing technique.

Patient Assessment

The patient's criteria for what they regard as »good or bad endoprosthetics« are undoubtedly the most important to them. However, their judgment has only very limited objective relevance. The patient's opinion is actually only relevant when dealing with »bad endoprosthetics«, i.e., if the patient complains about pain, or if the operated joint does not move well, dislocates repeatedly, or the leg length is not equal after the operation.

The patient should be educated to understand that the *time* of the follow-up examination plays an important role in assessing pain. During the first weeks after surgery, symptoms must be accepted up to a certain degree without having to question a rating of »good endoprosthetics«. These complaints normally disappear in the course of the first postoperative weeks completely, or at least they rapidly decrease.

The so-called warm-up or thigh pain with cement-free fixation of femur stems provided the material for many discussions in the 1980s. Such pain is triggered when getting up from a chair or climbing stairs, i.e., when the prosthesis stem in its bone bed is stressed by torsion. Admittedly, these pains also disappear after a few months in most cases. However, there is no doubt that they must be regarded as signs of insufficient stability of the prosthesis stem. It is known, after all, that pain that can be triggered by a forced internal rotation of the leg is the most reliable clinical sign of a loosened stem. The probability that a prosthesis, especially the femoral stem, is not loose is very high in asymptomatic patients, particularly during the first five to six years after operation. An analysis of 18,486 primary total hip arthroplasties was performed between 1976 and 2001 and recorded at the M.E. Müller Research Centre for Orthopaedic Surgery at the University of Berne/Switzerland to assess the validity of clinical procedures in diagnosing loosening of prosthetic components. It suggested that the necessity of periodic clinical and radiological follow-up examinations of asymptomatic patients during the first five to six years after operation is questionable, because test sensitivities for diagnosing loosening in a symptomatic patient are too low and, therefore, require radiological assessment. On the other hand, loosening of the cup often produces no pain and usually therefore is detected late [19, 22, 26, 27].

Surgeon Assessment: Beware of One-Dimensional Assessments!

When assessing hip-joint arthroplasty, one should never limit study to an isolated evaluation of a prosthesis model. Success or failure of an arthroplasty actually do not by any means depend just on the model, as one could assume based on the almost unmanageable number of publications on short-term, medium-term, and long-term results for the various models. A one-dimensional point of view is the most common cause for misjudging an arthroplasty! The verdict on a hip arthroplasty can and may only be pronounced under simultaneous and comprehensive consideration of the design, surface consistency, material, and operation and cementing technique.

Because good endoprosthetics can largely be equated with complication-free endoprosthetics, questions about the quality indicators of the arthroplasty play a less decisive role in the assessment than indications for its possible later failure. Thus, an assessment has mainly the goal of detecting the signs of an unfavourable prognosis or a potential loosening. Insight is principally offered by 1) the clinical result, and 2) the X-ray film.

Clinical Assessment

A reliable assessment – in other words, the quality control of a prosthesis system – should be made based on a complete documentation and analysis of all data relevant to a result. The IDES documentation (International Documentation and Evaluation System), as it was initiated and primarily worked out by M.E. Müller and officially recognised by the SICOT (Société Internationale de Chirurgie Orthopédique et de Traumatologie), is now used worldwide [12].

Scores

A number of hip-rating systems to assess function before and after hip replacement have been developed. In 1990 Callaghan and coworkers [5] assessed one hundred hips in patients with primary uncemented prosthesis up for one or two years. All collaborators who were involved in the study produced different results. There was not only no uniformity and objectivity but also no uniformity between the ratings and the patient's impressions. However, since the pre-operative functional class of the patients, as defined by Charnley [6] in 1979, significantly affected all ratings, they proposed to include the Charnley classes (A, B and C) in all rating systems. »A category-A patient is physically fit in all respects relating to function, with allowances for age, and without any defect other than the hip affected by arthritis«. »Category-B patients have both hips affected but otherwise they are physically fit for their age and no other factor exists to interfere with function«. »Category-C is reserved for conditions directly impairing the act of walking«. The nowadays – at least in the North American literature – most frequently used rating system of clinical evaluation before and after surgery is the Harris Hip Score, introduced in 1969 [10].

To assess the subjective outcome after total hip arthroplasty the »Western Ontario and McMaster University Osteoarthritis Index« (WOMAC) and the »MOS-36-item short form health survey« (SF-36) have been developed and have shown a sound statistical relationship between walking ability and their functional aspects [2].

Hip arthroplasty has the clinical goal of freeing the patient from pain and of normalizing the mobility of the arthritic joint. If possible, the patient should be able to enjoy this result until the end of his life without a re-operation. Absence of pain and presence of mobility are such dominant assessment criteria that it should really be sufficient to conduct a clinical evaluation based only on pain and the degree of hip flexion. Even in the simple rating system of Merle d'Aubigné [17] – probably the most commonly used »score« in orthopaedics overall, which takes into account the three criteria pain, mobility, and ability to walk – one could limit the assessment to the first two criteria mentioned, since ability to walk depends after all not only directly on pain perception and mobility but also on a number of other factors not related to the hip arthroplasty itself. One just has to consider patients with polyarthritis and polyarthrosis or heart failure, whose score is a priori worse than that of an otherwise healthy monoarthritic, due to non-implant related criteria, e.g., ability to walk (Charnley class C, see above).

Radiological Assessment of the Endoprosthesis

The main aim of radiological assessment of a THR is to determine signs of implant loosening which include migration, defects in the cement mantle and radiolucent zones (osteolyses and radiolucencies) at implant interfaces.

There are no positive clinical criteria for estimating longevity of an arthroplasty, since current absence of pain, good mobility, and ability to walk are by no means guarantees of future performance. For such prognosticating imaging methods are required. The native X-ray film is usually sufficient. In exceptional cases only, e.g., when an infection is suspected, a scintigram may be indicated.

For the radiological assessment of a hip arthroplasty, a principal differentiation has to be made between positive criteria indicating good endoprosthetics and negative criteria that have to be listed as signs of risk in regard to the permanence of the implant anchoring. When evaluating the X-ray film, a differentiation has, of course, to be made between cemented and non-cemented endoprostheses.

Para-Articular (Heterotopic) Ossifications

The degree of obvious para-articular ossifications that have occurred postoperatively is determined according to the internationally accepted classification by Brooker [4] (◻ Fig. 16.1). Brooker degrees I and II can be found in the overwhelming majority of hip arthroplasties; however, they have no relevance with regard to mobility limitation as a rule. This does not even regularly apply to Brooker degree III. Degree IV, however, is equivalent to a stiffening of the joint.

Positioning of the Implants

If the cup position is too vertical, increased abrasion at the cups upper, weight-bearing part and margins results; conversely, an overly pronounced anteversion position increases the danger of luxation. A varus misalignment of the prosthesis stem increases the risk of premature aseptic loosening due to intermittent overload of the main transmitting calcar area.

Migration

Tilting or sinking in of an implant (subsidence) over time – generally called »migration« – used to be regarded as a clear sign of a loosening process being underway [11, 18]. However, this does not apply to a »subsidence« of up to 5 mm for implants fixed according to the press-fit concept [15, 20, 24]. In contrast, a straight, wedge-shaped prosthesis stem (Müller straight stem [24], an Exeter [8], or MS-30 stem [28]) gains new stability with subsidence.

Subsidence of a cemented stem can be measured as the difference of the distance between the upper circumference of the prosthesis shoulder and the sclerotic line above the shoulder, in other words by measuring the expansion of the radiolucent line between the two (◻ Fig. 16.2).

Assessment of the Cement Mantle

There is no longer any doubt that the quality of the cement mantle, i.e., its biomechanically proper spatial distribution, continuity and intimacy of contact with the stem and surrounding bone as well its resistance to abrasion, are decisive for the permanence of a cemented prosthesis stem [28]. Mistakes in the cementing technique are mainly insufficient medial support, an insufficient, mostly a too thin, cement mantle with metal-bone contact, insufficient dove-tailing between cement and bone, and finally, an incorrect positioning of the implant.

Based partly on finite-element studies, but mainly from clinical experience, we know that the optimal cement mantle is asymmetric. It is thicker and thus stronger at *those* places where the forces are mostly transmitted, i.e., proximo-medially at the calcar femorale and at the prosthesis tip (Gruen zones 7, 5, and 3). The thickness of the cement mantle should not drop below 2 mm at any place if at all possible. It also should be complete, i.e., it should not allow metal-bone contact [7, 9, 21].

The risk of a metal-bone contact consists mainly in creating the opportunity for an unimpaired spreading of generated particles (polyethylene, bone cement) in the so-called »extended joint space« if there is a direct connection between the bone-cement and the metal-cement interface [27]. Enzymes (interleukins, necrosis factors, prostaglandins, etc.) excreted by the macrophages in the process of phagocytosis of the 1–10 µm sized particles lead to breakdown of the bone (osteolysis) and thus to loosening of the implant in its bone bed.

With cemented femoral stems, the focus is mainly on the cement mantle and its connections to the prosthesis stem, on the one hand, and to the bone, on the other hand. With implants fixated without cement, special emphasis is placed on the assessment of the surrounding bone structure. Of course, the physiological changes in bone shape, such as an expansion of the medullary channel and

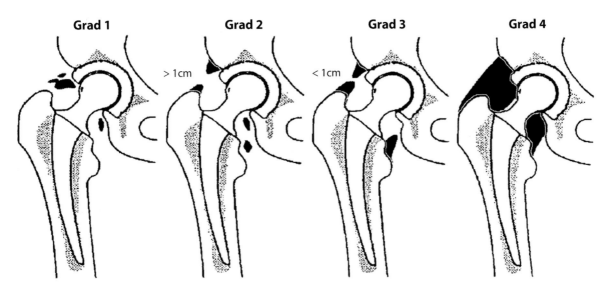

Grad 1   **Grad 2**   **Grad 3**   **Grad 4**

> 1cm   < 1cm

■ **Fig. 16.1.** Rating of para-articular ossifications according to Brooker et al. [4]

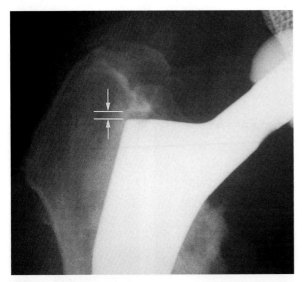

■ **Fig. 16.2.** Measurement of subsidence

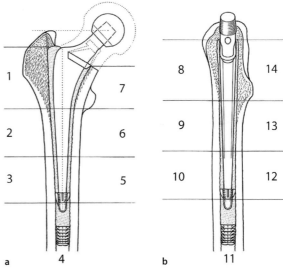

■ **Fig. 16.3. a** Zones 1–7, **b** zones 8–14 according to Gruen et al. [9]

thinning of the corticalis, as they occur with increasing age must also be included in the assessment since those changes also take place practically unimpaired in a femur supplied with an implant [23].

It is justifiably demanded that a cement mantle assessment should be made both in the antero-posterior and the axial beam path in order to be complete. The localisations critical in regard to a metal-bone contact are the zones 8 and 9 as they appear in the lateral image [3] (■ Fig. 16.3).

To create a cement mantle that completely surrounds the prosthesis stem, a stem number smaller than the reaming must already be selected during preoperative planning. The under-dimensioning of the stem compared to the cutting of the bone bed creates the space necessary for the cement mantle.

Gruen et al. (1979) [9] developed the now generally accepted method to locate osteolyses, radiolucent lines and fractures of the cement mantle in 7 zones, each on the a.-p. and axial view (■ Fig. 16.3). Barrack et al. in 1992 [1] emphasised the quality of cementing, and described four grades in postoperative radiographs:

A: complete filling of the medullary canal by bone cement, a so-called »white out« at the bone-cement interface,

B: slight radiolucency at the bone-cement interface,

C: radiolucency involving 50–99% of the bone-cement interface or a defective or incomplete cement mantle, and

D: definite radiolucency at the cement-bone interface of 100% in any projection, or a failure to fill the canal with cement such that the tip of the stem is not covered.

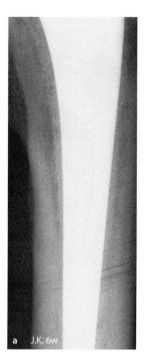
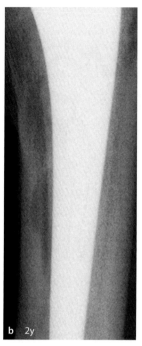
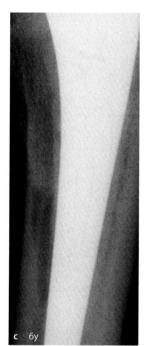
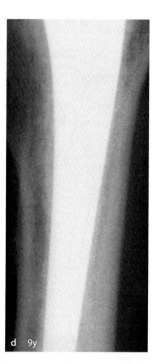

a   J.K. 6w   b   2y   c   6y   d   9y

☐ **Fig. 16.4. a** The postoperative X-ray film shows a radiolucency in zone 6 as a sign of insufficient pressurization during surgery (Barrack B) [1]. **b,c** (Condition at 2 and 6 years shown): Development of an oste- olysis with progression. **d** (Condition at 9 years shown): Between the 6th and 9th postoperative year no more progression. The patient died 11 years after surgery without having had pain

Osteolysis and Radiolucency

The surrounding bone is scanned for osteolysis. According to Joshi et al., we understand osteolysis to be »... a newly developed, cystic lesion with endosteal scalloping and/or migration which had not been seen on the immediate postoperative radiograph« [13]. Osteolysis is usually progressive and finally leads to loosening of the implant. Nevertheless, a wait-and-see approach is justified in case of smaller osteolyses, especially if there are no complaints (☐ Fig. 16.4). Now that polyethylene abrasion has been determined to be the main cause for the generation of particles, the extent of abrasion, especially on longer-term radiograph controls, is of interest for the further prognosis of the affected arthroplasty as a measure of the tribologic behaviour of the joint.

The cement-bone interface is scanned for radiolucent lines (☐ Fig. 16.5). Depending on their extent, we differentiate between potential, probable, and confirmed radiological loosening. Continuous radiolucencies around the cup in zones 1 to 3 according to DeLee and Charnley and continuous radiolucencies at the cement-bone or stem-bone interface are signs of definitive loosening [22]. The probability of loosening increases with the size of periprosthetic radiolucencies [16]. The most important prognostic factor for long-term survival of a cemented acetabular component are adequate cement mantle thickness and the absence of radiolucency in DeLee Charnley zone I on the

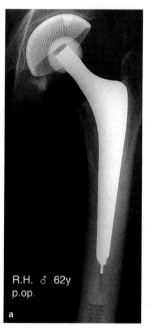
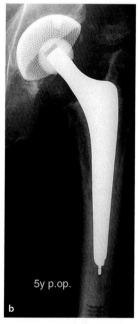

R.H. ♂ 62y
p.op.

a   5y p.op.   b

☐ **Fig. 16.5a,b.** Hybrid total prosthesis arthroplasty with cemented MS-30 stem and non-cemented press-fit cup. The postoperative X-ray image (**a**) shows radiolucency between cement mantle and cortical bone in zones 6 and 7 (Barrack B). The likely reason was insufficient pressurisation of the bone cement. Five years later (**b**), an increasing radiolucent line and newly appearing radiolucent line had occurred in zones 2 and 3. No pain, free mobility. Radiologically: increasing loosening, para-articular ossification Brooker degree I (compare with ☐ Fig. 16.1). Clinically: still excellent result

16

radiograph obtained after surgery [25]. A lucent line on the first postoperative film in zone I significantly increases the risk of loosening, up to 40 fold (■ Fig. 16.6).

Of course, the cement mantle is also examined for its intactness. Cement fractures are signs of accompanying loss of the metal-cement (debonding) and bone-cement mechanical interlock (loosening) (■ Fig. 16.7).

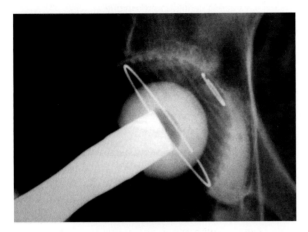

■ **Fig. 16.6.** Immediate postoperative radiograph of cemented socket with two typical mistakes. The acetabular component has been inserted incorrectly and pushed too far superiorly, as evidenced by a thick cement mantle medio-inferiorly (where it is not needed!) and a thin cement mantle (<1–2 mm) with radiolucent line in DeLee and Charnley zone I. This pattern is associated with a higher risk of failure

The reported prevalences of radiological loosening differ widely in the literature. Ling [15] found a variation between highest and lowest of 20! The reason of this variation is not only due to differences in prosthesis designs and quality of the operation and/or cementing technique but also due to the fact that the prevalence is directly related to the definition of radiological loosening of an implant and the unreliability of the interpretation of the X-ray films [22].

McCaskie et al. [16] measuring the level of inter- and intraobserver agreement in recording the appearance of lucent areas and migration of the prosthesis found, in general, a moderate intraobserver agreement but a poor interobserver agreement, similar to that expected by chance! This makes comparisons to be drawn between reports of different treatment modalities difficult or even impossible.

The Survival Time of a Hip Endoprosthesis

In accordance with the criteria of »Evidence Based Medicine«, the survivorship of an endoprosthesis – any revision being the endpoint – is from a clinical point of view the best defined criterion of quality or failure. The curves of Kaplan and Meier [14] have become standards for the assessment of hip arthroplasties and are the method for assessing data from the Scandinavian Implant Registers.

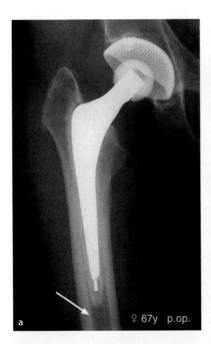
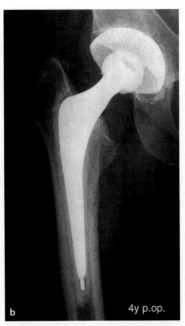
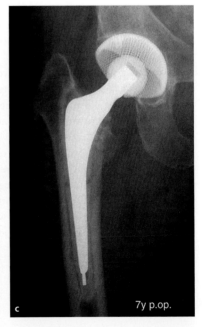

■ **Fig. 16.1a–c.** 67 years old female patient. **a** The postoperative X-ray film shows that the restrictor is obviously missing (*arrow*). As a consequence, pressurisation of the bone cement was insufficient and radiolucency can bee seen in zones 3, 5 and 7. **b** Four years postopera- tively the MS-30 stem had significantly subsided (with and within the cement mantle) and a transverse fracture of the cement mantle had developed. **c** Progressive radiolucency with definitive loosening at 7 years. The MS30 stem had to be revised

Conclusion and Summary

The pioneering times for endoprosthetics are over. Today's patients have a right to a surgeon adequately trained in endoprosthetics supplying them with endoprosthesis designs that have passed the test of time. Any change in mechanical design, of the surfaces, the material of an endoprosthesis, or of the operation technique must be thoroughly tested in the form of a prospective, if possible randomised study, and such an implant should really not be released until the benefit of the change has been shown in the form of improved results. In endoprosthetics, we have undoubtedly reached the asymptotic range of the success curve. Further progress will be increasingly harder to achieve. The standard endoprosthetics as reached by now has become the greatest obstacle for further progress! Good endoprosthetics is first of all an operation free from complications. The assessment of an endoprosthesis outcome has to consider all variables, in particular the patient's preoperative local and systemic status, design, surface characteristics, material, and operation or cementing technique, in their mutual influence and dependency: beware of one-dimensional assessments! The greatest variable is the surgeon. The quality of the cement mantle has a greater significance for assessing a cemented arthroplasty than the design of the prosthesis. The result of an assessment is no absolute measure. The assessment depends strongly on whether it is made in relation to the patient or the surgeon. These are two completely independent points of view, which in some cases may be diametrically opposed to each other. When assessing endoprosthetics, more emphasis must be placed on risk factors as predictive statements in regard to a later failure than on positive (mostly subjective) findings.

In summary: On the X-ray film, we therefore evaluate the cement mantle, the surrounding bone tissue and its reaction to the »foreign body cement and implant«, the boundary layers between cement and bone, as well as those between cement and metal stem of the prosthesis. Furthermore, we look for any obvious change in position compared to earlier images in the sense of tilting or subsidence. Subsidence can, however, be regarded as »second line of defense«, provided the »migration« takes place in the cement mantle itself (»subsidence within the cement mantle«) and not together with it (»with the cement mantle«) (see ❒ Fig. 16.3).

Take Home Messages

- ▬ A good joint arthroplasty means first of all no complications – aseptic loosening included.
- ▬ Survival of an arthroplasty depends on patient, surgeon and implant related factors. Principal implant related factors are 1. geometry (design, cement mantle thickness), 2. surface characteristics, 3. materials including choice of cement and 4. surgeon's cementing technique.
- ▬ Whether periodic (annual) follow-up examinations in an asymptomatic patient are necessary remains questionable, at least during the first 5 years.
- ▬ Clinical signs for diagnosing aseptic loosening in a symptomatic patient are insufficient. Therefore, radiological assessment is necessary.
- ▬ Clinical scores are unreliable indicators for quality assessment of an arthroplasty. For daily use, pain and mobility are sufficient clinical indicators.
- ▬ The radiological assessment for diagnosing implant loosening includes migration, defects and fractures of the cement mantle and signs of bone resorption: osteolysis and progressive radiolucencies.
- ▬ The radiological assessment of cemented stems must be done both on an a.-p. *and* lateral view!
- ▬ Subsidence of a straight, distally tapered femoral stem is usually not a sign of loosening.
- ▬ The prevalence of reported radiological aseptic loosening is not only due to actual, operative and the cementing technique effects but also to the definition of radiological loosening and the unreliability of the interpretation of the X-ray films.
- ▬ The greatest variable still is the surgeon!
- ▬ The quality of the cement mantle has a greater significance than the design of the prosthesis.

References

1. Barrack RL, Mulroy RD Jr, Harris WH (1992) Improved cementing techniques and femoral component loosening in young patients with hip arthroplasties, a 12 year radiographic review. J Bone Joint Surg 74-B:385–9
2. Boardman DL, Dorey F, Thomas BJ, Lieberman JR (2000) The Accuracy of Assessing total hip arthroplasty outcomes, J Arthroplasty 15:200–204
3. Breusch SJ, Lukoschek N, Kreutzer J, Brocai D, Gruen TA (2001) Dependency of cement mantle thickness on femoral stem design and centralizer. J Arthroplasty 16:648–657
4. Brooker AF, Bowerman JW, Robinson RA, Riley LH Jr (1973) Ectopic ossification following total hip replacement. Incidence and a method of classification. J Bone Joint Surg 55A:1629–1632
5. Callaghan JJ, Dysart SH, Savory CF, Hopkinson WJ (1990) Assessing the results of hip replacement, J Bone Joint Surg 72-B:1008–9
6. Charnley J (1979) Low friction arthroplasty of the hip. Theory and practice. Springer, Berlin Heidelberg New York

16

7. Ebramzadeh E, Sarmiento A, McKellop HA, Llinas A, Gogan W (1994) The cement mantle in total hip arthroplasty. J Bone Joint Surg 76A:77–87

8. Fowler JL, Gie GA, Lee AJC, Ling RSM (1988) Experience with the Exeter total hip replacement since 1970. Orthop Clin North Am 19:477–489

9. Gruen TA, McNeice GM, Amstutz HC (1979) Modes of failure of cemented stem-type femoral components. A radiographic analysis of loosening. Clin Orthop 141:17–27

10. Harris WH (1969) Traumatic arthritis of the hip after dislocation and acetabular fractures. Treatment by mold arthroplasty, J Bone Joint Surg 51 A:737–755

11. Harris WH, McGann WA (1986) Loosening of the femoral component after use of the medullary-plug cementing technique. Follow-up note with a minimum five-year follow-up. J Bone Joint Surg 68A:1064–1066

12. Johnston RC, Fitzgerald RH, Harris WH, Poss R, Müller ME, Sledge CB (1990) Clinical and radiographic evaluation of total hip replacement. J Bone Joint Surg 72A::161–168

13. Joshi RP, Eftekhar NS, McMahon DJ, Nercessian OA (1998) Osteolysis after Charnley primary low-friction arthroplasty. J Bone Joint Surg 80B:585–590

14. Kaplan EL, Meier P (1958) Nonparametric estimation from incomplete observations. J Am Stat Assoc 53:457–481

15. Ling RSM (1986) Observations on the fixation arthroplasty of the hip. Clin Orthop 210:80–96

16. McCaskie AW, Brown AR, Thompson JR, Gregg PJ (1996) Radiological evaluation of the interface after cemented total hip replacement. J Bone Joint Surg 78-B:191–194

17. Merle d'Aubigné R, Postel M (1954) Functional results of hip arthroplasty with acrylic prosthesis, J Bone Joint Surgery 36A:451–475

18. Mjöberg B, Selvik G, Hansson LI, Rosenqvist R, Oennerfält R (1986) Mechanical loosening of total hip prosthesis: a radiographic and roentgen stereophotogrammetric study. J Bone Joint Surg 68B:770–774

19. Morscher E, Schmassman A (1983) Failures of total hip arthroplasty and probable incidence of revision surgery in the future. Arch Orthop Trauma Surg 101:137–143

20. Morscher E, Wirz D (2002) Current state of cement fixation in THR. Acta Orthop Belg 68:1–12

21. Morscher E, Spotorno L, Mumenthaler A, Frick W(1995) The cemented MS-30-stem, In: E.W. Morscher (ed) Endoprosthetics. Springer Berlin New York, pp 211–219

22. Müller EM (1981) Acetabular Revision, in Proc. 9th open scientific meeting of the Hip Society. C.V. Mosby, St. Louis/USA, pp 46–56

23. Poss R, Staehlin P, Larson M (1987) Femoral expansion in total hip replacement. J Arthroplasty 2:259–264

24. Räber D, Czaja S, Morscher E (2001) Fifteen year results of the Müller CoCrNiMo straight stem. Arch Orthop Trauma Surg 121:38–42

25. Ritter MA et al. (1999) Radiological factors influencing femoral and acetabular failure in cemented Charnley total hip arthroplasty. J Bone Joint Surg [Br] 81-B:982–986

26. Röder C, Eggli S, Aebi M, Busato A (2003) The validity of clinical examination in the diagnosis of loosening of components in total hip arthroplasty. J Bone Joint Surg 85B:37–44

27. Schmalzried TP, Jasty M, Harris WH (1992) Periprosthetic bone loss in total hip arthroplasty. Polyethylene wear debris and the concept of the effective joint space. J Bone Joint Surg 74A:849–863

28. Wirz D, Zurfluh B, Goepfert B, Li F, Frick W, Morscher EW (2003) Results of in vitro studies about the mechanism of wear in the stem-cement interface of THR. In: GL Winters and MJ Nutt (eds): Stainless steels for medical and surgical applications, ASTM International (American Society for Testing Materials), West Conshohocken, PA, pp 222–234

Mistakes and Pitfalls with Cemented Hips

Götz von Foerster

Summary

More than any other factor it is the surgeon's operative performance which has the greatest influence on the long-term fate of a cemented total hip arthroplasty. Although most mistakes are forgiving, at least in the short term, the chances of success are compromised. In this chapter, the most common surgical errors and potential pitfalls, which can occur during the cementing process of stem and cup, are outlined.

Introduction

There is no doubt that when implanted with an optimal cementing technique cemented hip arthroplasties (THA) can achieve excellent long-term results. The surgeon's experience and technical ability is crucial for the success of the procedure.

Mistakes made during the cementing procedure rarely lead to immediate failure of the implant. This is one of the reasons why mistakes often remain undiscovered for a long time and are difficult to rectify. The weaknesses of faulty cementing technique do not become apparent until revealed by the long-term results of large case numbers. Although this suggests that even poor cementing techniques are forgiving this should not lead to a false conclusion.

The following questions must be considered:
- How long can hip arthroplasties survive when implanted with an optimal cementing technique?
- What are the cementing mistakes which shorten the survival of the implants?
- How serious must a mistake be in order to shorten the survival of an implant?

It is extremely difficult to pinpoint specific details here, therefore there is only one possible principle:

> Note: Every mistake in cementing technique shortens the survival of an implant and must be avoided.

We differentiate between two categories of cementing:
- primary cementing during primary joint arthroplasty,
- secondary cementing during revision surgery (modified bearing, larger implants).

The surgeon must ensure that all steps in the cementing procedure, i.e. preparation of the bone, mixing the cement, insertion at the correct time (timing!) and pressurisation of the cement, are carefully co-ordinated.

The Common Mistakes

The Cement Mantle

The aim is to achieve a complete and non-deficient cement mantle encompassing the entire implant. The cement mantle is defined by the correlation between the bone bearing, implant size and the position of the implant after implantation. The most common mistake is that the prosthesis stem is not implanted in a perfectly centred position. In many cases the implant is in a varus position and often there is contact between the metal tip of the implant and the bone (■ Fig. 17.1). The result is that at this point the cement mantle is too thin or not present at all. Osteolysis may result and later the implant tip migrates into the cortical bone and may cause fracture.

Valgus malpositioning is less frequent (■ Fig. 17.2), but is known to be more forgiving.

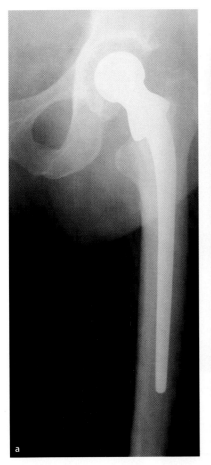
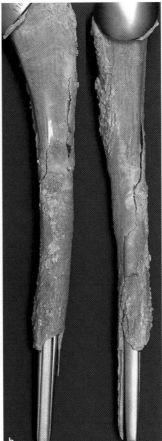
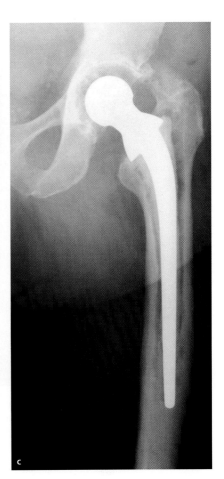

Fig. 17.1a–c. Prosthesis in varus position. Contact between metal and bone

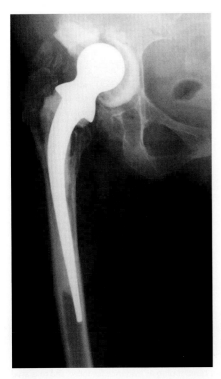

Fig. 17.2. Prosthesis in valgus position. Cement mantle incomplete

Another mistake which is often observed is incomplete filling of the femur with cement. The reason for this mistake is that the surgeon has failed to appropriately lavage and suction off all the fluid in the femur or to notice pockets of blood and air remaining in the cavity. As a consequence, air and blood entrapment with radiographically evident voids within the cement mantle or radiolucent lines at the cement-bone interface (visible on the first postoperative X-ray) may occur. This can result in prosthetic stem loosening from distal which leads to instability of the implant. The consequences of this mistake are, however, usually less dramatic than those of malpositioned implants.

If poor cementing technique and stem malpositioning are present as a combined surgical mistake, then early aseptic failure can result (Fig. 17.3). Figure 17.3 highlights a number of cardinal mistakes:

- The stem is in varus malalignment.
- This had led to a deficient cement mantle at the lateral stem tip (direct bone contact).
- The rounded distal tip of the cement mantle indicates residual blood entrapment above the cement restrictor and is evidence for poor intraoperative pressurisation.

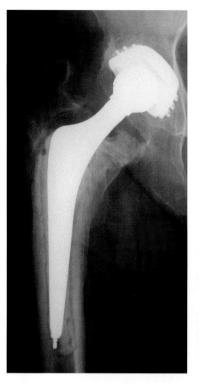
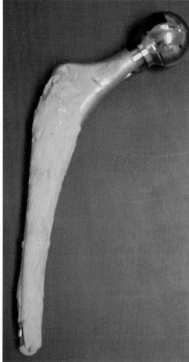
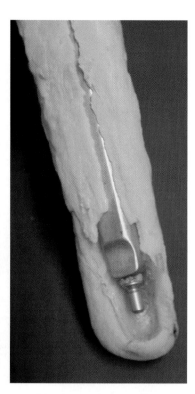

Fig. 17.3. Early aseptic loosening after 3 years which is unrelated to the implant type, but a consequence of poor surgical technique with a combination of varus stem malalignment and poor cement mantle (see text)

- The cement mantle is too thin (implant size!) and has cracked.
- At three years there is radiographic loosening with a complete radiolucent line at the cement bone interface.
- Radiographically the entire stem/cement complex has significantly subsided more than 5 mm (see stem shoulder!).
- The explanted specimen shows a smooth entire cement mantle as evidence for poor cementing technique. A smooth cement surface can only result, if no endosteal cancellous bone has been preserved and lavaged and if cement pressurisation was not or insufficiently done.

The Cement Restrictor

The cement restrictor in the distal femur plays a very important role. The restrictor must be inserted at exactly the right point using a longitudinally marked guide and the surgeon must check that it is firmly in position. If the restrictor is incorrectly placed, the cement spreads out over a long distance in the femoral medullary canal. This causes serious problems if revision is later necessary. These plugs of cement are extremely difficult to remove (Figs. 17.4 and 17.5).

Failure of the cement restrictor also results in reduced intramedullary pressure during the cementing process

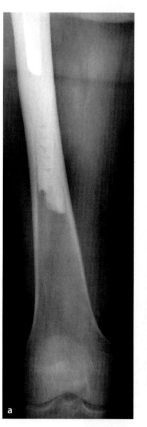
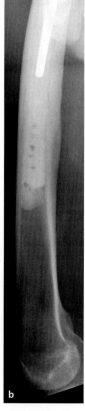

Fig. 17.4a,b. Long cement plug as evidence for failed and migrated cement restrictor

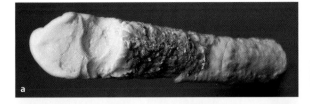

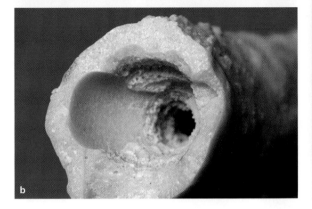

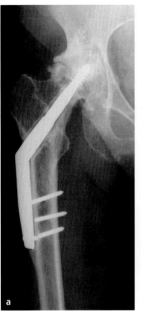

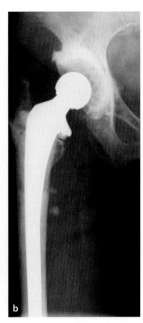

■ **Fig. 17.5a,b.** Distal cement plug specimens, difficult to remove at revision

■ **Fig. 17.6a,b.** Cement protrusion through screw holes

and thus to reduced penetration of the cement into the cancellous bone (bonding).

Cement Protrusion

There are various reasons for cement protrusion from the femoral medullary canal. During primary cementing, cement may protrude through unnoticed screw holes in patients, who had previous osteosynthesis, and can cause severe pain (■ Fig. 17.6).

Otherwise, cement protrusion usually happens during secondary cementing in revision surgery when cortical perforations occur (unnoticed), often in the critical region around the former implant tip (■ Fig. 17.7). This is because the affected areas were not sufficiently exposed during the operation. It is essential to ensure that the medullary canal is fully intact before cementing, particularly after osteosynthesis and removal of screws or during revision surgery.

For a while, some hospitals used additional material such as the Verhoewe »quiver« or osteosynthesis plating to close large defects at revision arthroplasty with extremely thick layers of cement (■ Fig. 17.8). This strategy did not lead to any improvement in the cement anchorage of a large defect. On the contrary, it only produced additional interfaces between the implant, cement, additional material and then the bone and therefore an increased risk of loosening, for example, when the material was subjected to greater stress than usual.

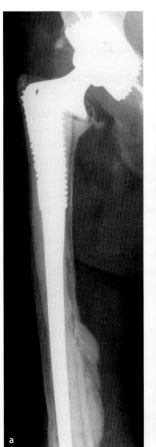

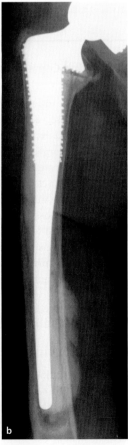

■ **Fig. 17.7a,b.** Cement protrusion through cortical perforation in revision surgery

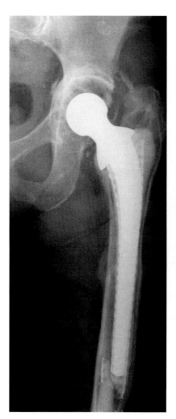
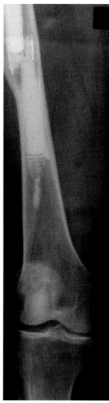
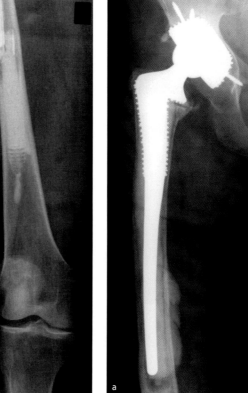
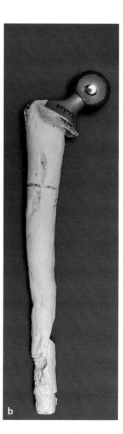

◻ **Fig. 17.8.** Stress fracture of a Verhoewe »quiver«

◻ **Fig. 17.9a,b.** Cementing a cementless hip is an unforgivable mistake

Cementing Cementless Hip Implants

Using cement to fix cementless implants in position is a frequently observed mistake. This happens when a suitable cemented implant is not available during surgery or when the surgeon is not aware of the consequences of cementing a cementless implant (◻ Fig. 17.9).

Cementing a cementless implant is in itself an uncomplicated procedure, but in revision cases removal of the cement is the exact opposite. A cemented cementless implant can only be removed together with the entire cement mantle. This often means that the femur has to be opened by fenestration or more extensive osteotomy. Cementing a cementless implant is therefore an unforgivable mistake.

Incomplete Removal of Cement at Revision Surgery

In certain situations in revision surgery (excluding infection cases) it is not always necessary to remove a firmly fixed cement mantle completely. It is possible to implant a new prosthesis in a distally well-preserved and firmly fixed cement mantle, especially if the prosthesis has a straight stem. If the surgeon decides to leave the cement mantle in place he must ensure that it really is intact and firm.

In patients with deep periprosthetic infection, however, all cement must be removed completely and thoroughly. Even the smallest cement fragments are most certainly colonised by bacteria and are bound to cause recurrence of infection (◻ Fig. 17.10).

When a joint is infected, even a firmly fixed cement mantle and distal cement plugs deep inside the femur must be completely removed. Otherwise, the procedure is doomed to failure with recurrent/persisting infection.

Cementing the Acetabular Cup

The fact that the long-term results of cemented cups are poorer than those of cemented stems could be attributed to the different type of bone bearing. The fact that cementless acetabular cups also have poorer long-term results than cementless stems would seem to confirm this conclusion.

Mistakes during the cementing of acetabular cups occur because the bone has been poorly prepared and/or the cement has been inadequately pressurised into the acetabulum. Correct and adequate pressurisation is only possible with the new instruments now available.

A further mistake is, that defects, especially in the centre of the acetabulum, are either not recognised or not sufficiently covered (with bone graft) and as a result

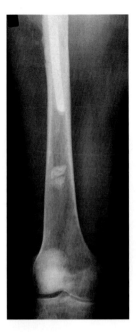

Fig. 17.10. Incomplete removal of cement in a case with deep infection

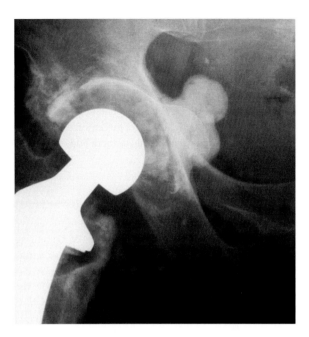

Fig. 17.11. Cement protrusion into the pelvis

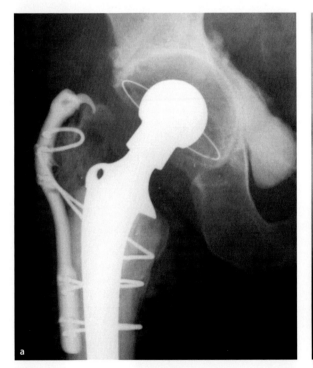

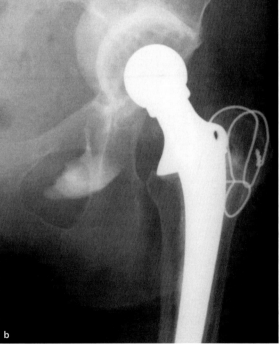

Fig. 17.12a,b. Inferior cement escape (**a**). Migration of disconnected cement fragment (**b**).

cement protrudes into the pelvis (**Fig. 17.11**). This can lead to serious complications such as vascular erosion and haemorrhaging, especially during later revision.

Inadequate handling and compression of cement also causes dispersion of small fragments of cement especially towards caudal. These are often not visible during surgery and are not discovered until later on the radiograph. For

this reason, meticulous inspection of the acetabulum after cementing is essential (**Fig. 17.12**). Protruding cement which is no longer connected firmly to the cement inside the acetabulum can migrate and endanger nerves and blood vessels.

Another cardinal mistake is filling the acetabular roof with cement in an area which is no longer contained.

In the course of time this cement is destined to fracture and slip away as it has no bone support (◪ Fig. 17.13).

It goes without saying that after the stem or cup have been cemented in position any surplus cement must be removed, otherwise this cement can later break off during joint movement. Small particles can penetrate into the acetabulum between the cup and head of the femoral stem where they can cause serious damage due to three body wear.

Conclusion

For expert cementing, surgeons must have comprehensive knowledge of and ability in the technique of cementing and carry out all the necessary checks to avoid or eliminate the mistakes described here.

To conclude, here are two notable examples. In the first case the cemented stem survived twelve years, which could be interpreted as evidence that even small amounts of cement in the right place can hold an implant in position for quite a long time (◪ Fig. 17.14).

The second case shows that although it may allow double mobility of the artificial femoral head in the cup and at the same time of the natural femoral head in the natural acetabulum, cementing implant components on an unsuitable base such as the »retained« femoral head after femoral neck fracture does not provide firm fixation for any length of time (◪ Fig. 17.15).

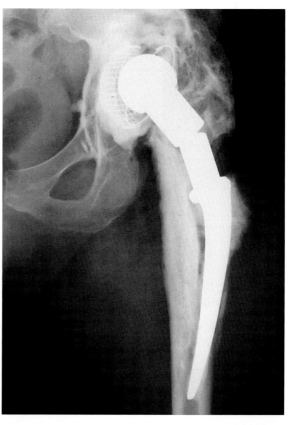

◪ **Fig. 17.14.** Despite small amounts of cement this implant was in position for 12 years

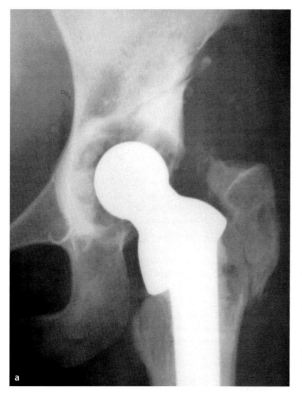

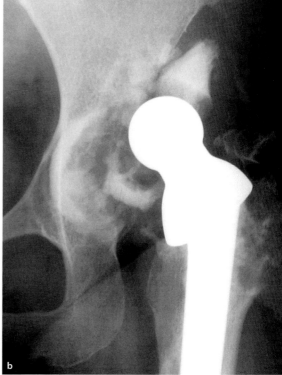

◪ **Fig. 17.13a,b.** Using cement in an uncontained area and roof defect will lead to failure. Cement has fractured and slipped away

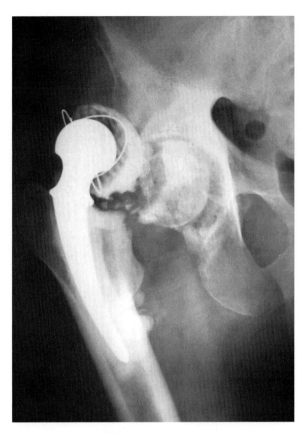

Fig. 17.15. »Too much mobility«

Take Home Messages

- Typical mistakes can occur during cemented THA and must be avoided.
- Too bulky stems and (varus) malalignment must be avoided.
- Thin and deficient cement mantles are the surgeons responsibility.
- Cement restrictor failure will result in poorer cement mantle and long distal cement plugs, which are difficult to remove.
- Cement protrusion through bone defects and screw holes can lead to pain and neurovascular complications.
- Remnant and free cement debris can migrate and cause problems.
- Do not cement implants designed for cementless fixation.
- Poor cementing technique at the acetabulum is less forgiving.
- Usage of cement in uncontained bone defects may lead to failure.
- Avoiding mistakes and performing perfect cementing technique are decisive for long-term implant survival.

Revision is Not Difficult!

Thorsten Gehrke

Summary

Aseptic and septic prosthesis exchange is a challenge for every surgeon. Intra- and postoperative complications are frequent and may have serious negative effects on the outcome of the operation. Suitable instruments and surgical techniques can, however, considerably lower the risk of complication. With the techniques described in this chapter and personal experience, readers will find that prosthesis exchange need not necessarily be a difficult procedure. Special emphasis is given to revisional surgery of cemented implants.

Preparation

During preparation for prosthesis exchange the possibility of septic loosening or periprosthetic infection must first of all be excluded as the cause of the patient's problem.

Diagnostics

Laboratory: CRP!, ESR, (leukocyte count).

> **Note:** CRP and ESR always rise postoperatively. CRP should return to normal after 2 to 3 weeks, while ESR may remain elevated for up to one year. Therefore, CRP monitoring is of decisive importance. The leukocyte count is of **no** or only small importance as this usually remains within the normal range.

Radiology: Plain X-rays in standardised planes, to scale if necessary.
Scintigraphy: Expensive, but does not yield very much useful information.

CT: Artifacts, used only for design of custom-made implants for large bone defects.
MRI: Artifacts, expensive, does not yield very much useful information. More suitable for assessment of soft tissues.

Arthrocentesis (Joint Aspiration)

Pathogen identification: Arthrocentesis or aspiration of joint fluid is the method of choice for obtaining a representative sample of fluid for successful detection and identification of pathogens.

The most suitable transport medium is the aspirated fluid itself. Swabs should not be used at all, culture tubes only in emergencies

 Note:
- Systemic antibiotic therapy must be discontinued 10–14 days prior to arthrocentesis.
- No local anaesthesia during arthrocentesis (antimicrobial effect).
- No irrigation or contrast media (diluting effect).
- Fluid samples must be cultured in the laboratory for at least 14 days.

General Preoperative Planning

Anaesthesia

- Clinical and anaesthesiologic assessment of operation risk,
- preoperative autologous blood or perioperative recovery and retransfusion,
- adequate quantity of additional donor blood,

- in case of long exchange operations preoperative administration of fibrinolysis inhibitors (e.g. Trasilol) is recommended. Cave: risk of anaphylactic shock!

Radiological Preparation

- Conventional X-rays in two or three planes in a standardised position are usually adequate.
- In some cases, X-rays may have to be taken with a radiopaque scale which allows exact definition of the film-focus distance, especially when special implants or megaprostheses (e.g. total femur replacement) are required.

Patient Information

- Risk of infection – about 5–8% during exchange operations,
- impaired wound healing requiring reoperation,
- damage to the sciatic and femoral nerves,
- severe haemorrhaging, especially in cases with acetabular implant protrusion into the pelvis,
- loss of function and stability in the muscles encompassing the hip,
- leg-length discrepancy,
- risk of fracture, intra- and postoperatively,
- rate of dislocation after aseptic and septic prosthesis exchange is markedly higher and is quoted in literature between 5 and 30%,
- increased risk of new aseptic loosening and also early loosening,
- range of movement may be restricted,
- partial weight-bearing is often necessary for up to 12 weeks.

Surgeon's Preparation

Choice of Implant

- Implants of different lengths and stem thicknesses must be at hand.
- Loss of bone substance, the possibility of intraoperative complications such as shaft fractures, perforations of the cortex, windows and destroyed pelvic bone must be taken into consideration when choosing the implant.
- Large defects in the pelvis can cause difficulties as here special acetabular components or rings and in some cases partial pelvis replacements may have to be implanted.
- If the pelvis is involved and there is a risk of injury to the iliac vessels or bladder, a vascular or abdominal surgeon or urologist should be present during surgery.

Approach

The following approaches are recommended for revision and exchange operations:

 Note:
Recommended approaches to the hip for prosthesis exchange:
- Posterior approach
- Transtrochanteric approach
- Anterolateral, transgluteal approach (Hardinge, Bauer)
- Transfemoral approach

Less suitable approaches to the hip for prosthesis exchange:
- Anterolateral approach (Watson-Jones)
- Anterior approach

The posterior approach offers a number of important advantages, also for revision surgery. Firstly, it avoids damage to the abductors which are the most important stabilising muscles for the pelvis in the frontal plane. Anterior neurovascular structures are rarely damaged and the sciatic nerve, which may lie very close to the site, can be easily palpated and monitored. This approach provides good exposure of the superior and postero-superior acetabular region which is the most frequent site of deficient bone stock and allows extensive reconstructive procedures. The surgeon can obtain almost complete exposure of the ilium by extending the incision proximally. The particular advantage is that, even if an extended trochanteric osteotomy is required or if an osteolytic proximal femur disintegrates, the vasto-gluteal sling remains intact, thus minimising the risk of proximal trochanter migration and gluteal weakness.

A clear disadvantage is the higher risk of dislocation, which can be reduced by careful orientation of the acetabular cup and reconstruction of the posterior soft tissues during wound closure.

Skin and Fascial Incision

- Old scars in the line of the skin incision should be excised. If a prior incision does not lie in this line, the surgeon should maintain sufficient distance between it and the new incision (■ Fig. 18.1).
- Crossing the old scar at an acute angle or deviating from it should be avoided.
- Fistulae should be integrated into the skin incision if possible and radically excised all the way to the joint. If fistulae lie too far anteriorly or posteriorly, they are handled by means of a separate incision.

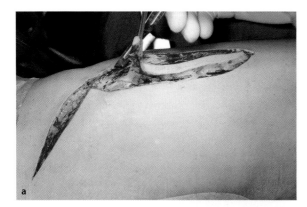

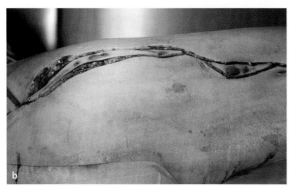

■ **Fig. 18.1a,b.** Previous incision scars must be excised. In infection (**b**) all sinus formations must also be included and excised

Biopsy

Biopsy material, preferably 5–6 samples, should be taken as a routine measure from all relevant areas of the operation site for microbiological evaluation.

> **Note:**
> Biopsy (routine):
> ▬ Joint capsule
> ▬ Entrance to femoral shaft
> ▬ Interior of femoral shaft
> ▬ Acetabular floor
>
> Biopsy (if necessary):
> ▬ Fistulae
> ▬ Abscesses

Removing Hip Implants (Cemented Stems)

Removing cemented stems is generally much easier and less invasive than removing cementless stems. Polished cemented stems are considered revision friendly, but textured stems, particularly those with a collar, can be difficult to remove.

The key to remove any cemented stem without risking fracture or avulsion of the greater trochanter is removal

of all accessible lateral cement around the shoulder of the stem prior (see below).

Instruments for Removing Cemented Stems

▬ Extraction instruments (■ Fig. 18.2):
  – system-specific extraction instruments,
  – punches,
  – taper extraction instrument (Nieder, from Waldemar Link, ■ Fig. 18.2, top),
  – box-type stem extractor for firmly fixed or non-modular heads (■ Fig. 18.2, bottom).
▬ Chisels (osteotomes) and graspers in different lengths and widths (■ Figs. 18.3 and 18.4):

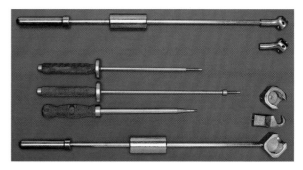

■ **Fig. 18.2.** Selection of instruments for stem extraction

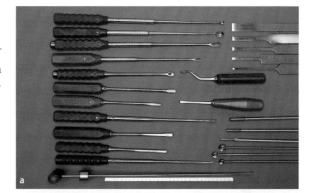

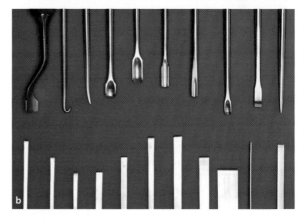

■ **Fig. 18.3a,b.** Osteotomes and chisels for cement removal in various sizes and thickness

> **Note:** All instruments must be long enough (up to 30 cm).

- osteotomes/cement chisels (long, flat),
- gouges (sharpened on the inside or outer edges),
- Lambotte chisels,
- angled (lug) chisel,
- hook-shaped chisel.

▬ Grasping instruments for cement fragment removal.

▬ Curetting instruments and taps with different diameters (■ Figs. 18.5 and 18.6):

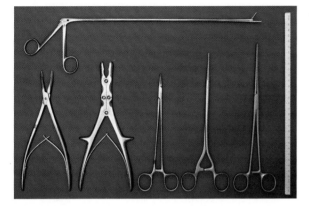

■ **Fig. 18.4.** A variety of special grasping instruments are required including bone nibblers, needle holder, long forceps and rongeurs

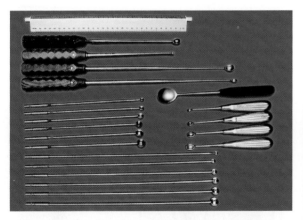

■ **Fig. 18.5.** A selection of instruments for curettage is necessary including curettes and ball headed reamers

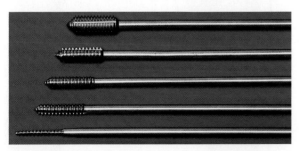

■ **Fig. 18.6.** Self-cutting cement extractors (taps) and long drills (not shown) for cutting a thread in the cement mantle and distal cement plug

- long curettes and sharp spoons (different lengths and sizes),
- ball headed reamers (∅ 8–16 mm) – reduced risk of canal perforation,
- cement taps for cement removal (technique see operative steps),
- pulsatile jet lavage.

Operative Steps

Implant Removal

▬ Remove all accessible bone cement between greater trochanter and implant shoulder to allow stem extraction and minimise the risk of trochanter fracture and avulsion (■ Fig. 18.7).

▬ Remove cement between implant collar and femoral cortex.

▬ Extract implant stem using stem-extraction instruments. If no collar is present, the Nieder extraction device (■ Fig. 18.8) can be used, which is firmly screwed onto the stem neck taper with sharp pointed screws denting into the metal taper.

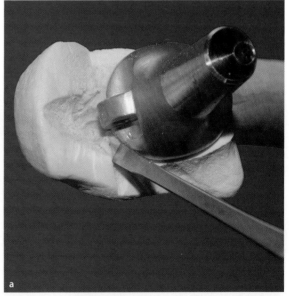

a

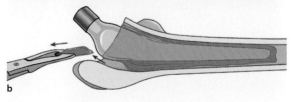

b

■ **Fig. 18.7a,b.** Removal of the cement between trochanter and shoulder of the prosthesis

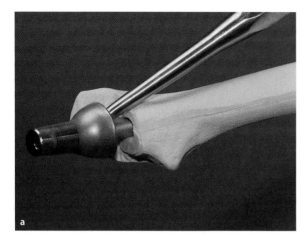

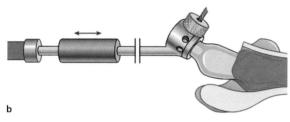

Fig. 18.8a,b. Stem removal of a collared stem with punch (**a**). Removal of collarless stem using the Nieder extraction device (**b**), where the neck taper is drilled and the device is firmly attached using pointed screws

Cement Removal

> **Note:** In aseptic revisions, there is often no need to removal all cement. Only the loose cement should be removed and often the distal cement plug can be kept and used as distal cement restrictor if a cemented revision is performed. More importantly, if both clinically and radiographically the cement-bone interface is still intact, a simple re-cementation into the old cement mantle can be performed by down-sizing the new implant. If revising to an uncemented implant all cement must be removed!

1. Remove all accessible proximal cement using narrow straight osteotomes with symmetrically honed blade.

> **Note:** To remove cement from the femoral medullary canal, the cement must always be split and chiselled away in a radial and longitudinal fashion (**Fig. 18.9**) to avoid perforating or damaging the cortex (**Fig. 18.10**).

2. Taps are used to remove a closed cement mantle from the distal cortical bone (**Fig. 18.10**). In the ideal case the cement mantle fractures on-bloc below the tap tip. In this fashion, the entire cement can be removed down to the distal cement plug.

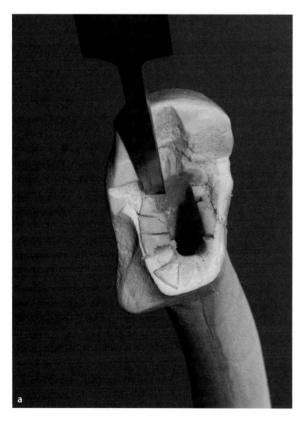

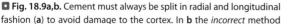

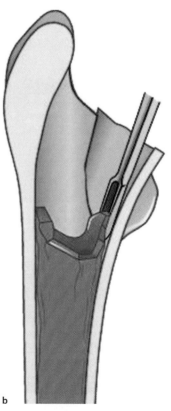

Fig. 18.9a,b. Cement must always be split in radial and longitudinal fashion (**a**) to avoid damage to the cortex. In **b** the *incorrect* method of using the osteotome between bone and cement is shown, which commonly results in a fracture of the surrounding cortex!

❯ **Note:** Always use the largest tap that the cement mantle will accommodate. The tap is »screwed« into the cement mantle cavity with a few turns until the surgeon feels resistance and hears an audible grinding sound. Taps are only practical when the cement mantle is circular and closed. If the mantle is open on one side, the tap can penetrate (via falsa) and may fracture the cancellous or cortical bone.

3. In between the stepwise cement mantle removal, it may be necessary to clean the endosteal canal surface and trim the cement edges to a similar level using ball headed reamers (■ Figs. 18.5 and 18.11) to facilitate the next step of cement extraction with the taps (■ Fig. 18.10).

4. The distal plug, if not removed with the last tap extraction, needs to be drilled using intramedullary drill guides to ensure a central canal for the taps (■ Fig. 18.12). In some situations, usage of the ultrasound cement melting device (Ultradrive, Biomet) can be helpful. However, the usage of ultrasound seems less favourable in infection due to the resulting cement smear and the risk of remnant cement smear within the endosteum.

5. After the cement has been completely removed, the wear membrane membrane lining the medullary canal is meticulously curetted.

6. During and after removal of cement, the femur must be inspected for possible perforation or fracture using a flexible probe (■ Fig. 18.13).

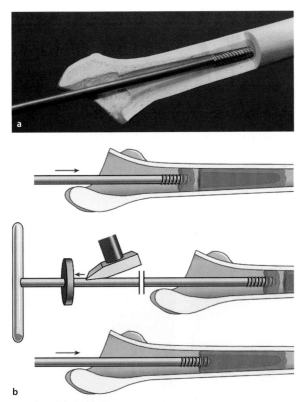

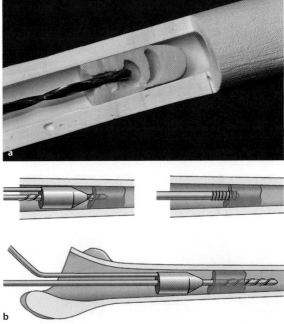

■ **Fig. 18.12a,b.** The distal cement plug can be drilled centrally and then removed by a tap (extractor)

■ **Fig. 18.10a,b.** Method or removing an intact cement mantle using taps. In the ideal case the cement mantle fractures on-bloc below the tip of the extractor tap

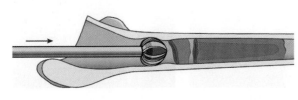

■ **Fig. 18.11.** Curettage of the medullary canal with a ball reamer to clean endosteal surface and to trim cement edges to same level before next step of cement mantle removal (see ■ **Fig. 18.10**)

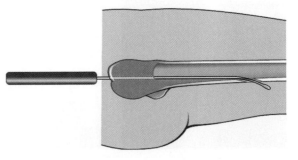

■ **Fig. 18.13.** Inspection of the femur using a flexible probe for possible damage

> **Note:** If there is a high risk that the cortical bone might be perforated due to extreme antecurvation of the femur or loose slivers of cement, the cement mantle should be removed through a cortical window (■ Fig. 18.14).

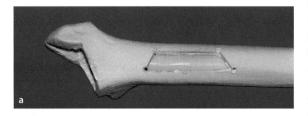

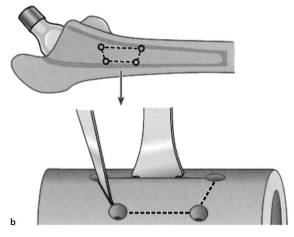

■ **Fig. 18.14a,b.** If necessary, the window should be located in the anterior femur. Drill holes will prevent extension of the fenestration. The saw cuts should be directed obliquely in a converging manner to create a cortical fragment, which can later be replaced with intrinsic stability

Special Situations and Tricks

Scenario 1: Cup Loosening With Well-Fixed Cemented Stem

In case of a socket revision with well-preserved femoral bone stock and well-fixed and intact cement–bone interface, it is sometimes useful to remove the stem to get better exposure of the acetabulum. In this situation, a polished tapered stem has the significant advantage of easy removal without destroying the cement mantle (■ Fig. 18.15). In this case, a simple re-cementation (cement-in-cement revision) is best. In those cases after exchanging the cup, the stem can be reinserted into the old cement mantle. The Exeter group reported five years' results of 189 patients with 100% survival by performing this method (► chapter 8.3).

Scenario 2: Removing Well-Integrated Cement or Cementless Stems

Removing well-integrated cement or cementless stems in infection can be difficult. The reason in many cases is that the infection affects only part of the bone–implant interface, while the rest of the implant is still integrated into the bone. Cementless implants with coarsely structured surfaces are especially likely to cause large bone defects during removal.

Very fine flexible osteotomes are useful in this scenario to loosen the bone–implant interface (■ Fig. 18.16). Via a cortical window the interface can be loosened using curved sawblades to cut around the implant circumference (■ Fig. 18.17).

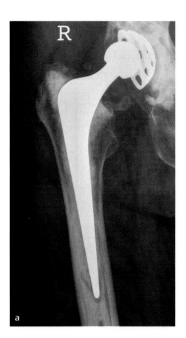

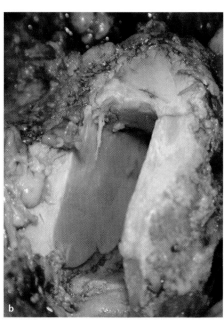

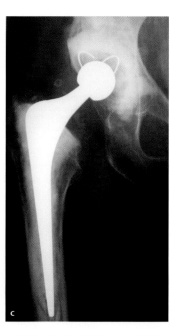

■ **Fig. 18.15a–c.** Cup loosening with a well fixed stem after 16 years (**a**). Radiographically the femoral cement-bone interface is intact and apart from two minor cement cracks the cement mantle is intact (**b**), allowing for simple stem cement-in-cement revision. Postoperative radiograph (**c**) show revised acetabulum with impaction grafting and preserved femoral cement which was not removed

> **Note:** When removing cementless stems the decision to open a window should be taken at a very early stage. In many cases, a window is the most time-saving and least invasive method. Windows should be located in the anterior femur (see ◘ Fig. 18.14).

After drilling a hole in the stem with a carbide-tipped drill bit, in most cases the stem can then be quite easily extracted using a pointed punch and a mallet.

Scenario 3: Removing Well-Cemented Cups

Removing cemented acetabular cups does not usually present any significant problems. Cups which are very loose are removed by drilling a hole in the centre of the cup with a 4.5 mm drill and extracted by retrograde application of a tap (◘ Fig. 18.18) or using a Moreland extractor (DePuy).

A crescent-shaped osteotome with a curved shaft is used to disrupt the polyethylene-cement interface of firmly fixed cups. If the cup cannot be removed with chisels, it must be cut into segments using a fine, sharp chisel/osteotomes (e.g. Lambotte chisel) using the central drill hole as the centre for the »cake segments«. The residual cement in the acetabular floor is divided into radial segments with an osteotome or scraped out with a sharp gouge.

Errors and Risks

When loosening the cup with a chisel, great care must be taken not to damage the bone especially near the roof of the acetabulum. No levering against acetabular bone!

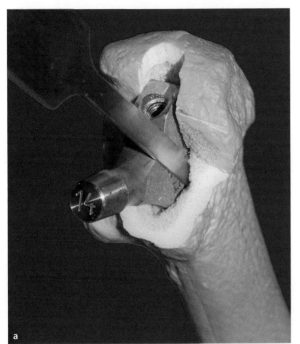

a

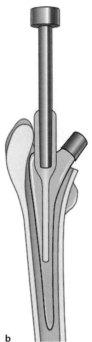

b

◘ **Fig. 18.16a,b.** Using fine, flexible osteotomes the interface of well ingrown implants can be loosened

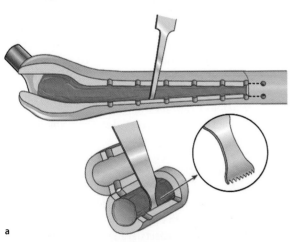

a

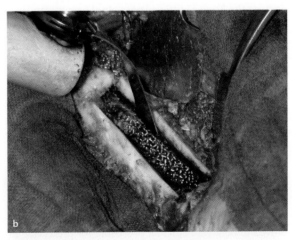

b

◘ **Fig. 18.17a,b.** The interface of well integrated implants can be loosened with curved saw blades via a cortical fenestration

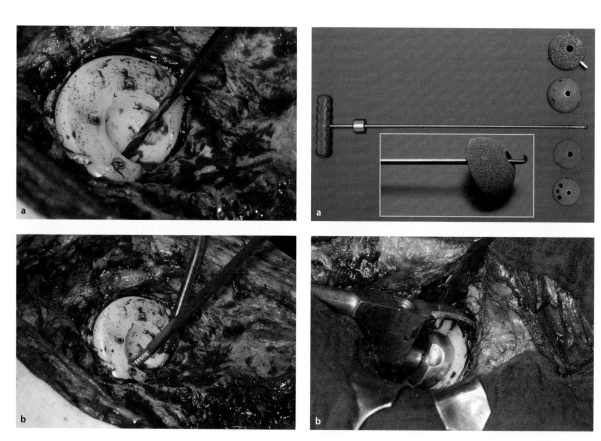

■ **Fig. 18.18a,b.** A drill hole is made (**a**) and a corresponding self-cutting tap is placed (**b**) in the dome of the cup, which allows removal of a loose cemented component

■ **Fig. 18.19a,b.** A hook can be useful to extract uncemented cups with a central hole (**a**). The new Zimmer cup explantation device utilizes centred curved blades to loosen the interface

Removing Cementless Acetabular Cups

After exposure of the cup rim, the polyethylene inlay is first levered out using a straight osteotome. Threaded or press-fit cups are loosened by circular chiselling around the using curved cup chisels while taking great care to damage the bone as little as possible. The cup can then be pulled out with a bone hook or by applying a few blows with a mallet (■ Fig. 18.19a) if the design has a central hole. A new and elegant method uses a cup extraction device (Zimmer), which utilised curved blades of varying sizes, which can be hammered around the acetabular component with the device centred within the PE inlay (■ Fig. 18.19b). This allows fairly atraumatic removal of ingrown sockets with preservation of bone stock.

Practical Tip

Retrograde extraction using a retrograde chisel hooked into the central drill-hole in the acetabular floor has proved to be a very efficient procedure for preserving as much bone as possible.

Re-Implantation of the Acetabular Cup

The principles of operative technique as used in primary THA (▶ chapter 2.1) also apply to the cemented cup re-implantation.

A   No significant loss of bone stock in the acetabulum (■ Fig. 18.20a):
1. ream to diameter of anterior and posterior wall with acetabular reamers,
2. for severe sclerosis use a high speed burr to expose bleeding cancellous bone,
3. drill anchoring holes with a 4.5 to 6 mm drill,
4. generous irrigation with the jet lavage,
5. implantation of a cemented socket using modern cementing techniques.

B   Cavernous defect with closed protrusion or minor floor defects (■ Fig. 18.20b,c)
1. as A),
2. impaction grafting of washed morcelised bone graft mixed with croutons,
3. if minor floor defects are present, these are first closed with structural bone graft (■ Fig. 18.20c).

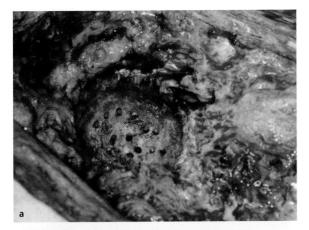

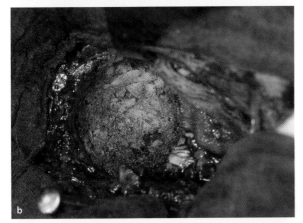

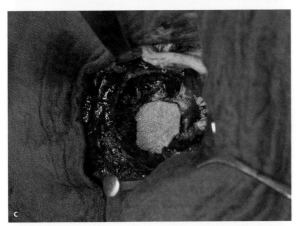

Fig. 18.20a–c. In »near primary« situation with well preserved bone a simple re-cementation can be carried out using modern cementing techniques is present stock. In cavitary defects and with marked socket sclerosis impaction grafting is required (**b**). In cases with a central floor defect a structural graft is necessary to contain the defect prior to impaction grafting (**c**)

After this impaction grafting with bone chips is carried out;

4. the acetabular cup is then cemented in place,
5. all larger defects with loss of roof or floor will require mesh or mostly acetabular cages.

Re-Implantation of the Stem

The choice of stem and stem length depends on preoperative planning, the bone defects found intraoperatively and the extent of remaining bone stock. As it is not always possible to assess the situation definitely in advance, the surgeon should ensure that a sufficient number of alternative implants will be at hand during the operation (see above). As a general rule, a simple re-cementation should only be carried out in an intact femoral tube if residual cancellous bone is present or if marked cortical thinning and osteoporosis make successful fixation of a press-fit uncemented stem unlikely. The distal cement plug should end immediately distal to the implant tip so that it does not impede reconstruction of the femur later.

The procedure for re-cementation is according to the rules of modern cementing techniques (► chapter 2.2), but often 120 g of cement are necessary.

Principles for Stem Re-Implantation in Infection

- Cemented stems should be used (antibiotic loaded cement!).
- The stem must be anchored at least 10 cm deep in healthy bone which is able to provide support for the implant.
- If the femur has been resected, the implant stem should be at least as long as the section of resected bone to achieve stable anchorage.
- If stable anchorage of the implant is not possible, a temporary long-stem prosthesis must first be implanted to act as a spacer. After infection has been eliminated this temporary implant can be exchanged for a total femur replacement.

> **Note:** The aim is to achieve adequate anchorage in healthy bone which is able to provide support for the implant. The stem should extend about 10 cm beyond the femoral defect. If the femur has been resected the implant stem should be at least as long as the section of resected bone.

Take Home Messages

- Appropriate planning is mandatory for all revisional hip surgery (approach, op-tactics, implant selection, expected complications).
- Always exclude infection with CRP and (!) joint aspiration.
- Excise previous scars (and in infection include sinus tracts in incision).
- The posterior approach is the most suitable approach for revision.

- An extensive selection of specialised instruments for stem extraction and cement removal must be available (appropriate length!).
- Polished and smooth cemented stems are more revision friendly.
- Uncemented stems are often »unfriendly«.
- Always remove all accessible lateral cement from the stem shoulder to prevent trochanter fracture/avulsion.
- During cement removal the cement must only be split in a longitudinal, radial fashion.
- A closed cement mantle can be removed using extracting self-cutting taps.
- In aseptic situation, where re-cementation is possible, not all cement needs to be removed (e.g a distal cement plug).
- In cases with an intact cement-bone interface a smaller stem size re-cemented into the preserved cement mantle.
- In infection all cement (and implants) must be removed.
- Windows are rarely require, but should be placed anteriorly.
- Special tricks using some special instruments are helpful in difficult situations.
- Re-implantation of cemented components follows the same principle as in primary arthroplasty, but often bone grafting is required.

18

Part VI   Future Perspectives

Chapter 19   Economic Evaluation of THA   – 360
                M. Ostendorf, H. Malchau

Chapter 20   The Future Role of Cemented
                Total Hip Arthroplasty   – 367
                H. Malchau, S.J. Breusch

Economic Evaluation of THA

Marieke Ostendorf, Henrik Malchau

Summary

In this era of cost containment, economic evaluation studies of medical technologies have become increasingly important in the competition for available healthcare resources.

This chapter describes the methodological criteria of economic evaluation studies and gives an overview of the available literature on economic evaluation studies in total hip arthroplasty (THA). Cemented THA has proven to be a very cost-effective treatment improving quality of life for many patients suffering from severe hip disease.

Introduction

Since World War II, medicine has experienced incredible growth [51]. Increased affluence, new technologies, and an ageing population have led to this unprecedented growth. Transplantation surgery, coronary artery bypass surgery, arthroscopic surgery and total joint replacement are examples of developments over the past 2 to 3 decades. These advances have increased the demand for healthcare and have produced a cost crisis in most countries of the developed world [8]. As such, healthcare interventions have come under increasing scrutiny. Coupled with the issue of cost concerns is the concept of quality assurance. Healthcare providers are interested in how good an intervention is and whether it is cost-effective [56]. Surgeons want to know which treatment has most benefit for their patients. Economic evaluation is increasingly used to inform decisions about which healthcare technologies are to be funded in collectively funded healthcare systems.

The outcomes movement has arisen from the issues of cost and quality assurance, but it has been given consider-able impetus by private health-management organisations that wish to provide quality medical care in a cost-effective manner [8]. These organisations have led the way in terms of developing practice guidelines, clinical pathways and cost-effectiveness research. Furthermore, healthcare providers have been examining individual procedures, such as total hip arthroplasty, in terms of cost-effective practice. Several studies found that total hip arthroplasty is one of the most cost-effective interventions known [37, 63].

Methodology in Economic Evaluations

To evaluate the cost-effectiveness of total hip arthroplasty, and particularly to compare it with other treatment modalities, it is necessary to use standardised cost and utility assessments. To understand these clinical epidemiology methodologies, it is necessary to be familiar with the terminology used.

Evaluation of different treatment regimens in terms of cost-effectiveness involves an economic assessment. This requires a calculation of the costs of the therapy or treatment being studied.

Often economic assessments are based on charges rather than actual costs. For instance, tertiary care centres that support costly, specialised programmes often have charges that are greater than community hospitals without these expensive services. It is obviously of great importance to determine the actual cost rather than the charge for a particular service. The calculation of costs includes both direct and indirect costs. Costs associated directly with the delivery of medical care include outpatient costs (drug costs, consultations costs), inpatient-related costs (hospital costs, surgical fees), and patient-specific costs (transportation costs, home-care service fees). Indirect costs include earnings a patient may have foregone while undergoing treatment or while affected by illness.

There are four different forms of economic evaluation studies:

- *Cost-identification studies* (minimisation studies) are considered the simplest form of healthcare economics evaluation by most health economists. This method considers only the inputs (or costs) of a given treatment strategy. The presumed goal of a cost-minimisation analysis is to find the least expensive way to achieve the same outcome. By definition a cost-minimisation analysis assumes that the outcomes of the treatments under consideration are equal, which is seldom the case [9].
- *Cost-effectiveness analysis* measures health outcomes in physical units, such as life years gained or cases successfully treated. No attempt is made to place a subjective value on the health outcomes that are reported.
- In *cost-utility analyses* outcomes of different treatments are expressed in terms of a single utility-based unit of measurement. Utility is a term used by health economists to describe the subjective level of well-being that people experience in different states of health. Measuring utilities allows valid comparisons among treatment options, and utilities are often used for the purpose of decision analysis.
- In *cost-benefit analysis* all inputs and outputs (such as health outcomes) are measured in monetary terms. Health consequences are valued by asking consumers what they would be willing to pay for health services that achieve a particular health outcome or state of health.

Measuring Outcome, Utility and Quality-Adjusted Life Years in Evaluation Studies

To study outcome after THA, a wide variety of measures is used to assess health-related quality of life. These can be divided into three different groups: disease-specific measures, generic (global) outcome measures and utility scores.

- *Patient-oriented* disease-specific questionnaires, such as the Western Ontario McMaster (WOMAC) Arthritis Index [5] and the Oxford Hip Score [17], measure quality of life experienced by the patient with regard to a special condition (hip disease). Clinical *disease-specific* measures, such as the Harris Hip Score and the Merle d'Aubigne Score (MdA), also measure disease-specific aspects but are filled out by the treating surgeon. It has become increasingly clear that clinical assessment of key aspects of outcome such as pain,

physical function and range of joint movement are often inaccurate and not reproducible [20]. They may also overly represent the concerns of the clinician, rather than those of the patient [16]. Disease-specific scores appear to generate a higher sensitivity to change in outcome of THA as compared to generic instruments [17]. It has been recommended to use the WOMAC and SF-36 in outcome assesment of THA. However, recently the Oxford Hip Score and the SF-12 showed excellent psychosomatic characteristics in the evaluation of THA [49].

- *Generic measurements* offer the possibility to assess health states over different disease categories, and in some cases to an age- and gender related population sample. A well-known, extensively used and tested generic measure in outcome research is the Short-Form 36 (SF-36) [62]. Other examples are the Nottingham Health Profile (NHP) and the Sickness Impact Profile (SIP) [18, 34].
- Some generic questionnaires, so-called multi-attribute *utility measures*, such as the EuroQol (EQ-5D) [22], the Quality of Well-Being index (QWB) [36], SF-6D [11] and the Health Utilities Index (HUI) [60] give the possibility to compare cost-utility between different interventions, which is important in this era of limited healthcare budgets [6, 10, 13, 59].

Quality-Adjusted Life Years

With this cost-utility approach, the cost of an intervention can be related to the number of quality-adjusted life years (QALYs), that is, a ratio between the cost and the effect of the treatment times the duration of the improvement. The life of an individual consists of two major components, (1) the quantity and (2) the quality of life. This can be demonstrated graphically: ◘ Figure 19.1 shows a life profile of an individual before and after THA [48]. The area between the two curves represents the QALY gained: increase in both the quantity and quality of life. This provides a single comprehensive measure of health improvement, which allows one to compare various treatments across different health disciplines. However, to measure clinical outcome it is recommended to use disease-specific and generic questionnaires as well. There has been some debate on the validity of the QALY principle, because the QALY utility values are based on opinions from the general population on a certain health state and might not represent patient preferences [35, 45].

Interventions costing less than $ 20,000.– per QALY are considered to be extremely cost-effective and should be utilised. Those interventions costing between $ 20,000.– and $ 100,000.– per QALY are moderately cost-effective and should be funded but require discussion. Interventions that cost more than $ 100,000.– per

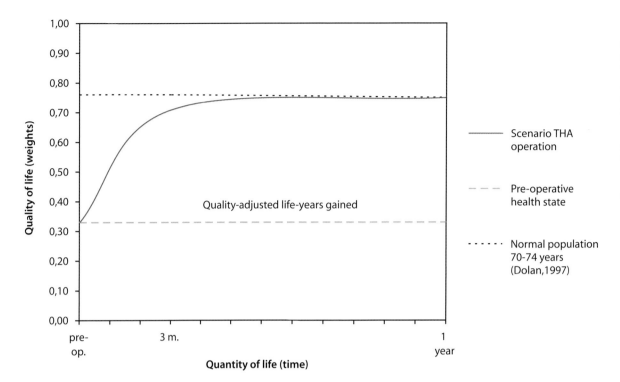

■ **Fig. 19.1.** Different scenarios for utility (EQ-5D$_{index}$) scores over time before and after THA [48]. The *black line* shows the development in mean utility scores pre- and post-surgery. The *grey dotted line* shows the mean preoperative utility score just before THA. The *black dotted* line shows the utility score for the general population in the age group 70–74 years (0.76) [19]. The area between the *black line* and the *grey dotted line* is the gain in quality-adjusted life-years (QALYs)

QALY might be effective but are extremely costly and require considerable analysis before being implemented [37]. In cost-effectiveness analysis, the relative value of an intervention as a health investment is defined by its cost-effectiveness ratio, obtained by dividing the net cost of the intervention by its net benefit [30]. Benefits are most often assessed in terms of QALYs. To improve the comparability and quality of studies, consensus-based recommendations guiding the conduct of cost-effectiveness analysis (CEA) have been developed [55, 61]. The recommendations include the use of the societal perspective in CEA analyses and the use of sensitivity analyses to test the robustness of the results [55]. Moreover, since comparisons are made in the present, measurements have to be adjusted for timing. This is because individuals have a positive rate of time preference. They prefer the desirable consequences of health improvements to occur earlier and the undesirable features, such as costs, later. Future effects and costs have therefore to be discounted to the present [42]. Also, the time horizon used in an economic evaluation study is important: the study should be long enough to capture all major resource implications and health effects associated with the procedure. In orthopaedics, interventions are often associated with costs and effects that occur in the long term, and hence assessment may extend far beyond the period for which

primary information is available. In such cases, mathematical models may be used to extrapolate from the intermediate to the final endpoints [12, 24, 26].

When the costs and effects of an intervention take many years to occur, modelling can be used to extrapolate the findings. It is also useful when diseases are characterised by multiple stages, when data and results need to be moved from one setting to another, or when research needs to compare two treatments which have been previously been individually assessed against a common option, such as a placebo. It should be kept in mind that models have shortcomings: those who develop and use them should pay particular attention to sources of information, underlying assumption and their overall validity. There are few studies in THA in which modelling has been used [12, 15, 24, 26].

Overview of Economic Evaluations in THA

To date, quite a few economic evaluations of THA have been performed [1–3, 26, 39, 43]. However, the hip-arthroplasty literature is deficient in methodologically sound economic evaluations [57]. Good quality economic evaluations of THA are important in the competition for healthcare resources made available for the procedure. In a study from Canada, Rorabeck et al. compared the costs of cemented versus cementless THA in a well-designed, prospective randomised study of 250 patients with osteo-arthritis of the hip. The authors reported similar costs per QALY in both groups (CA $ 17,915.– QALY gained for cemented versus CA $ 18,398.– for cementless) [54]. However, in a follow-up study they reported that the cemented prostheses required more revisions of the femoral component they had used than did the group with the cementless prostheses, with due consequences for the cost-effectiveness of the two prosthesis systems [38]. In a cost-utility study of THA, Chang et al. reported a cost-QALY gain of US $ 4,600.– less than that of coronary artery bypass surgery or renal dialysis [15]. In a Finnish study, Rissanen et al. prospectively compared costs and cost-effectiveness in THA and total knee arthroplasty (TKA) patients [52]. They found that on average, THA patients gained more in terms of health-related quality of life and the surgeries were more often cost-effective ($ 6,153.–/QALY) versus TKA ($ 10,413.–/QALY). Gillespie et al. compared potential cost-effectiveness of various new cemented prosthetic designs in an economic model [29]. They found that in young active THA patients a new (uncemented) prosthetic design would have to guarantee a 90% improvement in survivorship over 15 years and a 15% reduction in the cost of revision surgery to justify a price of 2 to 2.5 times that of »conventional« cemented components, such as the Charnley low friction arthroplasty, and still be cost-effective. In older patients, only a very small increase in the cost of a prosthesis could ever be justified, because of shorter life expectancy and high survivorship of the implant. Hence, there seems to be a strong economic case for tailoring the choice of prosthesis to specific patient subgroups [31, 32]. Similar findings were reported by Faulkner et al. [24]. Using Markov modelling, Briggs et al. stated that in setting the price for a new prosthesis, the manufacturer has a major determinant of the prosthesis' cost-effectiveness under control [12]. Further, they suggested that new implants with additional acquisition cost may be justified in younger patients if a reduction in revision rate of the order of 21–27% can be demonstrated.

The National Institute for Clinical Excellence (NICE) in the UK reviewed available evidence on the effectiveness and cost-effectiveness of alternative hip prostheses and concluded that prostheses should only be used in the NHS if they are able to demonstrate, using appropriate trial or observational data, 10 year revision rates of 10% or less, or rates consistent with that over a shorter period of not less than 3 years [23]. NICE's guidance also made clear the paucity of effectiveness data from appropriately powered randomised trials with sufficient follow-up to assess long-term revision rates. The Institute recognised that data on long-term revision rates would typically have to be identified in non-experimental studies, such as national registers [47].

Cost Reduction in THA

To reduce cost in THA (and improve outcome if possible), several measures have been taken. Hospital revenues for orthopaedic operations are not keeping pace with inflation or with rising hospital expenses, even more so for revision operations [4, 7, 26, 58]. Most profit has been made in reducing length of stay in the hospital, for instance by using special patient-management systems or clinical pathways [25, 32]. Another strategy has been to negotiate about implant prices with implant vendors, which reduced the price for hip implants with 32% [33, 46].

Of course, the reduction of revision rates in THA is a very important factor in reducing costs in (revision) THA. Revision operations compete for the same limited resources currently allocated to primary THA. As the number of patients with THA in situ rises, the number failing also rises. This is creating an epidemic of patients requiring revision operations, a veritable iatrogenic tidal wave [14]. The size of this wave and its timing depend on several factors, in particular, the life expectancy of the patients at the age they receive their first hip replacement and the longevity of the implant [50]. Apart from the fact that patients receiving THA may be younger than a decade ago patients are living longer, so the number of patients »at risk« with hips in place is rising even faster than might be predicted from the number of primary operations being performed. Apart from the surgical technique and the skill and experience of the operating surgeon, some THAs appear, as a result of their design, to last longer than others by a very significant amount [41]. Further, revision THA does not last as long as primary THA and patients undergoing early revision of their hip prosthesis appear to be at increased risk for further re-revision [21]. Pynsent et al. considered the idea of a lifetime care package to encapsulate the idea of quality when considering the purchasing of total hip arthroplasties [50]. Assumed that a primary THA costs £ 3500.– and a revision THA twice as much, they calculated that the additional premium on the best implant available at that time (in terms of revision rate) would be £ 630.– (1995 pounds). The premium payable on the same patient using the worst design would be £ 3080.–, thus illustrating the importance of quality in THA surgery.

Pre-Surgery Cost

Patients undergoing THA have substantial out-of-pocket costs pre-surgery, which fall dramatically over the first postoperative year [43]. Poorer preoperative functional status has been shown to be associated with a worse outcome at 6 months and 2 years after THA [27, 28]. Poorer pre-surgery health status predicted greater expenditure during the first postoperative year, with assistive equipment and alterations to the home being the major components [43]. While a direct cause and effect cannot be concluded from this observational study, the results suggest that earlier surgery or more aggressive attention to physical function pre- and postoperatively may improve outcomes and reduce costs from the patients' perspective.

Is has been shown that waiting times for THA are associated with loss in quality-adjusted life years for patients on the waiting list. With an average waiting time of 6 months, 21 QALYs are lost per 100 patients [48]. Apart from out-of pocket costs, there is no evidence yet in the literature that operating sooner is cost-saving for society. Because most patients receiving THA are no longer part of the working force, a major part of indirect costs is not relevant in this population. However, large costs are involved if one assumes that the consequence of not operating is severe disability which results in admission to a nursing home [15]. The fact that several studies showed that patients with worse preoperative health status never reach the postoperative level of patients with better preoperative health status might be an indication that patients should have been operated earlier in the disease process [28, 49].

Further, as patients become better informed and more aware of present treatment possibilities, they may be less inclined to accept their disability and prefer treatment in an earlier stage of their disease. This development, in combination with an ageing population and longer life expectancy will put further pressure on healthcare resources.

The Value of Data Collection (Hip Register)

Although previous reports have showed that THA ranks high among common healthcare interventions in terms of cost per quality of life year gained [44], to verify and test this assumption, it has been recommended that orthopaedic surgeons should begin to prospectively collect data regarding the costs and outcomes of THA. To help facilitate this goal, national total hip arthroplasty registries should begin to include economic variables in the outcome databases [40]. It is assumed that the Swedish National Hip Registry reduced the revision burden of THA in Sweden by 50%, which is equivalent to 11,630 revisions prevented the past 10 years. Expressed in cost savings, the register saved US$ 14,000,000.– per year (direct costs). To put it another way, the register becomes already cost-effective if the annual number of revisions is reduced by thirty-three, assumed that the register costs US$ 400,000.– per year and the direct cost for a revision THA is US$ 12,000.– [40].

As increasing constraints continue to be placed on scarce healthcare resources, it is incumbent on orthopaedic surgeons to show the true value of THA to our patients and to society [9].

Take Home Messages

- In this era of limited healthcare budgets and cost constraints, economic evaluation studies are important to show the relative value of medical technologies to society.
- Economic evaluation studies should meet some essential criteria regarding methodological quality, such as the use of the right utility measures, indication of the perspective of the study and the use of discounting and sensitivity analysis.
- Apart from the costs and effects of THA at the time of operation, long-term survival rates and outcomes are very important in the eventual cost-effectiveness of the procedure.
- Performing THA in a later stage of the disease process or after a long waiting time might be less cost-effective due to preventable loss in quality time for patients and increasing costs because of disability caused by hip disease.
- Cost of THA is reduced by shorter length of stay, lower implant prices, but most importantly by preventing revision.
- National arthroplasty registries have been shown to be cost-effective. Significant cost savings have been made by reducing the national revision burden.
- Based on current cost evaluation studies, cemented THA remains the treatment of choice. If more costly uncemented prostheses are to be cost-effective, 35–44% improvement in prosthesis survival in patients between 50–70 years would be needed versus 21–27% improvement in patients under 50 years [26].

References

1. Barber TC, Healy WL. The hospital cost of total hip arthroplasty. A comparison between 1981 and 1990. J Bone Joint Surg (Am) 1993;75:321–5
2. Barrack RL. Economics of revision total hip arthroplasty. Clin Orthop 1995:209–14
3. Baxter K, Bevan G. An economic model to estimate the relative costs over 20 years of different hip prostheses. J Epidemiol Community Health 1999;53:542–7
4. Bear B, Evans B, Salvati EA. Relationship of age to hospital and reimbursement in primary total hip arthroplasty: a two year comparative study at the hospital for special surgery. Abstract 1995:1–2
5. Bellamy N, Buchanan WW, Goldsmith CH, Campbell J, Stitt LW. Validation study of WOMAC: a health status instrument for measuring clinically-important patient-relevant outcomes following total hip or knee arthroplasty in osteoarthritis. J Orthop Rheumatol 1988;1:95–108
6. Blanchard C, Feeny D, Mahon JL, Bourne R, Rorabeck C, Stitt L, Webster-Bogaert S. Is the Health Utilities Index responsive in total hip arthroplasty patients? J Clin Epidemiol 2003;56:1046–54

7. Boardman DL, Lieberman JR, Thomas BJ. Impact of declining reimbursement and rising hospital costs on the feasibility of total hip arthroplasty. J Arthroplasty 1997;12:526–34

8. Bourne RB, Maloney WJ, Wright JG. An AOA critical issue. The outcome of the outcomes movement. J Bone Joint Surg Am 2004;86-A:633–40

9. Bozic KJ, Saleh KJ, Rosenberg AG, Rubash HE. Economic evaluation in total hip arthroplasty: analysis and review of the literature. J Arthroplasty 2004;19:180–9

10. Brazier J, Deverill M, Green C, Harper R, Booth A. A review of the use of health status measures in economic evaluation. Health Technol Assess 1999;4:1–164.

11. Brazier J, Roberts J, Deverill M. The estimation of a preference-based measure of health from the SF-36. J Health Econ 2002;21:271–92

12. Briggs A, Sculpher M, Britton A, Murray D, Fitzpatrick R. The costs and benefits of primary total hip replacement. How likely are new prostheses to be cost-effective? Int J Technol Assess Health Care 1998;14:743–61

13. Brooks R. EuroQol: the current state of play. Health Policy 1996;37:53–72

14. Bulstrode C. Keeping up with orthopaedic epidemics. Br Med J (Clin Res Ed) 1987;295:514

15. Chang RW, Pellisier JM, Hazen GB. A cost-effectiveness analysis of total hip arthroplasty for osteoarthritis of the hip. Jama 1996;275:858–65

16. Dawson J, Carr A. Outcomes evaluation in orthopaedics. J Bone Joint Surg Br 2001;83:313–5

17. Dawson J, Fitzpatrick R, Carr A, Murray D. Questionnaire on the perceptions of patients about total hip replacement. J Bone Joint Surg Br 1996;78:185–90

18. de Bruin AF, de Witte LP, Stevens F, Diederiks JP. Sickness Impact Profile: the state of the art of a generic functional status measure. Soc Sci Med 1992;35:1003–14

19. Dolan P. Modeling valuations for EuroQol health states. Med Care 1997;35:1095–108

20. Drake BG, Callahan CM, Dittus RS, Wright JG. Global rating systems used in assessing knee arthroplasty outcomes. J Arthroplasty 1994;9:409–17

21. Eisler T. On loosening and revision in total hip arthroplasty. Dept. of Orthopaedics, Stockholm Söder Hospital, Karolinska Institutet. Stockholm, 2003

22. EuroQol – a new facility for the measurement of health-related quality of life. The EuroQol Group. Health Policy 1990;16:199–208

23. Excellence NIfC. Guidance on the selection of prostheses for primary total hip replacement (www.nice.org.uk). London: National Institute for Clinical Excellence, 2000

24. Faulkner A, Kennedy LG, Baxter K, Donovan J, Wilkinson M, Bevan G. Effectiveness of hip prostheses in primary total hip replacement: a critical review of evidence and an economic model. Health Technol Assess 1998;2:1–133

25. Fisher DA, Trimble S, Clapp B, Dorsett K. Effect of a patient management system on outcomes of total hip and knee arthroplasty. Clin Orthop 1997:155–60

26. Fitzpatrick R, Shortall E, Sculpher M et al. Primary total hip replacement surgery: a systematic review of outcomes and modelling of cost-effectiveness associated with different prostheses. Health Technol Assess 1998;2:1–64

27. Fortin PR, Clarke AE, Joseph L et al. Outcomes of total hip and knee replacement: preoperative functional status predicts outcomes at six months after surgery. Arthritis Rheum 1999;42:1722–8

28. Fortin PR, Penrod JR, Clarke AE et al. Timing of total joint replacement affects clinical outcomes among patients with osteoarthritis of the hip or knee. Arthritis Rheum 2002;46:3327–30

29. Gillespie WJ, Pekarsky B, O'Connell DL. Evaluation of new technologies for total hip replacement. Economic modelling and clinical trials. J Bone Joint Surg (Br) 1995;77:528–33

30. Gold MR, Russell RB, Siegel JE, Weinsyein MC. Cost-Effectiveness in Health and Medicine. New York: Oxford University Press, 1996

31. Healy WL. Economic considerations in total hip arthroplasty and implant standardization. Clinical orthopaedics and related research 1995;311:102–8

32. Healy WL, Ayers ME, Iorio R, Patch DA, Appleby D, Pfeifer BA. Impact of a clinical pathway and implant standardization on total hip arthroplasty: a clinical and economic study of short-term patient outcome. J Arthroplasty 1998;13:266–76

33. Healy WL, Iorio R, Lemos MJ, Patch DA, Pfeifer BA, Smiley PM, Wilk RM. Single Price/Case Price Purchasing in orthopaedic surgery: experience at the Lahey Clinic. J Bone Joint Surg Am 2000;82:607–12

34. Hunt SM, McKenna SP, McEwen J, Backett EM, Williams J, Papp E. A quantitative approach to perceived health status: a validation study. J Epidemiol Community Health 1980;34:281–6

35. Johannesson M. On aggregating QALYs: a comment on Dolan. J Health Econ 1999;18:381–6

36. Kaplan RM, Anderson JP. A general health policy model: update and applications. Health Serv Res 1988;23:203–35

37. Laupacis A, Feeny D, Detsky AS, Tugwell PX. How attractive does a new technology have to be to warrent adoption and utilization? Tentative guidelines for using clinical and economic evaluations. Can.Med.Assoc.J. 1992;146:473–81

38. Laupacis A, Bourne R, Rorabeck C, Feeny D, Tugwell P, Wong C. Comparison of Total Hip Arthroplasty Performed with and without Cement: A Randomized Trial. J Bone Joint Surg Am 2002;84-A:1823-8

39. Lavernia CJ, Drakeford MK, Tsao AK, Gittelsohn A, Krackow KA, Hungerford DS. Revision and primary hip and knee arthroplasty. A cost analysis. Clinical orthopaedics and related research 1995;311:136–41

40. Malchau H, Herberts P, Eisler T, Garellick G, Soderman P. The Swedish Total Hip Replacement Register. J Bone Joint Surg Am 2002;84-A Suppl 2:2–20

41. Malchau H, Herberts P, Garellick G. Annual Report of the Swedish Total Hip Arthroplasty Registry. Gothenburg: Dept. Orthopaedics, Joint Replacement Unit, University of Gothenburg, 2004:1–62

42. Maniadakis N, Gray A. Health economics and orthopaedics. J Bone Joint Surg Br 2000;82:2–8

43. March L, Cross M, Tribe K, Lapsley H, Courtenay B, Brooks P. Cost of joint replacement surgery for osteoarthritis: the patients' perspective. J Rheumatol 2002;29:1006–14

44. Maynard A. Developing the health care market. Economic Journal 1991;101:1277–86

45. Neumann PJ, Zinner DE, Wright JC. Are methods for estimating QALYs in cost-effectiveness analyses improving? Med Decis Making 1997;17:402–8

46. Office NA. Hip replacements: getting it right first time. London, 2000

47. Office NA. Hip replacements: an update. London, 2003

48. Ostendorf M, Buskens E, Van Stel H, Schrijvers A, Marting L, Dhert W, Verbout A. Waiting for total hip arthroplasty: Avoidable loss in quality time and preventable deterioration. J Arthroplasty 2004;19:302–9

49. Ostendorf M, van Stel HF, Buskens E, Schrijvers AJ, Marting LN, Verbout AJ, Dhert WJ. Patient-reported outcome in total hip replacement. A comparison of five instruments of health status. J Bone Joint Surg Br 2004;86:801–8

50. Pynsent PB, Carter SR, Bulstrode CJ. The total cost of hip-joint replacement; a model for purchasers. J Public Health Med 1996;18:157–68

51. Relman AS. Assessment and accountability: the third revolution in medical care. N Engl J Med 1988;319:1220–2

52. Rissanen P, Aro S, Sintonen H, Asikainen K, Slatis P, Paavolainen P. Costs and cost-effectiveness in hip and knee replacements. A prospective study. Int J Technol Assess Health Care 1997;13:575–88

53 Ritten MA, Albohm MJ. Overview: maintaining outcomes for total hip arthroplasty. The past, present and future. Clin Orthop 1997:81–7

54. Rorabeck CH, Bourne RB, Laupacis A, Feeny D, Wong C, Tugwell P, Leslie K, Bullas R. A double-blind study of 250 cases comparing cemented with cementless total hip arthroplasty. Cost-effectiveness and its impact on health-related quality of life. Clin Orthop Rel Res 1994;298:156–64

55. Russell LB, Gold MR, Siegel JE, Daniels N, Weinstein MC. The role of cost-effectiveness analysis in health and medicine. Panel on Cost-Effectiveness in Health and Medicine. JAMA 1996;276:1172–7

56. Sackett DL, Rosenberg WM, Gray JA, Haynes RB, Richardson WS. Evidence based medicine: what it is and what it isn't. BMJ 1996;312:71–2

57. Saleh KJ, Gafni A, Saleh L, Gross AE, Schatzker J, Tile M. Economic evaluations in the hip arthroplasty literature: lessons to be learned. J Arthroplasty 1999;14:527–32

58. Sculco TP. The economic impact of infected joint arthroplasty. Orthopedics 1995;18:871–3

59. Shields RK, Enloe LJ, Leo KC. Health related quality of life in patients with total hip or knee replacement. Arch Phys Med Rehabil 1999;80:572–9

60. Torrance GW, Boyle MH, Horwood SP. Application of multi-attribute utility theory to measure social preferences for health states. Oper Res 1982;30:1043–69

61. Udvarhelyi I, Colditz G, Rai A, Epstein A. Cost-effectiveness and cost-benefit analyses in the medical lieteratre: are the methods being used correctly? Ann Intern Med 1992;116:238

62. Ware JE, Jr., Kosinski M, Bayliss MS, McHorney CA, Rogers WH, Raczek A. Comparison of methods for the scoring and statistical analysis of SF-36 health profile and summary measures: summary of results from the Medical Outcomes Study. Med Care 1995;33:AS264–79

63. Williams A. Seeking priorities in health care: an economist's view. J Bone Joint Surg (Br) 1991;73:365–7

The Future Role of Cemented Total Hip Arthroplasty

Henrik Malchau, Steffen J. Breusch

Future Burden of Ageing Population

The World Health Organisation estimates that in the next 20 years the elderly population will increase 4 fold, which will greatly increase the demand for total hip arthroplasty as the population seeks to remain more active [9]. Total hip arthroplasty has enjoyed tremendous success and has gained worldwide popularity, but with this continued growth comes an impending epidemic of failures necessitating revision surgery. This revision burden can be tempered by knowing which hip systems have enjoyed clinical success and those that have poor outcomes. The most effective data must be obtained by more prospective clinical trials comparing implants and using reproducible outcomes measurements. Other methods, including larger scale-joint registries as have been created in Sweden and Norway, have shown enormous utility in tracking the results of all implants placed in those countries. Registries such as these are significantly important in tracking the early, midterm and late results of many implants which are not reported in the literature but widely used today. Due to the enormous volume of patients being tracked in these registries, we can detect early component failures with relative ease. Therefore, it will be extremely important to implement similar registries throughout Europe as well as in the United States where huge volumes of unproven and newly designed hip systems are being implanted and are poorly tracked. The financial burden on society due to revision-hip surgery is extremely large and will continue to rise with the increasing number of hip replacements being done, but these costs can be dramatically cut with the implementation of a registry that can efficiently detect implants that are destined to fail in a timely manner.

Evaluation of New Implant Systems

The question which fixation technique is optimal and most durable has been debated for many years. Several new cements, implant designs and bearing surfaces have been introduced in the past 10–15 years, but surprisingly often without appropriate scientific, clinical documentation. The Bonelock cement, Capital hip system and heat-treat polyethylene (Hylamer) are only some examples, which have created major clinical problems with unacceptable failure rates. Decisions about medical treatment should be based on a careful appraisal of the best evidence available. In order to increase evidence-based decision-making in the evaluation of new surgical techniques and implants a stepwise introduction is necessary to expose as few patients as possible to the risk of failure.

The history of development of total hip arthroplasty could have been different if the introduction had been more careful and performed in a stepwise manner. Inferior properties would have been revealed earlier thus reducing the number of failures and allowing the necessary improvements. It is therefore desirable that the profession agree on a standardised way to introduce new implants.

Market Introduction

Based on the Swedish experience the following schedule for stepwise clinical introduction [4–7] of new implants is suggested (◘ Fig. 20.1):

- The *initial step* is a preclinical testing.
- The *first clinical step* is the open prospective and preferably randomised trial including a minimum of patients to obtain a valid evaluation. The strict rules

of prospective randomised trials should be addressed. In this first clinical level, high accuracy methods such as radiostereometric analysis (RSA) and dual energy X-ray absorptiometry (DEXA) are required to detect potential early problems. Within 6 months to 2 years these methods have the potential of identifying implants with inferior/superior fixation, extreme wear or unfavourable/favourable bone remodelling. Results from these methods determine if further clinical evaluation is worthwhile. It should be noted and underlined that all types of complication cannot be predicted and further follow up is necessary and should be done. If migration analysis is performed with conventional methods (less accurate than RSA), larger cohorts is needed, exposing more patients for potential risks.

- *Step 2:* If favourable results are obtained in step 1, the second step, a multi-centre trial exposing the new procedure to a broader aspect of the orthopaedic community can be initiated. The implant will then be exposed to various surgical techniques and hospital environments. In step-1 investigations there is a risk for susceptibility and performance bias as the inventors often perform these first introductory investigations. The protocol of the multi-centre study must be carefully prepared and agreed upon by all participating inventors. A sufficient number of patients must be included in order to allow statistical analysis. The witnessed or written patient consent is essential, as is an approval by ethical committee. The ultimate goal will be to make even the multi-centre trial randomised using a well-documented implant as the golden standard on baseline control.
- *Step 3* in the evaluation is a continuous quality control effected by register studies based on large population to reveal early or unusual and potential catastrophic complications. In a comparable small community, e.g. Sweden, the register should be nation-wide and include all units in a specific field.

The Benchmark

Based on existing figures, a chance of at least 92–95% can be promised to the average patient, requiring a total hip replacement, to still have their original implant after 10 years. This is a benchmark hard to beat. It is estimated that approximately 4330 patients are needed in a comparative study with a valid statistical approach (a = 0.05, power = 0.95) to show an improvement from 95% survival to 95.5%. It will therefore be difficult for any new implant or technology to prove that it will perform better than established designs with a long-term track record. However, there is always room for further improvement and we should continue to thrive to achieve better and even more consistent outcomes for our patients, but under controlled and scientific circumstances as outlined above.

Current »Trends« in THA

It is both intriguing and worrying with how much vehemence and marketing efforts new implant technologies drive both so-called »champion surgeons« or »opinion leaders« as well as the industry, often despite the lack of long-term evidence. It is long-term evidence, which is required before we can offer a new technique of implant to our patients. We not only stand on much firmer ground, but also owe this to our patients. It is not enough to »think« that the proposed method »may« be of benefit.

Currently, metal-on-metal resurfacing and minimally invasive hip surgery (MIS) are advocated, considered »trendy« and hence rapidly gained popularity. These are already included in treatment algorithms that lack scientific support [1, 2]. Yet, the public is led to believe that these »modern« methods are better. It will take decades to determine if the benefits of metal-on-metal bearings or MIS outweigh the associated risks [1, 3, 8]. Hence, it is

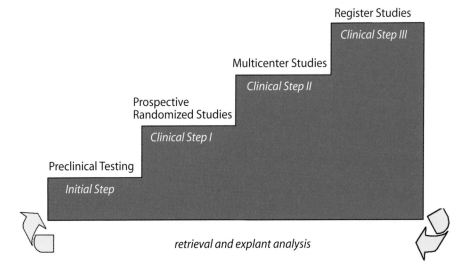

Fig. 20.1.

long to go before enough data will be available to draw any firm conclusions. The jury is still out!

Until then it is questionable whether these techniques should be offered on a larger scale and tested by the average arthroplasty surgeon and treatment centres, which lack the infrastructure to conduct clinical trials.

The Value of Cemented THA

It is not an issue in our opinion to further fuel the long and ongoing debate about uncemented or cemented fixation. The future arthroplasty surgeon needs to be familiar with both techniques. Based on the experience gained from cemented fixation over the past four decades, it is probably not unreasonable to state that this concept has been driven to a very high standard with reproducible outcome.

The basic science, operative technique and outcome data have been compiled for this book to give a comprehensive background of current knowledge and state of the art of cemented THA. It is a method – if performed well – which is highly successful, reproducible and cost-effective. It is based on this knowledge, that we believe that a well-performed cemented THA still remains the treatment of choice for the average patients with osteoarthritis of the hip over the age of 60–65 with average activity. Younger patients and those with high demand activity will have to accept a higher chance of earlier failure irrespective of the mode of fixation and choice of implant.

It is important to realise and accept, that surgical technique is most important and that the future for cemented THA should be seen in continued and improved training of young surgeons with an interest in arthroplasty.

References

1. Berry DJ. »Minimally invasive« total hip arthroplasty. J Bone Joint Surg 2005; 87-A:699–700
2. Carr AJ, Morris RW, Murray DW, Pynsent PB. Survival analysis in joint replacement surgery. J Bone Joint Surg 1993;75-B(2):178–82
3. Fehring TK, Mason JB. Catastrophic complications of minimally invasive hip surgery. J Bone Joint Surg 2005; 87-A:711–14
4. Gross M. Innovations in surgery. A proposal for phased clinical trials. J Bone Joint Surg 1993; 75B:351–354
5. Malchau H. On the importance of stepwise introduction of new hip implant technology. Thesis, Göteborg University, 1995
6. Malchau H. Introduction of orthopaedic devices to the marketplace. Presidential guest lecture The Hip Society, AAOS, Anaheim, USA, February 7, 1999
7. Malchau H. Introducing new technology: a stepwise algorithm. Spine 2000; 25(3): 285
8. Silva M, Heisel C, Schmalzried TP. Metal-on-metal total hip replacement. Clin Orthop 2005; 430:53–61
9. Woolf AD, Pfleger B. Burden of major musculoskeletal conditions. Bull World Health Org 2003;81:646–656

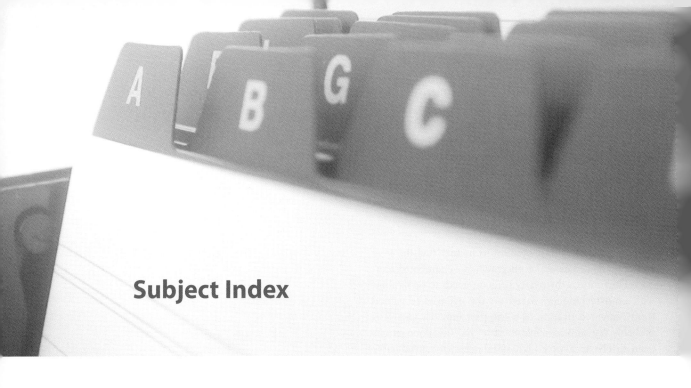

Subject Index

A

acetabular
- bone preparation 9, 10, 14, 16, 23, **24**, 27, **141–143**, 148, 265, 267, 325–329
- component 141, 260–267, 270–277, 282–285, 349
- dysplasia 40–44, 274
- floor graft 16, **20**, 21, 25, 27
- notch 5, 9, 14, 18, 22, 43
- pressurisation **24, 25**, 121, **164–167**, 210, 211, 263, 265, 268, 271
- roof (preparation) 5, 9, 16, **17–23**, 141, 208, 210, 215, 268–270
- roof graft 16, **44**, 49, 273–278
- technique 16–27, 206–208
acetabulum 40, 141, , 164–167, 212, 219, 268–273, 344–347
acrylic cement 52–59, 60–66, 67–78,, 83–85, 94, 102, 104, 118, 181, 221, 222
air entrapment 107, 115
ALAC »antibiotic loaded acrylic cement« 87, 357
alcoholic disinfectants 315
allergic reactions 69, 88, 108, 315, 317
ALVAL »aseptic lymphocytic vasculitis-associated lesions« 285
anatomical stem design 137, 172, 174, 242
anchoring holes 22, 23, 141, 142, 209, 209, 264, 268, 356
antegrade cement technique 150, 327, 328

anterior approach 3, 12, 14, 15
antero–lateral approach 3, 6, 8, 15, 29, 243, 246, 349
antibiotics 86f, 108, 313
- bone cement 53, 59, 86–91, 110, 115, 318
- clindamycin 88–91
- gentamicin **87–92,** 103, 110–112, 237, 240, 244, 318
- tobramycin 88, 90
- systemic 103, 105, 317–319
- vancomycin 88, 90, 317
antibiotic
- prophylaxis 317–319
- release 53, 86–91, 103, 107, 110
antibiotic-loaded acrylic cement (ALAC) 87, 357
- diffusion 87
- elution 87
- mechanical properties 90
- porosity 87
antiseptics 315
approach
- anterior 3, 12, 14, 15
- antero-lateral 3, 6, 8, 15, 29, 243, 246, 349
- posterior 3,10, 37, 42, 209, 230, 237, 256, 305, 349, 357
- transfemoral 349
- transgluteal 349
- transtrochanteric 349
- extended trochanteric osteotomy 42, 222, 228, 237, 256, 259, 276, 349
aseptic loosening 61,103, 105, 110, 119, 129, 168, 185, 216, 228, 229, 240, 242, 265, 269, 271, 274, 286, 295, 334, 338
- acetabulum 141, 207, 219, **260–265**, 269, 275
- femoral stem 187, 191, 192, 216, 224, 232, 238, 244, 247, 250, 257, 342
aseptic lymphocytic vasculitis-associated lesion (ALVAL) 285
aseptic revisions 16, 28, 61, 79, 84, 87, 94, 103, 104, 111, 126, 129, 137–142, 147, 149, 153, 159, 163, 185, 187, 192, 207, 217–219, 222–226, 230, 238, 244, 251, 260, 269, 275, 291, 319, 340, 348, 352, 357, 262
ASTM standard 68, 77, 78

B

backside polyethylene wear 261, 282
bacteria (l)
- biofilm 86, 91, 314, 319
- colonisation 53, 86, 68, 91, 104, 314
- contamination 313–316
- planctonic form 86
- resistance 86, 317
- sessile form 86, 91, 314
barium sulphate 54, 59, 80, 81, 115, 268
Barrack classification /cement grading 36, 129, 244, 245, 249, 336
bearing 67, 103, 187, 215, 261, 266, 279, 286, 367
- ceramic 262, 279, 285

– chemical structure   279
– hard   187, 260, 273
– mechanical properties   279
– metal on metal (MOM)   279, 283, 285, 368
– molecular weight   279
– polyethylene wear   273, 279, 283
– ultrahigh molecular weight polyethylene (UHMWPE)   279, **282–285**
benzoyl peroxide   52, 53, 54, 59
bioactive glass cements   67
bleeding   24, 120, 121, 126, 147, 155, 164, 211, 326
– back-bleeding   25, 32, 34, 35, 210
– bone   19, 22, 119, 120, 160, 356
– interface   16, 28, 147, 154, 167
– intraosseous   25, 164
– model   128, 167, 326
– pressure   120, 150, 160, 164
blood
– lamination   24, 164, 165
– loss   2, 24, 120, 210, 302, 303, 305, 306, 310, 317
bone-cement
bone cement (see also acrylic cement)
– bending strength   57, 60, 61, 80, 88, 115
– brittleness   67, 83
– creep   57, **60–63**, 66, 68, 71, 77, 79, 81, 83, 85, 98, 102, 171–174, 177, 182, 190, 204, 240
– damping factor   83, 84
– dynamic mechanical analysis (DMA)   84
– energy dissipation   84
– fatigue   53, 55, 57–61, 64–69, 75, 77, 78, 80–85, 94, 107–112, 115, 118, 205
– fatigue testing   77, 78, 80, 98, 102
– fume exposure   118
– gamma radiation   55, 79, 80, 82, 83, 85
– glass transition temperature   56, 57, 83, 84
– high viscosity   27, 58, 70, 72, 73, 80, 103, 104–106, 114–116, 146, 161–163, 326
– interface   55, 61, 93, 98, 102, 112, **118–121**, 123, 138, 140, 141, 143, 153, 163, 189, 210, 224, 249, 265, 268, 270–272, 326, 335
– isothermal microcalorimetry (IMC)   82
– low viscosity   33, 58, 69, 72, 73, 78, 80, 103, 104, 160–162, 326, 327

– mechanical properties   51, 60, 61, 63, 65, 66, 68, 69, **76–81**, 83, 88–91, 103, 107, 109, 116, 118, 155, 164
– medium viscosity   36, 72, 73, 78, 162, 163
– metal interface   80, 96, 102, 110, 111, 178, 189, 195
– mixing   32, 33, 36, 52, 54, 58, 68–78, 88, 90, 94, **107, 113**, 123, 147, 155–158, 162, 210, 340
– molecular weight   54, 55, 59, 67–69, 74, 79–85
– monomer   52, **54–56**, 58, 59, 69, 71, 73, 77, 81, 84, 87, 90, **93–97**, 102, 197, 108, 111, 113, 117, 123, 322, 323, 330, 331
– polymer   **52–59, 61–69**, 71, 73, **77–86**, 88, **93–97**, 102, 108, 109, 114, 117
– porosity   55, 58, 59, 61, 68, 87, 88, 94, **107–110**, 113, 115–118, 123, 158, 164, 189
– sterilisation   80, 82
– vacuum mixing   59, 69, 70, 93–97, 102, **107–111, 113–118**, 123, 147, 157
– viscoelasticity   83, 84
– viscosity   80, 103, 326
– water uptake   55, 56, 83, 96
– working behaviour   58, 59
– ZrO$_2$ 54, 69, 81
Bone-cement types
– Boneloc   **68, 69**, 72, 74–76, 78–85, **103**, 104, 106, 148, 149, 195, 367
– Cemex   **69**, 74–78
– CMW   **68, 69**, **72–74**, 76–78, 87, **103**, 111, 114, 155, 268
– Duracem   **69**, 82
– Osteopal   **68, 69**, 72, 74, 76–78, 87
– Palacos   24, 53, **68–83**, 85–87, 91, 92, **103**, 106, 109, 114, 115, 151, 155, 197, 217–219, 239, 240, 244, 269, 319, 326
– Palamed   **68, 69**, 72, 77, 78, 87, 92, 112, 114–116, 118, 155
– Simplex   **68, 69**, 72, 74–76, **78–85, 103**, 106, 111, 114–116, 118, 120, 121, 123, 155, 157, 210, 211, 217–219
– SmartSet HV   **68**, 76, 78, 155
– Sulfix-6   **68, 69**, 71, 72, 74, 76–78
bone grafting   16, **44**, 49, 273–278, 358
bone (pulsatile) lavage   16, 23, 24, 27, 28, 32, 33, 34, 36, 48, 69, **125–128**, 141, 142, 147–148, 150, 162–164, 230, 265, 267, **325–329**
bone preparation   16, 126, 148, 265, 340

– acetabular   9, 10, 14, 16, 23, **24**, 27, **141–143**, 148, 265, 267, 325–329
– femoral   28, 119, 121, 123, 125, **126–128**, 135–137, 242
bone-to-cement interface   55, 61, 93, 98, 102, 112, **118–121**, 123, 138, 140, 141, 143, 153, 163, 189, 210, 224, 249, 265, 268, 270–272, 326, 335
broaching   29–32, 129, 132, 137, 162, 197
Brooker classification   238, 241, 334, 336
Buchholz   86, 87 318

C

Calcar
– femorale   29, 131–133, 138, 140, 240, 334
– resorption   182, 233
canal flare index (CFI)   129, 131
cardiac arrest   304, 320, 321
cardiopulmonary complications   128, 304, **320–323**, 328, 331
cement (see also bone cement)
– application   16, 23–25, 28, 33, 125, 127, 128, 146–148, 150, 164, 264, 320, 326–329
– abrasion   168–170, 177, 234, 242
– to bone interface   55, 61, 93, 98, 102, 112, **118–121**, 123, 125, 138, 140, 141, 143, 153, 163, 189, 210, 224, 249, 265, 268, 270–272, 326, 335, 341
– crack   94, 101, 108, 110, 169, 171, 177, 249, 354
– creep   57, **60–63**, 66, 68, 71, 77, 79, 81, 83, 85, 98, 102, 171–174, 177, 182, 190, 204, 240, 282
– flow   160, 162
– fractures   143, 238, 244, 337
– gun   155–158
– -in-cement revision   187, 354
– interdigitation   26–28, 32, 36, 53, 125, 129, **141, 142**, 146, 147, 159, 182, 326–329
– laminations   33
– mantle   17, 25–28, 31, 32, 35, 51, 57, 80, 83–85, 98, 101, 109–111, 125, **128–140**, 143, 146,155, 169, 170–173, 182–188, 190, 196–198, 208, 212, 229, **231–240**, 242, 247, 249, 252, 258, 327, **334–338**, 340, 242, 344, 347, 351–354, 358

– mixing   32, 33, 36, 52, 54, 58, 68–78, 88, 90, 94, **107, 113,** 123, 147, 155–158, 162, 210, 340
– penetration   16, 23, 24, 28, 33, 34, 36, **125–129,** 138, 139, 141–144, **146–148,** 150, 155, **160–164,** 206, 209, 211, 271, 326, 328
– plug   342–244, 352, 357, 358
– protrusion   343, 345, 347
– to prosthesis interface   107, 109, 111, 189
– restrictor   32, 33, 48, 145–148, **150–153,** 162, 244, 268, **326–330,** 342, 347, 352
– toxicity   112, 286, 322, 329, 330, 322
cemented press-fit   101, 102, 137
cementing technique   10, 21, 28, 36, 44, 48, 59, 101, 102, 107, 113, 123, 129, 138, 141, 161, **235–237,** 242, 244, 264, 265, 284, 325, 332, 334, 337, 338, **340–342**
– acetabular   **24–26,** 142, 207, 210, 212, 264, 356
– femoral   **33–36,** 129, 147, 163
– modern   5, 6, 9, 15, 16, 28, 44, 59, 69, 108, 123, 129, 137, 141–143, **145–148,** 150–153, 158, 159, 164–166, 194, **210–212,** 237, 238, 244, 265, 328, 357
– first generation   69, **147,** 188, 229, 233, 263, 264
– second generation   69, **147,** 159, 167, 264, 267
– third generation   69, **147,** 194, 230, 233
centralizer   35, 125, 129, **131–140,** 147, 148, 172, 187, 198, 230, 231, 234, 236, 242–244, 246
centre of rotation   16–18, 21, 37, 42, 47, 263, 274, 275, 277
ceramic-on ceramic   262, 279, 285, 286
champagne flute   130, 131
Charnley
– classes   333, 334
– low-friction arthroplasty   50, 52, 102, 111, 138–144, 146, 149, 154, 163, 167, 191, 207, 208, **221–227,** 241, 262, 263, **268, 270,** 332, 363
– retractor   3, 4
– Sir John   52, 90, 98, 125, 146, 150, 161, 180, 191, 208, 262, 268, 271, 273, 316
Chiari osteotomy   273, 276
Clindamycin   88–91

collar   29, 102, 171, **172–175,** 182, 186, 190, 192–195, 205, 228, 241, 350, 351
compaction grafting   275
complications   187, 238, 258, 266, 291, 304, 307–311, 332, 338, 345, 347, 349, 357, 368
– cardiopulmonary   128, 304, **320–323,** 328, 331
– centralizer   136, 161
– infection   258, 317
– MIS   2, 369
– pain   187
– wound   2, 309
congenital dislocation hip (CDH)   **39–41,** 45, 222, 254, 255, 257, 259, **273–275**
containment   **17–19,** 27, 146, 150, 372
cortical index (CI)   129, 131, 139
cost reduction   363
cost-benefit analysis   361
cost-effectiveness analysis   298, 360, 361
cost-identification study   361
cost-utility analyses   293, 298, 361
cotyloplasty   274
creep   57, 68, 71, 79, 84, 171, 173, 240
cross-linked polyethylene   208, 226, 227, 260, 262, 267, 269, 279, **280–283,** 286
Crowe's grading system   38, 42, 256, 259, 274, 275
cup implantation   24–27, 207
curetting (instruments)   146, 351

D

debonding   110–112, 129, 168, 169, **171–173,** 177, 181–183, 190–193, 202–204, 239, 249, 337
deep vein thrombosis (DVT)   303, 306, 311, 320, 329, 331
delayed-type hypersensitivity (DTH)   285
DeLee-Charnley zone I   17, 26, 143, 144, 166, 245, 264, 269, 336, 337
design philosophy (stem)   168, 173–178, 181
– shape-closed   171, 175, 176, 181, 182, 190, 233 (taper slip)
– force-closed   170, 171, 174, 175, 182, 190, 233
developmental dysplasia of the hip (DDH)   17, 18, **37–40,** 42, 45, 46,

49, 50, 222, 233, **254–257,** 259, 273, **275–277**
dislocation
– hip   4, 6, 9, 13–15, 16, 18, 20, 25, 27, 42, 43, 45, 132, 185–187, 208, 219, 223, 229, 230, 233, 239, 242, 244, 256, 273, 276, 284, 292, 295–297
– congenital dislocation hip (CDH)   **39–41,** 45, 222, 254, 255, 257, 259, **273–275**
Dorr type   33, 129, 130, 131
dynamic mechanical analysis (DMA)   84
dysplasia   17, 18, **37–40,** 42, 45, 46, 49, 50, 222, 233, **254–257,** 259, 273, **275–277**

E

economic evaluation   297, 298, **360–364**
endosteal scalloping   137, 238, 244, 336
epidural anaesthesia   16, 28, 162, 303, 305, 309, 330
ethylene oxide (EO)   55, 80, 82, 83, 280
EuroQol (EQ-5D)   291–293, 361, 362
evidence based medicine   291, 293, 337, 366, 367
Exeter pressuriser   164–166, 209

F

face masks   316
fat embolism   28, 32, 33, 128, 153, 154, 304, **320–323, 326–329**
fatigue   53, 55, 57–61, 64–69, 75, 77, 78, 80–85, 94, 107–112, 115, 118, 205
– fractures   109, 115
– propagation   109
– testing   57, 77, 78, 80, 98, 102
– stress concentration   64, 84, 108, 109, 111, 171, 198
femoral
– pressurisation   **33, 34,** 128, 129, 145, **160–163,** 244
– seal   28, 34, 129, 163
– stem designs   29, 138, 170, 174, 180, 190, 241, 242, 247, 338
finite element analysis (FEA)   98, 110, 111, 126, 137, 139, 141, 142, 169, 170, 175, 177, 182, 334

first generation cementing technique
    69, 146, **147**, 188, 229, 233, 263, 264
flanged acetabular component   25,
    43, 142, **206–209**, 211–213, **265–267,**
    268–272
force-closed   170, 171, 174, 175, 182,
    190, 233
French paradox   249, 251, 253
fretting wear   184, 200

G

gamma radiation
– PMMA   55, 80,
– Polyethylene   280–282
general anaesthesia   303
generic questionnaire   361, 365
Gentamicin   **87–92,** 103, 110–112,
    237, 240, 244, 318
glass-ionomeric cements   6, 67, 68
glass transition temperature   56, 57,
    83, 84
graft augmentation   274
graft incorporation   274
Gruen zones   26, 28, 36, 125, 129,
    132–137, 162, 181, 200, 236, 238,
    240, 243–247, 334, 335
gun application   146, 155

H

hand hygiene   315
Harris hip score   238, 239, 244, 333,
    361
Hartofilakidis grading system   38, 40,
    50, 274, 275
heat
– necrosis   54, 74
– polymerisation   52, 54, 55, 58, 67,
    69, 74–78, 82, 322
– treatment   280, 281, 367
health utilities index (HUI)   361
hemiarthroplasty   187
heterotopic ossification (Brooker)   238,
    241, 334, 336
high
– false acetabulum   273
– hip centre   21, 274
– viscosity bone cement   27, 58, 70,
    72, 73, 80, 103, 104–106, 114–116,
    146, 161–163, 326

highly cross-linked polyethylene
    liners   260, 281, 283, 288
hip-rating systems   333
– Harris Hip Score   238, 239, 244, 333,
    361
– Merle, D'Aubigne, Postel   222, 269,
    333, 361
– Oxford hip questionnaire   244, 361
– SF 12   361
– SF 36   333, 361
host defence   313
hydrogen peroxide   82, 120, 124, 143,
    164, 167, 210
hydroxyapatite (HA)   88, 100, 205, 216,
    220, 241, 261
hypotension   303–305, 320, 322
hypotensive anaesthesia   16, 28, 143,
    162, 164

I

IDES documentation   237, 333
implant removal   351
implantation syndrome   322, 323,
    331
incisional drapes   315
inter-/intraobserver agreement   337
interface   107, 169, 184
– bone (to) cement   55, 61, 93, 98,
    102, 112, **118–121,** 123, 125, 138,
    140, 141, 143, 153, 163, 189, 208, 210,
    224, 249, 265, 268, 270–272, 326,
    335, 341
– polymer to monomer   93, 94, 102
– stem (to) cement   35, 66, 85, 109,
    129, **169–171,** 176, **181–184,** 188,
    192, 194, 196, 230, 233, 241, 242
International Documentation and
    Evaluation System (IDES)   237
intramedullary
– bleeding pressure   120, 150, 160,
    164 (see bleeding)
– drill guides   353
– plug   28, 69, 114, 129, 146–148,
    150–153, 163, 229, 230, 237, 327,
    328
– plug migration   151
– pressure   34, 147, **150–153,** 320,
    323, **325–329,** 342
ISO 5833   57–61, 68, 66, 68, **75–77,**
    88, 91
isothermal microcalorimetry (IMC)   82,
    85

J

jet-lavage (pulsatile, pressurised)   16,
    23, 28, 33, **127–129,** 143, 148, 162,
    164, 167, 244, 265, 267, 320, 326,
    328, 329, 351, 356
joint registry   61, 123, 124, 149, 154,
    163, 173, 191, 262, 264, 291, 297, 298,
    363, 364, 367

K

Kaplan-Meier survival   104, 146, 270,
    292, 337

L

laminar air-flow   316
lavage   16, 23, 24, 27, 28, 32, 34, 36,
    48, 51, 69, 120, **125–129,** 138, 139,
    143, 144, 147, 148, 153, 162, 164,
    210, 229, 230, 244, 264, 267, 320,
    325–329, 341, 342, 351, 356
leg length   3, 5, 6, 11, 29, 31, 37, 45,
    48, 185, 186, 188, 212, 254, 255, 258,
    259, 274, 332
– discrepancy   37, 45, 186, 349
liner exchange   16, 261
long-term
– follow-up   221, 227, 274, 277, 285
– outcome   2, 32, 38, 129, 136, 138, 146,
    190, 221, 227, 242, 260, 267, 277, 332
– properties   60, 61, 64, 66, 83, 164
– results   16, 40, 41, 61, 93, 113, 139,
    143, 146, 149, 167, 180, 185, 194, 219,
    242, 247, 250, 254, 260, 266, 275, 340
– survival   28, 40, 53, 66, 107, 108,
    111, 127, 141, 143, 182, 189, 223, 232,
    242, 273, 277, 336, 347, 364
loosening   190
– aseptic   61, 103, 105, 110, 119, 129,
    168, 185, 216, 228, 229, 240, 242,
    260–265, 269, 271, 274, 286, 295,
    334, 338
– septic   348
low
– friction arthroplasty   50, 52, 102,
    111, 138–144, 146, 149, 154, 163,
    167, 191, 207, 208, **221–227,** 241,
    262, 263, **268, 270,** 332, 363

– viscosity cement   33, 58, 69, 72,
  73, 78, 80, 103, 104, 160–162, 326,
  327
lubrication   283
lumbo-sacral plexus block   303

M

macroporosity   95, 107, 115
market introduction   368
mechanical interface strength   164
mechanical interlock   141, 337
mechanical properties
– antibiotic-loaded acrylic
  cements   90
– bearing   279
– bone cements   51, 60, 61, 63, 65, 66,
  68, 69, **76–81,** 83, 88–91, 103, 107,
  109, 116, 118, 155, 164
mechanical strength   67, 84, 88, 107,
  111, 113, 115
medium viscosity cement   36, 72, 73,
  78, 162, 163
Merle, D'Aubigne, Postel   222, 269,
  333, 361
Metal
– to-bone cement interface   80, 96,
  102, 110, 111, 178, 184, 189, 195
– /stem to bone contact   133, 137,
  172, 235, 236, 240, 334, 335
– -on-metal (MOM)   227, 279, 283,
  286, 288, 368
– -on-metal resurfacing   368
– -on-polyethylene (MOP)   283
methyl methacrylate (MMA)   52, 53,
  55, 59, 80, 82, 87, 112
micro-
– motion   169, 184, 192, 196,
– organism   313, 315
– porosity   107, 115, 157, 158
migration   169, 173, 177, 182
– femoral head   17, 20, 21, 38, 182,
  183
– fluid/particle   182, 184, 246
– plug/restrictor   150–153
– stem   119, 129, 132, 142, 169, **171–
  179,** 182, 183, 188, 190–194, 231,
  233, 238, 240, 247, 261, 334, 336, 338,
  345, 368
minimal inhibitory concentration
  (MIC)   86, 88
minimally invasive hip surgery
  (MIS)   2, 15, 243, 368

MIS   2, 15, 243, 368
mixing
– system   33, 58, 70, 107, **112–118,**
  155, **157–159,** 162, 340
– vacuum mixing system   59, 70, 71,
  95, 108, **111–118,** 123
– technique   32, 70, 107, 111, 113,
  115, 118
MMA   52, 53, 55, 59, 80, 82, 87, 112
modern
– cementing technique (see cementing technique)   10, 21, 28, 36, 44,
  48, 59, 101, 102, 107, 113, 123, 129,
  138, 141, 161, **235–237,** 242, 244,
  264, 265, 284, 325, 332, 334, 337,
  338, **340–342**
– generation cementing   148, 154,
  155
monomer   52, **54–56,** 58, 59, 69, 71,
  73, 77, 81, 84, 87, 90, **93–97,** 102,
  197, 108, 111, 113, 117, 123, 322, 323,
  330, 331
morbidity   2, 293, 302, 305, 307–309,
  311
mortality   285, 302, 322
multi-attribute utility measure   361
multi-media education   308
multimodal perioperative pain
  management   309
myocardial ischaemia   304

N

national implant register   61, 123, 124,
  149, 154, 163, 173, 191, 262, 264, 291,
  297, 298, 363, 364, 367
National Institute for Clinical Excellence
  (NICE)   363
nerve palsy   255, 259
NICE 363
nicotine-replacement therapy   309
N,N-dimethyl-p-toluidine (Dmpt)   53,
  54
nozzle
– cement   33, 34, 71, 72, 117, 122,
  155, 158, 162
– lavage   32, 33
normothermia   316
Norwegian register   79, 105, 110,
  216–219, 233, 261, 265, 297,
  316–318
Nottingham health profile (NHP)
  361

O

offset   20, 37, 45, 131, 171, 185, 230,
  242, 254, 258, 259, 276
Ogee cup   206, 208, 244, **268–272,**
  292
osteolysis   16, 61, 101, 109, 112, 125,
  128, 129, 136, 137, 139, 147, 170, 177,
  192, 219, **238– 242,** 245, **260–262,**
  279, 282, 284, 286, 292, 298, 334, 336,
  338, 340
Osteopal   **68, 69,** 72, 74, 76–78, 87
osteotomy
– acetabular   273, 276
– Chiari   273
– extended trochanteric   256, 276,
  349
– failed   229, 230
– femoral   37, 38, 40, 46–49, **254–259,**
  276
– neck   10, 29, 34, 162, 240
– oblique   256
– planar   47, 48
– previous   41, 42, 258
– rotational   41, 186
– shortening   41, 186, 254, 256, 259
– step-cut   256
– subtrochanteric   47, 256, 268, 276,
  332
– trochanteric   42, 133, 154, 222, 228,
  237, 268
Oxford hip questionnaire   244, 361

P

Palacos   24, 53, **68–83,** 85–87, 91, 92,
  103, 106, 109, 114, 115, 151, 155,
  197, 217–219, 239, 240, 244, 269,
  319, 326
Palamed   **68, 69,** 72, 77, 78, 87, 92,
  112, 114–116, 118, 155
patient-oriented disease-specific
  questionnaire   361
– Harris hip score   361
– Merle d'Aubigne score   361
– Oxford hip score   361
– WOMAC   361
peak
– intra-acetabular pressure   166, 206,
  271
– pressures   150, 164, 166, 206, 271
pelvic venous blood flow   303

peri-acetabular osteotomy   273, 278
perioperative
– antibiotic prophylaxis   317–319
– blood loss   2, 24, 120, 210, 302, 303,
   305, 306, 310, 317
– management   302
periprosthetic
– fracture   47, 136–138, 147, 187, 230,
   239, 244, 246, 258, 295, 296, 326
– infection   53, 86–89, 91, 313, 314,
   315, 316, 318, 344, 348
physical therapy evaluation   308
plug
– cement plug   342–244, 352, 357, 358
– intramedullary plug 28, 69, 114, 129,
   146–148, **150–153**, 163, 229, 230,
   237, 327, **328**
– migration   151
polished (tapered) stem   35, 66, 84, 98,
   103, 171, 175, 181–184, 187, 188, 191,
   204, 216, 227, 229, 233, 247, 249, 354
polishing wear   183
polyethylene
– polymer   279, 280
– sterilisation   280
– ultra high molecular weight PE   221,
   227, 265, 269, 279, 280, 287–290
– wear   25, 143, 144, 192, 219, 245,
   256, 260, 262, 267, 275, 282–284, 298
polymer
– bone cement   **52–59, 61–69**, 71, 73,
   77–86, 88, **93–97**, 102, 108, 109, 114,
   117
– polyethylene   279, 280
polymerization   27, 32, 35, 52, 54–59,
   67, 70–74, 77, 81, 83, 87, 93–96, 107,
   109, 112, 120, 123, 124, 162, 163, 167,
   209, 271, 322, 323
polymer-monomer interface   93, 94,
   102
polymethylmethacrylate (PMMA)
   (see also acrylic cement and bone
   cement)   25, 52–55, 59–61, 63–67,
   77, 78, 85–91, 93, 95, 98–100, 102,
   107, 109, 111, 115, 152, 153, 167, 169,
   172, 193, 198, 204, 222, 318
poor cementing technique   21, 129,
   141, 340–342, 347
porosity   55, 58, 59, 61, 68, 87, 88, 94,
   107–110, 113, 115–118, 123, 158,
   164, 189
– macro   95, 107, 115
– micro   107, 115, 157, 158
posterior approach   3, 10, 37, 42, 209,
   230, 237, 256, 305, 349, 357

postoperative
– care   302, 304, 305, 309
– physiotherapy   311
– transfusion   305
post-surgical femur   41, 45
pre-arthroplasty rehabilitation   308
pre-chilling   59, 93, 102
pre-cooling   70, 124
pre-heating (stem)   96, 111, 118, 119,
   123
preoperative planning   3, 20, 27, 29,
   36, 43, 131, 236, 310, 335, 348, 357
pre-packed bone cements   117
press-fit
– anchorage   101
– cement restrictor   151
– cemented   101, 102, 137, 238, 250
– concept/principle   101, 235, 236,
   240, 334
– HA   219
– PMMA   99
– uncemented   197, 204, 219, 240,
   261, 356, 357
pressure
– acetabular   **166**, 206, 271
– intramedullary   34, 147, **150–153**,
   320, 323, **325–329**, 342
– peak   150, 164, 166, 206, 271
pressurisation
– acetabular   **24, 25**, 121, **164–167**,
   210, 211, 263, 265, 268, 271
– cement   10, 17, 19, 24–27, 48, **119–
   123**, 127, **146–150**, 153, 155, 157,
   162, 164, 166, 206, 227, 228, 230,
   244, 250, 253, 304, **325–328**, 337,
   340, 342–344
– femoral   **33, 34**, 128, 129, 145,
   160–163, 244
– pre-pressurisation (cement)   93, 94,
   97
– sustained   24, 36, 128, 143, 166, 207,
   267, 326, 328
pressuriser   121, 122, 148, 166, 207
– acetabular   27, 121, 143, 164, 167,
   210
– Bernoski   165, 166
– Exeter   165, 166, 209, 211
– femoral   34, 147, 161
protrusio acetabuli   20, 21, 222, 230,
   274
proximal femoral seal   28, 34, 129, 163
pulmonary embolism (PE)   304, 320
pulsatile lavage   16, 23, 28, 33,
   127–129, 143, 148, 162, 164, 167, 244,
   265, 267, 320, 326, **328, 329**, 351, 356

Q

quality-adjusted life year   361–363
QALY   298, 361
quality of Well-Being index (QWB)
   361
QWB   361

R

radiation   269, **280**, 281, 285, **287–289**
radiographic
– analysis   133, 135, 139, 222, 241,
   246, 247, 291, 292, 339
– assessment   129, 139, 224, 241, 244,
   334
radiolucent lines   22, 119, 124,129,
   141, 142, 144, **166**, 211, 231, 238,
   244, 245, 247, 250, 253, 264, **335,
   336**, 342
radiolucency   2, 129, 143, 166, 201,
   209, 218, 263–265, **335–337**
radiopacifier   53–55, 67, 69, 115
radiostereometric/roentgenstereomet-
   ric analysis (RSA)   66, 110, 174, 182,
   183, 188–190, **192, 194**, 233, 234,
   246, 261, 339, 368,
rapid recovery protocol   307, 309–311
reaming   21, 22, 25, 28, 31, 43, 44, 126,
   138, 141, 142, 162, 197, 210, 236, 249,
   250, 274, 335
red cell salvage   305
rehabilitation   2, 3, **307–309**, 311
reinforcement rings   275
resorbable cements   67
restrictor   32, 33, 48, 145–148, **150–
   153,** 162, 244, 268, **326–330**, 342,
   347, 352
retrograde
– cement application   128, 146, 147,
   148, 162, 328, 329
– cementing technique   161, 328
revascularisation   93, 97, 99, 102
revision
– aseptic   16, 28, 61, 79, 84, 87, 94,
   103, 104, 111, 126, 129, 137–142,
   147, 149, 153, 159, 163, 185, 187, 192,
   207, 217–219, 222–226, 230, 238,
   244, 251, 260, 269, 275, 291, 319, 340,
   348, 352, 357, 262
– burden   292, **294, 295**, 297–299,
   364, 367

– rate   16, 84, 106, 111, 137, 139, 149, 185, 191, 192, 195, 235, 238, 239, 261, 263, 264, 268, 270, 272, 274, 285, 295, 298, 319, 263
– septic   91, 104, 105, 168, 233, 352
rheogoniometer   71, 72
Röhm   52
roof graft   16, **44**, 49, 273–278
rotational stability   29, 48, 132, 145, 170, 171, 192, **196, 198**, 201, 203, 204, 236, 242
RSA   66, 110, 174, 182, 183, 188–190, **192, 194**, 233, 234, 246, 261, 339, 368,

S

Scalloping (endosteal)   137, 238, 244, 336
second generation cementing techniques   69, **147**, 159, 167, 264, 267
self-locking cemented stems   101, 240
septic loosening   348
SF-36   333, 361
SF-6D   361
Shape-closed   **171, 175, 176**, 181, 182, 190, 233 (taper slip)
shear strength   61, 78, 118, 120, **124–127**, 138, 139, 147, 150, 161, 163, 181
shortening osteotomy   41, 48, 49, 186, 254, 256, 259
shrinkage   27, 55, 59, 67, **93, 96–98**, 102, 107, 109, 110, **123**
sickness impact profile (SIP)   361
Simplex   **68, 69**, 72, 74–76, **78–85, 103**, 106, 111, 114–116, 118, 120, 121, 123, 155, 157, 210, 211, 217–219
skin antiseptics   315
smoking
– cessation protocols   309
– intervention programme   309
snow flurry   323, 324
socket   5, 14, **16–21**, 23–27, 43, 141, 142, 187, **208–213**, 216, **260–267**, 270, 271, 275, 277, 337, 354, 356, 357
spinal
– anaesthesia   16, 28, 303, 305, 306, 309, 310, 329
– deformity   3, 38
stability
– anchoring   196, 204
– cement restrictor   32, 150–154
– heat (bone cement)   55, 82, 88

– implant   29, 110, 141, 142, 171, 177, 196, 311
– interface   100, 126
– joint   31, 286, 349
– mechanical   58, 272
– rotational   29, 48, 132, 145, 170, 171, 192, 196, 198, 201, 203, 204, 236, 242
staphylococcus aureus (MRSA)   90, 314, 317
staphylococcus epidermidis (MRSE)   317
stem
– design   29, 138, 170, 174, 180, 190, 241, 242, 247, 338
– fracture   181, 186, 191, 227, 228, 230, 232
– geometry   190, 191, 195, 204
– implantation/insertion   5, 10, **34–36**, 109, **122, 123**, 128, **161, 162**, 182, 186, 323, 325,
– malpositioning   341
– to-cement interface   35, 66, 85, 109, 129, **169–171**, 176, **181–184**, 188, 192, 194, 196, 230, 233, 241, 242
– subsidence   64, **66, 67**, 79, 84, 85, 88, 98, 175, 179, **182, 184**, 189, 190, 192–194, 196, 198, **230–234**, 238–240, 242, 244, 246, 247, 249, 258, 334, 335, 338
– varus position   31, 136, 137, 236, 340, 341
sterilisation
– bone cement   80, 82
– UHMWPE   280
stove pipe femur   33, 130, 131, 152, 153
stress
– relaxation   **60, 61, 63, 64**, 66, 79, **83–85**, 173, 174
– riser   47, 68, 77, 138, 236, 243, 258
strut grafts   257, 258
subchondral bone (plate)   21, 44, 141, 142, 167, 209, 264, 265, 270
subsidence   64, **66, 67**, 79, 84, 85, 88, 98, 175, 179, **182, 184**, 189, 190, 192–194, 196, 198, **230–234**, 238–240, 242, 244, 246, 247, 249, 258, 334, 335, 338
substained cement pressurisation   24, 36, 128, 143, 166, 207, 267, 326, 328
surgical errors   340
survivorship   337, 363
– acetabulum   141, 142, 207, 226, 227, 261, **263–266**, 269, 270, 272

– femur   180, 185, 187, 224, 226, 227, 232–234, 235, 238, 240, 247
– metal on metal   283, 285, 290
Swedish hip register   111, 128, 147, 191, 192, 194, 216, 265, 291, 298
syringe lavage   127, 128, 326

T

tapered stem design   26, 84, 146, 150, 161, 172, 175, 181–183, 187, 188, 194, 202, 216, 233, 239, 240, 242, 326, 354
templating   18, 31, 32, 26, 43, 153, 162, 197, 210, 243, 244, 327, 328
testing
– biomechanical   61, 63, 6, 72, 137, 190, 197
– cement gun   158, 159
– fatigue   57, 58, 68, 77, 181
– preclinical   367
– shear   78, 98, 102
– tensile   76, 77
– torsional   181, 197
theatre ventilation   316
thigh pain   186, 216, 250, 333
third-generation cementing techniques   69, **147**, 194, 230, 233
three interface characteristics   93
thrombo-embolism   303, 305
Tobramycin   88, 90
torsional stability   196, 204
transfemoral approach   349
transgluteal approach   230, 244, 349
transoesophageal echocardiography (TEE)   56, 322, 329
transosseous suture   6, 11
transtrochanteric approach   349
transverse deepening   17, 18, 20, 21
Trendelenburg gait   11, 37, 274
tricalciumphosphate (TCP)   100
Tromsdorff effect   74
true acetabulum   40, 42, 43, 273, 275, 276

U

UHMWPE   83, 221, 227, 265, 269, 279, 280, 287–290
ultra-clean air ventilation   316

ultrahigh molecular weight polyethylene (UHMWPE)   221, 227, 265, 269,
   279, 280, 287–290
unflanged acetabular component   25,
   27, 206, 207, 209, 264, 265, 270–272
utility score   361, 362

V

vacuum mixing
– bone cement   93, 107, 108, 113,
   155, 157
– system 59, 70, 71, 95, 108, **111–118**,
   123
vacuum technique   327
Vancomycin   88, 90, 317
Vancomycin-resistant enterococci
   (VRE)   317
varus position (stem)   31, 136, 137,
   236, 340, 341
viscoelasticity bone cement   83, 84
viscosity   58, 67, 80, 103, 119, 155
– high   27, 58, 70, 72, 73, 80, 103,
   104–106, 114–116, 146, 161–163, 326
– low   33, 58, 69, 72, 73, 78, 80, 103,
   104, 160–162, 326, 327
– medium   36, 72, 73, 78, 162, 163
visual analogue scale (VAS)   292, 293

W

wear   16, 61, 80, 183, 184, 196, 224,
   269, 274, 282,
– abrasive   183, 184, 188, 192, 204,
   282
– polyethylene   25, 143, 144, 192,
   219, 245, 256, 260, 262, 267, 275,
   282–284, 298
– particle   68, 175, 181, 192, 234, 242,
   246, 279, 282, 284, 286
WOMAC   333, 361
working behaviour (bone
   cements)   58, 59

Z

Zirconium 54, 59, 80, 109, 115
ZrO_2 54, 69, 81